New Diagnostic and Therapeutic Approaches for the Care of the Severely Injured Patient

New Diagnostic and Therapeutic Approaches for the Care of the Severely Injured Patient

Editors

Frank Hildebrand
Klemens Horst

MDPI • Basel • Beijing • Wuhan • Barcelona • Belgrade • Manchester • Tokyo • Cluj • Tianjin

Editors

Frank Hildebrand
University Hospital RWTH
Aachen
Germany

Klemens Horst
University Hospital RWTH
Aachen
Germany

Editorial Office
MDPI
St. Alban-Anlage 66
4052 Basel, Switzerland

This is a reprint of articles from the Special Issue published online in the open access journal *Journal of Clinical Medicine* (ISSN 2077-0383) (available at: https://www.mdpi.com/journal/jcm/special_issues/Diagnostic_Therapeutic_Approaches_Severely_Injured).

For citation purposes, cite each article independently as indicated on the article page online and as indicated below:

LastName, A.A.; LastName, B.B.; LastName, C.C. Article Title. *Journal Name* **Year**, *Volume Number*, Page Range.

ISBN 978-3-03943-777-1 (Hbk)
ISBN 978-3-03943-778-8 (PDF)

Cover image courtesy of University Hospital RWTH Aachen.

Contents

About the Editors

Frank Hildebrand, MHBA, studied human medicine at the Medical University of Hannover/Germany (MHH) from 1994 to 2001 and completed his doctoral thesis in 2001. He absolved his surgical training at MHH where he also started his scientific career. In 2006, he received the venia legendi (Habilitation) for surgery (MHH) and was appointed as Professor in 2010. From 2012 to 2017, Prof. Hildebrand held a Professorship for Posttraumatic Inflammation at the Department for Orthopaedic Trauma and Reconstructive Surgery at the University Hospital RWTH Aachen/Germany before he was appointed a W3-Professorship and head of the department in 2017. Professor Hildebrand is member of several associations such as national and international trauma and intensive care societies. Furthermore, he frequently reviews highly sophisticated research applications by the German Research Foundation (DFG) and acts as reviewer for various international recognized journals. His scientific work is frequently awarded by renowned institutions such as national and international trauma societies (i.e., Germany, Great Britain, USA and European Society).

Klemens Horst, MHBA, FEBS studied human medicine at the University Witten/Herdecke, Germany from 2004 to 2010 before he entered his surgical training at the Department for Orthopaedic Trauma and Reconstructive Surgery at the University Hospital RWTH Aachen/Germany. His doctoral thesis (2012) was followed by the venia legendi (Habilitation) for trauma and orthopaedic surgery in 2018. In 2017, he became a Fellow of the European Board of Surgeons (FEBS) and thereover is a member of several national and international trauma/surgical societies. In 2019, Priv.-Doz. Dr. Horst was elected into the section-board for "Surgical Research" by the German Society for Surgery. Furthermore, he acts as reviewer for several international recognized journals. His scientific work has been awarded by renowned institutions such as national and international trauma societies (i.e., Germany, USA and European Society).

Journal of
Clinical Medicine

MDPI

Editorial

New Diagnostic and Therapeutic Approaches for the Care of the Severely Injured Patient

Frank Hildebrand and Klemens Horst *

Department of Trauma and Reconstructive Surgery, University Hospital RWTH Aachen, 52074 Aachen, Germany; fhildebrand@ukaachen.de

* Correspondence: khorst@ukaachen.de

Received: 20 October 2020; Accepted: 23 October 2020; Published: 28 October 2020

Severe trauma remains a leading cause of death, especially in the younger population. Pre- and intrahospital diagnostic and therapeutic procedures according to well-established guidelines (e.g., Advanced Trauma Life Support® (ATLS®, American College of Surgeons, The Committee on Trauma, Chicago, IL, USA) are widely accepted to beneficially influence posttraumatic outcomes. However, the further assessment and treatment of severely injured patients still remain challenging due to a high variety of injury patterns and manifold patient-specific factors. The latter individual aspects (e.g., age, gender) have been shown to modulate the posttraumatic immune response, which in turn has a significant impact on the clinical course after severe trauma. To improve posttraumatic outcomes, further clinical and experimental research is needed to better understand the underlying pathomechanisms and to improve diagnostic and therapeutic strategies. This Special Issue of the Journal of Clinical Medicine therefore focuses on recent aspects of the management of severely injured patients. Based on data from clinical studies, pathomechanisms, new diagnostic and therapeutic approaches, as well as outcome observations are presented.

The ABCDE scheme represents the basis of the ATLS®-recommendations of the American College of Surgeons (ACS) Committee on Trauma. According to this algorithm, securing the airway (A-problem) and ensuring ventilation (B-problem) are the first priorities when approaching a severely injured patient. However, the establishment of a safe airway might be very difficult. In a monocentric, prospective study on a physician-staffed air ambulance, Macke et al. proved that C-MAC (Storz Medical, Tuttlingen, Germany) videolaryngoscopy in the prehospital setting was associated with significantly better first pass success for endotracheal intubation compared to direct laryngoscopy [1]. As lethal hemorrhage remains a leading cause of early death in severely injured patients, the maintenance or restoration of a hemodynamically stable situation (C-problem) is another priority of the ATLS concept. To estimate the risk of massive transfusion, Horst et al. introduced the modified Trauma-Induced Coagulopathy Clinical Score (mTICCS) as a new scoring system to identify patients in need of massive transfusion. Based on an analysis of a trauma registry, the authors successfully validated mTICCS against well-established and more sophisticated algorithms and found that it presents an useful tool to predict the need for massive transfusion early [2]. Focusing on neurological aspects (D-problem), Popp et al. validated a CT protocol with mandatory dedicated computer tomography angiography (CT-A) to detect cervical artery dissections in severely injured patients [3]. From the results of their monocentric, prospective study, the authors concluded that their imaging pathway is likely to reduce possible therapeutic delays. Peripheral neurological symptoms are mainly caused by injuries of the spinal column. Based on a retrospective analysis, Kobbe et al. support the concept of early spinal stabilization in severely injured patients with AOSpine B-/C-type injuries, especially of the thoracic spine. However, in AOSpine A-type injuries, the beneficial impact of early spinal stabilization seems to be overemphasized and the benefit should be weighed against the risk of patients' deterioration during early spinal stabilization [4].

Chest trauma is one of the most common injury types after severe trauma and also has a significant impact on the clinical course. A flail chest is a serious condition after chest trauma, however the optimal treatment (conservative vs. operative) for this kind of injury is not clarified. In their retrospective study, Niemann et al. did not find differences in clinical parameters (e.g., the duration of mechanical ventilation, analgesia requirements, pneumonia incidence) between conservatively and operatively treated patients. However, a prolongation of both the length of intensive care unit (ICU) stay and hospital treatment duration was observed in operatively treated patients [5]. In a further study with a retrospective design, Eckhardt et al. confirmed the relevance of chest trauma in the posttraumatic course (longer ventilation time, prolonged ICU stay, increased mortality) Interestingly, being overweight resulted in an independent mortality reduction in patients with severe chest trauma [6]. It was postulated that overweight-associated factors, such as nutritive advantages or a modulated posttraumatic immune response, might be responsible for the observed survival benefit [6].

Immunological alterations after severe trauma were also discussed by two other manuscripts of this Special Issue. In a clinical review, Kobbe et al. summarized the current knowledge about the neuroendocrine modulation of the immune system during trauma and sepsis and the potential arising therapeutic options [7,8]. Schindler et al. retrospectively investigated the relevance of traumatic brain injury (TBI) with or without concomitant injuries on systemic inflammation and other markers of neurological damage (e.g., S100b). They found that TBI is associated with a decreased interleukin expression. However, the diagnostic relevance of potential markers of neuronal damage seems to be limited [7,8]. Two other studies performed blood analyses in order to investigate posttraumatic changes in the humeral and cellular inflammatory response as well as in the complement and coagulation system [9,10]. In this context, Sturm et al. focused on the $CD4^+$ T lymphocyte population after severe trauma. They observed that the number of T-regulatory cells was decreased within this population; however, their inductiveness (e.g., by IL-10) was increased [9,10]. Vollrath et al. described a promising predictive value of C5a and thrombin-activatable fibrinolysis inhibitor (TAFI) levels for the development of sepsis [9,10]. Zechendorf et al. investigated ribonuclease (RNase) 1 and its antagonist (RNase inhibitor (RNH) 1 to determine the association of post-operative acute kidney injury (AKI) and in-hospital mortality [11]. RNase 1 belongs to the group of antimicrobial peptides that is elevated in septic patients and indicates the prediction of two or more organ failures. Both RNase1 and RNH1 may be therapeutically relevant and may represent biomarkers for post-operative AKI and in-hospital mortality [11]. Hesselink et al. concentrated on infections after trauma and described persistent inflammation, immunosuppression, and catabolism syndrome (PICS) as a potential explanation of recurrent infections. PICS was associated with prolonged hospitalization, many surgical procedures, and frequent readmissions. Therefore, PICS forms a substantial burden on the patient and the hospital, despite its low incidence [12].

Diverse studies of this Special Issue focused on severe trauma in the elderly population, which clearly underlines the increasing clinical importance of this topic. Stassen et al. found a high prevalence of sarcopenia among severely injured patients that was particularly pronounced in the older patients. As sarcopenia was also identified as a predictor of 30-day mortality, the clinical relevance of the identification of a low muscle mass via CT scan seems to be obvious [13]. Focusing on fragility fractures of the pelvis (FFP), Rommens et al. retrospectively found that even isolated fractures of the anterior pelvic ring without any involvement of the posterior ring (FFP Type I) were associated with relevant mortality, a loss of independence, restricted mobility, and a decreased quality of life. The authors concluded that pubic ramus fractures are indicators of the need to optimize the patient's general condition [14]. In fractures affecting the posterior pelvic ring, Hartensuer et al. explored in a retrospective study the safety, effect, and feasibility of percutaneous sacroiliac (SI) screws with and without augmentation. Cement augmentation seemed to reduce the complication risk in FFP patients and shorten their hospital stay, without increased specific complications or correlated neurological impairment [15]. In order to ensure the earliest possible mobilization after FFP, Pfeufer et al. were able to reliably detect the extremity load in patients with FFP with the help of an insole device [16].

They concluded that this technique might offer a great potential to improve the choice and time of treatment of FFP. In a study based on the "Trauma Registry DGU", Freigang et al. clearly showed that severe trauma also significantly affects the long-term outcomes of elderly patients with no improvement in their health-related quality of life (HRQoL) up to 24 months after trauma in patients ≥65 years [17].

Apart from injury pattern and specific patient groups, the treatment of severely injured patients is associated with high personnel and structural requirements. Therefore, the targeted and reasonable use of these resources is of upmost importance. Heinrich et al. showed in a retrospective analysis that slightly injured patients (Abbreviated Injury Scale (AIS) ≤ 1, Maximum Abbreviated Injury Scale (MAIS) ≤ 1 and Injury Severity Score (ISS) ≤ 3) might not need to complete a ≥24 h monitoring [18]. In the light of the economic use of resources, the importance of predicting risk factors associated with specific injury pattern as well as an analysis of the need for extended diagnostic procedures are presented by two further manuscripts of this Special Issue [19,20]. In a study using data from the "Trauma Registry DGU", Weber et al. defined the risk factors and accident mechanisms which are indicative of the presence of knee injuries and described a significant impact of this injury pattern on the clinical course [19,20]. Halvachizadeh et al. retrospectively investigated the significance of intraoperative computed tomography (CT) for the operative treatment of intra-articular fractures after severe trauma. They found that CT was associated with improved surgical results and concluded that the decrease in reoperations may justify its use, despite the higher CT-associated radiation dose [19,20].

Further studies of this Special Issue also focus on innovative therapeutic approaches. As patients with spinal cord injury (SCI) are likely to exhibit hemostasis disorders, Mackiewicz-Milewska et al. assessed the effects of different rehabilitation programs on hemostasis in patients with SCI. They found that a 4-week program was suggestive of positive results, more pronounced in the subacute and chronic state (≥3 to 6 months) rather than in the short term after SCI [21]. In severely injured patients, bony mal- or non-unions are a regularly observed complication. Wang et al. therefore investigated the possibility of an arthroscopy-assisted corrective osteotomy (AACO), reduction, internal fixation, and strut allograft augmentation for cases affecting the tibial plateau. The authors proved good radiological and clinical results [22]. Additionally scarring is a further common problem after severe injury. Joo et al. evaluated the effects of extracorporeal shock wave therapy (ESWT) on hypertrophic scars of the hand caused by burn injuries. They were able to prove that ESWT was effective in decreasing pain, suppressing hypertrophic scarring, and improving hand function [23]. In addition, the same study group showed that a virtual-reality (VR) based rehabilitation program is likely to be as effective as conventional rehabilitation programs for recovering function in a burned hand [24].

In conclusion, the presented articles reflect the current knowledge about the pathomechanisms associated with the impact of severe injury and its consequences for the further clinical course on the one hand and points out new insights in regard to diagnostic and therapeutic approaches in severely injured patients on the other hand. Furthermore, interesting aspects regarding future directions for the care of the severely injured patient are illustrated, and we hope you enjoy reading our selections of topics regarding the importance of investigating all aspects associated with severe trauma.

Author Contributions: F.H., K.H. have made a substantial, direct and intellectual contribution to the work, and approved it for publication. All authors have read and agreed to the published version of the manuscript.

Funding: This research received no external funding.

Conflicts of Interest: The authors declare no conflict of interest.

References

1. Macke, C.; Gralla, F.; Winkelmann, M.; Clausen, J.D.; Haertle, M.; Krettek, C.; Omar, M. Increased First Pass Success with C-MAC Videolaryngoscopy in Prehospital Endotracheal Intubation-A Randomized Controlled Trial. *J. Clin. Med.* **2020**, *9*, 2719. [CrossRef] [PubMed]
2. Horst, K.; Lentzen, R.; Tonglet, M.; Mert, Ü.; Lichte, P.; Weber, C.D.; Kobbe, P.; Heussen, N.; Hildebrand, F. Validation of the mTICCS Score as a Useful Tool for the Early Prediction of a Massive Transfusion in Patients with a Traumatic Hemorrhage. *J. Clin. Med.* **2020**, *9*, 945. [CrossRef] [PubMed]
3. Popp, D.; Thiedemann, C.; Baumler, W.; Ernstberger, A.; Alt, V.; Schicho, A. Modified Split-Scan Computed Tomography (CT) Diagnostics of Severely Injured Patients: First Results from a Level I Trauma Center Using a Dedicated Head-and-Neck CT-Angiogram for the Detection of Cervical Artery Dissections. *J. Clin. Med.* **2020**, *9*, 2568. [CrossRef] [PubMed]
4. Kobbe, P.; Krug, P.; Andruszkow, H.; Pishnamaz, M.; Hofman, M.; Horst, K.; Meyer, C.; Scheyerer, M.J.; Faymonville, C.; Stein, G.; et al. Early Spinal Injury Stabilization in Multiple-Injured Patients: Do All Patients Benefit? *J. Clin. Med.* **2020**, *9*, 1760. [CrossRef] [PubMed]
5. Niemann, M.; Graef, F.; Tsitsilonis, S.; Stockle, U.; Mardian, S. Retrospective Analysis of the Clinical Outcome in a Matched Case-Control Cohort of Polytrauma Patients Following an Osteosynthetic Flail Chest Stabilization. *J. Clin. Med.* **2020**, *9*, 2379. [CrossRef] [PubMed]
6. Eckhardt, T.; Horst, K.; Störmann, P.; Bläsius, F.; Hofman, M.; Herren, C.; Kobbe, P.; Hildebrand, F.; Andruszkow, H. Impact of Chest Trauma and Overweight on Mortality and Outcome in Severely Injured Patients. *J. Clin. Med.* **2020**, *9*, 2752. [CrossRef]
7. Kobbe, P.; Blasius, F.M.; Lichte, P.; Oberbeck, R.; Hildebrand, F. Neuroendocrine Modulation of the Immune Response after Trauma and Sepsis: Does It Influence Outcome? *J. Clin. Med.* **2020**, *9*, 2287. [CrossRef]
8. Schindler, C.R.; Lustenberger, T.; Woschek, M.; Störmann, P.; Henrich, D.; Radermacher, P.; Marzi, I. Severe Traumatic Brain Injury (TBI) Modulates the Kinetic Profile of the Inflammatory Response of Markers for Neuronal Damage. *J. Clin. Med.* **2020**, *9*, 1667. [CrossRef]
9. Vollrath, J.T.; Marzi, I.; Herminghaus, A.; Lustenberger, T.; Relja, B. Post-Traumatic Sepsis Is Associated with Increased C5a and Decreased TAFI Levels. *J. Clin. Med.* **2020**, *9*, 1230. [CrossRef]
10. Sturm, R.; Xanthopoulos, L.; Heftrig, D.; Oppermann, E.; Vrdoljak, T.; Dunay, I.R.; Marzi, I.; Relja, B. Regulatory T Cells Modulate CD4 Proliferation after Severe Trauma via IL-10. *J. Clin. Med.* **2020**, *9*, 1052. [CrossRef]
11. Zechendorf, E.; Gombert, A.; Bülow, T.; Frank, N.; Beckers, C.; Peine, A.; Kotelis, D.; Jacobs, M.J.; Marx, G.; Martin, L. The Role of Ribonuclease 1 and Ribonuclease Inhibitor 1 in Acute Kidney Injury after Open and Endovascular Thoracoabdominal Aortic Aneurysm Repair. *J. Clin. Med.* **2020**, *9*, 3292. [CrossRef]
12. Hesselink, L.; Hoepelman, R.J.; Spijkerman, R.; de Groot, M.C.; van Wessem, K.J.; Koenderman, L.; Leenen, L.P.; Hietbrink, F. Persistent Inflammation, Immunosuppression and Catabolism Syndrome (PICS) after Polytrauma: A Rare Syndrome with Major Consequences. *J. Clin. Med.* **2020**, *9*, 191. [CrossRef]
13. Stassen, R.C.; Reisinger, K.W.; Al-Ali, M.; Poeze, M.; Ten Bosch, J.A.; Blokhuis, T.J. High Prevalence of Sarcopenia in Older Trauma Patients: A Pilot Study. *J. Clin. Med.* **2020**, *9*, 2046. [CrossRef] [PubMed]
14. Rommens, P.M.; Hopf, J.C.; Herteleer, M.; Devlieger, B.; Hofmann, A.; Wagner, D. Isolated Pubic Ramus Fractures Are Serious Adverse Events for Elderly Persons: An Observational Study on 138 Patients with Fragility Fractures of the Pelvis Type I (FFP Type I). *J. Clin. Med.* **2020**, *9*, 2498. [CrossRef]
15. Hartensuer, R.; Lodde, M.F.; Keller, J.; Eveslage, M.; Stolberg-Stolberg, J.; Riesenbeck, O.; Raschke, M.J. Safety, Effect and Feasibility of Percutaneous SI-Screw with and without Augmentation–A 15-Year Retrospective Analysis on over 640 Screws. *J. Clin. Med.* **2020**, *9*, 2660. [CrossRef]
16. Pfeufer, D.; Becker, C.A.; Faust, L.; Keppler, A.M.; Stagg, M.; Kammerlander, C.; Böcker, W.; Neuerburg, C. Load-Bearing Detection with Insole-Force Sensors Provides New Treatment Insights in Fragility Fractures of the Pelvis. *J. Clin. Med.* **2020**, *9*, 2551. [CrossRef] [PubMed]
17. Freigang, V.; Müller, K.; Ernstberger, A.; Kaltenstadler, M.; Bode, L.; Pfeifer, C.; Alt, V.; Baumann, F. Reduced Recovery Capacity After Major Trauma in the Elderly: Results of a Prospective Multicenter Registry-Based Cohort Study. *J. Clin. Med.* **2020**, *9*, 2356. [CrossRef]

18. Heinrich, M.; Lany, M.; Anastasopoulou, L.; Biehl, C.; Szalay, G.; Brenck, F.; Heiss, C. Evidence of Prolonged Monitoring of Trauma Patients Admitted via Trauma Resuscitation Unit without Primary Proof of Severe Injuries. *J. Clin. Med.* **2020**, *9*, 2516. [CrossRef] [PubMed]
19. Weber, C.D.; Solomon, L.B.; Lefering, R.; Horst, K.; Kobbe, P.; Hildebrand, F.; DGU, T. Which Risk Factors Predict Knee Ligament Injuries in Severely Injured Patients?—Results from an International Multicenter Analysis. *J. Clin. Med.* **2020**, *9*, 1437. [CrossRef] [PubMed]
20. Halvachizadeh, S.; Berk, T.; Pieringer, A.; Ried, E.; Hess, F.; Pfeifer, R.; Pape, H.C.; Allemann, F. Is the Additional Effort for an Intraoperative CT Scan Justified for Distal Radius Fracture Fixations? A Comparative Clinical Feasibility Study. *J. Clin. Med.* **2020**, *9*, 2254. [CrossRef]
21. Mackiewicz-Milewska, M.; Cisowska-Adamiak, M.; Rosc, D.; Glowacka-Mrotek, I.; Swiatkiewicz, I. Effects of Four-Week Rehabilitation Program on Hemostasis Disorders in Patients with Spinal Cord Injury. *J. Clin. Med.* **2020**, *9*, 1836. [CrossRef]
22. Wang, J.Y.; Cheng, C.Y.; Chen, A.C.; Chan, Y.S. Arthroscopy-Assisted Corrective Osteotomy, Reduction, Internal Fixation and Strut Allograft Augmentation for Tibial Plateau Malunion or Nonunion. *J. Clin. Med.* **2020**, *9*, 973. [CrossRef]
23. Joo, S.Y.; Lee, S.Y.; Cho, Y.S.; Seo, C.H. Clinical Utility of Extracorporeal Shock Wave Therapy on Hypertrophic Scars of the Hand Caused by Burn Injury: A Prospective, Randomized, Double-Blinded Study. *J. Clin. Med.* **2020**, *9*, 1376. [CrossRef]
24. Joo, S.Y.; Cho, Y.S.; Lee, S.Y.; Seok, H.; Seo, C.H. Effects of Virtual Reality-Based Rehabilitation on Burned Hands: A Prospective, Randomized, Single-Blind Study. *J. Clin. Med.* **2020**, *9*, 731. [CrossRef]

Journal of
Clinical Medicine

MDPI

Article

The Role of Ribonuclease 1 and Ribonuclease Inhibitor 1 in Acute Kidney Injury after Open and Endovascular Thoracoabdominal Aortic Aneurysm Repair

Elisabeth Zechendorf [1,†], Alexander Gombert [2,†], Tanja Bülow [3], Nadine Frank [1], Christian Beckers [1], Arne Peine [1], Drosos Kotelis [2], Michael J. Jacobs [2], Gernot Marx [1] and Lukas Martin [1,*]

1 Department of Intensive Care and Intermediate Care, University Hospital RWTH Aachen, 52062 Aachen, Germany; ezechendorf@ukaachen.de (E.Z.); nfrank@ukaachen.de (N.F.); cbeckers@ukaachen.de (C.B.); apeine@ukaachen.de (A.P.); gmarx@ukaachen.de (G.M.)
2 European Vascular Center Aachen-Maastricht, University Hospital RWTH Aachen, 52062 Aachen, Germany; agombert@ukaachen.de (A.G.); dkotelis@ukaachen.de (D.K.); mjacobs@ukaachen.de (M.J.J.)
3 Department of Medical Statistics, University Hospital RWTH Aachen, 52062 Aachen, Germany; tbuelow@ukaachen.de
* Correspondence: lmartin@ukaachen.de; Tel.: +49-(0)-241-8037606
† Equally contributed authorship.

Received: 30 August 2020; Accepted: 12 October 2020; Published: 14 October 2020

Abstract: Acute kidney injury (AKI) is one of the most common post-operative complications and is closely associated with increased mortality after open and endovascular thoracoabdominal aortic aneurysm (TAAA) repair. Ribonuclease (RNase) 1 belongs to the group of antimicrobial peptides elevated in septic patients and indicates the prediction of two or more organ failures. The role of RNase 1 and its antagonist RNase inhibitor 1 (RNH1) after TAAA repair is unknown. In this study, we analyzed RNase 1 and RNH1 serum levels in patients undergoing open ($n = 14$) or endovascular ($n = 19$) TAAA repair to determine their association with post-operative AKI and in-hospital mortality. Increased RNH1 serum levels after open TAAA repair as compared with endovascular TAAA repair immediately after surgery and 12, 48, and 72 h after surgery (all $p < 0.05$) were observed. Additionally, elevated RNase 1 and RNH1 serum levels 12, 24, and 48 h after surgery were shown to be significantly associated with AKI (all $p < 0.05$). RNH1 serum levels before and RNase 1 serum levels 12 h after TAAA repair were significantly correlated with in-hospital mortality (both $p < 0.05$). On the basis of these findings, RNase 1 and RNH1 may be therapeutically relevant and may represent biomarkers for post-operative AKI and in-hospital mortality.

Keywords: thoracoabdominal aortic aneurysm; ribonuclease; ribonuclease inhibitor 1; biomarker; complex aortic surgery; acute kidney injury

1. Introduction

Thoracoabdominal aortic surgery is associated with several post-operative complications and increased mortality [1]. Mortality is 8.3% 30 days after open surgery and 5.8% after endovascular surgery [2]. Multiple organ failure is one of the dreaded post-operative complications after open and endovascular surgical treatment of thoracoabdominal aortic aneurysms (TAAA). Furthermore, acute kidney injury (AKI) is one of the most common organ failures after TAAA repair with an incidence between 13% and 42%. In addition to cardiovascular morbidity, AKI is associated with increased mortality [3–5]. AKI is diagnosed according to the Kidney Disease – Improving Global

Outcomes (KDIGO) criteria. According to KDIGO, AKI is diagnosed when serum creatinine increases by ≥0.3 mg/dl (26.5 µmol/l) within 48 h or ≥1.5-fold, or when there is a reduction in urine volume to <0.5 mL/kg/h over 6 h. The three stages of AKI (I–III) are based on the aforementioned criteria: In addition to urinary excretion, diagnosis of AKI is based on patient serum creatinine levels. However, serum creatinine is a controversial biomarker for the detection of impaired renal function due to its delayed increases and low sensitivity [6–8]. Therefore, the establishment of new clinically available and reliable biomarkers and therapeutic approaches for the treatment of AKI is necessary [9].

Ribonuclease (RNase) 1 is a host defense peptide of the innate immune system which is expressed ubiquitously in various tissues and body fluids [10]. The primary function of RNase 1 is the degradation of circulating double- and single-stranded RNAs [10]. In a previous study, we observed increased RNase 1 serum levels in septic patients as compared with healthy subjects. Furthermore, we demonstrated that RNase 1 serum concentrations indicated a prediction of dysfunction of two or more organs in septic patients [11]. RNase inhibitor 1 (RNH1) is also ubiquitously expressed as an inhibitor of RNase 1 in a variety of tissues that inhibits its activity by direct binding [12,13]. In a recent study, we detected increased RNH1 serum levels in septic patients, as well as elevated extracellular RNA [14]. However, the role of RNase 1 and RNH1 as biomarkers of AKI and in-hospital mortality in the setting of TAAA repair has not yet been investigated.

The aim of this study was to evaluate the role of RNase 1 and RNH1 as potential biomarkers, as well as therapeutic strategies for the prediction of post-operative AKI and in-hospital mortality in patients undergoing complex open and endovascular TAAA repair.

2. Experimental Section

2.1. Study Approval and Design

All serum samples were collected, in 2017, between January and December after approval by the internal ethics committee of the University Hospital Aachen (EK004/14). Written informed consent was obtained preoperatively from all subjects. After screening and exclusion of patients who met the exclusion criteria, including emergency procedures, age below 18 years, pregnancy, chronic kidney disease requiring permanent dialysis treatment, and ongoing immunosuppressive therapy, 33 patients were included in this study. Of these, 14 patients underwent open repair and 19 patients underwent endovascular TAAA repair (Figure 1). Demographic data, medical history, and daily physiological variables were obtained from patient records and electronic flowcharts at the bedside (IntelliSpace Critical Care and Anesthesia, Philips Healthcare, Andover, MA, USA). On the basis of serum creatinine levels and 24-h urine output detection during the first 72 h after surgery, AKI was defined according to the KDIGO criteria [9]. The trial is registered under the ClinicalTrials.gov number NCT03093857. The cohort of patients has been previously described in a recently published study [15].

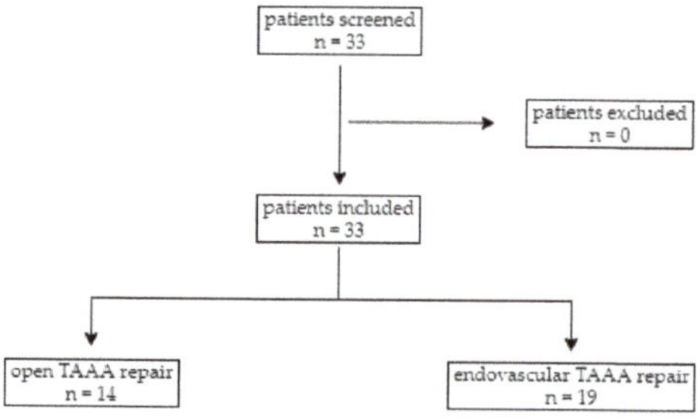

Figure 1. Screening and exclusion of patients.

2.2. Surgery

During open TAAA repair, different techniques were used to reduce intraoperative organ ischemia. Sequential aortic clamping, extracorporal circulation using distal aortic perfusion, and selective visceral perfusion are established methods to reduce organ damage during surgery [16,17] [18]. Renal perfusion was achieved using 4 °C tempered Custodiol® (Dr. Franz Köhler Chemie, Bensheim, Germany) [19]. In the case of endovascular TAAA repair, a contrast agent was carefully applied to avoid kidney failure, leading to a mean application of 65 ± 17 mL per endovascular procedure [20].

2.3. Serum Sampling

Serum samples were collected after patients were enrolled in the study at six different time points (before surgery, after admission to the intensive care unit (ICU), and 12, 24, 48, and 72 h after surgery). Serum samples were centrifuged at 3000 rpm for 10 min at room temperature after 10 min of coagulation. Samples were stored at −80 °C until RNase 1 and RNH1 serum levels were measured.

2.4. Human RNase Inhibitor 1 (RNH1) Enzyme-Linked Immunosorbent Assay

RNH1 serum levels were assessed using an ELISA designed by our research group. A 96-well plate was coated with 100 µL of diluted (2.5 µg/mL in PBS) capture antibody (#ABIN1342154, Abnova, Taipeh, Taiwan) and incubated at 4 °C overnight. After washing with 0.05% Tween in PBS for 3 min three times, the plate was blocked in blocking buffer containing 5% fat free milk and 10% HS for two h at room temperature. A standard series was prepared in a range from 0.78 to 100 ng/mL using a recombinant RNH1 Protein (#ABIN1318405, Abnova). After repeating the wash step, 100 µL of standard and samples were added to each well and incubated for 2 h at room temperature. Wells were subsequently aspirated and washed five times, followed by addition of 100 µL of diluted detection antibody with a working concentration of 1 µg/mL to each well. Next, the wells were aspirated, washed, and incubated, for 1 h, in 100 µL of an HRP-conjugated goat anti-rabbit antibody (#31460, Thermo Fisher Scientific, Bedford, MA, USA). The wash step was repeated, and the TMB substrate solution was added and incubated, for 5 to 20 min, at room temperature protected from light before the reaction was stopped with 2 N sulfuric acid. The optical density was determined at a wavelength of 450 nm using a plate reader (Tecan Group, Männedorf, Switzerland). For statistical analysis, GraphPad 7 (GraphPad Inc., San Diego, CA, USA) was used.

2.5. Human Ribonuclease (RNase) 1 Enzyme-Linked Immunosorbent Assay

Levels of RNase 1 in human serum were determined using a commercial ELISA kit (#SEK13468, Sino Biological Inc., Peking, China) according to the manufacturer's instructions. For analysis, the optical density was measured at 450 nm using a microplate reader (Tecan).

2.6. Endpoints

To investigate the role of RNase 1 and RNH1 in AKI after TAAA repair, especially to analyze differences between open and endovascular TAAA repair, we examined preoperative renal function in relation to RNase 1 and RNH1 serum levels. In order to analyze only preoperative kidney function, patients with preexisting kidney disease (defined as preoperative serum creatinine >1.25 mg/dL according to the cut-off used in the Cleveland Clinic foundation score [21]) were excluded. Furthermore, we investigated the relationship between RNase 1 and RNH1 serum levels and in-hospital mortality in patients undergoing open and endovascular TAAA repair, as well as the differences in these two surgical techniques.

The association of serum levels of RNase 1 and RNH1 was also investigated with post-operative endpoints, such as ICU stay, sepsis and inflammatory markers C-reactive protein (CRP), procalcitonin (PCT), and interleukin-6 (IL-6). Sepsis is defined as a life-threatening organ dysfunction that is identified by a 2-point increase in SOFA score (sequential (sepsis-related) organ failure assessment) [22].

2.7. Statistical Analysis

Continuous data are presented as box-whisker plots. Lines inside the boxes represent the median and the pluses represent the mean. The box is defined by Q1 and Q3. The whiskers range from Q1 to Q1 + 1.5 ∗ (Q3 − Q1) and Q3 to Q3 − 1.5 ∗ (Q3 − Q1), with observations outside of the whiskers shown as points classified as outliers. Categorical data are presented as absolute frequencies and percentages. RNase 1 and RNH1 serum levels are visualized over time again as box-whisker plots. To compare patient characteristics between open TAAA repair and endovascular TAAA repair, unpaired t-tests were used. For each point in time, a univariable logistic regression model was applied to assess the association between the outcome variables AKI (yes/no) and in-hospital mortality (died/survived) with RNase 1 and RNH1 serum levels.

The diagnostic quality of RNase 1 and RNH1 serum levels with respect to AKI and in-hospital mortality was evaluated for each point in time using the receiver operating characteristic (ROC) analysis. Sensitivity (Se), specificity (Sp), positive and negative likelihood ratio (LR+ and LR−), area under the curve (AUC), and the optimal cut-off value according to the Youden index were given in addition to the ROC curves for each time point and the respective diagnostic variable.

A monotone correlation between RNase 1 and RNH1 and perioperative variables was evaluated using Spearman correlation coefficient. Due to the various sample sizes, the reliability of the correlation coefficient was assessed through the p-value testing for a correlation coefficient different from 0. For all Spearman correlation coefficients statistically significant different from 0, the respective *p*-value has been stated. A Spearman correlation coefficient above 0.3 is considered to be an indicator for a moderate correlation, and above 0.5 to be a strong monotone correlation.

The level of significance was set at 5%. No adjustments were made for multiple comparisons due to the exploratory nature of this study. Statistical analyses were performed using SAS software version 9.4 (SAS Institute, Cary, NC, USA) and R, version 3.6.1. ROC analysis was performed using MedCalc, version 19.2.5.

3. Results

3.1. Study Population

The median age of patients undergoing endovascular TAAA repair (74 (69–78)) was significantly higher than those undergoing open TAAA repair (51 (37–65)) (p < 0.001). Pre-operative renal insufficiency was observed in three patients undergoing open (21.4%) and in two patients undergoing endovascular TAAA repair (10.5%). Ten patients undergoing open (71.4%) and seven (36.8%) undergoing endovascular TAAA repair developed post-operative AKI as diagnosed according to the KDIGO classification criteria. All details of patient characteristics can be found in Table 1.

Table 1. Patient characteristics.

	Open TAAA Repair (n = 14)	Endovascular TAAA Repair (n = 19)	*p*-Value
Age (year) (IQR)	51 (37–65)	74 (69–78)	<0.001
Male sex (%)	8 (57.1)	9 (47.4)	0.593
BMI (kg/m^2) (IQR)	25.7 (20.6–30.6)	25.4 (21.5–27.1)	0.600
Diabetes mellitus (%)	2 (14.3)	4 (21.1)	0.685
Smoker (%)	4 (28.6)	8 (42.1)	0.440
Operation time (min) (IQR)	312.5 (295.5–474.5)	392.0 (280.0-460.0)	0.908
LOS ICU (days) (IQR)	5 (4–21)	3 (6–2)	0.075
LOS in-hospital (days) (IQR)	27 (19–38)	15 (9–35)	0.190
In-hospital mortality (%)	2 (14.3)	4 (21.1)	0.631
Pre-operative renal insufficiency (%)	3 (21.4)	2 (10.5)	0.4039
Post-operative acute kidney injury (%)	10 (71.4)	7 (36.8)	0.051

Data are presented as n (%) or median (IQR). Unpaired t-test (two-tailed) was used for statistical analysis. IQR, interquartile ranges (Q1–Q3); BMI, body mass index; LOS, length of stay; ICU, intensive care unit.

3.2. Ribonuclease (RNase) 1 Serum Levels

We first investigated serum levels of RNase 1 in patients undergoing open or endovascular TAAA repair. RNase 1 concentrations decreased in patients undergoing open TAAA repair from 56.9 ± 44.4 ng/mL before surgery to 40.4 ± 17.5 ng/mL 24 h after surgery (Figure 2). Forty-eight hours after surgery, RNase 1 serum levels increased so that a concentration of 71.1 ± 45.9 ng/mL was reached 72 h after surgery (Figure 2). In patients undergoing endovascular TAAA repair, RNase 1 serum levels increased over time from 46.78 ± 26.7 ng/mL to 77.86 ± 37.2 ng/mL (Figure 2). When comparing the two groups, no significant difference was detected (Figure 2).

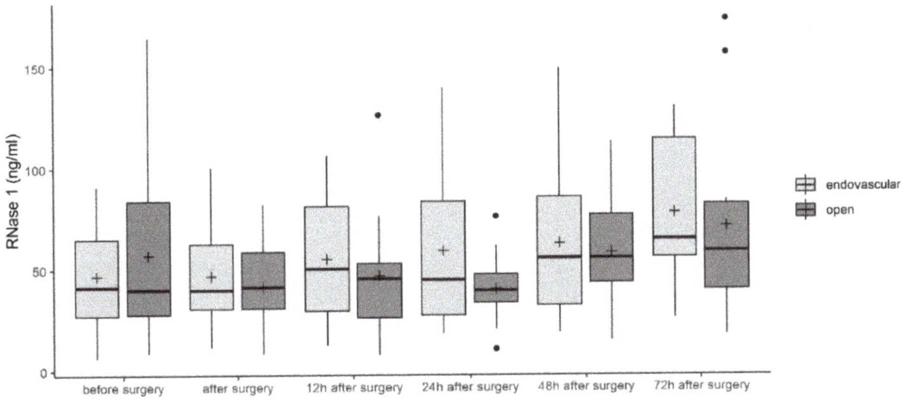

Figure 2. Ribonuclease (RNase) 1 serum levels in patients undergoing open or endovascular thoracoabdominal aortic aneurysm (TAAA) repair. Data are presented as box-whisker plots. Lines inside the boxes represent the median and the pluses represent the mean. The box is defined by Q1 and Q3. The whiskers range from Q1 to Q1 + 1.5 ∗ (Q3 − Q1) and Q3 to Q3 − 1.5 ∗ (Q3 − Q1), with observations outside of the whiskers shown as points classified as outliers. Unpaired t-test (two-tailed) was used for statistical analysis of the two groups. RNase 1, ribonuclease 1.

3.3. RNase Inhibitor 1 (RNH1) Serum Levels

As described before, RNH1 is an antagonist of RNase 1 and inhibits its enzymatic activity by direct binding. Therefore, we next investigated serum levels of RNH1 in patients undergoing TAAA repair. In contrast to RNase 1 serum concentrations, we detected increased RNH1 concentrations from 8.3 ± 6.9 ng/mL and 4.2 ± 4.5 ng/mL before open and endovascular TAAA repair to 18.9 ± 5.9 ng/mL and 11.5 ± 10.3 ng/mL, respectively, 12 h after surgery (Figure 3). Afterwards, RNH1 serum concentrations decreased to 13.0 ± 7.3 ng/mL and 5.5 ± 4.3 ng/mL 72 h after open and endovascular TAAA repair, respectively (Figure 3). Before surgery, no significant differences between the two groups were observed. After surgery and 12, 48, and 72 h after admission to the ICU, significantly increased RNH1 serum levels were observed after open TAAA repair as compared with endovascular TAAA repair (all $p < 0.05$, Figure 3).

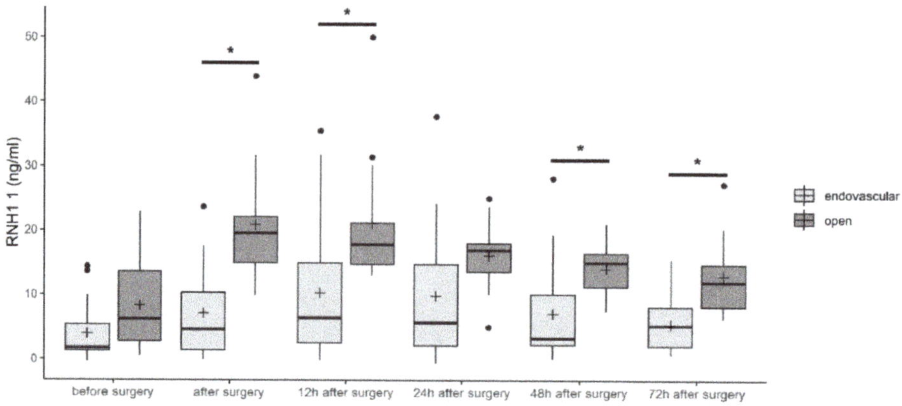

Figure 3. RNase inhibitor 1 (RNH1) serum levels in patients undergoing open or endovascular TAAA repair. Data are presented as box-whisker plots. Lines inside the boxes represent the median and the pluses represent the mean. The box is defined by Q1 and Q3. The whiskers range from Q1 to Q1 + 1.5 ∗ (Q3 − Q1) and Q3 to Q3 − 1.5 ∗ (Q3 − Q1), with observations outside of the whiskers shown as points classified as outliers. Unpaired *t*-test (two-tailed) was used for statistical analysis of the two groups. * $p < 0.05$; RNH1, RNase inhibitor 1.

3.4. Correlation of RNase 1 and RNH1 with Acute Kidney Injury (AKI)

Analyzing the effect from RNase 1 and RNH1 serum levels on the probability of suffering AKI with a univariable logistic regression model for each point in time, RNase 1 showed a statistically significant effect 12 h after surgery ($p = 0.0327$, OR = 1.035) and 48 h after surgery ($p = 0.0144$, OR = 1.045, Figure 4A). Higher RNH1 serum levels conveyed a statistically significant higher probability of experiencing AKI 12 h after surgery ($p = 0.0199$, OR = 1.129), 24 h after surgery ($p = 0.0435$, OR = 1.106), and 48 h after surgery ($p = 0.0194$, OR = 1.178, Figure 4C).

Regarding a correlation between RNase 1 and AKI, focusing on all patients suffering from post-operative AKI according to the KDIGO classification, a test accuracy of 0.702–0.750 was observed (Figure 4B). From 24 h to 48 h after surgery, the sensitivity reached 93.33–100%, and the specificity was 56.25–62.50% (Figure 4B). RNH1 showed good test accuracy for post-operative AKI with an AUC between 0.702 and 0.790 for all time points after surgery (Figure 4C). Upon admission to the ICU, the test accuracy was 0.781, with a sensitivity of 85.71% and a specificity of 81.25%. Further details can be found in the Supplementary Materials Tables S1 and S2.

While assessing the predictive abilities of RNase 1 and RNH1 for AKI separated in KDIGO 0 (n = 16) and 3 (n = 4), a favorable test accuracy for RNase 1 measured 48 h after TAAA surgery was observed (AUC 0.969, sensitivity 100%, specificity 87.5%, Table 2).

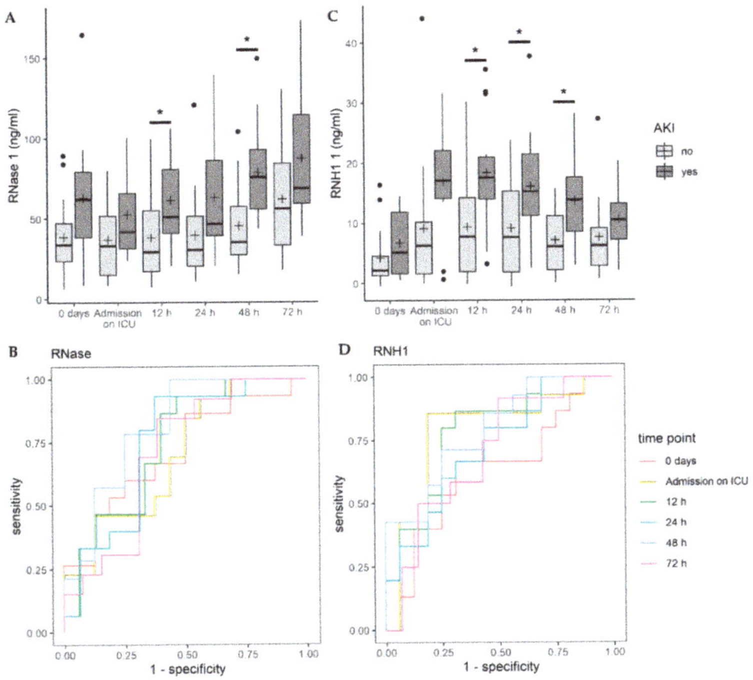

Figure 4. The correlation of (**A**) RNase 1 and (**C**) RNH1 with acute kidney injury (AKI). Data are presented as box-whisker plots. Lines inside the boxes represent the median and the pluses represent the mean. The box is defined by Q1 and Q3. The whiskers range from Q1 to Q1 + 1.5 ∗ (Q3 − Q1) and Q3 to Q3 − 1.5 ∗ (Q3 − Q1), with observations outside of the whiskers shown as points classified as outliers. ROC analysis of the diagnostic accuracy of (**B**) RNase 1 and (**D**) RNH1 serum levels for acute kidney injury in patients undergoing endovascular or open TAAA repair. * $p < 0.05$; RNase, ribonuclease; RNH1, RNase inhibitor 1.

Table 2. RNASE to predict AKI (stadium = 0) vs. AKI (stadium = 3).

Time of Measurement	Optimal Cut-Off (Youden Index)					AUC
	Cut-Off (ng/mL)	Sensitivity (%)	Specificity (%)	LR+	LR−	
0 days n = 20	≥57.64	75.00 [19.4, 99.4]	81.25 [54.4, 96.0]	4.00	0.31	0.828 [0.595, 0.957]
Admission on ICU n = 20	≥31.00	100.00 [39.8, 100.0]	50.00 [24.7, 75.3]	2.00	-	0.672 [0.429, 0862]
12 h n = 19	≥61.42	75.00 [19.4, 99.4]	86.67 [59.5, 98.3]	5.63	0.29	0.817 [0.575, 0.954]
24 h n = 20	≥32.81	100.00 [39.8, 100.0]	62.50 [35.4, 84.8]	2.67	-	0.797 [0.560, 0.941]
48 h n = 20	≥67.81	100.00 [39.8, 100.0]	87.50 [61.7, 98.4]	8.00	-	0.969 [0.779, 1.000]
72 h n = 17	≥62.28	100.00 [39.8, 100.0]	69.23 [38.6, 90.9]	3.25	-	0.904 [0.663, 0.992]

3.5. Correlation of RNase 1 and RNH1 with In-Hospital Mortality

Analyzing the effect of RNase 1 and RNH1 serum levels on in-hospital mortality with a univariable logistic regression model for each point in time, RNase 1 showed a statistically significant effect 12 h after surgery ($p = 0.018$, OR = 1.048, Figure 5A). For higher RNH1 serum levels, a statistically significant higher probability to die was observed at 0 days ($p = 0.0414$, OR = 1.174, Figure 5C).

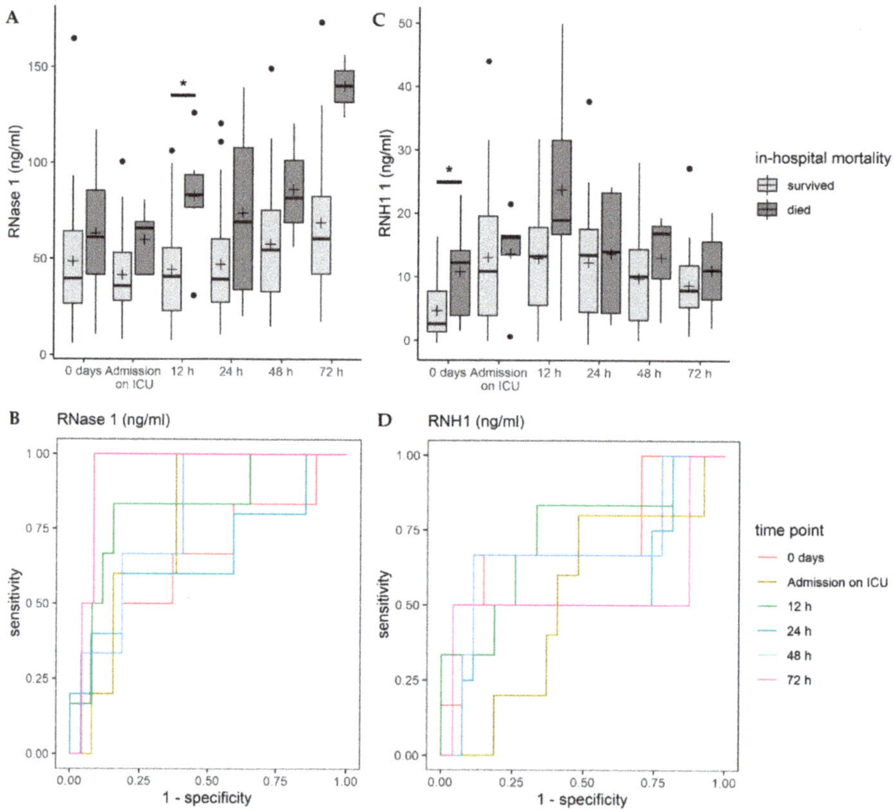

Figure 5. The correlation of (**A**) RNase 1 and (**C**) RNH1 with in-hospital mortality. Data are presented as box-whisker plots. Lines inside the boxes represent the median and the pluses represent the mean. The box is defined by Q1 and Q3. The whiskers range from Q1 to Q1 + 1.5 ∗ (Q3 − Q1) and Q3 to Q3 − 1.5 ∗ (Q3 − Q1), with observations outside of the whiskers shown as points classified as outliers. ROC analysis of the diagnostic accuracy of (**B**) RNase 1 and (**D**) RNH1 serum levels for in-hospital mortality in patients undergoing endovascular or open TAAA repair. * $p < 0.05$; RNase, ribonuclease; RNH1, RNase inhibitor 1.

The test accuracy of RNase 1 to predict in-hospital mortality increased over time, reaching 0.938 72 h after surgery, with a sensitivity of 100% and a specificity of 91.67% (Figure 5B). A moderate predictive accuracy for in-hospital mortality and RNH1 was also observed (Figure 5D). All details can be found in Tables S3 and S4.

3.6. Correlation of RNase 1 and RNH1 with Perioperative Variables

A Spearman correlation statistically significant different from 0 of RNase 1 and SOFA-Score was observed 48 and 72 h after surgery ($p = 0.02$ and 0.03, respectively), indicating a strong monotone correlation. Regarding the length of stay in the ICU, a statistically significant correlation different from 0 was observed for RNase 1 levels 48 h after surgery ($p = 0.01$), indicating a moderate monotone correlation. Statistically significant correlations different from 0 for several time points of RNH1 measurement and all assessed parameters were observed. Further correlations of RNase 1 and RNH1 with variables are shown in Tables 3 and 4. Although other than the pointed correlation coefficients of RNase 1 and RNH1 indicated moderate or strong correlations, for example, RNase 1 and PCT before surgery, the sample size for these markers were insufficient to make reliable conclusions about the magnitude of the correlation.

Table 3. Spearman's correlation coefficient for RNase 1 and perioperative variables. The number of included patients is shown below the coefficient. If the coefficient was statistically significantly different from 0, a *p*-value is stated below the number.

	Before Surgery	After Surgery	12 h After Surgery	24 h After Surgery	48 h After Surgery	72 h After Surgery
SOFA Score	x	0.20292 (n = 6)	0.22965 (n = 31)	0.25394 (n = 29)	0.57451 (n = 15) (*p* = 0.0251)	0.73193 (n = 8) (*p* = 0.0390)
Leucocytes	−0.03862 (n = 33)	0.14354 (n = 30)	−0.07718 (n = 32)	−0.02492 (n = 28)	0.37221 (n = 22)	0.40294 (n = 16)
PCT	−0.86603 (n = 3)	0.00000 (n = 9)	0.20843 (n = 20)	0.24527 (n = 24)	0.33636 (n = 11)	0.26190 (n = 8)
CRP	0.22086 (n = 32)	0.10000 (n = 9)	0.00351 (n = 19)	−0.01342 (n = 18)	0.01072 (n = 15)	0.20000 (n = 15)
IL-6	(n = 1)	−0.08571 (n = 6)	0.54545 (n = 12)	0.00000 (n = 12)	0.54286 (n = 6)	(n = 1)
LOS ICU	0.04169 (n = 33)	0.11124 (n = 31)	0.05597 (n = 32)	0.22260 (n = 32)	0.46103 (n = 30) (*p* = 0.0103)	0.36988 (n = 26)

SOFA, sequential (sepsis-related) organ failure assessment; PCT, procalcitonin; CRP, C-reactive protein; IL, interleukin; LOS, length of stay; ICU, intensive care unit.

Table 4. Spearman's correlation coefficient for RNH1 and perioperative variables. The number of included patients is shown below the coefficient. If the coefficient was statistically significantly different from 0, a *p*-value is stated below the number.

	Before Surgery	After Surgery	12 h After Surgery	24 h After Surgery	48 h After Surgery	72 h After Surgery
SOFA Score	x	−0.72471 (n = 6)	0.31193 (n = 32)	0.41576 (n = 29) (*p* = 0.0249)	0.32676 (n = 15)	−0.11119 (n = 7)
Leukocytes	−0.03996 (n = 33)	−0.15045 (n = 31)	−0.32879 (n = 33)	−0.36971 (n = 28)	−0.04123 (n = 22)	0.27857 (n = 15)
PCT	0.86603 (n = 3)	0.69457 (n = 9) (*p* = 0.0379)	0.41986 (n = 20)	0.52142 (n = 24) (*p* = 0.0090)	0.60000 (n = 11)	0.60714 (n = 7)
CRP	−0.05668 (n = 32)	−0.13333 (n = 9)	−0.43333 (n = 19)	0.23220 (n = 18)	0.54334 (n = 15) (*p* = 0.0363)	0.43736 (n = 14)
IL-6	(n = 1)	0.54286 (n = 6)	0.23776 (n = 12)	0.75524 (n = 12) (*p* = 0.0045)	0.08571 (n = 6)	(n = 1)
LOS ICU	0.20422 (n = 33)	0.18342 (n = 32)	0.20371 (n = 33)	0.21947 (n = 31)	0.40419 (n = 30) (*p* = 0.0267)	0.44018 (n = 26) (*p* = 0.0244)

SOFA, sequential (sepsis-related) organ failure assessment; PCT, procalcitonin; CRP, C-reactive protein; IL, interleukin; LOS, length of stay; ICU, intensive care unit.

4. Discussion

Thoracoabdominal aortic surgery is associated with post-operative complications and increased mortality [1]. Multiple organ failure is one of the dreaded post-operative complications after open and endovascular surgical treatment of thoracoabdominal aortic aneurysms (TAAA). AKI is one of the feared post-operative complications. Due to the absence of reliable biomarkers, such as serum creatinine, the establishment of new clinically available and reliable biomarkers and therapeutic approaches for the treatment of AKI is essential. In this study, we measured the RNase I and RNH1 levels in open and endovascular TAAA repair to determine their association with post-operative AKI. We showed, for the first time, that RNase 1 and its antagonist RNH1 play a role in open and endovascular TAAA repair and are associated with post-operative AKI and in-hospital mortality.

Thoracoabdominal aortic surgery is associated with a high mortality rate; the literature describes a mortality of 8.3% 30 days after open surgery and 5.8% after endovascular surgery [2]. In this study population, we detected a higher mortality rate of 14.3% after open surgery and 21.1% after endovascular surgery (Table 1), due to the fact that Greenberg and colleagues had examined a larger patient population. They analyzed samples from more than five years and in total they included 724 patients [2]. We investigated a collective of only 33 patients (Table 1). Furthermore, the number of patients with a type 2 TAAA was relatively high for this small study and urgent cases were also included in this study.

As a consequence of TAAA repair, open surgery may be related to an increased rate of organ damage, while endovascular TAAA repair leads to post-implantation syndrome and severe endothelial damage, both of which result in release of danger-associated molecular patterns (DAMPs). Extracellular RNA (eRNA) represents one of these DAMPs. Extracellular RNA binds to both TLR 3 and 7, inducing increased production of pro-inflammatory cytokines, such as tumor necrosis factor alpha, by translocation of nuclear factor kappa B [23,24]. This leads to an increased inflammatory reaction and results in organ dysfunction, such as AKI. Zhou and Yang described the involvement of eRNA in kidney failure [25]. RNase 1 recognizes pathogenic RNA and degrades it [10]. Therefore, increased release of RNase 1 after TAAA repair is expected. Indeed, we detected increased RNase 1 in the serum of patients after TAAA repair up to 72 h after surgery (Figure 2). An antagonist of RNase 1, RNH1 protects the cytosolic compartments from the toxic effects of RNases, however, this also has the consequence of inhibiting their antimicrobial properties [26]. In previous studies by this group, we also detected increased RNH1 and RNase 1 levels in serum of septic patients as compared with healthy subjects [11,14]. In line with these findings, we observed increased RNH1 serum levels after open and endovascular TAAA repair (Figure 3). After open TAAA repair, increased RNH1 serum levels were detected as compared with serum levels after endovascular TAAA repair (Figure 3). However, for RNase 1 serum levels, there was no difference between open and endovascular TAAA repair (Figure 2).

Martin et al. reported that elevated RNase 1 serum levels in patients with sepsis indicated dysfunction of two or more organs [11]. In line with Martin et al., we demonstrated that patients with increased RNase 1 serum levels, 12 and 48 h after surgery, exhibited a higher probability of suffering AKI (Figure 4). Additionally, Martin et al. demonstrated that patients with renal dysfunction experienced significantly higher RNase 1 levels as compared with those without renal dysfunction [11]. Indeed, we also found that patients with higher RNase 1 serum levels, 48 h after surgery, suffered a higher probability of stage 3 than stage 1 AKI (Table 2). Furthermore, we demonstrated that patients with higher RNH1 serum levels, 12, 24, and 48 h after surgery, also exhibited a higher probability of suffering AKI (Figure 4). Twelve hours after TAAA repair, we observed that RNase 1 serum levels correlated with in-hospital mortality (Figure 5). This may be due to the fact that the highest mean RNH1 serum levels were measured 12 h after surgery (15.34 ± 11.29). On the basis of these findings, it can be assumed that RNase 1 is strongly inhibited by RNH1 at this time, which means that RNase 1 is unable to cleave eRNA. This results in an increased inflammatory response and may be associated with organ dysfunction, which may explain the increased mortality at this time point.

Next, we investigated the correlation of RNase 1 and RNH1 with perioperative variables. We found, for the first time, that RNase 1 serum levels had a strong monotone correlation with 48 and 72 h time points after surgery, and RNH1 serum levels had a moderate monotone correlation 24 h after surgery with SOFA score (Tables 3 and 4). The length of stay in the ICU had a moderate monotone correlation with RNase 1 serum levels 48 h after surgery and with RNH1 serum levels 48 and 72 h after surgery (Tables 3 and 4). On the basis of these findings, RNase 1 and RNH1 serum levels may have the potential to predict post-operative sepsis, and thus the length of a hospital stay.

5. Limitation and Conclusions

Since our investigation is limited to a small patient collective with a variation in the number of measurements of some variables, further investigations with a larger collective must be aimed at to underline our results. Moreover, our measurements were limited to RNase 1 and RNH1 serum levels, the analysis of eRNA concentrations in serum would be helpful to confirm the findings of this study.

In conclusion, our data show, for the first time, that open TAAA repair results in significantly increased RNH1 serum levels as compared with endovascular TAAA repair, after admission to the ICU and 12, 48, and 72 h after surgery. We found that RNase 1 serum levels 12 and 48 h after surgery and RNH1 serum levels 12, 24 and 48 h after surgery showed a statistically significantly higher probability of suffering AKI. Furthermore, we demonstrated, for the first time, that RNH1 exhibits good test accuracy for post-operative AKI. In addition, higher RNase 1 serum levels 12 h after surgery and increased RNH1 serum levels on day 0 convey a significantly higher probability for in-hospital mortality. On the basis of these findings, RNase 1 and RNH1 may be therapeutically important and may represent biomarkers for post-operative AKI and in-hospital mortality.

Supplementary Materials: The following are available online at http://www.mdpi.com/2077-0383/9/10/3292/s1, Table S1: Test accuracy of RNase 1 and AKI according to the KDIGO classification for all patients suffering from AKI, Table S2: Test accuracy of RNH 1 and AKI according to the KDIGO classification for all patients suffering from AKI, Table S3: Test accuracy of RNase 1 and in-hospital mortality, Table S4: Test accuracy of RNH 1 and in-hospital mortality.

Author Contributions: Conceptualization, E.Z., L.M., and A.G.; methodology, E.Z., T.B., N.F., and C.B.; validation E.Z., L.M., and A.G.; formal analysis, T.B.; investigation, E.Z., L.M., and A.G.; resources, A.G., E.Z., L.M., and G.M.; data curation, E.Z., L.M., and A.G., T.B.; writing—original draft preparation, E.Z.; writing—review and editing, E.Z., L.M., A.G., T.B. and A.P.; visualization, T.B.; supervision, M.J.J.; D.K. and G.M.; project administration, E.Z. and A.G.; funding acquisition, E.Z. and L.M. All authors have read and agreed to the published version of the manuscript.

Funding: This research was funded by an intramural grant to E.Z. (START 131/19) and a grant of the German Research Foundation to L.M. (DFG, MA 7082/3-1).

Conflicts of Interest: The authors declare no conflict of interest. The funders had no role in the design of the study; in the collection, analyses, or interpretation of data; in the writing of the manuscript, or in the decision to publish the results.

References

1. Riambau, V.; Bockler, D.; Brunkwall, J.; Cao, P.; Chiesa, R.; Coppi, G.; Czerny, M.; Fraedrich, G.; Haulon, S.; Jacobs, M.J.; et al. Editor's choice—Management of descending thoracic aorta diseases: Clinical practice guidelines of the european society for vascular surgery (ESVS). *Eur. J. Vasc. Endovasc. Surg.* **2017**, *53*, 4–52. [CrossRef]
2. Greenberg, R.K.; Lu, Q.; Roselli, E.E.; Svensson, L.G.; Moon, M.C.; Hernandez, A.V.; Dowdall, J.; Cury, M.; Francis, C.; Pfaff, K.; et al. Contemporary analysis of descending thoracic and thoracoabdominal aneurysm repair: A comparison of endovascular and open techniques. *Circulation* **2008**, *118*, 808–817. [CrossRef] [PubMed]
3. Thakar, C.V. Perioperative acute kidney injury. *Adv. Chronic Kidney Dis.* **2013**, *20*, 67–75. [CrossRef]
4. Chertow, G.M.; Burdick, E.; Honour, M.; Bonventre, J.V.; Bates, D.W. Acute kidney injury, mortality, length of stay, and costs in hospitalized patients. *J. Am. Soc. Nephrol.* **2005**, *16*, 3365–3370. [CrossRef]

5. Drews, J.D.; Patel, H.J.; Williams, D.M.; Dasika, N.L.; Deeb, G.M. The impact of acute renal failure on early and late outcomes after thoracic aortic endovascular repair. *Ann. Thorac. Surg.* **2014**, *97*, 2027–2033. [CrossRef]
6. Nickolas, T.L.; Schmidt-Ott, K.M.; Canetta, P.; Forster, C.; Singer, E.; Sise, M.; Elger, A.; Maarouf, O.; Sola-Del Valle, D.A.; O'Rourke, M.; et al. Diagnostic and prognostic stratification in the emergency department using urinary biomarkers of nephron damage: A multicenter prospective cohort study. *J. Am. Coll. Cardiol.* **2012**, *59*, 246–255. [CrossRef] [PubMed]
7. Moran, S.M.; Myers, B.D. Course of acute renal failure studied by a model of creatinine kinetics. *Kidney Int.* **1985**, *27*, 928–937. [CrossRef]
8. Kellum, J.A.; Prowle, J.R. Paradigms of acute kidney injury in the intensive care setting. *Nat. Rev. Nephrol.* **2018**, *14*, 217–230. [CrossRef]
9. Lamb, E.J.; Levey, A.S.; Stevens, P.E. The kidney disease improving global outcomes (kdigo) guideline update for chronic kidney disease: Evolution not revolution. *Clin. Chem.* **2013**, *59*, 462–465. [CrossRef] [PubMed]
10. Koczera, P.; Martin, L.; Marx, G.; Schuerholz, T. The ribonuclease a superfamily in humans: Canonical rnases as the buttress of innate immunity. *Int. J. Mol. Sci.* **2016**, *17*, 1278. [CrossRef]
11. Martin, L.; Koczera, P.; Simons, N.; Zechendorf, E.; Hoeger, J.; Marx, G.; Schuerholz, T. The human host defense ribonucleases 1, 3 and 7 are elevated in patients with sepsis after major surgery—A pilot study. *Int. J. Mol. Sci.* **2016**, *17*, 294. [CrossRef]
12. Futami, J.; Tsushima, Y.; Murato, Y.; Tada, H.; Sasaki, J.; Seno, M.; Yamada, H. Tissue-specific expression of pancreatic-type rnases and rnase inhibitor in humans. *DNA Cell Biol.* **1997**, *16*, 413–419. [CrossRef] [PubMed]
13. Dickson, K.A.; Haigis, M.C.; Raines, R.T. Ribonuclease inhibitor: Structure and function. *Prog. Nucleic Acid Res. Mol. Biol.* **2005**, *80*, 349–374. [PubMed]
14. Zechendorf, E.; O'Riordan, C.E.; Stiehler, L.; Wischmeyer, N.; Chiazza, F.; Collotta, D.; Denecke, B.; Ernst, S.; Muller-Newen, G.; Coldewey, S.M.; et al. Ribonuclease 1 attenuates septic cardiomyopathy and cardiac apoptosis in a murine model of polymicrobial sepsis. *JCI Insight* **2020**, *5*. [CrossRef] [PubMed]
15. Averdunk, L.; Rückbeil, M.V.; Zarbock, A.; Martin, L.; Marx, G.; Jalaie, H.; Jacobs, M.J.; Stoppe, C.; Gombert, A. Slpi—A biomarker of acute kidney injury after open and endovascular thoracoabdominal aortic aneurysm (taaa) repair. *Sci. Rep.* **2020**, *10*, 3453. [CrossRef]
16. Mommertz, G.; Sigala, F.; Langer, S.; Koeppel, T.A.; Mess, W.H.; Schurink, G.W.; Jacobs, M.J. Thoracoabdominal aortic aneurysm repair in patients with marfan syndrome. *Eur. J. Vasc. Endovasc. Surg.* **2008**, *35*, 181–186. [CrossRef]
17. Jacobs, M.J.; Schurink, G.W. Open repair in chronic type b dissection with connective tissue disorders. *Ann. Cardiothorac. Surg.* **2014**, *3*, 325–328.
18. Jacobs, M.J.; Elenbaas, T.W.; Schurink, G.W.; Mess, W.H.; Mochtar, B. Assessment of spinal cord integrity during thoracoabdominal aortic aneurysm repair. *Ann. Thorac. Surg.* **2002**, *74*, S1864–S1866. [CrossRef]
19. Tshomba, Y.; Baccellieri, D.; Mascia, D.; Kahlberg, A.; Rinaldi, E.; Melissano, G.; Chiesa, R. Open treatment of extent iv thoracoabdominal aortic aneurysms. *J. Cardiovasc. Surg.* **2015**, *56*, 687–697.
20. Canyigit, M.; Cetin, L.; Uguz, E.; Algin, O.; Kucuker, A.; Arslan, H.; Sener, E. Reduction of iodinated contrast load with the renal artery catheterization technique during endovascular aortic repair. *Diagn. Interv. Radiol.* **2013**, *19*, 244–250. [CrossRef]
21. Thiele, R.H.; Isbell, J.M.; Rosner, M.H. Aki associated with cardiac surgery. *Clin. J. Am. Soc. Nephrol.* **2015**, *10*, 500–514. [CrossRef] [PubMed]
22. Singer, M.; Deutschman, C.S.; Seymour, C.W.; Shankar-Hari, M.; Annane, D.; Bauer, M.; Bellomo, R.; Bernard, G.R.; Chiche, J.D.; Coopersmith, C.M.; et al. The third international consensus definitions for sepsis and septic shock (sepsis-3). *JAMA* **2016**, *315*, 801–810. [CrossRef] [PubMed]
23. Chen, C.; Feng, Y.; Zou, L.; Wang, L.; Chen, H.H.; Cai, J.Y.; Xu, J.M.; Sosnovik, D.E.; Chao, W. Role of extracellular rna and tlr3-trif signaling in myocardial ischemia-reperfusion injury. *J. Am. Heart Assoc.* **2014**, *3*, e000683. [CrossRef] [PubMed]
24. Feng, Y.; Chen, H.; Cai, J.; Zou, L.; Yan, D.; Xu, G.; Li, D.; Chao, W. Cardiac rna induces inflammatory responses in cardiomyocytes and immune cells via toll-like receptor 7 signaling. *J. Biol. Chem.* **2015**, *290*, 26688–26698. [CrossRef]

25. Zhou, Y.; Yang, J. Extracellular rna in renal diseases. *ExRNA* **2019**, *1*, 5. [CrossRef]
26. Abtin, A.; Eckhart, L.; Mildner, M.; Ghannadan, M.; Harder, J.; Schroder, J.M.; Tschachler, E. Degradation by stratum corneum proteases prevents endogenous rnase inhibitor from blocking antimicrobial activities of rnase 5 and rnase 7. *J. Investig. Dermatol.* **2009**, *129*, 2193–2201. [CrossRef]

Publisher's Note: MDPI stays neutral with regard to jurisdictional claims in published maps and institutional affiliations.

Journal of
Clinical Medicine

MDPI

Article

Impact of Chest Trauma and Overweight on Mortality and Outcome in Severely Injured Patients

Thurid Eckhardt [1], Klemens Horst [1], Philipp Störmann [2], Felix Bläsius [1], Martijn Hofman [1], Christian Herren [1], Philipp Kobbe [1], Frank Hildebrand [1] and Hagen Andruszkow [1,*]

1 Department for Trauma and Reconstructive Surgery, University Hospital Aachen, Pauwelsstr. 30, 52074 Aachen, Germany; thurid.eckhardt@rwth-aachen.de (T.E.); khorst@ukaachen.de (K.H.); fblaesius@ukaachen.de (F.B.); mhofman@ukaachen.de (M.H.); cherren@ukaachen.de (C.H.); pkobbe@ukaachen.de (P.K.); fhildebrand@ukaachen.de (F.H.)

2 Department for Trauma and Reconstructive Surgery, University Hospital Frankfurt am Main, Theodor-Stern-Kai 7, 60590 Frankfurt, Germany; philipp.stoermann@kgu.de

* Correspondence: handruszkow@ukaachen.de; Tel.: +49-(0)241-80-36076

Received: 27 June 2020; Accepted: 16 August 2020; Published: 26 August 2020

Abstract: The morbidity and mortality of severely injured patients are commonly affected by multiple factors. Especially, severe chest trauma has been shown to be a significant factor in considering outcome. Contemporaneously, weight-associated endocrinological, haematological, and metabolic deviations from the norm seem to have an impact on the posttraumatic course. Therefore, the aim of this study was to determine the influence of body weight on severely injured patients by emphasizing chest trauma. A total of 338 severely injured patients were included. Multivariate regression analyses were performed on patients with severe chest trauma (AIS ≥ 3) and patients with minor chest trauma (AIS < 3). The influence of body weight on in-hospital mortality was evaluated. Of all the patients, 70.4% were male, the median age was 52 years (IQR 36–68), the overall Injury Severity Score (ISS) was 24 points (IQR 17–29), and a median BMI of 25.1 points (IQR 23–28) was determined. In general, chest trauma was associated with prolonged ventilation, prolonged ICU treatment, and increased mortality. For overweight patients with severe chest trauma, an independent survival benefit was found (OR 0.158; $p = 0.037$). Overweight seems to have an impact on the mortality of severely injured patients with combined chest trauma. Potentially, a nutritive advantage or still-unknown immunological aspects in these patients affecting the intensive treatment course could be argued.

Keywords: chest trauma; weight disorders; overweight; obesity; outcome

1. Introduction

Trauma is known to be a leading public health concern, with approximately 16,000 deaths worldwide due to various injuries each day [1]. In Western civilizations, severe trauma is the main cause of death among 15- to 44-year-olds [2]. Consequently, trauma contributes to the highest incidence of years of potential life lost, generating a large economic impact [1].

Severe chest trauma has been identified as one of the most frequent injury patterns, in addition to being a crucial prognostic factor and a leading cause of death after trauma [1]. Recent studies revealed extended periods of mechanical ventilation and length of ICU stay for severely injured patients with thoracic injuries [3]. Furthermore, severe chest trauma has been shown to be associated with the development of diverse complications (e.g., multiple organ dysfunction syndrome (MODS) and an increase of mortality by approximately 25% considering all trauma-related deaths) [3,4].

Meanwhile, obesity and overweight are constantly rising in modern society, leading to a growing public concern worldwide. Two-thirds of the adult population in the United States are known to be overweight or obese. In Europe, the incidence of obesity is increasing simultaneously, currently with 20% of European citizens considered to be obese [5]. Excess weight disorders represent risk factors for many diseases, such as hypertension, arthritis, heart disease, diabetes mellitus, and cancer. Even though the association between these chronic conditions and obesity has been investigated, varying results have been reported concerning the consequences of weight disorders on complications and outcome following trauma [6,7]. While some studies reveal increased mortality in underweight and obese patients, contemporary analyses indicate no impact of body weight [8,9]. Although these studies analysed the influence of weight disorders on outcome in trauma patients in general, little is known about the effects of body weight, particularly focusing on chest trauma as one of the most common injury patterns after trauma.

Therefore, the present study intended to evaluate the impact of different weight entities on the posttraumatic course of traumatized patients with a focus on chest trauma.

2. Experimental Section

The present study follows the guidelines of the revised World Medical Association Declaration of Helsinki in 1975 and its latest amendment in 2013 (64th general meeting). Ethical approval was obtained from the Ethics Committee of the Medical Faculty of the RWTH Aachen University (EK 346/15).

2.1. Study Design and Inclusion Criteria

A retrospective analysis of traumatized patients admitted to the RWTH Aachen University Hospital (level I trauma centre) between 2010 and 2015 was performed. Hospital charts were studied to acquire standardised documentation of the clinical course from first contact with the responsible physicians until discharge or death in the hospital. The collected data included information on demographics, pattern of injury, comorbidities, preclinical and clinical management, procedures, laboratory findings, and outcome. To ensure the highest possible data quality, all parameters were immediately reviewed for plausibility. The inclusion criteria for the present study were an Injury Severity Score (ISS) ≥ 9 and patient age ≥ 18 years. Minor injury patients (ISS < 9) aged < 18 and patients who deceased on-scene were excluded.

2.2. Injury Distribution and Injury Severity

To evaluate the thoracic injury distribution, the 2005 revised and 2008 updated versions of the Abbreviated Injury Scale (AIS) were used [10]. The AIS is an anatomy-based severity scoring system that classifies injuries by body region. Each injury is assigned an AIS score on a six-point scale according to importance, from 1 (minor) to 6 (unsurvivable) [11]. In the present study, relevant severe chest trauma was defined by an AIS score ≥ 3, while minor chest trauma was defined by an AIS score < 3. Consequently, patients without chest trauma (AIS $= 0$) were included in this group.

The AIS score is the basis for the calculation of the Injury Severity Score (ISS), determining the overall injury distribution. To calculate the ISS, identification of the three most seriously injured body regions is necessary. The highest AIS score for each of these regions is squared and summed up to a total score [10].

Furthermore, multiple prognostic scores were compared with the observed outcome to allow the examination of different injury patterns and severity between the respective subgroups. The investigated scores contained the anatomic injury-based New Injury Severity Score (NISS) [12].

2.3. In-Hospital Complications and Mortality

The severity of multiple organ dysfunction was measured using the Multiple Organ Dysfunction Score (Marshall MODS) [13]. This score mirrors organ dysfunction by using simple physiologic measures of dysfunction in six organ systems. It correlates with the highest risk of ICU and hospital mortality [13]. Additionally, the total number of deaths during the entire clinical stay was determined to note the in-hospital mortality.

2.4. Body Mass Index (BMI)

Weight disorders were assessed using the body mass index (BMI), an index of weight for height, which is defined as weight in kilograms divided by the square of height in metres (kg/m^2) [14]. The population was subsequently classified into four groups based on the BMI using the classification of the World Health Organization as follows: BMI < 20 kg/m^2 (underweight), BMI 20–25 kg/m^2 (normal weight), BMI 25–30 kg/m^2 (overweight), and BMI > 30 kg/m^2 (obesity). Body weight and height were measured at hospital admission.

2.5. Statistical Analysis

Data were analysed using the Statistical Package for the Social Sciences (SPSS 25, IBM Inc., Somers, NY, USA). Continuous values are presented as median with 25 and 75 interquartile ranges (25/75-IQR), while developments are presented with counts and percentages. Differences between the groups were evaluated with nonparametric Mann–Whitney U tests for continuous data, while Pearson's chi-square test was used for categorical values. To verify the impact of chest trauma and weight disorders on outcome, multivariate logistic regression analyses were performed. Odds ratios (ORs) with 95% confidence interval (95%-CI) were noted. A two-sided p-value < 0.05 was considered to be significant.

3. Results

A total of 338 patients admitted to the RWTH University Hospital between 2010 and 2015 fulfilled the inclusion criteria. Table 1 provides a demographic overview according to the presence of severe chest trauma, including data on age, gender, BMI, injury distribution, and mortality. In general, the median age was 52 years (IQR 36–68), and 238 patients were male (70.4%). In total, 92.3% suffered from blunt and 7.7% from penetrating injuries, and the most common cause was traffic accident (66.4%).

Table 1. Demographic overview according to the presence of severe chest trauma.

	Overall	Group I	Group II	p-Value
Number of patients (n)	338	137	201	-
Age (median 25/75-IQR)	52 (36–68)	49.0 (38–62)	52 (34–72)	0.175
Male (%)	70	75	67	0.113
ISS (median 25/75-IQR)	24 (17–29)	27.0 (18–34)	24 (17–25)	<0.001
AIS head (median 25/75-IQR)	3.5 (0–4)	1.0 (0–3)	4.0 (3.0–5.0)	<0.001
BMI (median 25/75-IQR)	25.1 (23–28)	25.7 (24–28)	24.8 (23–28)	0.042
Underweight (n)	30	13	17	
Normal weight (n)	146	54	92	
Overweight (n)	119	53	66	
Obesity (n)	43	20	23	
MODS (%)	26.3	30.3	20.1	<0.001
Mortality (%)	24.3	32.3	12.4	<0.001
Duration of ventilation (h) (median 25/75-IQR)	48 (2–258)	70 (10–222)	25 (0–287)	0.022
Duration of ICU treatment (days) (median 25/75-IQR)	11 (1–23)	17 (9–29)	6 (2–17)	<0.001
Length of stay (days) (median 25/75-IQR)	16 (7–27)	17 (10–29)	14 (5–25)	0.008

IQR: Interquartile range; BMI: Body mass index; MODS: Multiple Organ Dysfunction Score (Marshall MODS).

3.1. Chest Trauma

A total of 137 patients with severe chest trauma (group I) and 201 patients with minor chest trauma (group II) were analysed.

3.2. Impact of BMI and Chest Trauma

Multivariate logistic regression analysis revealed a survival benefit for patients with severe chest trauma in association with overweight compared with patients with only minor chest trauma and obesity or normal weight (Table 2: OR 0.158; p = 0.037). Furthermore, the severity of traumatic brain injury was shown to have an impact on mortality (OR 1.822, $p = 0.001$). Age, gender, and the overall injury severity had no influence on mortality, according to this statistical model.

Table 2. Multivariate regression analysis of patients with Abbreviated Injury Scale (AIS) chest ≥ 3 referring to mortality.

	Regression Coefficient	Odds Ratio (OR)	95% Confidence Interval (95%-CI)	*p*-Value
Age (years)	0.027	1.028	0.988–1.069	0.172
Gender (male)	−0.218	0.804	0.232–6.671	0.799
Overweight	−1.847	**0.158**	**0.028–0.892**	**0.037**
Obesity	0.030	1.094	0.203–5.885	0.917
ISS (per point)	0.057	1.059	0.989–1.133	0.102
AIS head	0.600	**1.822**	**1.102–3.013**	**0.019**
Constant	−6.148	–	–	<0.001

Normal weight was set as a categorical reference group for regression analysis between the BMI groups. The significant variables were in bold.

In contrast, the aforementioned survival benefit of overweight could not be noted for patients with only minor chest trauma (Table 3). For these patients, age and injury severity were determined as influencing factors for mortality.

Table 3. Multivariate regression analysis of patients with AIS chest < 3 referring to mortality.

	Regression Coefficient	Odds Ratio (OR)	95% Confidence Interval (95%-CI)	*p*-Value
Age (years)	**0.028**	**1.028**	**1.009–0.048**	**0.004**
Gender (male)	0.387	1.472	0.684–3.166	0.323
Overweight	−0.311	0.733	0.334–1.607	0.438
Obesity	−0.282	0.755	0.234–2.434	0.637
ISS (per point)	**0.068**	**1.071**	**1.023–1.120**	**0.003**
AIS head	0.341	1.407	1.096–1.806	0.007
Constant	−4.928	-	-	0.007

Normal weight was set as a categorical reference group for regression analysis between the BMI groups. The significant variables were in bold.

4. Discussion

The present study was designed to evaluate the influence of different weight entities on outcome in severely injured patients, with emphasis on chest trauma. To the best of our knowledge, the presented results were the first to focus on this specific injury pattern in multiple trauma patients.

Our main results can be summarized as follows:

1. Severe chest trauma was associated with prolonged treatment and in-hospital complications.
2. Subgroup analysis revealed overweight to be an independent survival factor in patients with severe chest trauma. In contrast, this aspect was not proven for severely injured patients with only minor chest trauma.

The treatment of trauma patients represents a clinical challenge, particularly in the case of associated severe chest trauma. Epidemiologic data indicate a high coincidence of severe chest trauma in severely injured patients, with consistent rates during the last several decades [15,16].

Analysing patients with only minor chest trauma, we found a positive correlation between mortality and Glasgow Coma Scale (GCS), AIS head, ISS, and age. Overall mortality in this group was slightly elevated compared with that in a corresponding study by Bayer et al. [17]. The reason could be the exclusion of patients with severe head injury in their analysis. Regarding the mean ISS for multiple trauma patients with an AIS chest < 3, no significant difference could be detected.

Additionally, the total length of stay and the limited need for mechanical ventilation in patients without severe chest trauma compared with minor chest trauma patients coincided.

A recently performed prospective study by Grubmüller et al. investigated the impact of severe chest trauma on severely injured patients, showing a significantly increased rate of in-hospital complications like organ failure and respiratory failure [18]. Consistent with that analysis, the presented study found increased incidence of MODS ($p < 0.001$; r = 0.849). Similar results were also found in several other studies examining the influence of chest trauma on multiple organ dysfunction [16,19]. Respiratory insufficiency and hemodynamic failure represent the major causes of deaths in patients with severe chest trauma, resulting in mortality rates of up to 25% [20,21]. This underlines the results of other studies showing that chest trauma is one of the most important concomitant injuries in severely injured patients having an impact on mortality [16,19,22]. Accordingly, we also found a significantly higher mortality rate for patients with an AIS chest ≥ 3 compared with patients with an AIS chest < 3. However, not all studies found an influence of severe chest trauma on mortality [18]. Potential reasons for these divergent results might be the exclusion of all patients with penetrating chest trauma and a lower overall mortality rate in the study of Grubmüller et al. [18]. The aforementioned impact of severe chest trauma on the posttraumatic clinical course is also mirrored by a prolongation of both duration of ventilation and ICU treatment in our study. In accordance with our results, Bayer et al. also revealed a correlation between an increased AIS chest score and a prolonged intubation period ($p = 0.005$) [17]. Moreover, Lin et al. found a significant association between severe chest trauma and prolonged ICU treatment ($p < 0.003$) [23]. It might be summarized that the results of the presented study on the impact of chest trauma on mortality and the clinical course are in line with those of the vast majority of studies in the current literature.

Overweight and obesity are steadily increasing in modern society. In accordance with international data, only 45.6% of our study population presented with a normal weight [24]. In general, a BMI > 30 has been described as increasing the risk for the development of multiple organ failure with an associated prolongation of the length of ICU and overall in-hospital treatment [25]. Relevant medical comorbidities related to weight disorders have been supposed to be the most likely risk factors for postsurgical and posttraumatic complications [26]. A prospective study by Goulenok et al. analysed severely injured patients, focusing on two body weight groups, BMI < 25 and >25. The authors revealed an increased mortality during ICU treatment for the second group [27]. In this respect, the present study generated four study groups according to the established BMI definition in order to investigate the impact of different weight entities on mortality [28]. We feel it is safe to argue that the current WHO classification offers a more precise predictive validity compared with the aforementioned BMI graduation by Goulenok [25]. In this context, the presented subgroup analysis revealed overweight (BMI 25–30) to be an independent survival factor in severely injured patients with concomitant chest trauma. This main result is supported by previous observations by Mica et al., who found a protective effect of a BMI between 25 and 30 points on the Systemic Inflammatory Response Syndrome (SIRS) and sepsis after severe trauma in general. Furthermore, they found the mortality rate to be decreased in the overweight BMI group compared with that in normal-weight patients (7.2% vs. 8.8%; $p < 0.001$). Significant differences in the clinical course, like duration of ICU treatment, duration of ventilation, and overall hospital stay, were not found. In contrast to the presented study, Mica et al. did not focus on a specific injury distribution like chest trauma [29,30]. The present study could therefore be argued to focus on potential outcome variables after trauma being more valid, with greater emphasis on different injury patterns and weight entities.

However, currently, only Fatica et al. investigated a potential association between chest trauma and body mass index in severely injured patients [22]. In their retrospective study with 233 thoracic trauma patients, obesity (defined as a BMI > 25) increased mortality independently of overall injury severity in chest trauma patients. Additionally, hospital admission rate, length of hospital stay, and injury severity were significantly increased for patients with a BMI > 25 [22]. However, as the present study defined overweight and obesity more precisely compared with Fatica et al., we were able to specify these results, indicating that obesity but not overweight seems to be associated with adverse outcome, whereas overweight was identified as an independent survival factor after severe trauma with severe chest trauma. In this context, a nutritive advantage for overweight patients during the prolonged intensive care course might represent a feasible explanation [31].

Additionally, a shielding impact of fatty tissue on inflammatory reactions following trauma, supressing an excessive immune response, should be considered. The reason for this could be the protective effect of oestrogens produced by aromatase activity in adipocytes as well as the immunomodulatory effect of adiponectin, which can lead to endotoxin tolerance and lower susceptibility to generalized inflammation [32,33]. Whilst patients with a BMI > 30 often suffer from chronic medical comorbidities and present with higher mortality rates after severe trauma, overweight patients with a BMI ranging from 25 to 30 points rarely present with severe medical conditions and can therefore benefit from the protective effect of the additional fatty tissue.

In patients with only minor chest trauma, no advantage for overweight patients was noted. The reason for this could be the different pattern of injury and different injury characteristics for the respective weight entities [34,35]. Additionally, the lung represents a primary target organ due to the inflammatory response after multiple trauma and could therefore be more predisposed to secondary damage in patients with chest trauma [15]. Studying the obesity-related inflammatory profile could provide additional insight.

Interpretation of the presented results should consider the limitations of this study. First, this study is limited by its retrospective design. Furthermore, BMI was the only parameter used for body weight since it represents the most widely accepted parameter in current literature analysing trauma populations [7,36]. Our two groups (AIS $\geq$ 3 vs. AIS < 3) differed considerably on the extent of injury severity, measured by the ISS (ISS 27 $\pm$ 11 Gr. I vs. 23 $\pm$ 8 Gr. II, $p < 0.001$) and the incidence of head trauma (AIS 1.7 $\pm$ 2 Gr. I vs. 3.4 $\pm$ 2 Gr. II, $p < 0.001$). In order to consider the divergent groups statistically, a multivariate regression analysis was performed.

Notwithstanding these limitations, this study offers new aspects regarding morbidity and mortality in severely injured patients, emphasizing different weight entities with concomitant chest trauma. In this respect, a BMI ranging from 25 to 30 seems to alter the clinical course, and its protective effects must be investigated in future studies.

5. Conclusions

Based on the presented analysis, the presence of severe chest trauma in severely injured patients has a considerable impact on the clinical course. Furthermore, divergent weight entities seem to affect this impact on outcome. The treatment of severely injured patients should therefore reflect the presence of overweight or obesity, assessing this influencing factor correctly during the clinical course.

Author Contributions: H.A. and F.H. initiated and conceptualized the study. T.E. collected the data, validated the data, performed the statistical analysis, interpreted the results, and prepared the original draft. H.A., F.H., K.H., M.H., F.B., P.S., C.H., and P.K. supervised the study, supported the interpretation of the data and results, and corrected the original draft. All authors have read and agreed to the published version of the manuscript.

Funding: This research received no external funding.

Conflicts of Interest: The authors declare no conflict of interest.

References

1. Lecky, F.E.; Bouamra, O.; Woodford, M.; Alexandrescu, R.; O'Brien, S.J. Epidemiology of Polytrauma. In *Damage Control Management in the Polytrauma Patient*; Pape, H.-C., Peitzman, A., SCHWAB, C.W., Giannoudis, P.V., Eds.; Springer New York: New York, NY, USA, 2010; pp. 13–24. ISBN 978-0-387-89507-9.
2. The global burden of injuries. *Am. J. Public Health* **2000**, *90*, 523–526. [CrossRef]
3. Andruszkow, H.; Schweigkofler, U.; Lefering, R.; Frey, M.; Horst, K.; Pfeifer, R.; Beckers, S.K.; Pape, H.-C.; Hildebrand, F. Impact of Helicopter Emergency Medical Service in Traumatized Patients: Which Patient Benefits Most? *PLoS ONE* **2016**, *11*, e0146897. [CrossRef] [PubMed]

4. Bakowitz, M.; Bruns, B.; McCunn, M. Acute lung injury and the acute respiratory distress syndrome in the injured patient. *Scand. J. Trauma Resusc. Emerg. Med.* **2012**, *20*, 54. [CrossRef] [PubMed]
5. Doak, C.M.; Wijnhoven, T.M.A.; Schokker, D.F.; Visscher, T.L.S.; Seidell, J.C. Age standardization in mapping adult overweight and obesity trends in the WHO European Region. *Obes. Rev.* **2012**, *13*, 174–191. [CrossRef] [PubMed]
6. Byrnes, M.C.; McDaniel, M.D.; Moore, M.B.; Helmer, S.D.; Smith, R.S. The effect of obesity on outcomes among injured patients. *J. Trauma* **2005**, *58*, 232–237. [CrossRef] [PubMed]
7. Hoffmann, M.; Lefering, R.; Gruber-Rathmann, M.; Rueger, J.M.; Lehmann, W. The impact of BMI on polytrauma outcome. *Injury* **2012**, *43*, 184–188. [CrossRef]
8. Maheshwari, R.; Mack, C.D.; Kaufman, R.P.; Francis, D.O.; Bulger, E.M.; Nork, S.E.; Henley, M.B. Severity of injury and outcomes among obese trauma patients with fractures of the femur and tibia: A crash injMury research and engineering network study. *J. Orthop. Trauma* **2009**, *23*, 634–639. [CrossRef]
9. Osborne, Z.; Rowitz, B.; Moore, H.; Oliphant, U.; Butler, J.; Olson, M.; Aucar, J. Obesity in trauma: Outcomes and disposition trends. *Am. J. Surg.* **2014**, *207*, 387–392. [CrossRef]
10. Baker, S.P.; O'Neill, B.; Haddon, W.; Long, W.B. The injury severity score: A method for describing patients with multiple injuries and evaluating emergency care. *J. Trauma Acute Care Surg.* **1974**, *14*, 187–196. [CrossRef]
11. Civil, I.D.; Schwab, C.W. The Abbreviated Injury Scale, 1985 Revision: A Condensed Chart For Clinical Use. *J. Trauma Inj. Infect. Crit. Care* **1988**, *28*, 87–90. [CrossRef]
12. Osler, T.; Baker, S.P.; Long, W. A modification of the injury severity score that both improves accuracy and simplifies scoring. *J. Trauma Acute Care Surg.* **1997**, *43*, 922–925, discussion 925-6. [CrossRef] [PubMed]
13. Marshall, J.C.; Cook, D.J.; Christou, N.V.; Bernard, G.R.; Sprung, C.L.; Sibbald, W.J. Multiple organ dysfunction score: A reliable descriptor of a complex clinical outcome. *Crit. Care Med.* **1995**, *23*, 1638–1652. [CrossRef] [PubMed]
14. Blackburn, H.; Jacobs, D. Commentary: Origins and evolution of body mass index (BMI): Continuing saga. *Int. J. Epidemiol.* **2014**, *43*, 665–669. [CrossRef]
15. Huber-Wagner, S.; Qvick, M.; Mussack, T.; Euler, E.; Kay, M.V.; Mutschler, W.; Kanz, K.-G. Massive blood transfusion and outcome in 1062 polytrauma patients: A prospective study based on the Trauma Registry of the German Trauma Society. *Vox Sang.* **2007**, *92*, 69–78. [CrossRef] [PubMed]
16. Horst, K.; Andruszkow, H.; Weber, C.D.; Pishnamaz, M.; Herren, C.; Zhi, Q.; Knobe, M.; Lefering, R.; Hildebrand, F.; Pape, H.-C. Thoracic trauma now and then: A 10 year experience from 16,773 severely injured patients. *PLoS ONE* **2017**, *12*, e0186712. [CrossRef]
17. Bayer, J.; Lefering, R.; Reinhardt, S.; Kühle, J.; Zwingmann, J.; Südkamp, N.P.; Hammer, T. Thoracic trauma severity contributes to differences in intensive care therapy and mortality of severely injured patients: Analysis based on the TraumaRegister DGU®. *World J. Emerg. Surg.* **2017**, *12*, 43. [CrossRef]
18. Grubmüller, M.; Kerschbaum, M.; Diepold, E.; Angerpointner, K.; Nerlich, M.; Ernstberger, A. Severe thoracic trauma—Still an independent predictor for death in multiple injured patients? *Scand. J. Trauma Resusc. Emerg. Med.* **2018**, *26*, 6. [CrossRef]
19. Veysi, V.T.; Nikolaou, V.S.; Paliobeis, C.; Efstathopoulos, N.; Giannoudis, P.V. Prevalence of chest trauma, associated injuries and mortality: A level I trauma centre experience. *Int. Orthop.* **2009**, *33*, 1425–1433. [CrossRef]
20. Dewar, D.C.; Tarrant, S.M.; King, K.L.; Balogh, Z.J. Changes in the epidemiology and prediction of multiple-organ failure after injury. *J. Trauma Acute Care Surg.* **2013**, *74*, 774–779. [CrossRef]
21. Hildebrand, F.; Weuster, M.; Mommsen, P.; Mohr, J.; Fröhlich, M.; Witte, I.; Keibl, C.; Ruchholtz, S.; Seekamp, A.; Pape, H.-C.; et al. A combined trauma model of chest and abdominal trauma with hemorrhagic shock—Description of a new porcine model. *Shock* **2012**, *38*, 664–670. [CrossRef]
22. Fatica, F.; Geraci, G.; Puzhlyakov, V.; Modica, G.; Cajozzo, M. The effect of body mass index on chest trauma severity and prognosis. *Ann. Ital. Chir.* **2017**, *88*, 289–391. [PubMed]
23. Lin, F.C.-F.; Tsai, S.C.-S.; Li, R.-Y.; Chen, H.-C.; Tung, Y.-W.; Chou, M.-C. Factors associated with intensive care unit admission in patients with traumatic thoracic injury. *J. Int. Med. Res.* **2013**, *41*, 1310–1317. [CrossRef] [PubMed]
24. Durgun, H.M.; Dursun, R.; Zengin, Y.; Özhasenekler, A.; Orak, M.; Üstündağ, M.; Güloğlu, C. The effect of body mass index on trauma severity and prognosis in trauma patients. *Ulus. Travma Acil Cerrahi Derg.* **2016**, *22*, 457–465. [CrossRef] [PubMed]

25. Andruszkow, H.; Veh, J.; Mommsen, P.; Zeckey, C.; Hildebrand, F.; Frink, M. Impact of the body mass on complications and outcome in multiple trauma patients: What does the weight weigh? *Mediat. Inflamm* **2013**, *2013*, 345702. [CrossRef] [PubMed]
26. Ciesla, D.J.; Moore, E.E.; Johnson, J.L.; Burch, J.M.; Cothren, C.C.; Sauaia, A. Obesity increases risk of organ failure after severe trauma. *J. Am. Coll. Surg.* **2006**, *203*, 539–545. [CrossRef]
27. Goulenok, C.; Monchi, M.; Chiche, J.-D.; Mira, J.-P.; Dhainaut, J.-F.; Cariou, A. Influence of overweight on ICU mortality: A prospective study. *Chest* **2004**, *125*, 1441–1445. [CrossRef] [PubMed]
28. WHO Regional Office for Europe. Body Mass Index—BMI. Available online: https://www.euro.who.int/en/health-topics/disease-prevention/nutrition/a-healthy-lifestyle/body-mass-index-bmi (accessed on 25 August 2020).
29. Mica, L.; Vomela, J.; Keel, M.; Trentz, O. The impact of body mass index on the development of systemic inflammatory response syndrome and sepsis in patients with polytrauma. *Injury* **2014**, *45*, 253–258. [CrossRef] [PubMed]
30. Mica, L.; Keller, C.; Vomela, J.; Trentz, O.; Plecko, M.; Keel, M.J. The impact of body mass index and gender on the development of infectious complications in polytrauma patients. *Eur. J. Trauma Emerg. Surg.* **2014**, *40*, 573–579. [CrossRef]
31. Jeevanandam, M.; Young, D.H.; Schiller, W.R. Obesity and the metabolic response to severe multiple trauma in man. *J. Clin. Investig.* **1991**, *87*, 262–269. [CrossRef]
32. Zacharioudaki, V.; Androulidaki, A.; Arranz, A.; Vrentzos, G.; Margioris, A.N.; Tsatsanis, C. Adiponectin promotes endotoxin tolerance in macrophages by inducing IRAK-M expression. *J. Immunol.* **2009**, *182*, 6444–6451. [CrossRef]
33. Choudhry, M.A.; Bland, K.I.; Chaudry, I.H. Trauma and immune response—Effect of gender differences. *Injury* **2007**, *38*, 1382–1391. [CrossRef] [PubMed]
34. Chuang, J.-F.; Rau, C.-S.; Kuo, P.-J.; Chen, Y.-C.; Hsu, S.-Y.; Hsieh, H.-Y.; Hsieh, C.-H. Traumatic injuries among adult obese patients in southern Taiwan: A cross-sectional study based on a trauma registry system. *BMC Public Health* **2016**, *16*, 275. [CrossRef]
35. Brown, C.V.R.; Velmahos, G.C. The consequences of obesity on trauma, emergency surgery, and surgical critical care. *World J. Emerg. Surg.* **2006**, *1*, 27. [CrossRef] [PubMed]
36. Kraft, R.; Herndon, D.N.; Williams, F.N.; Al-Mousawi, A.M.; Finnerty, C.C.; Jeschke, M.G. The effect of obesity on adverse outcomes and metabolism in pediatric burn patients. *Int. J. Obes.* **2012**, *36*, 485–490. [CrossRef] [PubMed]

Journal of
Clinical Medicine

MDPI

Article

Increased First Pass Success with C-MAC Videolaryngoscopy in Prehospital Endotracheal Intubation—A Randomized Controlled Trial

Christian Macke *, Felix Gralla, Marcel Winkelmann, Jan-Dierk Clausen, Marco Haertle, Christian Krettek and Mohamed Omar

Trauma Department, Hannover Medical School, Carl-Neuberg-Strasse 1, 30625 Hanover, Germany; felix.gralla@st.ovgu.de (F.G.); winkelmann.marcel@mh-hannover.de (M.W.); Clausen.Jan-Dierk@mh-hannover.de (J.-D.C.); haertle.marco@mh-hannover.de (M.H.); krettek.christian@mh-hannover.de (C.K.); omar.mohamed@mh-hannover.de (M.O.)

* Correspondence: macke.christian@mh-hannover.de; Tel.: +49-511-532-2050

Received: 28 June 2020; Accepted: 20 August 2020; Published: 22 August 2020

Abstract: Endotracheal intubation (ETI) with direct view laryngoscopy (DL) is the gold standard for airway management. Videolaryngoscopy (VL) can improve glottis visualization, thus facilitating ETI. The aim of this monocentric, randomized, prospective study on a physician staffed German air ambulance is to compare DL and VL for ETI in terms of number of attempts and time as well as visualization of the glottis in a prehospital setting in a physician-based rescue system in adult patients. A power analysis was performed à priori. We used consecutive on-scene randomization with a sealed envelope system for the DL and VL-group. Successful ETI with first pass success was significantly more frequent with VL than DL and three seconds faster. The percentage of glottis opening and the Cormack & Lehane classification were significantly better with VL than DL. Regarding improved first pass success in ETI with the VL, we would recommend the use of VL for prehospital airway management in physician-based rescue systems.

Keywords: airway management; intubation; laryngoscopy; video; prehospital care; rescue helicopter; air ambulance

1. Introduction

A difficult airway with a "cannot intubate—cannot ventilate" situation is a potentially fatal issue and a challenge for every physician [1]. Up to date, there is no simple reliable test for prediction of a difficult airway, therefore it is often impossible to perform the available tests in an emergency situation because of the missing opportunity for a structured evaluation of these factors.

In a physician based rescue system the gold standard in airway management should be endotracheal intubation (ETI). However, even in the routine elective surgery situation Adnet and colleagues reported a high rate of minor difficulties in ETI (37%) in a consecutive trial [2]. Additionally, Timmermann et al. could demonstrate a failure rate of right bronchus or esophageal intubation from emergency medical services in Germany of 10% and 6% in 2006 [3].

The question remains: How can we perform a safe ETI in the prehospital setting? A possible tool to manage the airway problem and establish a secure airway is the videolaryngoscope (VL) [4,5].

Loughan and co-workers found no significant difference for VL and direct view laryngoscopy (DL) in elective surgery [6]. Otherwise, a Cochrane review with 7044 participants undergoing elective surgery found moderate evidence for a reduction of failed intubation and laryngeal/airway trauma for VL and improved laryngeal view [7]. However, there was no evidence for a reduction in first pass success. In contrast, Pieters and colleagues showed in a meta-analysis of 1329 elective patients with known difficult airways a significant improvement even for the experienced anesthetist for first-pass success, laryngeal view, and a reduction of mucosal trauma [8]. Unfortunately, nearly all of these studies are performed as in-hospital studies with known sobriety anesthesia, complete medical history, and known risk factors.

In the past years some studies for prehospital videolaryngoscopy were published [9–11]. However, the results are quite distributed, ranging from only 48% first pass success rate up to 86% with different videolaryngoscopes. However, all of these studies are performed in air ambulance settings with experienced anesthesiologists as prehospital care physicians. They are on the one hand not representative for the common prehospital physician in Germany [12]. On the other hand, anesthetists are highly trained in direct laryngoscopy and therefore tend to have a lack of motivation to use this device as a new standard [13,14].

Therefore, the aim of this study was a comparison of DL and VL with regard to first-pass success and time of attempts as well as glottis visualization in a prehospital setting in a physician-based rescue system in adult patients. We hypothesized that VL will lead to a higher first pass success rate and a better visibility of the glottis for non-anesthetist prehospital physicians.

2. Experimental Section

Ethical approval was obtained by the ethical board of Hannover Medical School with the registration number 2016–7268. In accordance with the requirements of the ethical approval, informed consent was obtained after recovery of the patient. In case of death or permanent disability consent was obtained from relatives.

Prior to study, a power analysis with sample size calculation was performed for the first pass success rate. For 80% quality with a significance level of $p < 0.05$ the sample size was set to 76 patients per group, resulting in a total patient number of 152, assuming a first pass success rate of 80% in the DL [15] and 95% in the VL group [16].

We performed a prospective, consecutive, and randomized enrolment of all adult patients with indication for intubation on the air ambulance from 04/2017–01/2019 (Figure 1 Flow Chart).

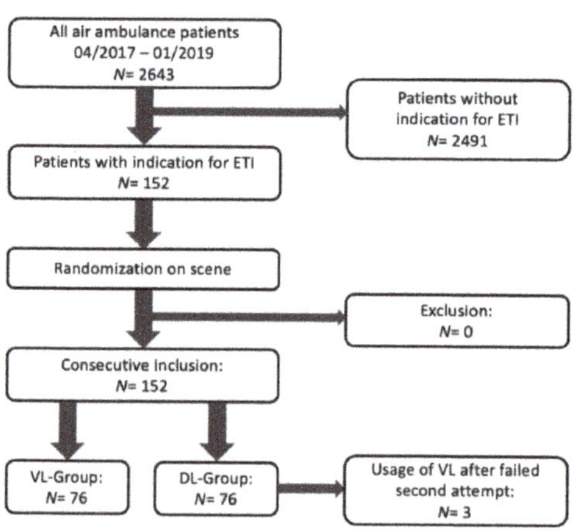

Figure 1. Flow-Chart of patient enrollment.

2.1. Primary Outcome

First pass success rate in comparison of DL vs. VL.

2.2. Secondary Outcome

Visualization of the glottis in comparison of DL vs. VL.

Comparison of success rate of less experienced physicians with <100 intubations (LEP) vs. experienced physicians with >100 intubations (EP).

Inclusion criteria: Age ≥ 18 years; Necessity of endotracheal intubation.

Exclusion criteria: Age < 18 years.

2.3. *Intubation and Staff*

Intubations were performed with rapid-sequence induction in all patients >GCS 3 in a team approach of a physician with the help of a HEMS paramedic. In patients with GCS 3 the intubation was conducted without drugs. The treating physician had free choice of induction drug, but was instructed to use a relaxant according to our standard operating procedures.

2.3.1. Physician

In contrast to most other German air ambulances all our physicians are experienced trauma surgeons with an additional qualification for prehospital care. The experienced group had an experience > 100 intubations (EP) prior to this study, the less experienced group < 100 intubations (LEP) in total.

2.3.2. HEMS Paramedic

The Helicopter Emergency Medical Service paramedics are specially trained and are qualified to prepare ETI as well as support the physician during the intubation procedure. In this study the HEMS paramedic conducted the documentation, drug administration, and time measurement.

2.4. *Randomization*

Immediately after the decision for endotracheal intubation the HEMS paramedic pulled a sealed, opaque envelope with the randomized method and prepared the equipment for intubation. The physician only knew the method right before the intubation. The envelopes were prepared with a consecutive numbered standardized protocol (see measured parameters) in advance by author FG, who was not involved in the treatment of the patients.

2.5. *Airway Management Problems*

In case of ETI problems with DL the physician was allowed to change the method to VL anytime but had to switch to VL after the second fail with DL. Other back-up systems were also available (laryngeal tube, bag-mask-ventilation, surgical airway).

2.6. *Laryngoscope*

The standard laryngoscope was a Vital View II LED from GE, Boston, Massachusetts, USA with single use blades, whereas the videolaryngoscope was the C-MAC® PM from Storz Medical, Tuttlingen, Germany with multi-use blades (Macintosh II-IV, D-Blade). The videolaryngoscope has been available on the air ambulance since 2016. Moreover, every physician had a briefing into the usage prior to the study and had to conduct at least ten intubations on an airway trainer.

2.7. *Measured Parameters*

All of these parameters were documented on a standardized protocol after performing the intubation:

- Assumed intubation problems (facial trauma, limited mouth opening (<2.5 cm), no neck, rigid collar during intubation, fluid in pharynx (vomit/blood)).
- Indication (resuscitation/CPR (cardiopulmonary resuscitation), trauma-resuscitation/trauma-CPR, musculoskeletal trauma, neurologic, burns, pulmonary, drowning).
- Site (floor, ambulance stretcher, sitting position, inside helicopter, other).

- Lighting conditions (poor, good, too bright).
- Necessary or applied relaxation with induction.
- Oxygen saturation before, during and after intubation.
- Best sight of glottis with percentage of glottis opening (POGO-Score) and Cormack-Lehane Score (CL) I–IV.
- Time for intubation measured by the HEMS paramedic with a stopwatch from taking off the mask to either tube blocking and detectable end-tidal CO_2 or putting back the mask.
- In case of videolaryngoscopy usage: whether the monitor or direct laryngoscopy was used. In all cases the monitor was used.
- Number of attempts with video- or direct view laryngoscopy.
- Blade size and type (Macintosh II-IV, D-Blade).
- Correctness of intubation proofed by auscultation and capnography.
- Necessity of alternative airway management.

2.8. Statistical Analysis

Statistical analysis was performed with SPSS 25 (IBM). For dichotomous variables the Fisher's-Exact-Test was used, and for mean variables the Mann-Whitney-U-Test after checking for normal distribution. Significance level was set to $p < 0.05$.

3. Results

3.1. General Patient Data

Median age of the patients was 68 years (Q1:Q3; 55:78) and they were predominantly male ($n = 113$ (74.3%) vs. $n = 39$ (25.7%)). No alternative airway was necessary in any of the 152 cases. Thirty-four patients (22.4%) died at the scene of ETI, all other patients were brought to hospital alive ($n = 118$ (77.6%)). All patients, including the deceased, had a documented detectable end-tidal CO_2. There were no differences in basic parameters in both groups. The site of intubation was as follows: stretcher of an ambulance car ($n = 79$ (52.0%)), ground ($n = 72$ (47.4%)), sitting position in a car due to entrapment ($n = 1$ (0.7%)). This was handled without difficulties in the first attempt with VL. For distribution of indications for ETI see also Table 1.

Table 1. Indication for endotracheal intubation (ETI) in the study population.

Indication	Number (n (%)) Total	Number (n (%)) VL	Number (n (%)) DL
Resuscitation/CPR	70 (46.1%)	29 (38.2%)	41 (53.9%)
Trauma-resuscitation/Trauma-CPR	14 (9.2%)	10 (13.2%)	4 (5.3%)
Musculoskeletal trauma	47 (30.9%)	27 (35.5%)	20 (26.3%)
Neurologic	11 (7.2%)	6 (7.9%)	5 (6.6%)
Burns	5 (3.3%)	1 (1.3%)	4 (5.3%)
Pulmonary	4 (2.6%)	2 (2.6%)	2 (2.6%)
Drowning	1 (0.7%)	1 (1.3%)	0 (0.0%)

CPR: cardiopulmonary resuscitation; VL: videolaryngoscopy; DL: direct view laryngoscopy.

There were no differences in the DL and VL group in view of lighting conditions, medical indication, intubation site, as well as necessary or applied relaxation. All patients with GCS > 3 had a relaxant administered with induction. Possible intubation problems—defined as facial trauma, limited mouth opening (<2.5 cm), no neck, rigid collar during intubation, fluid in pharynx (vomit/blood)—were found in 50% of the patients in each group (Table 2). There were no significant differences regarding the above mentioned assumed possible intubation problems between DL and VL group.

Table 2. Comparison of videolaryngoscopy (VL) and laryngoscopy (DL) of possible intubation problems.

	VL (*n* (%; 95%-CI))	DL (*n* (%; 95%-CI))	*p*-Value
Number	76	76	-
Rigid collar during ETI	19 (25%; 15–35)	11 (14%; 6–23)	0.15
No neck patient	12 (16%; 7–24)	8 (11%; 3–18)	0.47
Mid facial trauma	10 (13%; 5–21)	8 (11%; 3–18)	0.80
Bleeding/aspiration	10 (13%; 5–21)	12 (16%; 7–24)	0.82
Limited mouth opening	6 (8%; 2–14)	3 (4%; −1–8)	0.49
Assumed intubation problems	42 (55%; 44–67)	39 (51%; 49–63)	0.75

We aimed to evaluate the oxygen saturation before, during, and after intubation. Unfortunately, only in $n = 71$ (46.7%) cases these parameters were documented sufficiently. Nearly all cases were unproblematic intubations in the first attempt with a desaturation no more than ten per cent. Especially in CPR situations the values were poorly documented or not measurable.

3.2. Experienced vs. Less Experienced Physicians

No difference was found between the group of experienced physicians and less experienced physicians for all parameters. The groups were distributed equally with 48% (47/98) VL usage for the EP and 54% (29/54) VL ($p = 0.6$) usage for the LEP.

3.3. First Pass Success Rate

No alternative airway management had to be used in any of the 152 patients. Table 3. Displays the success rate in relation to the number of attempts. VL resulted in 95% successful ETI at the first attempt compared to 79% with DL. All of the four unsuccessful first attempts with VL were interrupted attempts because of massive aspiration and/or pharyngeal bleeding before placing the tube, and subsequent necessity for suction, whereas only three of the 16 s attempts with DL group were related to this issue. The others were due to visibility problems. All aspirations or bleedings, except for one aspiration in group DL and one in group VL after induction respectively, occurred before the first intubation attempt and were not due to induction or intubation. Moreover, 100% (76/76) in the VL group had a correctly placed tube after two attempts, whereas only 96% (73/76) in the DL group were placed successfully at the second attempt.

Table 3. Number of attempts for VL and DL.

Attempts	VL (*n*, (%; 95%-CI))	DL (*n*, (%; 95%-CI))	*p*-Value
1st attempt successful	72 (95%; 90–100)	60 (79%; 70–88)	0.007
2nd attempt successful	4 (100%; 100)	13 (81%; 60–103)	1.0
3rd attempt successful	0 (0%)	2 (67%; −77–210)	not applicable
4th attempt successful	0 (0%)	1 (100%; 100)	not applicable

Of the three patients with a second failed attempt with DL two could be intubated successfully (67%) with VL in the first attempt. Only one patient with a Cormack-Lehane Score of IV needed a second VL attempt.

The number needed to treat (NNT) for the first pass success with VL was 6.3, and the absolute risk reduction was 0.16.

3.4. ETI Time and Glottic View

Median ETI time at the first attempt of VL and DL was 15.5 s (Q1:Q3; 10:20) and 18.5 s (Q1:Q3; 12.5:24.5) ($p = 0.01$). See Table 4. For all attempts.

Table 4. Duration in relation to number of attempts for VL and DL in seconds (s).

Attempts	VL (s) as Median (Q1:Q3)	DL (s) as Median (Q1:Q3)	p-Value
1st attempt	15.5 (10:20)	18.5 (12.5:24.5)	0.01
2nd attempt	15 (9.0:25.0)	15 (10:20)	0.89
3rd attempt	n. a.	12 (10.5:18.5)	n. a.
4th attempt	n. a.	30	n. a.

Overall, VL leads to a significantly better glottic view in the first attempt (Table 5).

Table 5. Visibility of glottic opening in the first and second attempt for VL and DL.

Dependence on 1st Attempt	VL	DL	p-Value
POGO-Score (%), median (Q1:Q3)	100 (90:100)	65 (30:90)	<0.001
Cormack & Lehane, median (Q1:Q3)	1 (1:2)	2 (2:2)	<0.001
Dependence on 2nd Attempt	**VL**	**DL**	**p-Value**
POGO-Score (%), median (Q1:Q3)	72.5 (51.25:90)	20 (0:62.5)	0.04
Cormack & Lehane, median (Q1:Q3)	2 (2:2)	2 (2:3.75)	0.29

POGO: percentage of glottis opening.

4. Discussion

This prospective, consecutive and randomized study compared the success rate of the video-laryngoscopic ETI with the conventional ETI in a preclinical setting of a German air ambulance.

The primary goal was to address the question whether the first pass success, meaning an successful ETI in the first attempt, was higher in the VL group, as it is well-known that more than one attempt for ETI in an emergency situation is a significant predictor for adverse events [17].

In our study we demonstrated a first-pass success rate of 79% with DL and 95% with VL, which is comparable to the existing literature for DL but better for VL in the prehospital setting [10,11]. The first pass success rate for in-hospital emergency ETI ranges from 75% to 85% with DL [15,18,19], and up to 96% with VL [16,20,21]. Mackie and colleagues could demonstrate that first pass success could be significantly increased from 59.2 to 85.1% with the C-MAC video-laryngoscope in 163 emergency intubations by emergency registrars [22]. Moreover, the complication rate dropped from 28.9 to 16.1% in their study.

A possible reason for the higher success rates with VL might be improved glottis visibility, as it is long known for DL that a better view leads to higher success rates [23]. Piepho and colleagues demonstrated in 52 patients with a Cormack & Lehane grade III an improvement with VL in 94% of the patients [24] and Sulser and his co-workers reported a significantly better Cormack & Lehane grade for VL in a randomized trial in an emergency department [25], although they were not able to demonstrate a higher first-pass success rate as they had a first-pass success of almost 100% in both groups. One possible explanation for these findings could be that all of the intubations were performed by three very experienced anesthesiology consultants under favorable conditions in an emergency department. However, this is not the usual setting for out of hospital ETI and the majority of prehospital active emergency physicians in Germany are not that well experienced, since only about 25% are consultants [12].

We aimed to evaluate the desaturation during intubation as oxygen saturation is a crucial factor during intubation [26]. Bodily and colleagues found in their study of $n = 265$ rapid sequence inductions in an emergency department a desaturation in 35.5%, but had to exclude 99 patients from their study due to unavailable data, although they used electronic data acquisition [26]. Unfortunately, our documentation here is not adequate with data only recorded in 46.7% of cases. It should also be mentioned that all intubations were performed in a team approach with reduced resources. Especially in CPR situations with only a team of two persons the possibility for documentation is not always possible without endangering the patient. In our cohort more than half of the patients were patients with CPR/Trauma-CPR with an initial GCS of 3. Moreover, the time for intubation was quite short, so that desaturation was unlikely.

These points demonstrate the difficulty in transferring data from emergency in-hospital situations to the rough environment in the prehospital setting.

Furthermore, it should be mentioned that the type of videolaryngoscope could have an influence on first pass success, too. Ruetzler and colleagues found different success rates in a comparison of five different videolaryngoscopes in a training situation in which C-MAC performed very well in difficult airway situations [27]. Cavus et al. however, found the C-MAC only comparable to the A.P.Advance but better than the KingVision [11].

Thus, the results for videolaryngoscopy with 95% first pass success could be linked to the type of videolaryngoscope employed. Another possibility could be the profession of the physicians: all of the physicians are trauma surgeons with training in arthroscopy. They are used to perform complex triangulation on a 2D screen. Maybe this expertise helps in performing ETI with VL.

In this study there was no difference between well-experienced physicians with more than 100 ETIs and less-experienced physicians. Referring to Mackie and colleagues LEP probably were able to intubate with high success rates with VL [22] and the success rates with DL are comparable to other physician-based preclinical ETI rates with DL [19]. Because of the study design with focus on comparison of VL and DL, preplanned patient number in both groups for this particular question would be too small to answer it with high statistical power. On the other hand, we had no necessity for an alternative airway in any of the 152 patients, and even two out of three patients (67%) with two failed DL attempts could be intubated with VL at the first try.

Another finding of our study was the three-seconds-faster ETI with VL. The absolute time seems quite fast with 16 and 19 s, respectively. Different authors reported intubation times around 30 s [6,25]. However, it is difficult to compare the absolute time for intubation procedure as the definition of beginning and ending differs vastly. Moreover, we are convinced—in accordance with the literature—that time is not as crucial as the first-pass-success, as long as there is no desaturation with hypoxia during intubation [7,15].

4.1. Limitations, Strength, and Generalizability

There are limitations to this study. First, the study was only performed on one air ambulance in Germany with physicians experienced in prehospital care, which limits the results to physician-based prehospital care with the use of rapid-sequence induction. Moreover, all of the physicians are trauma surgeons without any anesthesiological background, which limits the generalizability of this study.

On the other hand, this could be a strength as well. Only half of the physicians had performed more than 100 intubations in their medical career. However, the results of this study are comparable to other anesthesiological studies where only experienced anesthesiologists performed emergency intubations, but better regarding videolaryngoscopy [5,9,10]. Furthermore, our group of physicians is very homogenous with relatively low experience in ETI from 50 to 300 in total. This represents the German reality in prehospital care even better than well-experienced anesthesiologic consultants would do [12]. With regard to the relatively low experience in ETI of our physicians and the high rate of patients without the need for rapid-sequence-induction, this study may be applicable for paramedics as well.

A further strength of this prehospital study with prospective randomization is the consecutive inclusion of the participants without any loss of recruitment or exclusion of patients.

Moreover, we performed a prior power analysis and assumed a distribution of 80% (DL) and 95% (VL) first pass success for an 80% quality. It should be mentioned that we assumed the different values based on one review and meta-analysis of Park et al. [15] which deals with intubations in emergency departments. Furthermore, because of a lack of high-volume studies or wide distribution regarding the success rates of videolaryngoscopy in emergency situations, we used Aziz et al. [16] to estimate the success rate of videolaryngoscopy. This study is a retrospective in-hospital study. It could be debated whether this is transferrable to our study. Otherwise, the prior power analysis correlates very closely with our results.

4.2. Summary

We could demonstrate a significantly better first pass success, a better glottic view and a slightly faster ETI with VL. Since most of the prehospital active emergency physicians in Germany are not very experienced in ETI [12] and younger and less experienced physicians benefit most from VL [20,22], we would recommend videolaryngoscopy as primary device for ETI in prehospital care at least in a physician-based system.

5. Conclusions

In this prehospital randomized study comparing videolaryngoscopy and direct laryngoscopy we showed a significant advantage of videolaryngoscopy in view of success at the first attempt in prehospital endotracheal intubation. Therefore, we recommend videolaryngoscopy as the primary device for airway management with endotracheal intubation in the prehospital setting in a physician-based rescue system. Since the completion of this study we use videolaryngoscopy as the primary device in our own air ambulance.

Author Contributions: Conceptualization, C.M. and M.O.; data curation, C.M., M.W., and M.O.; formal analysis, C.M., F.G., M.W., J.-D.C., M.H., and M.O.; investigation, C.M., F.G., M.W., J.-D.C., M.H., and M.O.; project administration, C.M. and M.O.; resources, C.M. and M.O.; supervision, C.M. and M.O.; validation, C.M.; visualization, C.M., F.G., M.W., J.-D.C., and M.O.; writing—original draft, C.M.; writing—review and editing, C.M., F.G., M.W., J.-D.C., M.H., C.K., and M.O. All authors have read and agreed to the published version of the manuscript.

Funding: This research received no external funding.

Acknowledgments: This study was awarded the Evidence Based Medicine Prize 2019 of the German Society for Orthopedics and Trauma (DGOU). The authors want to thank all physicians and HEMS paramedics of the air ambulance Christoph 4 for their support during this study. Moreover, we want to thank Justin Bender for his help with English correction.

Conflicts of Interest: The authors declare no conflict of interest.

References

1. Lavery, G.; McCloskey, B.V. The difficult airway in adult critical care. *Crit. Care Med.* **2008**, *36*, 2163–2173. [CrossRef] [PubMed]
2. Adnet, F.; Racine, S.; Borron, S.W.; Clemessy, J.L.; Fournier, J.L.; Lapostolle, F.; Cupa, M. A survey of tracheal intubation difficulty in the operating room: A prospective observational study. *Acta Anaesth. Scand.* **2001**, *45*, 327–332. [CrossRef]
3. Timmermann, A.; Russo, S.G.; Eich, C.; Roessler, M.; Braun, U.; Rosenblatt, W.H.; Quintel, M. The Out-Of-Hospital Esophageal and Endobronchial Intubations Performed by Emergency Physicians. *Anesth. Analg.* **2007**, *104*, 619–623. [CrossRef]
4. Aziz, M.F.; Brambrink, A.M.; Healy, D.W.; Willett, A.W.; Shanks, A.; Tremper, T.; Jameson, L.; Ragheb, J.; Biggs, D.A.; Paganelli, W.C.; et al. Success of Intubation Rescue Techniques after Failed Direct Laryngoscopy in Adults: A Retrospective Comparative Analysis from the Multicenter Perioperative Outcomes Group. *Anesthesiology* **2016**, *125*, 656–666. [CrossRef]
5. Bernhard, M.; Bax, S.N.; Hartwig, T.; Yahiaoui-Doktor, M.; Petros, S.; Bercker, S.; Ramshorn-Zimmer, A.; Gries, A. Airway Management in the Emergency Department (The OcEAN-Study)-A prospective single centre observational cohort study. *Scand. J. Trauma Resusc. Emerg. Med.* **2019**, *27*, 20. [CrossRef]
6. Loughnan, A.; Deng, C.; Dominick, F.; Pencheva, L.; Campbell, D. A single-centre, randomised controlled feasibility pilot trial comparing performance of direct laryngoscopy versus videolaryngoscopy for endotracheal intubation in surgical patients. *Pilot Feasibility Stud.* **2019**, *5*, 50. [CrossRef]

7. Lewis, S.R.; Butler, A.; Parker, J.; Cook, T.; Schofield-Robinson, O.; Smith, A. Videolaryngoscopy versus direct laryngoscopy for adult patients requiring tracheal intubation: A Cochrane Systematic Review. *Br. J. Anaesth.* **2017**, *119*, 369–383. [CrossRef]
8. Pieters, B.M.A.; Maas, E.H.A.; Knape, J.T.A.; Van Zundert, A.A.J. Videolaryngoscopy vs. direct laryngoscopy use by experienced anaesthetists in patients with known difficult airways: A systematic review and meta-analysis. *Anaesthesia* **2017**, *72*, 1532–1541. [CrossRef]
9. Trimmel, H.; Kreutziger, J.; Fitzka, R.; Szuts, S.; Derdak, C.; Koch, E.; Erwied, B.; Voelckel, W.G. Use of the glidescope ranger video laryngoscope for emergency intubation in the prehospital setting: A Randomized Control Trial. *Crit. Care Med.* **2016**, *44*, e470–e476. [CrossRef] [PubMed]
10. Kreutziger, J.; Hornung, S.; Harrer, C.; Urschl, W.; Doppler, R.; Voelckel, W.G.; Trimmel, H. Comparing the McGrath Mac Video Laryngoscope and Direct Laryngoscopy for Prehospital Emergency Intubation in Air Rescue Patients. *Crit. Care Med.* **2019**, *47*, 1362–1370. [CrossRef] [PubMed]
11. Cavus, E.; Janssen, S.; Reifferscheid, F.; Caliebe, A.; Callies, A.; von der Heyden, M.; Knacke, P.G.; Doerges, V. Faculty Opinions recommendation of Videolaryngoscopy for Physician-Based, Prehospital Emergency Intubation: A Prospective, Randomized, Multicenter Comparison of Different Blade Types Using A.P. Advance, C-MAC System, and KingVision. *Anesth. Analg.* **2018**, *126*, 1565–1574. [CrossRef] [PubMed]
12. Luckscheiter, A.; Lohs, T.; Fischer, M.; Zink, W. Preclinical emergency anesthesia: A current state analysis from 2015–2017. *Anaesthesist* **2019**, *68*, 270–281. [CrossRef] [PubMed]
13. Cook, T.M.; Boniface, N.; Seller, C.; Hughes, J.; Damen, C.; Macdonald, L.; Kelly, F.E. Universal videolaryngoscopy: A structured approach to conversion to videolaryngoscopy for all intubations in an anaesthetic and intensive care department. *Br. J. Anaesth.* **2018**, *120*, 173–180. [CrossRef] [PubMed]
14. Wu, T.-Y. Education: The last mile to universal videolaryngoscopy. *Br. J. Anaesth.* **2018**, *120*, 1431–1432. [CrossRef]
15. Park, L.; Zeng, I.; Brainard, A.H. Systematic review and meta-analysis of first-pass success rates in emergency department intubation: Creating a benchmark for emergency airway care. *Emerg. Med. Australas.* **2016**, *29*, 40–47. [CrossRef]
16. Aziz, M.; Healy, D.; Kheterpal, S.; Fu, R.F.; Dillman, D.; Brambrink, A.M. Routine Clinical Practice Effectiveness of the Glidescope in Difficult Airway Management. *Anesthesiology* **2011**, *114*, 34–41. [CrossRef]
17. Sakles, J.C.; Chiu, S.; Mosier, J.; Walker, C.; Stolz, U. The importance of first pass success when performing orotracheal intubation in the emergency department. *Acad. Emerg. Med.* **2013**, *20*, 71–78. [CrossRef]
18. Powell, E.K.; Hinckley, W.R.; Stolz, U.; Golden, A.J.; Ventura, A.; McMullan, J.T. Abstract 4: Predictors of Definitive Airway sans Hypoxia/Hypotension on First Attempt (DASH 1A) Success in Traumatically Injured Patients Undergoing Prehospital Intubation. *Prehosp. Emerg. Care* **2019**, *7*, 1–8. [CrossRef]
19. Guihard, B.; Chollet-Xémard, C.; Lakhnati, P.; Vivien, B.; Broche, C.; Savary, D.; Ricard-Hibon, A.; Cassou, P.-J.M.D.; Adnet, F.; Wiel, E.; et al. Effect of Rocuronium vs Succinylcholine on Endotracheal Intubation Success Rate Among Patients Undergoing Out-of-Hospital Rapid Sequence Intubation: A Randomized Clinical Trial. *JAMA* **2019**, *322*, 2303–2312. [CrossRef]
20. Min, B.C.; Park, J.E.; Lee, G.T.; Kim, T.; Yoon, H.; Cha, W.C.; Shin, T.G.; Song, K.J.; Park, M.; Han, H.; et al. C-MAC Video Laryngoscope versus Conventional Direct Laryngoscopy for Endotracheal Intubation During Cardiopulmonary Resuscitation. *Medicina* **2019**, *55*, 225. [CrossRef]
21. Eberlein, C.M.; Luther, I.S.; Carpenter, T.A.; Ramirez, L.D. First-Pass Success Intubations Using Video Laryngoscopy Versus Direct Laryngoscopy: A Retrospective Prehospital Ambulance Service Study. *Air Med. J.* **2019**, *38*, 356–358. [CrossRef] [PubMed]
22. Mackie, S.; Moy, F.; Kamona, S.; Jones, P. Effect of the introduction of C-MAC videolaryngoscopy on first-pass intubation success rates for emergency medicine registrars. *Emerg. Med. Australas.* **2019**, *32*, 25–32. [CrossRef] [PubMed]
23. Wilson, P.M.E.; Spiegelhalter, P.D.; Robertson, F.J.A.; Lesser, F.P. Predicting Difficult Intubation. *Br. J. Anaesth.* **1988**, *61*, 211–216. [CrossRef] [PubMed]
24. Piepho, T.; Fortmueller, K.; Heid, F.M.; Schmidtmann, I.; Werner, C.; Noppens, R.R. Performance of the C-MAC video laryngoscope in patients after a limited glottic view using Macintosh laryngoscopy. *Anaesthesia* **2011**, *66*, 1101–1105. [CrossRef] [PubMed]

25. Sulser, S.; Ubmann, D.; Schlaepfer, M.; Brueesch, M.; Goliasch, G.; Seifert, B.; Spahn, D.R.; Ruetzler, K. C-MAC videolaryngoscope compared with direct laryngoscopy for rapid sequence intubation in an emergency department. *Eur. J. Anaesth.* **2016**, *33*, 943–948. [CrossRef] [PubMed]
26. Bodily, J.B.; Webb, H.R.; Weiss, S.J.; Braude, D.A. Incidence and Duration of Continuously Measured Oxygen Desaturation During Emergency Department Intubation. *Ann. Emerg. Med.* **2016**, *67*, 389–395. [CrossRef]
27. Ruetzler, K.; Imach, S.; Weiss, M.; Haas, T.; Schmidt, A.R. Comparison of five video laryngoscopes and conventional direct laryngoscopy: Investigations on simple and simulated difficult airways on the intubation trainer. *Anaesthesist* **2015**, *64*, 513–519. [CrossRef]

Journal of
Clinical Medicine

MDPI

Article

Safety, Effect and Feasibility of Percutaneous SI-Screw with and without Augmentation—A 15-Year Retrospective Analysis on over 640 Screws

René Hartensuer [1,*], Moritz F. Lodde [1], Jonas Keller [1], Maria Eveslage [2], Josef Stolberg-Stolberg [1], Oliver Riesenbeck [1] and Michael J. Raschke [1]

1 Department of Trauma-, Hand- and Reconstructive Surgery, University of Muenster, 48149 Münster, Germany; moritz.lodde@ukmuenster.de (M.F.L.); j_kell13@uni-muenster.de (J.K.); Josef.Stolberg-Stolberg@ukmuenster.de (J.S.-S.); oliver.riesenbeck@ukmuenster.de (O.R.); michael.raschke@ukmuenster.de (M.J.R.)

2 Institute of Biostatistics and Clinical Research, University of Muenster, 48149 Münster, Germany; maria.eveslage@ukmuenster.de

* Correspondence: hartensuer@uni-muenster.de; Tel.: +49-251-83-59204

Received: 24 June 2020; Accepted: 14 August 2020; Published: 17 August 2020

Abstract: Background: Minimally invasive sacroiliac-screw (SI-screw) fixation of the pelvis is used in energy trauma (Arbeitsgemeinschaft für Osteosynthesefragen (AO) classified) and fragility fractures (Fragility Fracture of the Pelvis (FFP) classified). However, available clinical data are based on small case series and biomechanical data seem to be contradictory. Methods: The present single center retrospective cohort study investigated percutaneous SI-screw fixation and augmentation over 15 years. Groups were compared concerning the general epidemiological data, mobilization, complication rates, duration of stay, and safety of SI-screw insertion. Multivariable analyses were performed using logistic regression. Results: Between 2005 and March 2020, 448 patients with 642 inserted SI-screws were identified. Iatrogenic neurological impairment was documented in 2.47% and correlated with screw misplacement. There was an increased complication risk in patients with AO type C over patients with AO type B and in FFP II over FFP III/IV patients. Cement-augmented FFP patients showed a 25% reduced stay in hospital and a reduced complication risk. Cement-associated complications were seen in 22% without correlation to neurologic impairment. Conclusions: The present study confirms the safety and usability of percutaneous SI-screw fixation, despite specific risks. Cement augmentation seems to reduce the complication risk in FFP patients and shorten hospital stay for some reasons, without increased specific complications or correlated neurological impairment.

Keywords: sacroiliac-screw; SI-screw; percutaneous operation; augmentation; pelvic ring; fragility fracture; 3-D navigation

---

1. Introduction

Percutaneous sacroiliac-screw (SI-screw) fixation is considered to be the "gold standard" for the treatment of posterior pelvic ring fractures since it was described in 1973 [1]. However, there is still a considerable risk of iatrogenic injury to the lumbo-sacral nerve roots, the superior gluteal artery and the iliac vessels [2]. These complications can be caused by K-wire or screw mal-positioning during insertion. The rate of mal-positioning is still reported to be approximately 5% [3,4]. Nevertheless, the advantages over open techniques are obvious and some authors consider percutaneous SI-screw fixation to be the only minimally invasive technique to stabilize the posterior pelvic ring [5]. Traditionally, pelvic injuries are considered to be associated with an immense traumatic impact, often associated with other severe injuries. An increasing number of cases, however, resulted from low energy trauma associated with osteoporosis in the geriatric population. Different classifications are available to rate these injuries. One common classification was introduced by Tile [6] and is included into the AO classification systematics [7]. To prevent complications, early mobilization is one reason for surgery. Despite the increasing usage of the minimally invasive SI-screw technique, knowledge is still limited. Recent reviews are based on small case series, biomechanical investigations, and technical reports, so far [8,9].

The rising numbers of fractures to the pelvis occurs in the aging population. Here is an increasing incidence of fractures to the pelvis as a result of low impact and associated with an advanced frailty status [10]. It seems to be crucial to distinguish between these two entities. The so-called fragility fractures are described to differ in terms of morphology and injury mechanisms from high-energy pelvic injuries. The grade of instability in these fractures may increase over time [11]. In 2013 Rommens and Hofmann proposed a new classification for the fragility fractures of the pelvis (FFP) [12]. The FFP classification is reported to allow moderate intra- and inter-rater reliability [13]. A disproportionately high in-hospital mortality rate with these, in supposedly less severely injured patients, is reported [14]. Pain reduction and rapid return to mobility are the main treatment goals in these patients [15]. Eckardt et al. described a good functional outcome after percutaneous screw stabilization in patients suffering fragility fractures of the pelvis [16]. They investigated 50 patients with a mean age of 79 years. They described a 1-year mortality of 10% and an additional loss of independency in 13%. Furthermore, they reported on one intraoperative screw misplacement, one severe intraoperative bleeding and one post-operatively detected misplaced screw with ischial pain. Moreover, implant loosening in over 30% with 18% of patients requiring revision surgery is reported [16]. Despite the wide usage of percutaneous SI-screw fixation for the treatment of pelvic ring fractures, this technique remains insufficient for the anchorage of the screws inside the sacrum in cases of severe osteoporosis. To gain increased anchoring, Tjardes et al., as well as Müller and Fuchtmeier, suggested cement augmentation [17,18], which was described by Wähnert et al. using cannulated perforated SI-screws [19]. To data, few data are available on this topic. A recent systematic review by König et al. found eleven studies. Out of these, five were case series and the other six were biomechanical cadaveric studies [9]. They concluded that, based on few clinical case series with relatively low numbers of patients and available biomechanical data, the augmentation of SI-screws was safe and effective. However, the biomechanical results on the effect of augmentation are contradictory. Some authors found no difference between the augmentation of sacroiliac-screw and conventional sacroiliac-screw fixation [20–22]. Others report on improved biomechanical stability due to cement augmentation [23–25]. Clinical data again are only available from small case series. The number of patients ranges from 8 to 34 [19,26–29]. König et al. concluded in their review that there were no larger case series, prospective data or randomized trials available [9]. To our knowledge, these important contributions to estimate the clinical impact are still missing.

We were able to retrospectively investigate percutaneous SI-screw fixation and augmentation in a large number of patients treated over the last 15 years. These single center retrospective observational data should provide an important contribution to the remaining uncertainty about risk, safety and immediate effects of SI-screw fixation, with and without augmentation.

2. Experimental Section

This is a retrospective, single-center cohort study. From January 2005 to March 2020, patients were identified by operation and procedure coding (OPS) (5-790.0d, 5-79a.0e, 5-79b.0e, 5-83b.20, 5-83b.21) using the hospital database. Individual case review was performed for each case, including digitally available imaging. Retrospective data acquisition included age, sex, numbers of SI-screws, cement augmentation, classification of injury, Patient Clinical Complexity Level (PCCL) [30], American Society of Anesthesiologists (ASA) score, Charlson Comorbidity Index (CCI) [31], body mass index (BMI), duration of in-hospital stay, major and minor complications, screw-associated complications, cement=associated complications, mobility at time of discharge, usage of intraoperative 3D scan, usage of intraoperative navigation and postoperative peripheral neurological complications. All documented complications were recorded and rated to be minor or major complications.

An overview is given in Table 1. All cases were re-classified using available imaging or the description of morphology. Descriptive analysis was performed including all patients providing the required data. The number of included patients for distinct analysis was provided where appropriate. An overview is given in the result section (Figure 1). Pelvic ring fractures caused by high-energy trauma were classified using the Arbeitsgemeinschaft für Osteosynthesefragen (AO) Classification [7]. All fractures caused by minor trauma were classified using the FFP classification [12]. By doing so, we were able to distinguish between high- and low-energy trauma in our data set. Screw-associated complications distinguished between the non-perforation of cortical bone, less than 3.6 mm (mild) and more or equal than 3.6 mm (severe), regardless of potential clinical significance. This grading was chosen in context with the used 7.3 mm and 7.5 mm screws. Cement-associated complications were defined to include all cement extrusions outside the bony sacrum, regardless of potential clinical significance. Clinically obvious problems, like postoperative peripheral neurological impairment, were recorded and reported separately.

Table 1. Minor and major complications.

Minor Compilation	Major Complication
• Hypertensive derailment	• Inguinal hernia incarcerated postoperatively
• Delayed wound healing	• Cerebral hemorrhage postoperatively
• Infections (UTIs [1], pneumonia, other infections without severe clinical impact)	• Postoperative fracture dislocation
	• Intraoperative resuscitation
• Postoperative atrial fibrillation	• Death
• Postoperative anemia	• Implant failure requiring revision surgery
• Pain described to be the reason of delayed discharge	• Heavy intraoperative bleeding [2]
• Superficial wound infections	• Acute kidney failure (AKIN)
• Hematoma (without revision)	• Persistent postoperative neurological impairment until discharge [3]
• Temporary neurological impairment [1]	• Postoperative cerebral insult
• Postoperative angioedema	• Wound infection requires revision surgery
• New diagnosis of restless leg syndrome	• Postoperative pulmonary artery embolism
• Early loosening of external supraacetabular fixator	• Postoperative wound-related hemorrhage
• Pain beyond a period of about 6 months	• Postoperative severe hematoma with revision surgery
	• Postoperative positive Trendelenburg sign

[1] Urinary tract infection; [2] intraoperative transfusion or description of severe bleeding in the surgeon's report; [3] Postoperative peripheral neurological impairment is reported separately.

Statistical analyses were performed using the SAS® software version 9.4 for Windows (SAS Institute, Cary, NC, USA). Data are described using the median and interquartile range (Q1–Q3) or the absolute and relative frequencies. Groups were compared concerning the complication rates (i.e., proportion of patients with at least one major/minor complication) using Fisher's exact test. Multivariable analyses were performed using logistic regression. Results are reported as odds ratios (OR) and the corresponding 95% confidence intervals. Groups were compared concerning the ordinal and continuous variables using the Mann–Whitney *U* test. Linear regression was used to analyze the duration of hospital stay, which was log-transformed because of its skewed distribution. Therefore, the results are reported in terms of ratios concerning the geometric mean and corresponding 95% confidence intervals. Missing data are indicated for each analysis in the results section.

The study was approved from the local ethical committee (Ref.#2020-409-f-S).

3. Results

Between 2005 and March 2020, 448 patients with 642 inserted SI-screws were identified. The median age was 57.93 years (Q1:40.97; Q3:77.16). Overall sex distribution f/m was 249/199 (56%/44%). Median age of males was 49.72 years (Q1:31.07; Q3:65.84); median age of females was 70.90 years (Q1:48.83; Q3:81.59).

One hundred and twenty-four patients (27.68%) were classified as AO B, 176 patients (39.29%) as AO C, 117 patients (26.12%) as FFP II, nine patients (2.01%) as FFP III and 22 patients (4.91%) as FFP IV. There was an obvious difference in age and sex between the trauma categories. The median age in AO B patients was 49.35 years (Q1 31.04; Q3 64.71). In AO C patients the median age was 46.49 years (Q1 28.50; Q3 60.98). The median age in FFP II patients was 80.16 years (Q1 73.09; Q3 85.36), in FFP III patients 71.61 years (Q1 65.96; Q3 81.88) and in FFP IV patients 76.31 years (Q1 69.90; Q3 80.81), respectively.

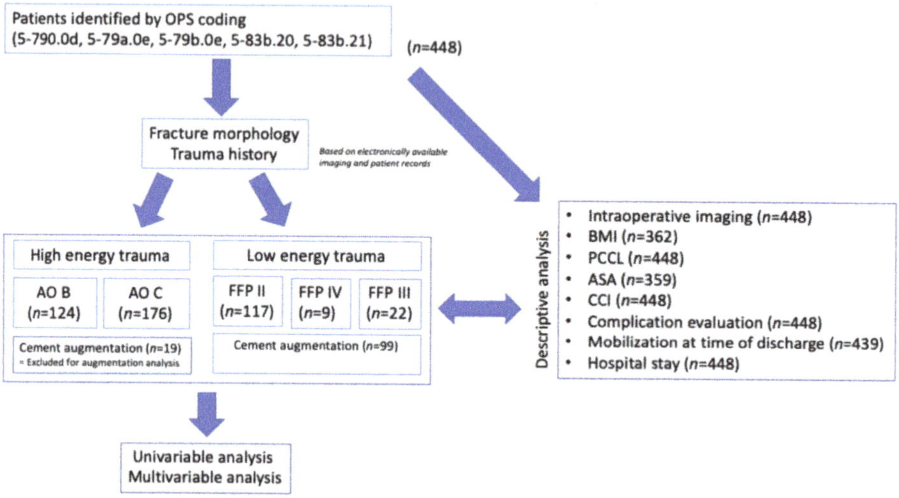

Figure 1. Schematic overview of the included cases according to the STrengthening the Reporting of OBservational studies in Epidemiology (STROBE) recommendations [32]. High-energy trauma was excluded from the analysis of augmentation. No follow-up was performed. Reduced numbers represent missing data in available sources. In all cases, a clinical report and a distinct radiological report or imaging was available. In cases of available electronic imaging, classification was performed by the authors. Patients without a history of high-energy trauma were re-classified using the fragility fractures of the pelvis (FFP) classification (FFP II—non-displaced posterior ring fracture; FFP III—displaced unilateral posterior pelvic ring fracture; and FFP IV—displaced bilateral posterior pelvic ring fracture). OPS = operation and procedure coding; AO = Arbeitsgemeinschaft für Osteosynthesefragen; FFP = Fragility fractures of the pelvis; BMI = Body mass index; PCCL = Patient Clinical Complexity Level; ASA = American Society of Anesthesiologists score; CCI = Charlson Comorbidity Index.

Sex distribution in both AO groups ($n = 300$) was f/m 39.67%/60.33% and in all FFP groups ($n = 148$) f/m 87.84%;12.16%, respectively. The different distribution of age separated by sex is presented in Figure 2.

BMI calculation was possible in 362 patients. Median BMI was 24.49 (Q1: 22.28; Q3: 27.68) ranging from 15.76 (min) to 50.70 (max). No differences between males and females were found.

A single screw was inserted in 282 (63.09%) patients, two screws in 145 (32.44%) patients and more than two screws in 20 (4.47%) patients. Intraoperative 3D imaging was documented in 69%. Consecutively, in 31%, intraoperative conventional 2D fluoroscopic imaging was documented. Out of the 305 cases in which 3D imaging was documented, one single scan was performed in 246 cases (80.66%), two scans were documented in 47 (15.40%) cases and three scans were documented in 12 cases (0.04%). Navigation was used in 141 cases (31.69%). Intraoperative 3D scans performed for image acquisition to perform 3D navigation was not counted for the above presented interoperative 3D imaging. Out of the navigated cases, five cases of 2D navigation were documented. All the others were 3D navigated.

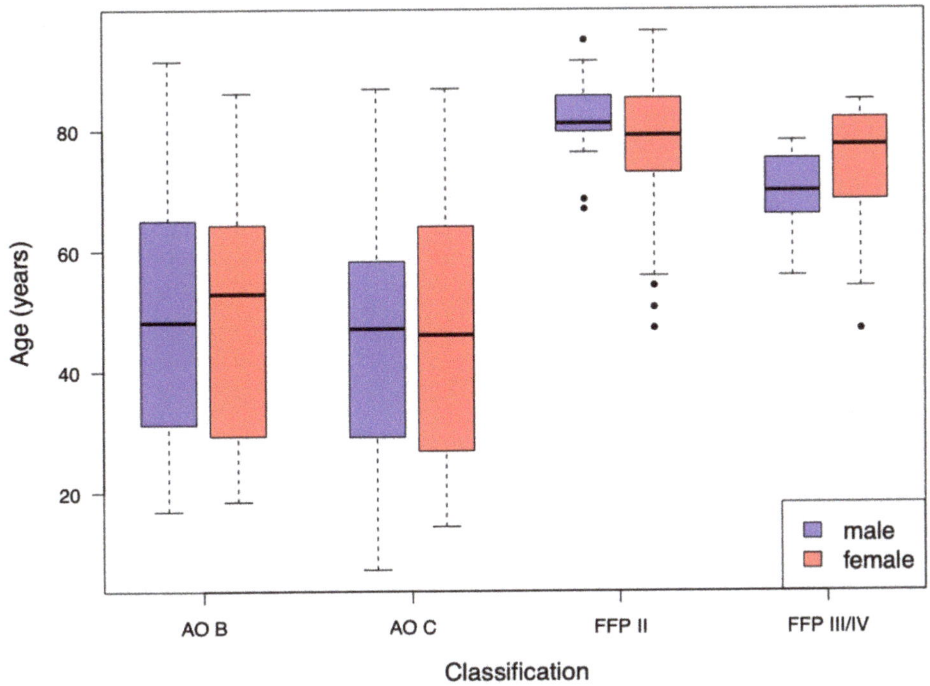

Figure 2. Descriptive analysis of age separated by sex in the different classification patterns. Dots indicating outliers.

Overall documented PCCL coding was distributed with two peaks. PCCL 0 was found in 101 cases (22.54%), whereas PCCL 1 and PCCL 2 were documented only in 22 (4.91%) and 44 (9.82%) cases, respectively. Another peak was seen in PCCL 3 and PCCL 4 with 117 (26.12%) and 100 (22.32%), respectively. PCCL 5 was found in 51 cases (11.38%) and PCCL 6 in 13 (2.90%). The majority of cases were rated ASA 2 and 3 (ASA 1: 18.66%; ASA 2: 45.68%; ASA 3: 33.70%; ASA 4: 1.95%), whereas the majority of cases presented a CCI of 0 (CCI 0: 64.29%; CCI 1:15.18%; CCI 2: 10.04%; CCI 3: 5.36%; CCI 4: 2.01%; CCI 5: 1.79%; CCI 6: 0.89%; CCI 7: 0.45%). The median age in the cases with CCI 0 was 48.13 years (Q1: 29.31; Q3:63.90) whereas the median age in CCI 1–7 was higher than 70 years. In all patients, the major and minor complications were seen more frequently in males. Major complication rate (patients with at least one complication presented in Table 1) in males (17.09%) was twice as much compared to that in females (8.84%) ($p = 0.0097$). Moreover, minor complications occurred more often in males (29.65%) than in females (20.56%) ($p = 0.0278$). Multivariable regression analysis also shows a reduced risk of major complications in females compared to males (OR 0.538), an increased risk in AO C compared to AO B (OR 3.516) with a comparable risk between FFP II and AO B (OR 0.819). Furthermore, we found a considerable increased risk of FFP III/IV over AO B (OR 4.137) and even increased compared to AO C (OR 1.176). Odds ratios with 95% confidence limits for major complications are illustrated and presented in Figure 3a. The analysis for minor complications revealed comparable results illustrated and presented in Figure 3b. Since FFP group was predominant in augmented cases, a separate analysis on this group will be provided separately to facilitate comparability.

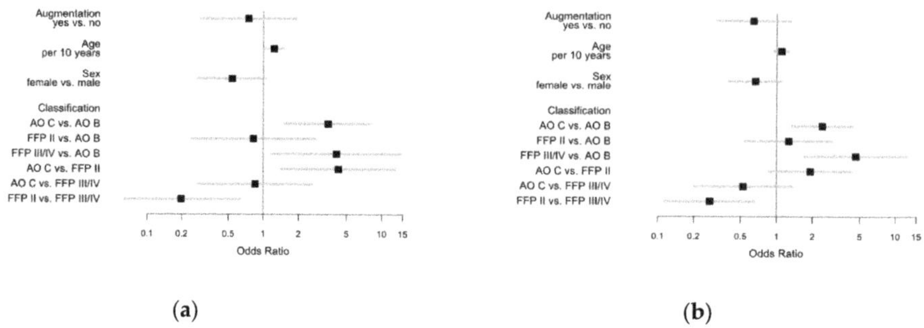

Figure 3. Odds ratios with 95% Wald confidence limits for (**a**) major complications (augmented vs. non-augmented 0.742; female vs. male: 0.538; AO C vs. AO B: 3.516; FFP II vs. AO B: 0.819; FFP III/IV vs. AO B: 4.137; AO C vs. FFP II: 4.293; AO C vs. FFP III/IV: 0.850; FFP II vs. FFP III/IV: 0.198) and (**b**) minor complications (augmented vs. non-augmented 0.642; female vs. male: 0.665; AO C vs. AO B: 2.423; FFP II vs. AO B: 1.263; FFP III/IV vs. AO B: 4.624; AO C vs. FFP II: 1.918; AO C vs. FFP III/IV: 0.524; FFP II vs. FFP III/IV: 0.273).

3.1. Safety of SI-Screw Insertion

Out of the 642 inserted SI-screws in 448 patients, the review of correct placement was possible for 422 patients (604 screws). Correct screw placement was accounted for in 385 patients (91.23%), whereas minor screw displacement was found in 19 patients (4.5%) and major displacement was seen in 13 patients (3.08%). In five cases, revision surgery was performed (1.18%). Iatrogenic neurological impairment after surgery was documented in 11/446 patients (2.47%). In eight cases, neurological deficit was present at the time of discharge, and in three cases, temporary impairment with recovery at time of discharge was documented. Despite the screw misplacement, 5/37 (13.51%) of the consecutive neurological deficits were found in this cohort. However, neurologic complications were correlated with screw misplacement (p = 0.0001). There was no difference concerning the observed rate of misplaced screws between the conventional placement (8.05%) and the 3D navigated screw insertion (9.24%). In this context, no reduction of screw-related complications using 3D navigation was seen (p = 0.3076) in our collective. The median BMI in patients with screw misplacement was 26.09 mg/m^2 (Q1 23.37; Q3 29.22) compared to a median BMI of 24.49 mg/m^2 (Q1 22.22; Q3 27.44) in patients without screw-related complications (p = 0.0938).

3.2. Analysis of AO-Classified Patients

Median duration of hospital stay in AO B patients was 15 days (Q1 8; Q3 24.5) and obviously shorter compared to 21 days (Q1 13; Q3 34) in the AO C patients. PCCL 0 and 1 was seen predominantly in the AO group. In the AO B group (n = 124), mobilization until discharge was performed using Crutches in 69.35%. Rollator or walking frame was necessary in 9.68%, a wheelchair in 11.29% whereas no adequate mobilization until discharge was documented in 8.87%. No information about mobilization was found in 0.81%. In the AO C group (n = 176), the rate of cases that were able to use crutches was obviously lower (45.45%). In this group, 26.70% required a wheelchair at the time of discharge, whereas 8.52% were mobilized using a rollator or walking frame. In 16.47%, no adequate mobilization was possible. In the remaining 2.84%, no information about mobilization was documented. As already shown, there was an obviously increased risk for developing a major or minor complication in AO C patients compared to the AO B patients presented in Figure 3.

3.3. Analysis of FFP-Classified Patients

In FFP II, the median duration of stay was 8 days (Q1 5; Q3 12), in FFP III 7 days (Q1 7; Q3 8) and in FFP IV 12 days (Q1 10; Q3 18). Overall, 52.03 % of FFP patients were mobilized using a rollator or walking frame. In addition, 29.73% were able to use crutches until discharge. In 7.43%, mobilizing was only possible using a wheelchair, and in 8.79%, mobilization was not successful until discharge. Data on mobilization were missing in the remaining 2.03%. There was no obvious coherence between mobilization and age except for bedridden cases. Median age in this population was about 5 to 10 years older. Details are provided in Table 2. There was no obvious influence of PCCL on the duration of stay except very high PCCL scores 5–6. Details are presented in Table 3.

Table 2. Mobilization at time of discharge.

	Free Mobilization	Rollator/Walking Frame	Wheelchair	Crutches/Walking Stick	Bedridden	No Information
Median age (years)	86.17	80.16	75.45	76.53	84.72	–
Q 25%	56.48	75.46	66.48	64.81	69.01	–
Q 75%	87.80	84.14	84.95	83.96	85.65	–
FFP II	2 (1.71%)	60 (51.28%)	7 (5.98%)	37 (31.62%)	9 (7.69%)	2 (1.71%)
FFP III	–	1 (11.11%)	1 (11.11%)	6 (66.67%)	–	1 (11.11%)
FFP IV	1 (4.55%)	16 (72.73%)	3 (13.64%)	1 (4.55%)	1 (4.55%)	–

Table 3. Duration of stay (number of days) after surgery and the occurrence of major complications in dependence of PCCL.

	PCCL					
	0–1	2	3	4	5–6	Total
n	33	18	50	37	10	148
Median (d)	9	5.5	8	9	25	8
Q 25%	5	4	5	6	16	5
Q 75%	12	8	11.5	15	32	13.5

PCCL: Patient Clinical Complexity Level.

Major complications in FFP II group were found in 7/117 (5.98%) compared to 2/9 (22.22%) in FFP III and 5/22 (22.73%) in FFP IV. We found 14 major complications in 148 patients in these groups. Moreover, minor complications occurred less in FFP II 20/117 (17.09%) compared to 4/9 (44.44%) in the FFP III and 9/22 (40.91%) in the FFP IV group. Due to similar complication rates in FFP III and FFP IV with relatively low numbers, FFP III and IV were merged for some analysis. In this case, the group is presented as FFP III/IV. There was an obvious difference between the FFP II and the FFP III/IV group, in the occurrence of at least one minor or major complication. Complication rate in the FFP II group was 27/117 (23.08%) compared to 17/31 (54.84%) in the FFP III/IV group. Multivariable regression analysis revealed a reduced risk for major complications with augmentation vs. none (OR 0.598), and a slightly reduced risk for females over males, also in the isolated analysis of FFP groups (OR 0.974). Furthermore, there was an increased risk in FFP III/IV compared to FFP II (OR 4.679), illustrated in Figure 4a. Comparable effects could be detected for minor complications. Further information is illustrated and presented in Figure 4b.

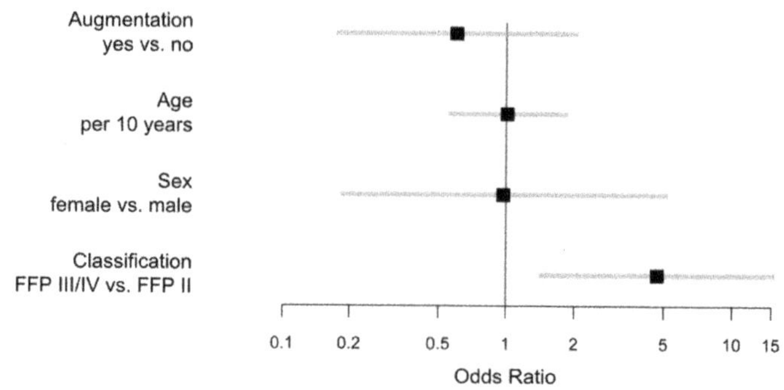

(**a**)

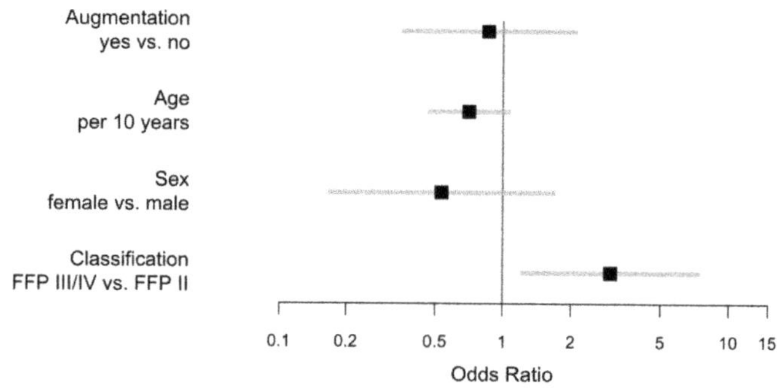

(**b**)

Figure 4. Odds ratios with 95% Wald confidence limits for (**a**) major complications (augmented vs. non-augmented: 0.598; female vs. male: 0.974; FFP III–IV vs. FFP II: 4.679) and (**b**) minor complications (augmented vs. non-augmented: OR 0.862; female vs. male: OR 0.532; FFP III–IV vs. FFP II: OR 3.006).

3.4. Effect and Safety of SI-Screw Augmentation

Augmentation was performed in 118 patients (26.34%). Out of these, 49 cases (41.53%) were treated with unilateral and 69 (58.47%) with bilateral augmentation. Augmentation was mainly performed in FFP-classified fractures (66.89% augmented vs. 6.33% in AO, p <0.0001). For further investigation regarding augmentation, only FFP-classified cases would be included. No statistical differences in BMI between the augmented (median: 24.01, Q1:21.41; Q3:26.57) and non-augmented patients (median: 24.69, Q1: 22.49; Q3: 27.76) were found.

FFP patients with augmented SI-screws showed a higher ASA scoring than the non-augmented (47.3% ASA 3–4 in patients with augmented SI-screws vs. 30.8% in patients without augmentation, $p = 0.0391$). Moreover, CCI was higher in the augmented group compared to the non-augmented (20.8% CCI >3 vs. 10.3%, $p = 0.150$).

Univariate regression revealed a 25% (ratio augmented vs. non-augmented 0.744, 95%CI 0.585–0.945, $p = 0.0157$) reduced time from surgery to discharge (unilateral: median 8 days; bilateral median 7 days; non-augmented median 11 days) in the augmented cases. There were no statistical differences between the unilateral and bi-lateral augmentation (Figure 5).

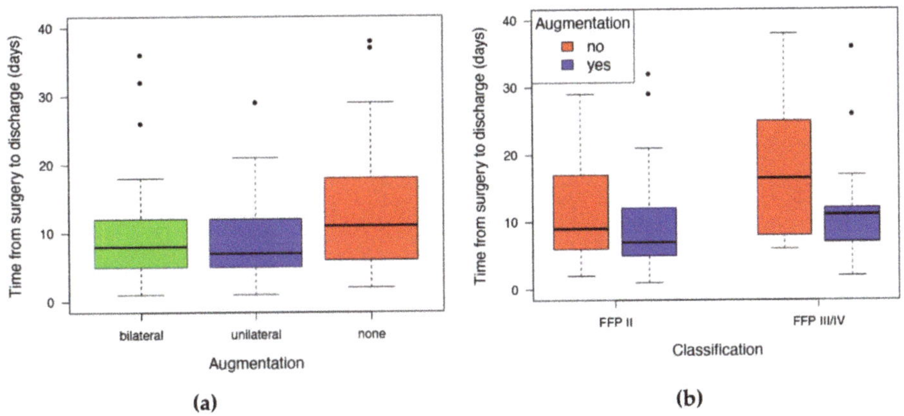

Figure 5. Postoperative duration of stay in the FFP cases: (**a**) bi-lateral and unilateral showing about a 25% shorter stay in hospital compared to the non-augmented group; (**b**) differentiation between the FFP II and FFP III/IV also shows the effect of augmentation with earlier discharge after augmentation. Dots indicating outliers.

Mobilization of the FFP patients after surgery was possible in 91.03%. Mobilization in dependence of augmentation showed a higher rate of cases mobilized with a rollator or walking frame, whereas in the non-augmented group, an obvious higher rate of mobilization with crutches was detectable ($p = 0.0736$). Details are provided in Table 4.

Table 4. Mobilization at time of discharge in dependence of augmentation.

	Free Mobilization	Crutches/Walking Stick	Rollator/Walking Frame	Wheelchair	Bedridden	No Information
Unilateral augmentation	2 (6.06%)	10 (30.30%)	18 (54.55%)	1 (3.03%)	2 (6.06%)	-
Bilateral augmentation	-	12 (18.18%)	39 (59.09%)	7 (10.61%)	6 (9.09%)	2 (3.03%)
No augmentation	1 (2.04%)	22 (44.9%)	20 (40.82%)	3 (6.12%)	2 (4.08%)	1 (2.04%)
In 3 cases, no information about mobilization could be found.						

There was no statistical difference in the occurrence of major complications between the augmented and non-augmented FFP cases (8/99 vs. 6/49 patients, $p = 0.5513$). Moreover, minor complications were not different with and without augmentation (20/99 vs. 13/49 patients, $p = 0.407$). In FFP patients, neither a difference was seen between female and male for major complications (2/18 m vs. 12/130 f, $p = 0.680$) nor for minor complications (6/18 m vs. 27/130 f, $p = 0.236$). Interestingly, major and minor complications occurred less in FFP II (major: 7/117, 5.98%; minor: 20/117, 17.09%) compared to FFP III/IV (major: 7/31, 22.58%; minor: 13/31, 41.94%). This difference was statistically noticeable for major complications ($p = 0.0108$) and minor complications ($p = 0.006$).

Univariable regression revealed a reduced risk of major complications in augmented FFP cases for bilateral augmentation (OR 0.850) and unilateral augmentation (OR 0.224) compared with no augmentation. A similar effect was explored concerning the minor complications for bilateral augmentation (OR 0.746) and unilateral augmentation (OR 0.615), shown in Figure 6.

Cement-associated complications were seen in 26/118 cases (22%). Out of these, spinal extravasation was detected in 3/118 cases (2.5%) and foraminal extravasation was seen in 2/118 cases (1.7%). All other cement extrusions were without correlations to neurologic structures and no cardio-vascular relevance was documented. Neurologic complications were correlated with documented screw misplacement (Section 3.1.), but not with cement complications ($p = 0.3936$).

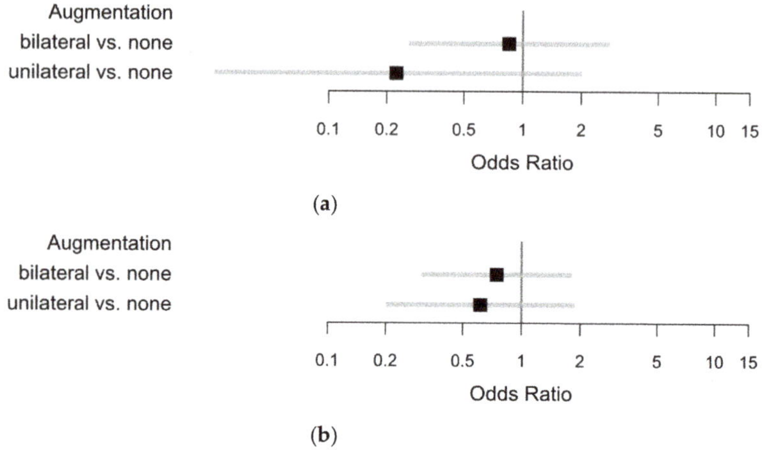

Figure 6. Univariable analysis of augmentation concerning (**a**) major complications; and (**b**) minor complications.

4. Discussion

Percutaneous SI-screw insertion in our department was performed over the last 15 years. In consequence, we were able to report on 448 patients with 642 inserted SI-screws. To our knowledge, this is the largest clinical study on this topic, so far. We have not investigated any alternative treatment options. For that reason, no comparative conclusion can be provided in this study.

A retrospective, single-center cohort study on 102 traumatic patients was reported by Pishnamaz et al. [33]. Misplacement in conventional placed screws is reported to be between 8.8–12.4% [4,33,34] in conventionally techniques and 3.6–4.9 % using 3D navigation [4,35]. We found correct screw placement in 91.23%, whereas minor screw displacement (<3.6 mm) occurred in 4.5% and major displacement was seen in 3.08%. The neurological sequel of screw mal-positioning was reported to be up to 18% [2]. Our results confirm this by 13.51% of consecutive neurological deficits. Furthermore, peripheral neurologic complications were correlated with screw misplacement ($p = 0.0001$).

The rate of mal-positioning is reported to be reduced in 3D navigated techniques [34,36]. We cannot confirm this from our results and found no statistical differences between the conventional SI-screw insertion and 3D navigation in this context. This is in accordance with a report from the German Pelvic Trauma Registry [4]. However, the investigated time period potentially included some surgical and technical evolutions. For that reason, it is difficult to generally reject potential advantages of 3D navigation based on our results. However, our data contribute to the general judgement that percutaneous SI-screw osteosynthesis is considered to be safe in general, but technically demanding with specific risks [2,36,37].

Most reports on screw misplacement and safety report on traumatic pelvic fractures [2,4,33–36]. The present study does not differentiate between traumatic and fragility fractures in this specific context. However, the mechanisms of injuries and its pathology are considered to be different [38]. For that reason, we used a differentiated method to evaluate and report our results. To avoid confusion, "traumatic fractures", resulting from high energy, were classified using the AO classification [6,7] and fragility fractures were classified using the FFP classification [12]. Doing so, we were able to report on both entities separately, but also together where appropriate. In addition to reporting on obvious screw-related complications, multivariable regression analysis revealed that women may have a reduced risk compared to men in developing complications. These findings contradict review-based reports on equal odds for complications in spinal surgery [39]. We also found an increased complication risk and a longer stay in hospital in patients with AO C fractures compared to AO B fractures.

These findings were expected and are consistent with current literature [40]. The distribution between AO B type and AO C type may be different to other epidemiologic reports [41]. This effect is potentially explained by the fact that only patients who received SI screw fixation were included in this study. We also revealed more complications and increased hospitalization time in FFP III/IV compared to FFP II. This is consistent with the anticipated increase in severity and instability within the classification [11,12]. Therefore, the usage of both classifications in our study are consistent. We found more complications and a longer stay in hospital in AO C patients compared to AO B. Interestingly, FFP II fractures showed a risk for complications comparable with AO B patients, whereas FFP III and IV revealed an increased risk for complications, even increased over AO C. Taking into account that there is a possibility of progression of fracture severity reported [42,43], further information seems to be mandatory which patients suffering FFP I or II fractures will heal conservatively, and which preferably should be offered early in the surgery to prevent progression. This is probably one of the most important questions in this field to be answered in the near future.

One additional option to potentially increase screw anchorage in reduced bone quality is cement augmentation. Höch et al. investigated in-screw augmentation in a prospective observational study of 34 patients and reported this technique to be effective and safe [27]. However, a recent review showed that there was little evidence in this field [9]. They reported that the confirmation of safety and effectiveness was based on only few clinical case series with relatively low numbers of patients. They concluded that based on available literature, augmented SI-screw techniques need to be considered to be experimental with unclear clinical benefit [9]. Our results on a relatively large number on patients may contribute to fill this gap of knowledge. No increase in specific complications was seen after the augmentation compared with non-augmented comparable patients. A reduced risk for general complications in the augmented group was seen, instead. Cement-associated complications were seen in 5.82%. This seems to be relatively low in comparison with recently published leakage rates of 14.7% in kyphoplasty [44]. Fragility fractures of the pelvis are reported to be associated with intense and immobilizing pain [11]. This immobilization may cause additional complications. Van Dijk et al. reported a complication rate of 20.2% after the fracture of the pubic ramus [45]. To prevent prolonged immobilization, surgery might facilitate mobilization. We found that immediate mobilization was possible in more than 90% after surgery. Augmented patients were predominately mobilized with a rollator or walking frame, whereas in the non-augmented group, a higher rate of mobilization with crutches was observed. Even if there was no statistically evident effect on the kind of mobilization, univariate regression revealed a 25% reduced time from surgery to discharge in the augmented group. Furthermore, multivariable regression revealed a potentially reduced risk for both minor and major complications, whereas no increased screw-related complication rates were seen between the augmented and non-augmented collective. Due to only 14 major complications in FFP groups, the statistical conclusiveness of multivariable analysis for major complications in these groups (shown in Figure 3) may be limited. However, the results are consistent with other findings presented in this study. Even in consideration of a selection bias in the surgeon's decision for augmentation, it is conjecturable that this was made in potentially lower bone quality and inferior patient conditions, which is supported by higher ASA and CCI scoring in the augmented group. This would even enhance the shown effect. To the best of our knowledge, this effect was not reported previously and would complement the shown safety with a potential benefit. The reason for this effect remained unclear. Osterhoff described that in a biomechanical study, the mode and dynamics of failure changed due to cement augmentation. However, they found no advantages in terms of screw motion or cycles to failure [21]. This is consistent with other biomechanical studies in which cement augmentation does not prevent from screw loosening and implant failure [22]. Other factors like the stabilization of the anterior pelvic ring potentially influence this mid- and long-term outcome, with a potentially additive effect. However, this was not investigated in this study.

To date, the benefit of cement augmentation in SI-screw osteosynthesis is considered to be unclear and the usage therefore to be experimental [9]. Our data conclude the safe and beneficial usage of cement augmentation of SI-screws in selected patients.

5. Conclusions

Percutaneous SI-screw osteosynthesis is confirmed to be safe for traumatic pelvic ring fractures and fragility fractures of the pelvis in general. However, this technique remains technically demanding with specific risks. The potential neurological sequel of screw mal-positioning reported previously was confirmed. Cement augmentation was shown to be safe and effective. We have not found increased specific complications or correlated neurological impairment in this context. Augmentation seems to reduce the risk of general complications in FFP patients. Furthermore, augmented FFP patients have a shorter hospital stay. Based on our results, the augmentation of percutaneous SI-screw osteosynthesis cannot be considered to be experimental with uncertain benefit anymore.

Author Contributions: Conceptualization, M.J.R. and R.H.; data curation, R.H., M.E., J.K.; formal analysis, O.R., M.E., R.H.; investigation, R.H., O.R., J.S.-S., J.K., M.F.L.; methodology, R.H., O.R., J.S.-S., M.E., J.K., M.F.L.; validation, R.H., J.S.-S., O.R. and M.J.R.; writing—original draft preparation, R.H.; writing—review and editing, O.R., J.S.-S., J.K., M.F.L., M.E.; visualization, M.E., R.H.; supervision, M.J.R.; project administration, M.J.R., R.H.; All authors have read and agreed to the published version of the manuscript.

Funding: No funding was received for this work.

Acknowledgments: The authors want to thank Moritz Freistühler for the support in identifying included cases.

Conflicts of Interest: The authors declare no conflict of interest.

References

1. Vidal, J.; Allieu, Y.; Fassio, B.; Adrey, J.; Goalard, C. Spondylolisthesis: Reduction with Harrington's rods. *Rev. Chir. Orthop. Reparatrice Appar. Mot.* **1973**, *59*, 21–41. [PubMed]
2. Iorio, J.A.; Jakoi, A.M.; Rehman, S. Percutaneous Sacroiliac Screw Fixation of the Posterior Pelvic Ring. *Orthop. Clin. N. Am.* **2015**, *46*, 511–521. [CrossRef]
3. Wang, J.-Q.; Wang, Y.; Feng, Y.; Han, W.; Su, Y.-G.; Liu, W.-Y.; Zhang, W.-J.; Wu, X.-B.; Wang, M.-Y.; Fan, Y.-B. Percutaneous Sacroiliac Screw Placement: A Prospective Randomized Comparison of Robot-assisted Navigation Procedures with a Conventional Technique. *Chin. Med. J.* **2017**, *130*, 2527–2534. [CrossRef]
4. Zwingmann, J.; Sudkamp, N.P.; Konig, B.; Culemann, U.; Pohlemann, T.; Aghayev, E.; Schmal, H. Intra-and postoperative complications of navigated and conventional techniques in percutaneous iliosacral screw fixation after pelvic fractures: Results from the German Pelvic Trauma Registry. *Injury* **2013**, *44*, 1765–1772. [CrossRef] [PubMed]
5. Mendel, T.; Radetzki, F.; Wohlrab, D.; Stock, K.; Hofmann, G.O.; Noser, H. CT-based 3-D visualisation of secure bone corridors and optimal trajectories for sacroiliac screws. *Injury* **2013**, *44*, 957–963. [CrossRef] [PubMed]
6. Tile, M. Acute Pelvic Fractures: I. Causation and Classification. *J. Am. Acad. Orthop. Surg.* **1996**, *4*, 143–151. [CrossRef] [PubMed]
7. Meinberg, E.G.; Agel, J.; Roberts, C.S.; Karam, M.D.; Kellam, J.F. Fracture and Dislocation Classification Compendium-2018. *J. Orthop. Trauma* **2018**, *32* (Suppl. 1), S1–S170. [CrossRef]
8. Alvis-Miranda, H.R.; Farid-Escorcia, H.; Alcala-Cerra, G.; Castellar-Leones, S.M.; Moscote-Salazar, L.R. Sacroiliac screw fixation: A mini review of surgical technique. *J. Craniovertebral Junction Spine* **2014**, *5*, 110–113. [CrossRef]
9. König, A.; Oberkircher, L.; Beeres, F.J.P.; Babst, R.; Ruchholtz, S.; Link, B.-C. Cement augmentation of sacroiliac screws in fragility fractures of the pelvic ring-A synopsis and systematic review of the current literature. *Injury* **2019**, *50*, 1411–1417. [CrossRef]
10. Ravindrarajah, R.; Hazra, N.C.; Charlton, J.; Jackson, S.H.D.; Dregan, A.; Gulliford, M.C. Incidence and mortality of fractures by frailty level over 80 years of age: Cohort study using UK electronic health records. *BMJ Open* **2018**, *8*, e018836. [CrossRef]
11. Rommens, P.M.; Wagner, D.; Hofmann, A. Fragility Fractures of the Pelvis. *JBJS Rev.* **2017**, *5*. [CrossRef] [PubMed]
12. Rommens, P.M.; Hofmann, A. Comprehensive classification of fragility fractures of the pelvic ring: Recommendations for surgical treatment. *Injury* **2013**, *44*, 1733–1744. [CrossRef] [PubMed]

13. Pieroh, P.; Hoch, A.; Hohmann, T.; Gras, F.; Mardian, S.; Pflug, A.; Wittenberg, S.; Ihle, C.; Blankenburg, N.; Dallacker-Losensky, K.; et al. Fragility Fractures of the Pelvis Classification: A Multicenter Assessment of the Intra-Rater and Inter-Rater Reliabilities and Percentage of Agreement. *J. Bone Jt. Surg. Am.* **2019**, *101*, 987–994. [CrossRef] [PubMed]
14. Verbeek, D.O.; Ponsen, K.J.; Fiocco, M.; Amodio, S.; Leenen, L.P.H.; Goslings, J.C. Pelvic fractures in the Netherlands: Epidemiology, characteristics and risk factors for in-hospital mortality in the older and younger population. *Eur. J. Orthop. Surg. Traumatol.* **2018**, *28*, 197–205. [CrossRef] [PubMed]
15. Benzinger, P.; Riem, S.; Bauer, J.; Jaensch, A.; Becker, C.; Buchele, G.; Rapp, K. Risk of institutionalization following fragility fractures in older people. *Osteoporos. Int.* **2019**, *30*, 1363–1370. [CrossRef] [PubMed]
16. Eckardt, H.; Egger, A.; Hasler, R.M.; Zech, C.J.; Vach, W.; Suhm, N.; Morgenstern, M.; Saxer, F. Good functional outcome in patients suffering fragility fractures of the pelvis treated with percutaneous screw stabilisation: Assessment of complications and factors influencing failure. *Injury* **2017**, *48*, 2717–2723. [CrossRef]
17. Muller, F.; Fuchtmeier, B. [Percutaneous cement-augmented screw fixation of bilateral osteoporotic sacral fracture]. *Unfallchirurg* **2013**, *116*, 950–954. [CrossRef]
18. Tjardes, T.; Paffrath, T.; Baethis, H.; Shafizadeh, S.; Steinhausen, E.; Steinbuechel, T.; Rixen, D.; Bouillon, B. Computer assisted percutaneous placement of augmented iliosacral screws: A reasonable alternative to sacroplasty. *Spine (Phila. Pa. 1976)* **2008**, *33*, 1497–1500. [CrossRef]
19. Wahnert, D.; Raschke, M.J.; Fuchs, T. Cement augmentation of the navigated iliosacral screw in the treatment of insufficiency fractures of the sacrum: A new method using modified implants. *Int. Orthop.* **2013**, *37*, 1147–1150. [CrossRef]
20. Hoch, A.; Schimpf, R.; Hammer, N.; Schleifenbaum, S.; Werner, M.; Josten, C.; Bohme, J. Biomechanical analysis of stiffness and fracture displacement after using PMMA-augmented sacroiliac screw fixation for sacrum fractures. *Biomed. Tech. (Berl.)* **2017**, *62*, 421–428. [CrossRef]
21. Osterhoff, G.; Dodd, A.E.; Unno, F.; Wong, A.; Amiri, S.; Lefaivre, K.A.; Guy, P. Cement Augmentation in Sacroiliac Screw Fixation Offers Modest Biomechanical Advantages in a Cadaver Model. *Clin. Orthop. Relat. Res.* **2016**, *474*, 2522–2530. [CrossRef] [PubMed]
22. Gruneweller, N.; Raschke, M.J.; Zderic, I.; Widmer, D.; Wahnert, D.; Gueorguiev, B.; Richards, R.G.; Fuchs, T.; Windolf, M. Biomechanical comparison of augmented versus non-augmented sacroiliac screws in a novel hemi-pelvis test model. *J. Orthop. Res.* **2017**, *35*, 1485–1493. [CrossRef] [PubMed]
23. Oberkircher, L.; Masaeli, A.; Bliemel, C.; Debus, F.; Ruchholtz, S.; Kruger, A. Primary stability of three different iliosacral screw fixation techniques in osteoporotic cadaver specimens-a biomechanical investigation. *Spine J.* **2016**, *16*, 226–232. [CrossRef] [PubMed]
24. Grechenig, S.; Gänsslen, A.; Gueorguiev, B.; Berner, A.; Müller, M.; Nerlich, M.; Schmitz, P. PMMA-augmented SI screw: A biomechanical analysis of stiffness and pull-out force in a matched paired human cadaveric model. *Injury* **2015**, *46*, S125–S128. [CrossRef]
25. Suero, E.M.; Greiner, A.; Becker, C.A.; Cavalcanti Kußmaul, A.; Weidert, S.; Pfeufer, D.; Woiczinski, M.; Braun, C.; Flatz, W.; Böcker, W.; et al. Biomechanical stability of sacroiliac screw osteosynthesis with and without cement augmentation. *Injury* **2020**. [CrossRef]
26. Collinge, C.A.; Crist, B.D. Combined Percutaneous Iliosacral Screw Fixation With Sacroplasty Using Resorbable Calcium Phosphate Cement for Osteoporotic Pelvic Fractures Requiring Surgery. *J. Orthop. Trauma.* **2016**, *30*, e217–e222. [CrossRef]
27. Hoch, A.; Pieroh, P.; Henkelmann, R.; Josten, C.; Bohme, J. In-screw polymethylmethacrylate-augmented sacroiliac screw for the treatment of fragility fractures of the pelvis: A prospective, observational study with 1-year follow-up. *BMC Surg.* **2017**, *17*, 132. [CrossRef]
28. Konig, M.A.; Hediger, S.; Schmitt, J.W.; Jentzsch, T.; Sprengel, K.; Werner, C.M.L. In-screw cement augmentation for iliosacral screw fixation in posterior ring pathologies with insufficient bone stock. *Eur. J. Trauma Emerg. Surg.* **2018**, *44*, 203–210. [CrossRef]
29. Sandmann, G.H.; Stockle, U.; Freude, T.; Stuby, F.M. Balloon Guided Cement Augmentation of Iliosacral Screws in the Treatment of Insufficiency Fractures of the Sacrum—Description of a New Method and Preliminary Results. *Acta Chir. Orthop. Traumatol. Cech.* **2018**, *85*, 85–88.
30. Franz, D.; Kaufmann, M.; Siebert, C.H.; Windolf, J.; Roeder, N. Orthopedic and trauma surgery in the German DRG System 2007. *Unfallchirurg* **2007**, *110*, 270–280. [CrossRef]

31. Charlson, M.; Szatrowski, T.P.; Peterson, J.; Gold, J. Validation of a combined comorbidity index. *J. Clin. Epidemiol.* **1994**, *47*, 1245–1251. [CrossRef]
32. Von Elm, E.; Altman, D.G.; Egger, M.; Pocock, S.J.; Gotzsche, P.C.; Vandenbroucke, J.P.; Initiative, S. The Strengthening the Reporting of Observational Studies in Epidemiology (STROBE) statement: Guidelines for reporting observational studies. *J. Clin. Epidemiol.* **2008**, *61*, 344–349. [CrossRef] [PubMed]
33. Pishnamaz, M.; Dienstknecht, T.; Hoppe, B.; Garving, C.; Lange, H.; Hildebrand, F.; Kobbe, P.; Pape, H.C. Assessment of pelvic injuries treated with ilio-sacral screws: Injury severity and accuracy of screw positioning. *Int. Orthop.* **2016**, *40*, 1495–1501. [CrossRef] [PubMed]
34. Grossterlinden, L.; Rueger, J.; Catala-Lehnen, P.; Rupprecht, M.; Lehmann, W.; Rucker, A.; Briem, D. Factors influencing the accuracy of iliosacral screw placement in trauma patients. *Int. Orthop.* **2011**, *35*, 1391–1396. [CrossRef] [PubMed]
35. Ghisla, S.; Napoli, F.; Lehoczky, G.; Delcogliano, M.; Habib, N.; Arigoni, M.; Filardo, G.; Candrian, C. Posterior pelvic ring fractures: Intraoperative 3D-CT guided navigation for accurate positioning of sacro-iliac screws. *Orthop. Traumatol. Surg. Res.* **2018**, *104*, 1063–1067. [CrossRef]
36. Thakkar, S.C.; Thakkar, R.S.; Sirisreetreerux, N.; Carrino, J.A.; Shafiq, B.; Hasenboehler, E.A. 2D versus 3D fluoroscopy-based navigation in posterior pelvic fixation: Review of the literature on current technology. *Int. J. Comput. Assist. Radiol. Surg.* **2017**, *12*, 69–76. [CrossRef]
37. Falzarano, G.; Rollo, G.; Bisaccia, M.; Pace, V.; Lanzetti, R.M.; Garcia-Prieto, E.; Pichierri, P.; Meccariello, L. Percutaneous screws CT guided to fix sacroiliac joint in tile C pelvic injury. Outcomes at 5 years of follow-up. *SICOT-J.* **2018**, *4*, 52. [CrossRef]
38. Rommens, P.M.; Wagner, D.; Hofmann, A. Do We Need a Separate Classification for Fragility Fractures of the Pelvis? *J. Orthop. Trauma* **2019**, *33* (Suppl. 2), S55–S60. [CrossRef]
39. Schoenfeld, A.J.; Reamer, E.N.; Wynkoop, E.I.; Choi, H.; Bono, C.M. Does Patient Sex Affect the Rate of Mortality and Complications After Spine Surgery? A Systematic Review. *Clin. Orthop. Relat. Res.* **2015**, *473*, 2479–2486. [CrossRef]
40. Hermans, E.; Biert, J.; Edwards, M.J.R. Epidemiology of Pelvic Ring Fractures in a Level 1 Trauma Center in the Netherlands. *Hip Pelvis* **2017**, *29*, 253–261. [CrossRef]
41. Falzarano, G.; Medici, A.; Carta, S.; Grubor, P.; Fortina, M.; Meccariello, L.; Ferrata, P. The orthopedic damage control in pelvic ring fractures: When and why-a multicenter experience of 10 years' treatment. *J. Acute Dis.* **2014**, *3*, 201–206. [CrossRef]
42. Ueda, Y.; Inui, T.; Kurata, Y.; Tsuji, H.; Saito, J.; Shitan, Y. Prolonged pain in patients with fragility fractures of the pelvis may be due to fracture progression. *Eur. J. Trauma Emerg. Surg.* **2019**. [CrossRef] [PubMed]
43. Rommens, P.M.; Arand, C.; Hopf, J.C.; Mehling, I.; Dietz, S.O.; Wagner, D. Progress of instability in fragility fractures of the pelvis: An observational study. *Injury* **2019**, *50*, 1966–1973. [CrossRef] [PubMed]
44. Chen, C.; Fan, P.; Xie, X.; Wang, Y. Risk Factors for Cement Leakage and Adjacent Vertebral Fractures in Kyphoplasty for Osteoporotic Vertebral Fractures. *Clin. Spine Surg.* **2020**. [CrossRef]
45. Van Dijk, W.A.; Poeze, M.; Van Helden, S.H.; Brink, P.R.; Verbruggen, J.P. Ten-year mortality among hospitalised patients with fractures of the pubic rami. *Injury* **2010**, *41*, 411–414. [CrossRef] [PubMed]

Journal of
Clinical Medicine

MDPI

Article

Modified Split-Scan Computed Tomography (CT) Diagnostics of Severely Injured Patients: First Results from a Level I Trauma Center Using a Dedicated Head-and-Neck CT-Angiogram for the Detection of Cervical Artery Dissections

Daniel Popp [1], Claudius Thiedemann [1], Wolf Bäumler [2], Antonio Ernstberger [1,3], Volker Alt [1] and Andreas Schicho [2,*]

1 Department of Trauma Surgery, University Medical Centre Regensburg, D-93053 Regensburg, Germany; daniel.popp@ukr.de (D.P.); Claudius.Thiedemann@stud.uni-regensburg.de (C.T.); antonio.ernstberger@ukr.de (A.E.); volker.alt@ukr.de (V.A.)
2 Department of Radiology, University Medical Centre Regensburg, D-93053 Regensburg, Germany; wolf.baeumler@ukr.de
3 Department of Trauma and Hand surgery, Hospital Osnabrück, D-49076 Osnabrück, Germany
* Correspondence: andreas.schicho@ukr.de

Received: 29 June 2020; Accepted: 6 August 2020; Published: 8 August 2020

Abstract: Introduction: Traumatic cervical artery dissections are associated with high mortality and morbidity in severely injured patients. After finding even higher incidences than reported before, we decided to incorporate a dedicated head-and-neck computed tomography angiogram (CT-A) in our imaging routine for patients who have been obviously severely injured or, according to trauma mechanism, are suspected to be severely injured. Materials and Methods: A total of 134 consecutive trauma patients with an ISS ≥ 16 admitted to our level I trauma center during an 18 month period were included. All underwent standardized whole-body CT in a 256-detector row scanner with a dedicated head-and-neck CT-A realized as single-bolus split-scan routine. Incidence, mortality, patient and trauma characteristics, and concomitant injuries were recorded and analyzed in patients with carotid artery dissection (CAD) and vertebral artery dissection (VAD). Results: Of the 134 patients included, 7 patients had at least one cervical artery dissection (CeAD; 5.2%; 95% CI 1.5–9.0%). Six patients (85.7%) had carotid artery dissections, with one patient having a CAD of both sides and one patient having a CAD and contralateral VAD combined. Two patients (28.6%) showed a VAD. Overall mortality was 14.3%, neurologic morbidity was 28.6%. None of the patients showed any attributable neurologic symptoms on admission. The new scanning protocol led to further 5 patients with suspected CeAD during the study period, all ruled out by additional magnetic resonance imaging with angiogram (MRI/MR-A). Conclusion: A lack of specific neurologic symptoms on admission urges the need for a dedicated imaging pathway for severely injured patients, reliable for the detection of cervical artery dissections. Although our modified CT protocol with mandatory dedicated CT-A led to false positives requiring additional magnetic resonance imaging, it likely helped reduce possible therapeutic delays.

Keywords: cervical artery dissection; vertebral artery; carotid artery; polytrauma; severely injured; computed tomography

1. Introduction

Overlooked injuries in severely injured patients are feared complications in the acute care of patients. Euler et al. were able to show that in 25% of cases at least one diagnosis remains undiscovered in severely injured patients [1]. With a mortality rate of up to 33% and a neurological morbidity rate of up to 38%, traumatic carotid artery dissections and vertebral artery dissections are serious injuries in complex and severely injured patients [2–4]. The majority of these diseases remain initially asymptomatic, which might lead to a missed diagnosis [3,4] and avoidable delays in therapy such as anticoagulation, surgery, or endovascular treatment by thrombectomy or stenting. Traumatic cervical vessel dissections may result from rapid movement, both acceleration and deceleration, of the head in relation to the neck in any axis or blunt trauma.

In the daily routine, a contrast-enhanced multidetector computed tomography (CT) of the head, neck, thorax, abdomen, and pelvis according to the S3 guideline is used in severely and multiply injured patients and offers a demonstrable survival advantage [5], even when the mean injury severity score (ISS) was greater than that in patients without standardized imaging.

However, there are no specific guidelines on how to identify vascular injuries in the neck area as accurately as possible. In the current S3 guidline for the care of severely injured patients, for example, only vague recommendations for head-and-neck injuries are made [6]. Even highly experienced trauma surgeons, based on case history and clinical examination, miss ~50% of blunt injuries, stressing the need for standardized protocols and algorithms for imaging in trauma patients [7]. As a consequence, especially for head-and-neck injuries, more liberal screening criteria are discussed [8,9]. Technically, the diagnosis is challenging because characteristic imaging features can be difficult to detect because of the small size of intracranial and cervical arteries. Thus, multimodal imaging is often needed to safely confirm the diagnosis. Other than computed tomography angiogram (CT-A) and magnetic resonance angiography (MR-A) as the most widely used modalities for the detection of cervical artery pathologies, DSA (digital subtraction angiography) is considered the gold standard but is the most invasive option, requiring femoral arterial access and catheter placement in the cervical vessels, which is associated with a risk of hemorrhage and stroke. Ultrasound is the most inexpensive modality and can be performed at the bedside, but its diagnostic accuracy highly depends on the knowledge and experience of the user.

In single-bolus contrast-enhanced whole-body CT scans, traumatic lesions of the carotid and vertebral arteries often go unrecognized because of the low arterial contrast and contrast-enhanced parallel veins and soft tissues. Beam hardening artifacts at the skull base further worsen the detectability of such lesions, which mostly are discreet. If suspicion is raised, further diagnostic work-up is needed fast, causing additional radiation and contrast-agent dose in case of a CT-angiogram (CT-A) and time, cost, and delay in therapy of concomitant injuries. There is no widely accepted standard for addressing this dilemma in between overdiagnostics firsthand or missed diagnosis and stepped-up diagnostics later on. As a first step, the implementation of a non-dedicated angiogram revealed incidences of 6.5% for cervical artery dissection (CeAD), which were above reported values of 1.7% and 4.9% [8,10].

We thus decided that any patient qualified for a standard trauma CT scan, who has either been obviously severely injured or, according to trauma mechanism, is suspected to be severely injured, will receive a dedicated head-and-neck CT-A in between the non-contrast-enhanced brain scan and the delayed phase whole-body scan. As any injury to the head-and-neck region, especially vessel injuries such as carotid (CAD) or vertebral artery dissections (VAD), is of highest relevance for mortality, morbidity, and immediate therapeutic decisions, we accepted the additional radiation and contrast-agent trade-off based on an interdisciplinary consensus in our trauma center; this decision is in accordance with current recommendations of the Deutsche Röntgengesellschaft (German Radiology Society, [11]). After 18 months using the new single-bolus split-scan imaging approach, we here report the first results from our level I trauma center.

2. Materials and Methods

For this study, all patients admitted to the emergency room of our level I trauma center requiring a whole-body CT scan since November 2018 with an ISS ≥ 16 after complete diagnostic work-up were included. The decision for the CT scan is based upon the trauma mechanism and assumptions of its severity, e.g., based on estimated driving speed in car accidents, ejection from vehicle, falling from a great height (>3 m), burial trauma, death of co-driver, the observable injuries and circulation parameters in the emergency room, patient's age, and assumed frailty, in accordance with national recommendations and guidelines as cited above. The decision is made by the leading trauma surgeon and radiologist on duty as a consensus. In November 2018, the whole-body CT scanning protocol was modified to a single-bolus split-scan approach including a dedicated contrast-enhanced head-and-neck CT-A triggered in the Aorta ascendens. The aim of this modification was to further optimize the detection rate of cervical artery dissections as we already had a non-dedicated head-and-neck angiogram as a mandatory component of our scanning protocol [4] with fixed-delay scanning.

The independent Ethics Committee at the Regensburg University confirmed that, for this specific scientific project, no dedicated ethics approval or commission's opinion was necessary according to our applicable laws and guidelines. The consultation was filed under no. 20-1914-104.

2.1. CT Scan Protocol

All patients were examined using a 2 × 128-detector row dual-energy scanner (SOMATOM Definition Flash; Siemens Healthcare GmbH, Erlangen, Germany), fulfilling the requirements stated in the national S3 guideline "Polytrauma/Schwerverletzten—Behandlung" [6].

First, a non-contrast-enhanced scan of the neurocranium was acquired in 0.75 mm slices (360 mAs, 120 kV, pitch 0.55, increment 0.75 mm, and field of view 230 mm). The second scan is the contrast-enhanced head-and-neck CT-A, triggered in the A. ascendens. It reaches from the aortic arch covering the outlets of the supra-aortic branches up to the vertex. The volume and concentration of the contrast agent used (Accupaque 350, GE Healthcare Europe GmbH, Freiburg, Germany) were standardized to a total of 120 mL, with 12 injected for the head-and-neck CT-A. The contrast agent injection was followed by a flush with 20 mL of saline, both contrast agent and saline flush were injected with rates of 3.5 mL/s. ECG-gating is not routinely used in our protocol. The third scan was a venous phase delayed scan, covering the thorax, abdomen, pelvis, and upper half of the thigh; in select cases, the scan length was modified to cover the knees. It was scanned with a fixed delay of 30 s after the CT-A. The standard field of view was 500 mm, the slice thickness was 5.0 mm, the increment was 5.0 mm, the pitch was 0.60, kV and mAs were calculated and set automatically (CARE kV and CARE Dose; Siemens Healthcare GmbH) based on the scan topogram. A soft-tissue kernel with medium edge attenuation (B26f medium) was used for the calculation of axial, coronal, and sagittal views of the head and neck. Additional thick-slab axial maximal intensity projection (MIP) was rendered (10 mm) axial, sagittal, and coronal. Additional reconstructions were rendered using a B60f kernel for lung tissue (axial), a B60f sharp kernel for bones (axial and coronal, additional sagittal for spine), and a B30f kernel for soft tissue (axial, additional coronal for abdomen). Further reconstructions were calculated on the radiologists' discretion depending on the findings or suspicions drawn from the standard datasets.

Image interpretation was performed using a standard three-monitor workstation using the Syngo and Syngo.via picture archiving and communication system (PACS; Siemens Healthcare GmbH, Erlangen, Germany). All imaging studies were read and validated by a board-certified radiologist. Additional magnetic resonance angiography (MR-A) and/or ultrasound were performed if the diagnosis of a cervical artery dissection remained unclear after the CT-A. Both MR-A and ultrasound were not mandatory parts of our diagnostic routine in the time period covered in this study.

2.2. Statistical Analysis

For statistical calculations, analysis, and plotting, GraphPad Prism Version 5.00a for Mac (GraphPad Software, Inc., La Jolla, CA, USA) and Microsoft Excel Version 16.38 (Microsoft Corporation, Redmond, WA, USA) were used. Arising from the observational character of this study, mainly, descriptive statistics was used. We did not calculate comparative statistics due to the small cohort size. Demographics and injury severity were compared against the cohort of all severely injured patients recorded in our database and/or the cohort of patients with CeAD before the most recent modification of our CT scan protocol, as reported before [4]. We calculated the confidence interval for proportions using a confidence level of 0.95. For prevalence or incidence proportions, in addition to the normal approximation interval, we calculated the Wilson score interval as it supports better results, especially for smaller samples and for edge proportions near 0 or 1 as in our case using R (V4.0.2, R Project, Vienna, Austria).

3. Results

Since introduction of our new CT scan protocol, 134 severely injured patients with an ISS ≥ 16 underwent the standardized whole-body computed tomography including a dedicated head-and-neck CT-A. Thereof, 7 patients were found with at least one cervical artery dissection (5.2%; 7/134). Six patients (85.7%; 6/7) had carotid artery dissections, with one patient having a CAD of both sides, and one patient having a CAD and contralateral VAD combined. Two patients (28.6%; 2/7) showed a VAD. ISS and mean age as well as gender distribution were comparable to past time frames (Table 1).

Table 1. Cohort characteristics depending on the diagnostic approach for the detection of cervical artery dissections (CeAD).

	CeAD W/O Dedicated Scan Protocol	CeAD W/Mandatory Angiogram	CeAD W/Dedicated CT-A
N (*n*)	53 of 1178	15 of 230	7 of 134
Rate of CeAD (%)	4.5	6.5	5.2
CI95	0.033; 0.057	0.033; 0.097	0.015; 0.090
Wilson score interval (CI95)	0.035; 0.058	0.040; 0.110	0.026; 0.104
ISS (mean)	39	35	33
Age (mean)	48	51	48
Sex (m/f)	36/17	10/5	5/2

CI95 = 95% confidence interval; ISS = Injury Severity Score; CT-A = computed tomography angiogram.

Another five patients underwent additional MRI including MR-A after CT with CT-A, which did not confirm a suspected cervical artery dissection. In 2 out of 7 cases with CT-A-diagnosed CeAD reported here, MRI confirmed the diagnosis. In 5 cases, CT-A diagnosis required no further imaging work-up. In all, 3 of 7 patients had an ultrasound of the extracranial vessels but none was able to identify the dissection; two of them had an MR-A-confirmed diagnosis of CeAD.

On admission, none of the patients showed any neurologic symptoms attributable to a CeAD. Five patients were put on anticoagulation (71.4%), two patients were not eligible for anticoagulation due to either intracerebral hemorrhages or a severe distraction-flexion-type spinal fracture C4–7. Two patients developed serious neurologic symptoms (aphasia, hemiparesis) due to carotid artery dissections, yielding a morbidity of 28.6%. One patient died, yielding a mortality of 14.3%.

The trauma mechanism was a fall from large height in one case (14.3%) and traffic accidents in all other cases (4 car accidents, 1 motor-scooter, 1 e-bike; 85.7%). Concomitant spinal fractures were found in 4 cases (57.1%). One patient had a complex midface fracture reaching into the skull, one patient had no fracture of the spine or thorax (Figure 1). Three patients had fractures of upper third ribs (42.9%).

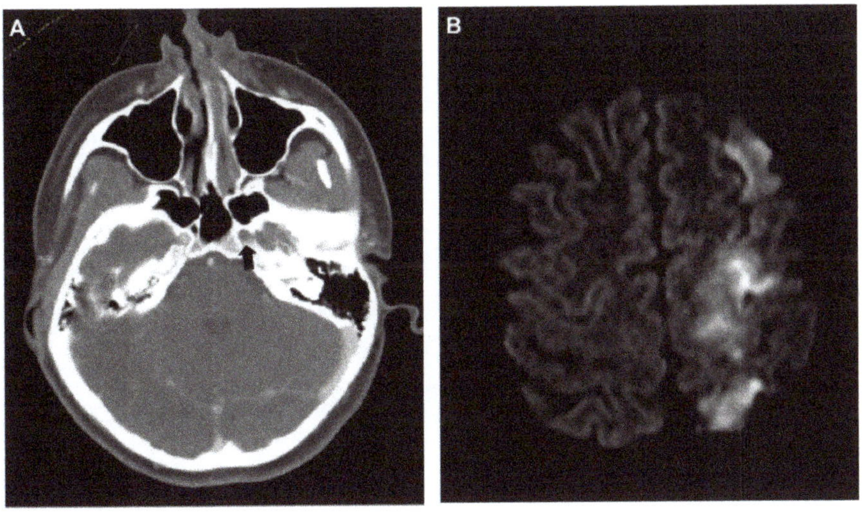

Figure 1. Dissection of the left internal carotid artery (ICA) with severe neurologic sequelae. (**A**) Axial computed tomography angiogram (CT-A) of the skull base shows no contrast agent in the ICA within the foramen carotideum on the left (black arrow). (**B**) Same-day magnetic resonance imaging (MRI) (diffusion weighted imaging (DWI), b800) shows ipsilateral infarction of the anterior and middle cerebral artery territories.

4. Discussion

In severely injured patients, rates of cervical artery dissections are reported to be as low as 0.9% based on ultrasound [12] and said to occur in around 1% of patients with blunt trauma [13]. Recently, we found a six-fold higher rate of 6.5% in our level I trauma center population by making a head-and-neck angiogram a mandatory component in the CT scan protocol for severely injured patients admitted to the emergency room [4]. This led to the idea, that further optimization of our scan protocol could yield even higher rates of cervical artery dissections and lower rates of non-diagnosed cases of cervical artery dissection, as a relevant proportion never shows any neurologic symptoms but is at risk for severe sequelae firsthand. We thus switched our scan protocol to a single-bolus split-scan scheme, which enabled integrating a dedicated head-and-neck CT-A into our diagnostic routine. Moreover, 18 months after implementing the new protocol into daily routine of care, we now can report a rate of 5.2%, which is lower than the 6.5% reported before, but higher than the 4.5% from the time we did not use a scanning protocol optimized for the detection of cervical artery dissections and still five-fold the value estimated overall for blunt traumata [13]. At the same time, we had 7 cases with an additional MRI/MR-A; five in patients with suspected dissection based on the CT-A, which all were negative; two in patients with a certain diagnosis of cervical artery dissection after CT-A with the primary intent of revealing the cerebral and cerebellar ischemic impacts.

Different conclusions can be drawn from the observations made: first, the true rate of cervical artery dissections in severely injured patients is likely to be in between our reported values of 6.5 and 5.2% in our trauma center and seems to vary rather widely within different populations as reported from different trauma centers worldwide; the Wilson score interval, which is a variant of the normal approximation 95% confidence interval more suitable for small sample sizes and edge proportions near 0 as in our case, yields a 95% CI range between 2.6% and 10.4% for CeAD in this cohort.

Second, dedicated CT-A did not lead to more dissections revealed in our cohort but did elicit uncertain or suspicious cases requiring additional imaging (Figure 2).

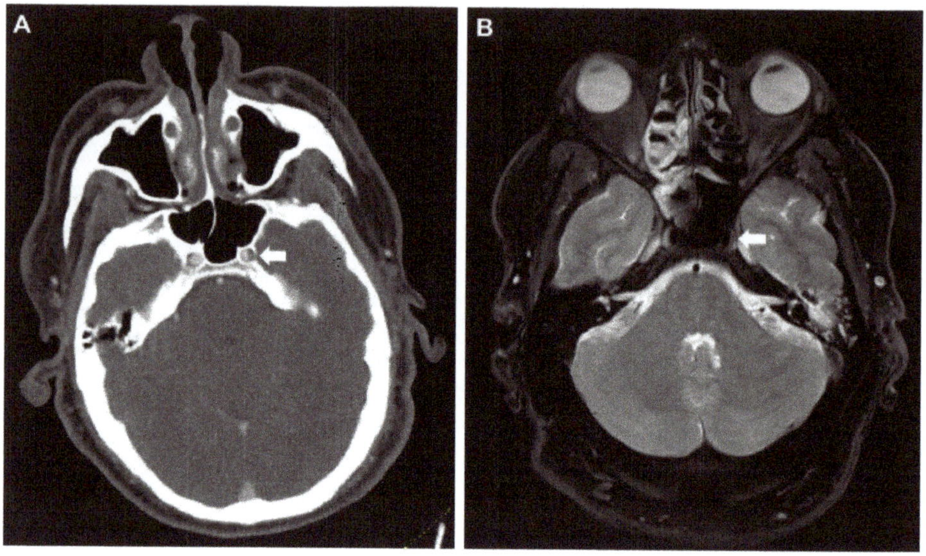

Figure 2. False-positive CT-A raising suspicion for an intramural hematoma of the left internal carotid artery (ICA) in its petrosal segment. (**A**) Axial CT-A of the skull base shows caliber asymmetry of the left ICA in the foramen carotideum (white arrow). (**B**) MR (proton-density fat saturated) rules out a wall hematoma. Asymmetry is presumably caused by the carotid plexus of nerves and sympathetics from the superior cervical ganglion (white arrow). MR, magnetic resonance.

Third, the most powerful predictor for cervical artery dissections seems to be any kind of high kinetic trauma mechanism, especially traffic accidents including cars, motorcycles/-scooters, bikes, and e-bikes, which is also true for aortic arch injuries due to a "whiplash"-type motion of fast deceleration and re-acceleration [14,15]. Some fractures should raise high suspicion toward cervical artery injuries, such as fractures of the cervical spine, skull base and/or complex midface fractures, or upper third rib (costae 1–4) fractures. Nonetheless, devastating dissections without an accompanying fracture are possible (Figure 1).

Fourth, large multicenter or registry-based studies are required to accurately assess cervical artery dissection risk factors, outcomes, and characteristics, as it will remain a low-incidence injury and rates between 1% [13] and 6.5% [4] are reported repeatedly.

Fifth, multimodal work-up of suspicious cases is highly relevant as with a dedicated head-and-neck CT-A a tendency toward false positives can be seen. With ultrasound, which often is used as the first add-on diagnostic due to fast availability and low cost, false negatives are very likely [12], being unable to safely rule out any CeAD and, as in our cases reported here, not being able to confirm CeAD either. Influence of dedicated training of ultrasound examiners or compulsory use of state-of-the-art techniques such as b-flow or contrast-enhanced ultrasound should be elaborated.

Despite the low incidence, the diagnosis of any artery dissection has to be made fast due to the severe consequences from any therapeutic delay, especially in cervical vessels as central nervous ischemia or embolization can lead to devastating and irreversible neurologic sequelae. In a population aged 45 and younger, 20% of ischemic strokes are due to traumatic and non-traumatic CeAD [12]. Moreover, blunt carotid injury has been associated with a higher stroke rate in general (up to 60%) and mortality rate (19–43%) [16]. In cases of cervical artery dissections, besides open surgery, recanalization via flow diverting or covered stenting of the carotid artery can be an option [17,18], with successful cases reported even for the vertebral arteries [19]. Anticoagulation should be established to prevent thrombus formation and embolization. However, in patients with ISS 16 and above, the majority show fractures, bleedings, or abdominal organ lacerations, which might stand in contradiction to systemic anticoagulation [20]. In these cases, an individual interdisciplinary treatment regime needs to be defined balancing possible benefits and risks. Crönlein et al. mentioned accordingly that there is no specific guideline for diagnosis and treatment established when it comes to severely injured patients, which is applicable to our patient collective [21]. Current recommendations from the German society for radiology suggest implementing differentiated scanning protocols, adjusted for dose and/or time; both include a cervical CT-A [11] despite the lack of larger trials or investigations addressing the topic of imaging optimization in the care of severely injured patients.

Injuries of the carotid or vertebral artery are reportedly associated with both high mortality rates and neurological morbidity rates, as again seen in the cohort reported here. In severely injured patients, diagnoses and decisions only based on history and clinical examination are prone to error with missed injuries in up to 47%. As none of the patients with CeAD in this population showed symptoms hinting specifically at a cervical vessel injury on admission, these diagnoses most likely would have gone unrecognized until the development of neurologic symptoms. Interestingly, a significant number of (66–73%) patients with blunt carotid injury may be asymptomatic upon initial presentation, developing delayed neurologic symptoms anywhere from 1 h to 7 days after injury. The onset of ischemic events can range from a few minutes to 31 days after injury, with the majority (82%) occurring within the first 7 days [9,22].

This delay in therapy needs to be avoided under all circumstances as secondary worsening or complications such as cerebral embolization could be prevented. Occlusive CeAD, multiple CeAD, and vertebral artery dissections result in an increased risk for delayed stroke, as reported by Lichy et al. [23].

Comparing the rates reported here with larger studies, our values are above those of others, possibly resembling missed injuries due to non-specific imaging protocols. Nevertheless, our values are lower than those reported from clinically preselected cohorts and our own past cohort. As a comparison, Lee et al. report an average annual incidence rate for CeAD of any cause of 2.6 per 100,000 population (95% CI, 1.86 to 3.33) [24]. Major trauma has an estimated incidence rate of 22.5 per 100,000 population in Germany [25], which leads us to an estimated incidence rate of 1.2 per 100,000 population (95% CI, 0.33 to 2.02) for CeAD in severely injured patients assuming our latest rate of 5.2%.

Limitations

As cervical artery dissections are highly relevant for the severely injured individual admitted to any emergency room, we wanted to report here the first results from our modifications of our diagnostic routine with the intent to nurture further discussions on the best diagnosis and treatment regimes in these uncommon but regularly to be seen cases. Thus, some relevant limitations are inherent to our study design.

First, as a single-center study reporting from an 18 month period, only few cases could be found and included. This needs to be addressed by further multicenter or registry-based examinations. As a direct consequence, we decided to report descriptive statistics and to not include comparative statistics, as this could tempt readers to draw conclusions that are not backed by sufficient data as this is a preliminary report. Second, in our level I trauma center, severely injured patients are admitted at a rate above the nationwide average in both severity and frequency, due to geographic and strategic reasons within the local emergency medicine services. Considering this, other hospitals will likely find lower or even higher incidences of CeAD in their population. Third, the true incidence of cervical artery dissections still remains unknown; no case showed neurologic symptoms on admission, some dissections remain clinically inapparent (3 out of 7 in this study), and a definite multimodality diagnostic work-up for suspected cases or even all severely injured patients is not yet established. In consequence, further studies should address the question of true incidence of CeAD by multimodality work-up including MR-A. However, capped capacities for additional MR-A work-up especially in smaller hospitals is another limitation that needs to be considered in setting up a diagnostic pathway for severely injured individuals.

The sensitivity (64–100%), specificity (67–100%), positive predictive value (65–100%), and negative predictive value (70–100%) of CT-A for the detection of CeAD compared with those of DSA vary widely with later studies indicating values close to those of DSA due to essential technical improvements made in the last few years [26,27]. MR-A has a sensitivity of 50–100%, specificity of 29–100%, positive predictive value of 43–100%, and negative predictive value of 89% compared to those of DSA [28]; especially for the smaller vertebral arteries, MRI yields diagnostic accuracy below that of CT-A because of the limited spatial resolution in many MRI/MR-A protocols. With modern scanners, the highest spatial resolution of MRI is at the same level as that of CT. Limited availability and long duration of the image acquisition in combination with physical restrictions (metal implants, narrow gantry) still makes MRI/MR-A not an option for first-line diagnostics in cases of suspected traumatic CeAD, as it is recommended as an initial test in non-trauma cases by the American Stroke Association (ASA) and American College of Radiology (ACR) [29].

One key finding of the results reported here is the need for a diagnostic routine in severely injured patients that is able to reliably detect cervical artery injuries, as none of the patients covered in the recent 18 month period showed symptoms on admission. Whenever possible, we put patients with CeAD on anticoagulation based on a case-by-case interdisciplinary consensus. Whether the low morbidity and mortality in comparison to cohorts reported before can be attributed to our imaging pathway cannot be answered from this study reasonably due to the limitations discussed before. As a first measure, any suspected case of cervical artery dissection should be ruled out by MRI/MR-A and/or qualified ultrasound within a defined and short timeframe (e.g., 2 h) based on the high mortality and morbidity risk in un- or delayed diagnosed cervical artery dissections.

5. Conclusions

Modification of the trauma imaging routine to include a dedicated head-and-neck CT-A realized as a single-bolus split-scan protocol showed an incidence of 5.2% for cervical artery dissections after the first 18 months under operation, which is slightly below values reported before, as are both mortality (14.3%) and morbidity (28.6%) in this cohort. We repeatedly encountered false-positive findings requiring further diagnostic work-up with MR-A. Ultrasound did not help substantially to make or rule out the diagnosis of CeAD in our setting. Further studies will need to address the value of multimodality diagnostics and the role of state-of-the-art ultrasound techniques for extra- and intracranial vessel diagnostics. As none of the detected cases of cervical artery dissections showed neurologic symptoms on admission, a reliable, fast, and multimodal imaging pathway for the detection of cervical artery dissections in severely injured patients is of utmost importance in trauma centers of any size to avoid any therapeutic delay.

Author Contributions: Conceptualization, A.S.; data curation, C.T. and A.E.; formal analysis, D.P., W.B. and A.S.; funding acquisition, V.A.; investigation, D.P. and A.S.; methodology, D.P. and A.E.; project administration, A.E. and A.S.; resources, C.T.; software, C.T.; supervision, V.A.; validation, D.P., V.A. and A.S.; visualization, A.S.; writing—original draft, D.P. and A.S.; writing—review and editing, D.P., W.B. and A.S. All authors have read and agreed to the published version of the manuscript.

Funding: This research received no external funding.

Conflicts of Interest: The authors declare no conflict of interest.

References

1. Euler, S.A.; Kastenberger, T.; Attal, R.; Rieger, M.; Blauth, M.; Petri, M. Do we still need autopsy in times of modern multislice computed tomography?—Missed diagnoses in the emergency room. *Arch. Orthop. Trauma Surg.* **2017**, *137*, 43–47. [CrossRef] [PubMed]
2. Fabian, T.C.; Patton, J.H.; Croce, M.A.; Minard, G.; Kudsk, K.A.; Pritchard, F.E. Blunt carotid injury. Importance of early diagnosis and anticoagulant therapy. *Ann. Surg.* **1996**, *223*, 513–525. [CrossRef] [PubMed]

3. Alimi, Y.; Di Mauro, P.; Tomachot, L.; Albanese, J.; Martin, C.; Alliez, B.; Juhan, C. Bilateral dissection of the internal carotid artery at the base of the skull due to blunt trauma: Incidence and severity. *Ann. Vasc. Surg.* **1998**, *12*, 557–565. [CrossRef] [PubMed]
4. Schicho, A.; Luerken, L.; Meier, R.; Ernstberger, A.; Stroszczynski, C.; Schreyer, A.; Dendl, L.M.; Schleder, S. Incidence of traumatic carotid and vertebral artery dissections: Results of cervical vessel computed tomography angiogram as a mandatory scan component in severely injured patients. *Ther. Clin. Risk Manag.* **2018**, *14*, 173–178. [CrossRef] [PubMed]
5. Caputo, N.D.; Stahmer, C.; Lim, G.; Shah, K. Whole-body computed tomographic scanning leads to better survival as opposed to selective scanning in trauma patients: A systematic review and meta-analysis. *J. Trauma Acute Care Surg.* **2014**, *77*, 534–539. [CrossRef]
6. Polytrauma/Schwerverletzten-Behandlung. Available online: http://www.awmf.org/leitlinien/detail/ll/012-019.html (accessed on 7 August 2020).
7. Beal, A.L.; Ahrendt, M.N.; Irwin, E.D.; Lyng, J.W.; Turner, S.V.; Beal, C.A.; Byrnes, M.T.; Beilman, G.A. Prediction of blunt traumatic injuries and hospital admission based on history and physical exam. *World J. Emerg. Surg.* **2016**, *11*, 46. [CrossRef]
8. Grabowski, G.; Robertson, R.N.; Barton, B.M.; Cairns, M.A.; Webb, S.W. Blunt Cerebrovascular Injury in Cervical Spine Fractures: Are More-Liberal Screening Criteria Warranted? *Glob. Spine J.* **2016**, *6*, 679–685. [CrossRef]
9. Geddes, A.E.; Burlew, C.C.; Wagenaar, A.E.; Biffl, W.L.; Johnson, J.L.; Pieracci, F.M.; Campion, E.M.; Moore, E.E. Expanded screening criteria for blunt cerebrovascular injury: A bigger impact than anticipated. *Am. J. Surg.* **2016**, *212*, 1167–1174. [CrossRef]
10. Fleck, S.K.; Langner, S.; Baldauf, J.; Kirsch, M.; Kohlmann, T.; Schroeder, H.W.S. Incidence of blunt craniocervical artery injuries: Use of whole-body computed tomography trauma imaging with adapted computed tomography angiography. *Neurosurgery* **2011**, *69*, 615–624. [CrossRef]
11. Braunschweig, R. Protokollempfehlungen der AG Bildgebende Verfahren des Bewegungsapparats (AG BVB) zur Ganzkörper-CT mehrfach verletzter bzw. polytraumatisierter Patienten. *Fortschr Röntgenstr* **2017**, *189*, 997–1014.
12. Mutze, S.; Rademacher, G.; Matthes, G.; Hosten, N.; Stengel, D. Blunt cerebrovascular injury in patients with blunt multiple trauma: Diagnostic accuracy of duplex Doppler US and early CT angiography. *Radiology* **2005**, *237*, 884–892. [CrossRef] [PubMed]
13. Redekop, G.J. Extracranial carotid and vertebral artery dissection: A review. *Can. J. Neurol. Sci.* **2008**, *35*, 146–152. [CrossRef] [PubMed]
14. Schicho, A.; Lürken, L.; Meier, R.; Stroszczynski, C.; Schreyer, A.; Dendl, L.M.; Schleder, S. Non-penetrating traumatic injuries of the aortic arch. *Acta Radiol.* **2018**, *59*, 275–279. [CrossRef] [PubMed]
15. Schicho, A. Vascular Geometry as a Risk Factor for Nonpenetrating Traumatic Injuries of the Aortic Arch. *PLoS ONE* **2017**, *12*, e0180066. [CrossRef]
16. Richardson, J.D.; Simpson, C.; Miller, F.B. Management of carotid artery trauma. *Surgery* **1988**, *104*, 673–680. [CrossRef]
17. Martinelli, O.; Venosi, S.; BenHamida, J.; Malay, A.; Belli, C.; Irace, F.G.; Gattuso, R.; Frati, G.; Gossetti, B.; Irace, L. Therapeutical options in the management of carotid dissection. *Ann. Vasc. Surg.* **2016**. [CrossRef]
18. Baptista-Sincos, A.P.W.; Simplício, A.B.; Sincos, I.R.; Leaderman, A.; Neto, F.S.; Moraes, A.; Aun, R. Flow-diverting Stent in the Treatment of Cervical Carotid Dissection and Pseudoaneurysm: Review of Literature and Case Report. *Ann. Vasc. Surg.* **2018**, *46*, 372–379. [CrossRef]
19. Murai, Y.; Matano, F.; Yokobori, S.; Onda, H.; Yokota, H.; Morita, A. Treatment Strategies of Subarachnoid Hemorrhage from Bilateral Vertebral Artery Dissection: A Case Report and Literature Review Focusing on the Availability of Stent Placement. *World Neurosurg.* **2017**, *106*. [CrossRef]
20. Schulman, S.; Kearon, C. The subcommittee on control of anticoagulation of the scientific and standardization committee of the international society on thrombosis and haemostasis Definition of major bleeding in clinical investigations of antihemostatic medicinal products in non-surgical patients. *J. Thromb. Haemost.* **2005**, *3*, 692–694. [CrossRef]
21. Crönlein, M.; Sandmann, G.H.; Beirer, M.; Wunderlich, S.; Biberthaler, P.; Huber-Wagner, S. Traumatic bilateral carotid artery dissection following severe blunt trauma: A case report on the difficulties in diagnosis and therapy of an often overlooked life-threatening injury. *Eur. J. Med. Res.* **2015**, *20*. [CrossRef]

22. Biousse, V.; D'Anglejan-Chatillon, J.; Touboul, P.J.; Amarenco, P.; Bousser, M.G. Time course of symptoms in extracranial carotid artery dissections: A series of 80 patients. *Stroke* **1995**, *26*, 235–239. [CrossRef] [PubMed]
23. Lichy, C.; Metso, A.; Pezzini, A.; Leys, D.; Metso, T.; Lyrer, P.; Debette, S.; Thijs, V.; Abboud, S.; Kloss, M.; et al. Predictors of Delayed Stroke in Patients with Cervical Artery Dissection. *Int. J. Stroke* **2015**, *10*, 360–363. [CrossRef] [PubMed]
24. Lee, V.H.; Brown, R.D.; Mandrekar, J.N.; Mokri, B. Incidence and outcome of cervical artery dissection: A population-based study. *Neurology* **2006**, *67*, 1809–1812. [CrossRef] [PubMed]
25. Debus, F.; Lefering, R.; Frink, M.; Kühne, C.A.; Mand, C.; Bücking, B.; Ruchholtz, S. Anzahl der Schwerverletzten in Deutschland. *Dtsch. Arztebl. Int.* **2015**, *112*, 823–829. [CrossRef]
26. Elijovich, L.; Kazmi, K.; Gauvrit, J.Y.; Law, M. The emerging role of multidetector row CT angiography in the diagnosis of cervical arterial dissection: Preliminary study. *Neuroradiology* **2006**, *48*, 606–612. [CrossRef]
27. Vertinsky, A.T.; Schwartz, N.E.; Fischbein, N.J.; Rosenberg, J.; Albers, G.W.; Zaharchuk, G. Comparison of multidetector CT angiography and MR imaging of cervical artery dissection. *Am. J. Neuroradiol.* **2008**, *29*, 1753–1760. [CrossRef]
28. Provenzale, J.M.; Sarikaya, B. Comparison of test performance characteristics of MRI, MR angiography, and CT angiography in the diagnosis of carotid and vertebral artery dissection: A review of the medical literature. *Am. J. Roentgenol.* **2009**, *193*, 1167–1174. [CrossRef]
29. Brott, T.G.; Halperin, J.L.; Abbara, S.; Bacharach, J.M.; Barr, J.D.; Bush, R.L.; Cates, C.U.; Creager, M.A.; Fowler, S.B.; Friday, G.; et al. Guideline on the management of patients with extracranial carotid and vertebral artery disease. *Vasc. Med.* **2011**, *16*, 35–77. [CrossRef]

Journal of
Clinical Medicine

MDPI

Article

Load-Bearing Detection with Insole-Force Sensors Provides New Treatment Insights in Fragility Fractures of the Pelvis

Daniel Pfeufer †, Christopher A. Becker *,†, Leon Faust, Alexander M. Keppler, Marissa Stagg, Christian Kammerlander, Wolfgang Böcker and Carl Neuerburg

Department of General, Trauma and Reconstructive Surgery, University Hospital, Ludwig-Maximilians-University Munich, 81377 Munich, Germany; daniel.pfeufer@med.uni-muenchen.de (D.P.); leon.faust@med.uni-muenchen.de (L.F.); alexander.keppler@med.uni-muenchen.de (A.M.K.); marissa.stagg@med.uni-muenchen.de (M.S.); christian.kammerlander@med.uni-muenchen.de (C.K.); wolfgang.boecker@med.uni-muenchen.de (W.B.); carl.neuerburg@med.uni-muenchen.de (C.N.)

* Correspondence: christopher.becker@med.uni-muenchen.de; Tel.: +49-(0)89-44-000; Fax: +49-(0)89-440-078-899

† These authors contributed equally to this work.

Received: 30 June 2020; Accepted: 3 August 2020; Published: 6 August 2020

Abstract: Background: Due to an aging society, more and more surgeons are confronted with fragility fractures of the pelvis (FFPs). The aim of treatment of such patients should be the quickest possible mobilization with full weight-bearing. Up to now however, there are no data on loading of the lower extremities in patients suffering FFPs. We hypothesized to find differences in loading of the lower limbs. Methods: 22 patients with a mean age of 84.1 years were included. During gait analysis with insole-force sensors, loading on the lower extremities was recorded during early mobilization after index fracture. Results: Especially the average peak force showed differences in loading, as the affected limb was loaded significantly less {59.78% (SD ± 16.15%) of the bodyweight vs. 73.22% (SD ± 14.84%) (p = <0.001, effect size r = 0.58)}. Furthermore, differences in loading in between the fracture patterns of FFPs were observed. Conclusion: This study shows that it is possible to reliably detect the extremity load, with the help of an insole device, in patients presenting with fragility fractures of the pelvis. There is great potential to improve the choice and time of treatment with insole-force sensors in FFPs in future.

Keywords: pelvic fracture; fragility fractures; pelvic ring; pelvic ring fracture; insole-force sensors; weight-bearing; geriatric fracture

1. Introduction

Fragility fractures of the pelvis (FFP) are one of the challenges in geriatric traumatology. The incidence of pelvic fragility fractures is steadily increasing, especially in the age group over 80 years [1]. In contrast to pelvic fractures of younger adults, which are usually caused by high-energy trauma such as severe road accidents, pelvic fragility fractures are caused by low-energy trauma, for instance a domestic fall. This can be primarily explained by reduced bone density and limited ligamentous stability in elderly patients [2]. There are two problems with the care of fragility fractures of the pelvis in older patients: first, the treatment of pelvic fractures is generally very demanding, even for experienced surgeons. This is made more difficult by reduced bone quality in the elderly. Secondly, older patients frequently present with various comorbidities, polypharmacy and muscle atrophy (sarcopenia), which aggravates frailty [3,4]. In these patients immobilization is a severe threat, as prolonged bedrest is associated with poor function at 2 months, and worsened survival at 6 months in elderly trauma patients [5]. Accordingly, the goal in diagnosing and treating these patients must be to make a decision as quickly as possible regarding surgery or conservative therapy, so that they can be mobilized and return to their daily activity with compensated pain status. This means that significant complications such as pneumonia, thrombosis and further muscle loss can be avoided during hospital stay and after discharge [6].

Differentiation of the fragility fractures of the pelvis can be made using the FFP classification by Rommens et al. [7–9]. Type FFP1 fractures are stable fractures that only affect the anterior pelvic ring. Type FFP2 are characterized by undisplaced fractures of the posterior pelvic ring, with type FFP3 showing displaced fractures on the posterior pelvic ring. In type FFP2 and FFP3, the anterior pelvic ring is usually also affected. Type FFP4 fractures are bilateral dislocated posterior pelvic ring fractures [8].

Diagnosing fragility fractures of the pelvis is difficult and in many cases the patients complain about pain, especially during movement [7]. Often there is no history of falls or trauma, or the patient cannot remember it due to dementia or cognitive impairment and the correct diagnosis might be delayed by this.

The pelvic CT scan is the work horse in diagnosing FFP, as it commonly shows the bony structures and cortical fracture lines which are often overseen in conventional radiographs [10]. Still MRI has great advantages as it can visualize bone marrow alterations such as edema or bone bruise. With 100% sensitivity for bone marrow alterations the MRI is proven to be the gold standard over conventional CT with 65–75% of sensitivity [11,12]. In daily clinical routine CT scans are usually ordered first and MRI is only performed when pain persists during mobilization.

A relatively new approach for diagnosing bone marrow edema in FFPs are dual-energy CT scans. Palm et al. describe in a recently published study that dual-energy CT scans are on par with MRI for sensitivity and specificity in diagnosing fragility fractures of the pelvis [13].

According to Rommens' recommendation, FFP1 fractures should be treated primarily with a conservative approach. In principle, FFP2 fractures are also treated without surgery, while surgery is only recommended if there is no pain compensation and sufficient mobilization within one week. Surgical intervention is frequently recommended for type FFP3 and FFP4 fractures [8].

In cases in which it remains unclear which choice of treatment is best, and as an attempt to monitor mobilization outcomes in FFP patients, the use of new biosensor recorders to assess the ability of load-bearing can be beneficial. Thus, wearable insoles offer a novel and unique technology to gather metrics of gait in a potentially more clinically relevant way [14,15]. Wearable insoles have been used in different situations, such as aftercare of hip fracture patients [16,17] to measure weight-bearing and collect gait analysis data in elderly patients.

The purpose of this study was to evaluate the ability of a wearable insole sensor device to measure gait parameters in geriatric patients with FFPs. Further we sought to determine if the device was suitable and sensitive enough to identify potential subtle changes between the measures of different fracture patterns and treatment approaches.

2. Materials and Methods

2.1. Study Design and Participants

After receiving approval from the ethics committee (Ethikkommission bei der LMU München Ref.-No.: 19–292), a prospective observational trial was conducted to evaluate if it was possible to measure a difference between the fractured limb and the unaffected limb in patients that had suffered a fragility fracture of the pelvis. Patients seen for an FFP were considered for the study. Inclusion criteria were FFP I-IV, age > 70 years and a signed written consent. All subjects gave their informed consent for inclusion before they participated in the study. The study was conducted in accordance with the Declaration of Helsinki.

Those patients with a Minimal Mental State Exam (MMSE) lower than 27 were excluded in the present preliminary study approach in order to validate feasibility of the novel gait analysis approach for FFPs and to reduce differences in loading triggered by cognitive impairment and gait balance disorders. Immobility prior to the fracture or an additional fracture, even of the upper extremity, was an exclusion criterion. After the informed consent form was signed, the patients completed gait analysis using the Loadsol insole sensor device by Novel (Munich, Germany). Insole sensors were fitted into the shoe of each participant according to their appropriate shoe size (Figure 1). All sensors communicated via Bluetooth with an iPad (Apple, Inc., Cupertino, CA, USA). The decision to operate or not was made by three experienced consultants and the geriatrician in charge. For the operative patients, the measurement was done between 4–7 days post-operative. Standardized pain medication regimen according to WHO treatment guidelines was used for all patients. During gait analysis no local pain catheter was in use. Those patients who received conservative treatment for their fractures performed analysis 4–7 days after diagnosis. All patients were allowed the walking aid of their choice during measurement.

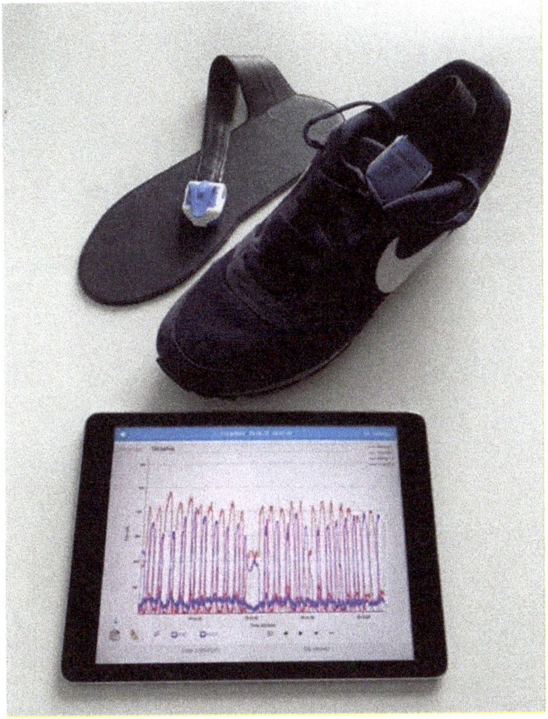

Figure 1. Setup of the Loadsol® insole sensor device.

2.2. Insole-Force Sensors

Loadsol® by Novel, was used in this study and has been shown to be a valid and reliable tool for wireless plantar force measurement in hopping, walking, and running [18]. Several studies were able to prove very similar results concerning the measurement with Loadsol® compared to force plates [19,20].

The distance for the measurement was fixed at 40 m for all participants. Some of the FFP patients were not able to walk the whole distance due to persistent pain, in these patients the average loading was recorded on a walking distances as much as tolerated. The measurement included starting from a chair, level walking the distance, turning, and returning to the chair. Peak force, average loading rate and step count were measured and recorded for each foot separately (Figure 2). The insole devices are designed to cover the entire plantar surface of the foot and record the plantar force up to 200 Hz (Figure 3).

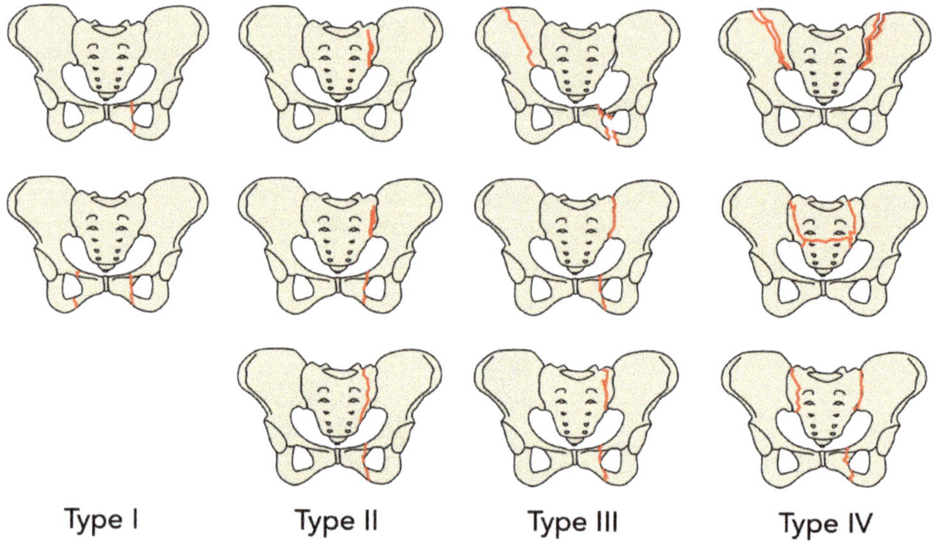

Figure 2. Comprehensive classification of fragility fractures of the pelvis according to Rommens and Hofmann [7]. Figure 1 is adapted from Ueda, Y. et al. [9] with permission from Springer Nature, 2020. FFP type I: anterior injury only. FFP type II: non-displaced posterior injury. FFP type III: displaced unilateral posterior injury. FFP type IV: displaced bilateral posterior injury.

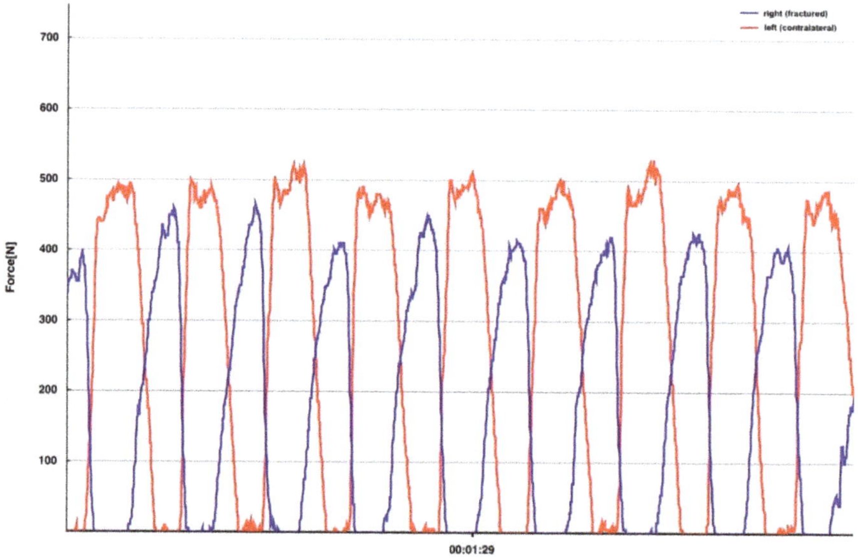

Figure 3. Displays the load in newton of the fractured side (blue graph) and the contralateral healthy side (red graph). Time in minutes is shown on the x-axis, while the y-axis represents force in newton. In this excerpt, 8 exemplary gait cycles are depicted.

The max peak force is the main outcome in this gait analysis. Percent peak force is the percentage of the peak force of the affected side compared to the total body weight in Newtons. The percent load rate is measured as the percentage of the loading rate (N/s) of the affected side compared to the unaffected side. Percent load rate is measured as the percentage of the loading rate (N/s) of the affected side compared to the unaffected side. The loading rate of the feet was measured in Newtons per seconds. The loading rate is calculated as

$$LR = \frac{(F80 - F20)}{(t80 - t20)} \tag{1}$$

where F20 and t20 are the Force in Newton (N) and time in second (s), measured when the force is at 20% of the heel impact peak. F80 and t80 are subsequently the force in Newton and time in seconds when the force is at 80% of the heel impact peak. An 11-point pain scale (0–10) was used to assess pain while walking and pain while resting. Additionally, the parker mobility score (PMS) and Barthel Index (BI) were collected from each patient.

2.3. Statistical Analysis

To check all data for normal distribution in advance of the analysis, the Shapiro–Wilk-Test was performed. Depending on the result of this test, either the Mann-Whitney-U-Test or the t-Test was used to identify significant differences between groups. When comparing FFP I and FFP IV patients the Mann-Whitney-U-Test was used for the percent avg. peak force and the *t*-Test was used for the percent max. peak force. Furthermore, the Wilcoxon rank sum test was performed to analyze the differences in the percent avg. peak force and the percent max. peak force comparing the fractured and the contralateral limb of each patient. To calculate the effect size of this test, the formula $r = \frac{Z}{\sqrt{n}}$ (Z = Z-Score, n = sample size) was used. The level of significance was set at $p < 0.05$. Patient characteristics were acquired using descriptive statistics.

Graphs and statistical analysis were calculated with IBM SPSS Statistics Version 25 (IBM Germany GmbH, Ehningen, Germany).

3. Results

Overall, 22 consecutive FFP patients were included within the trial with a mean age of 84.09 years (SD ± 5.98, range 73–95 years). 90.9% of the patients were female (20 female/2 male) with an overall mean weight of 58.66 kg (SD ± 8.04 kg), a mean BMI of 22.45 kg/m^2 (SD ± 3.35 kg/m^2) and a mean ASA Score of 2.68 (SD ± 0.65) (Table 1).

Table 1. Population Characteristics.

Characteristic	Mean ± SD
Age	84.09 ± 5.98
Female sex, *n* (%)	20 (90.9)
Weight (kg)	58.66 ± 8.04
BMI (kg/m^2)	22.45 ± 3.35
ASA Score	2.68 ± 0.65

The fractures presented were classified according to the FFP classification with the following distribution: FFP I (n = 3, 13.6%), FFP II (n = 13, 59.1%), FFP III (n = 1, 4.5%) and FFP IV (n = 5, 22.7%). For an easier understanding of the results we pooled the FFP subtypes together in their main groups. Of all patients included, a total of n = 13 patients were treated conservatively (59.1%) over n = 9 patients with an operative treatment (40.9%) (Table 2).

Table 2. FFP Classification and Treatment.

FFP Type	*n* (%)
FFP I	3 (13.6)
FFP II	13 (59.1)
FFP III	1 (4.5)
FFP IV	5 (22.7)
Treatment	
Surgery	13 (59.1)
Conservative	9 (40.9)

The first set of analyses investigated whether we could find a difference in weight-bearing between the fractured side and the contralateral unaffected side. As seen in the percent Avg. Pf., the patients loaded the limb ipsilateral to the fractured side of the pelvis significantly less, with a mean of 59.78% (SD ± 16.15%) of the bodyweight in comparison to the contralateral limb with 73.22% (SD ± 14.84%) of the bodyweight (p = <0.001, effect size r = 0.58). A comparison of the percent Max. Pf. showed that the patients put a significantly lower maximum load on the affected limb with 75.10% (SD ± 13.64%) of the bodyweight, as opposed to the contralateral limb with 87.77% (SD ± 13.80%) of the bodyweight (p = <0.001, effect size r = 0.50) (Table 3).

Table 3. Comparison fractured vs. contralateral limb: gait analysis.

Parameter	Limb	Mean ± SD	*p*-Value	*r*—Effect Size
Avg. Pf. (% of bodyweight)	Fractured	59.78 ± 16.15	<0.001	0.58
	Contralateral	73.22 ± 14.84		
Max. Pf. (% of bodyweight)	Fractured	75.10 ± 13.64	<0.001	0.50
	Contralateral	87.77 ± 13.80		

A descriptive analysis of the gait parameters collected for each group of the FFP fracture types showed that the patients of each group loaded their affected side differently.

In view of the percent Avg. Pf. the patients with an FFP type I fracture loaded the affected side with 84.89% of the bodyweight (SD ± 23.14%), FFP type II patients reached a mean of 56.18% (SD ± 13.26%), 54.09% were measured for the FFP type III patient and 55.21% (SD ± 5.01%) in the FFP type IV group. Moreover, the percent Max. Pf. showed differences between the FFP groups examined (FFP I: 96.62% ± 21.99%, FFP II: 73.52% ± 8.80%, FFP III: 63.15% and FFP IV: 68.55% ± 7.59%). However, no such clear tendency can be seen in the percent Loading Rate (FFP I: 79.18% ± 63.94% vs. FFP II: 65.46% ± 23.24% vs. FFP III: 75.30% vs. FFP IV: 67.78% ± 19.43%), especially comparing FFP II and IV (Table 4).

Table 4. Overall gait analysis.

Parameter	FFP I	FFP II	FFP III	FFP IV
Avg. Pf. (% of bodyweight)	84.89 ± 23.14	56.18 ± 12.26	54.09	55.21 ± 5.01
Max. Pf. (% of bodyweight)	96.62 ± 21.99	73.52 ± 8.80	63.15	68.55 ± 7.59
Percent Loading Rate (%)	79.18 ± 63.94	65.46 ± 23.24	75.30	67.78 ± 19.43

Concerning ASA score, Barthel Index and Parker Mobility Score there was no deterioration detectable with regards to an increasing FFP type (Table 5).

Table 5. Subgroup Characteristics.

Score	FFP I	FFP II	FFP III	FFP IV
ASA	2.67 ± 1.16	2.62 ± 1.64	3	2.80 ± 0.84
BI	65.00 ± 27.84	49.23 ± 13.20	75	67.00 ± 10.37
PMS	3.33 ± 1.16	2.23 ± 1.64	3	2.40 ± 1.14

Drawn from the descriptive analysis above, another promising finding was that the patients with a low grade FFP I fracture put a significantly higher load on their affected limb than the patients with a high grade FFP IV fracture. The percent Avg. Pf. in the FFP I group had a mean of 84.89% (SD ± 23.14%) in contrast to a mean percent Avg. Pf. of 55.21% (SD ± 5.01%) in the FFP IV group ($p = 0.036$). Furthermore, there was a significant difference in the percent Max. Pf. between both groups with a mean of 96.62% (SD ± 21.99%) in the FFP I group, versus a mean of 68.55% (SD ± 7.59%) in the FFP IV group ($p = 0.035$) (Table 6).

Table 6. FFP I vs. FFP IV.

Parameter	FFP I	FFP IV	*p*-Value
Avg. Pf. (% of bodyweight)	84.89 ± 23.14	55.21 ± 5.01	0.036
Max. Pf. (% of bodyweight)	96.62 ± 21.99	68.55 ± 7.59	0.035

Beyond this finding, a comparison of the FFP I group, with fractures limited to the anterior pelvic ring, and the remaining groups FFP II-IV, with an obligate involvement of the posterior pelvic ring, resulted in a significant difference. Again, patients with a low grade FFP I fracture put a higher load on the affected limb than patients with a more severe FFP II-IV fracture. This was detectable in both the Avg. Pf. (FFP I: 84.89% ± 23.14% vs. FFP II-IV: 55.93% ± 11.11%, $p = 0.002$) and the Max. Pf. (FFP I: 96.62% ± 21.99% vs. FFP II-IV: 71.66% ± 8.58%, $p = <0.001$) (Table 7).

Table 7. FFP I vs. FFP II-IV.

Parameter	FFP I	FFP II-IV	*p*-Value
Avg. Pf. (% of bodyweight)	84.89 ± 23.14	55.93 ± 11.11	0.002
Max. Pf. (% of bodyweight)	96.62 ± 21.99	71.66 ± 8.58	<0.001

4. Discussion

The results of this study show that a wearable insole-force sensor was sensitive enough to detect differences in load-bearing between the affected and contralateral side, in patients that suffer a fragility fracture of the pelvis (FFP). In this analysis of FFP patients, the average peak force was the most sensitive gait parameter to detect differences in gait. This gait parameter is easy to understand, as it is the force between foot and shoe, which is measured in newtons and can be detected with different types of sensors [21]. The wearable insole device may prove to be a suitable technology to use in a clinical setting, even if this preliminary data only gives an idea of what this system is capable of.

The first important finding is that we detected the fractured side correctly in 100 percent of the patients. This is not as trivial as it sounds, considering that the clinical picture, radiological morphology and stability range widely [22]. A FFP, which is often difficult to detect correctly with a conventional X-ray [10] and therefore a more sensitive CT Scan is often recommended, can be detected correctly with an insole device. Although classification of FFPs and therapy recommendations have been proven, classification of FFP subtypes involving a complete non-displaced or displaced sacral fracture showed relatively poor inter-/intraobserver reliability which limits the usefulness of the FFP classification for both clinical and research purposes [23]. Thus, the present findings give an idea of how sensitive load-bearing detection and the clinical measurement of load can be used as a clinical tool.

It is likely that these fractures cause pain due to micro movements in the fracture zone, and therefore the patients try to reduce loading the fractured side. This goes along with the anatomical description of the FFP, where a higher FFP classification indicates a more unstable fracture type [24]. Referring to the fracture pattern and taking under consideration the degree of resulting instability, a conservative or operative treatment is generally recommended.

The second main finding is that the fractured side is loaded significantly less. The average Peakforce applied to the fractured side is significantly lower on the affected side than on the contralateral. Similar findings were described in previous studies using load measuring insoles to detect the plantar force in lower limb fractures [16,17,25]. To the best of our knowledge the present study is the first to investigate the use of a mobile insole sensor in fragility fractures of the pelvis.

A sub-analysis of FFP1 to FFP4 shows another promising finding; the patients with FFP I fractures put a significantly higher load on the fractured side than the patients with an FFP IV fracture. This sub-analysis gives an insight on how the load-bearing between different grades of pelvic instability are measurable with the insole sensor. Anterior versus posterior injuries also seem to have different load-bearing patterns. This is in line with the classification of Rommens and Hofmann, as they assume higher instability with higher fracture classification. In the present study patients suffering only anterior fractures load significantly more weight on the fractured side than patients suffering from combined anterior and posterior pelvic ring fractures.

The basic presumption is that early mobilization should be facilitated, and therefore a surgical intervention might be needed in higher degree FFPs. On the other hand, the recommendation for FFP2 is to be reevaluated within 5–7 days after the fracture was diagnosed and if the patient is still not mobile, surgery may be necessary. An insole sensor as a sensitive clinical tool might facilitate this process in future. Cut off values which would lead to surgical intervention or allow for conservative treatment cannot be determined in this comparatively small sample size. This will be of interest as the clinical pathway to find the right treatment for a patient suffering from an FFP is still under construction. Given the relative ease of measurement of parameters of gait, this could become a clinically usable instrument in future.

Early mobilization under pain treatment is the primary therapy goal in FFP 1 and 2, as geriatric trauma patients have a significantly increased mortality risk due to immobilization [5]. Thus, a multidisciplinary team of physiotherapists, geriatricians, nurses, and surgeons should conclude therapy decision in patients suffering FFPs. The early decision whether a conservative or surgical approach is needed, can be chosen through previous full mobilization and significantly reduces complications [26]. This should include physiotherapy treatment under pain-dependent full load [2].

The therapy decision is currently based on an individual assessment of the mobility of the patient. Physiotherapists and nurses who work closely with the patient can get very different impressions regarding mobility. Therefore, a wearable load measuring device such as the Loadsol, could be used to additionally measure the load applied to the fractured side.

This study is limited to early post-operative/post fracture time and the results cannot be extrapolated beyond the first week at this time. However, as the first week of early mobilization is the most important time frame, this is likely the best timing for the measurement, although a continuous measurement over the first 6 weeks should be the goal [5]. Although gait analysis with an insole-force sensor has proven its feasibility to provide additional insights in FFPs, the present study contains some limitations. Furthermore, data of the present study remains preliminary while the sample size is still small. Also patients with an MMSE < 27 were excluded from the present study although this remains a condition frequently observed in elderly patients suffering from FFPs we aimed to reduce loading differences triggered by cognitive impairment and gait balance disorders. Only one wearable insole design was evaluated, and while the sensor used in this study shows a high validity and is easy to use [18–20,27], there are other products on the market (e.g., Mediologic, Tekscan, Pedar) that could offer similar measurements, and may merit further study [21].

Future studies should also focus on how to find cut off values and how to differentiate between unstable and stable fractures and choice of surgical treatment by load measuring devices.

5. Conclusions

The present study primarily proved feasibility of insole-force sensors that provide new treatment insights in fragility fractures of the pelvis. Gait analysis detected the fractured side correctly in 100 percent of the patients, while the limb where the FFPs were located was loaded significantly less compared to the healthy contralateral side. Furthermore, patients having suffered a low grade FFP I put significantly higher load on the fractured side than patients presenting with an FFP IV fracture. Additionally, differences in loading were observed when comparing fractures affecting the anterior pelvic ring only, compared to combined anterior and posterior pelvic ring fractures. Although gait analysis with an insole-force sensor has proven its feasibility to provide additional treatment insights in FFPs, future studies should focus on how to find cut off values for conservative vs. surgical treatment and how to differentiate between the choice of surgical treatment.

Author Contributions: Conceptualization, D.P. and C.A.B. and C.N.; Methodology, D.P. and L.F.; Validation, D.P., M.S. and C.A.B.; Statistical Analysis, L.F., M.S., W.B.; Investigation, C.A.B. and A.M.K.; Writing—Original Draft Preparation, D.P., C.A.B., L.F., A.M.K., C.K. and C.N.; Writing—Review & Editing, W.B., M.S., C.K., C.N., D.P. and C.A.B.; Supervision, C.N. and C.K.; Project Administration, C.N., C.K., W.B., C.A.B. and D.P. All authors have read and agreed to the published version of the manuscript.

Funding: This research received no external funding.

Conflicts of Interest: The authors declare no conflict of interest.

References

1. Andrich, S.; Haastert, B.; Neuhaus, E.; Neidert, K.; Arend, W.; Ohmann, C.; Grebe, J.; Vogt, A.; Jungbluth, P.; Rösler, G.; et al. Epidemiology of pelvic fractures in Germany: Considerably high incidence rates among older people. *PLoS ONE* **2015**, *10*, e0139078. [CrossRef] [PubMed]
2. Oberkircher, L.; Ruchholtz, S.; Rommens, P.M.; Hofmann, A.; Bücking, B.; Krüger, A. Osteoporotic pelvic fractures. *Dtsch. Ärzteblatt Int.* **2018**, *115*, 70–80. [CrossRef] [PubMed]
3. Höch, A.; Pieroh, P.; Gras, F.; Hohmann, T.; Märdian, S.; Holmenschlager, F.; Keil, H.; Palm, H.-G.; Herath, S.C.; Josten, C.; et al. Age and "general health"-beside fracture classification-affect the therapeutic decision for geriatric pelvic ring fractures: A German pelvic injury register study. *Int. Orthop.* **2019**, *43*, 2629–2636. [CrossRef] [PubMed]
4. Liem, I.S.; Kammerlander, C.; Suhm, N.; Blauth, M.; Roth, T.; Gosch, M.; Hoang-Kim, A.; Mendelson, D.; Zuckerman, J.; Leung, F.; et al. Identifying a standard set of outcome parameters for the evaluation of orthogeriatric co-management for hip fractures. *Injury* **2013**, *44*, 1403–1412. [CrossRef]
5. Siu, A.L.; Penrod, J.D.; Boockvar, K.S.; Koval, K.; Strauss, E.; Morrison, R.S. Early ambulation after hip fracture: Effects on function and mortality. *Arch. Intern. Med.* **2006**, *166*, 766–771. [CrossRef]
6. Reito, A.; Kuoppala, M.; Pajulammi, H.; Hokkinen, L.; Kyrölä, K.; Paloneva, J. Mortality and comorbidity after non-operatively managed, low-energy pelvic fracture in patients over age 70: A comparison with an age-matched femoral neck fracture cohort and general population. *BMC Geriatr.* **2019**, *19*, 315. [CrossRef]
7. Rommens, P.M.; Hofmann, A. Comprehensive classification of fragility fractures of the pelvic ring: Recommendations for surgical treatment. *Injury* **2013**, *44*, 1733–1744. [CrossRef]
8. Rommens, P.M.; Wagner, D.; Hofmann, A. Minimal invasive surgical treatment of fragility fractures of the pelvis. *Chirurgia* **2017**, *112*, 524. [CrossRef]
9. Ueda, Y.; Inui, T.; Kurata, Y.; Tsuji, H.; Saito, J.; Shitan, Y. Prolonged pain in patients with fragility fractures of the pelvis may be due to fracture progression. *Eur. J. Trauma Emerg. Surg.* Available online: https://link.springer.com/article/10.1007%2Fs00068-019-01150-0 (accessed on 8 April 2020). [CrossRef]
10. Tosounidis, G.; Wirbel, R.; Culemann, U.; Pohlemann, T. Fehleinschätzung bei vorderer Beckenringfraktur im höheren Lebensalter. *Unfallchirurg* **2006**, *109*, 678–680. [CrossRef]

11. Grangier, C.; Garcia, J.; Howarth, N.R.; May, M.; Rossier, P. Role of MRI in the diagnosis of insufficiency fractures of the sacrum and acetabular roof. *Skeletal Radiol.* **1997**, *26*, 517–524. [CrossRef] [PubMed]
12. Soles, G.L.S.; Ferguson, T.A. Fragility fractures of the pelvis. *Curr. Rev. Musculoskelet. Med.* **2012**, *5*, 222–228. [CrossRef] [PubMed]
13. Palm, H.-G.; Lang, P.; Hackenbroch, C.; Sailer, L.; Friemert, B. Dual-energy CT as an innovative method for diagnosing fragility fractures of the pelvic ring: A retrospective comparison with MRI as the gold standard. *Arch. Orthop. Trauma Surg.* **2020**, *140*, 473–480. [CrossRef] [PubMed]
14. Crea, S.; Donati, M.; De Rossi, S.M.M.; Oddo, C.M.; Vitiello, N. A wireless flexible sensorized insole for gait analysis. *Sensors* **2014**, *14*, 1073–1093. [CrossRef]
15. Chesnin, K.J.; Selby-Silverstein, L.; Besser, M.P. Comparison of an in-shoe pressure measurement device to a force plate: Concurrent validity of center of pressure measurements. *Gait Posture* **2000**, *12*, 128–133. [CrossRef]
16. Braun, B.J.; Bushuven, E.; Hell, R.; Veith, N.T.; Buschbaum, J.; Holstein, J.H.; Pohlemann, T. A novel tool for continuous fracture aftercare—Clinical feasibility and first results of a new telemetric gait analysis insole. *Injury* **2016**, *47*, 490–494. [CrossRef]
17. Kammerlander, C.; Pfeufer, D.; Lisitano, L.A.; Mehaffey, S.; Böcker, W.; Neuerburg, C. Inability of older adult patients with hip fracture to maintain postoperative weight-bearing restrictions. *JBJS* **2018**, *100*, 936–941. [CrossRef]
18. Burns, G.T.; Zendler, J.D.; Zernicke, R.F. Validation of a wireless shoe insole for ground reaction force measurement. *J. Sports Sci.* **2019**, *37*, 1129–1138. [CrossRef]
19. Peebles, A.T.; Maguire, L.A.; Renner, K.E.; Queen, R.M. Validity and repeatability of single-sensor loadsol insoles during landing. *Sensors* **2018**, *18*, 4082. [CrossRef]
20. Seiberl, W.; Jensen, E.; Merker, J.; Leitel, M.; Schwirtz, A. Accuracy and precision of loadsol® insole force-sensors for the quantification of ground reaction force-based biomechanical running parameters. *Eur. J. Sport Sci.* **2018**, *18*, 1100–1109. [CrossRef]
21. Price, C.; Parker, D.; Nester, C. Validity and repeatability of three in-shoe pressure measurement systems. *Gait Posture* **2016**, *46*, 69–74. [CrossRef] [PubMed]
22. Rommens, P.M.; Ossendorf, C.; Pairon, P.; Dietz, S.-O.; Wagner, D.; Hofmann, A. Clinical pathways for fragility fractures of the pelvic ring: Personal experience and review of the literature. *J. Orthop. Sci.* **2015**, *20*, 1–11. [CrossRef] [PubMed]
23. Krappinger, D.; Kaser, V.; Kammerlander, C.; Neuerburg, C.; Merkel, A.; Lindtner, R.A. Inter- and intraobserver reliability and critical analysis of the FFP classification of osteoporotic pelvic ring injuries. *Injury* **2019**, *50*, 337–343. [CrossRef]
24. Rommens, P.M.; Arand, C.; Hopf, J.C.; Mehling, I.; Dietz, S.O.; Wagner, D. Progress of instability in fragility fractures of the pelvis: An observational study. *Injury* **2019**, *50*, 1966–1973. [CrossRef] [PubMed]
25. Pfeufer, D.; Zeller, A.; Mehaffey, S.; Böcker, W.; Kammerlander, C.; Neuerburg, C. Weight-bearing restrictions reduce postoperative mobility in elderly hip fracture patients. *Arch. Orthop. Trauma Surg.* **2019**, *139*, 1253–1259. [CrossRef]
26. van Dijk, W.A.; Poeze, M.; van Helden, S.H.; Brink, P.R.G.; Verbruggen, J.P.A.M. Ten-year mortality among hospitalised patients with fractures of the pubic rami. *Injury* **2010**, *41*, 411–414. [CrossRef]
27. Renner, K.E.; Williams, D.B.; Queen, R.M. The reliability and validity of the Loadsol® under various walking and running conditions. *Sensors* **2019**, *19*, 265. [CrossRef]

Journal of
Clinical Medicine

MDPI

Article

Evidence of Prolonged Monitoring of Trauma Patients Admitted via Trauma Resuscitation Unit without Primary Proof of Severe Injuries

Martin Heinrich [1,2,*], Matthias Lany [1], Lydia Anastasopoulou [1,2], Christoph Biehl [1,2], Gabor Szalay [1], Florian Brenck [3] and Christian Heiss [1,2]

1 Department of Trauma, Hand and Reconstructive Surgery, University Hospital Giessen, 35392 Giessen, Germany; Matthias.Lany@chiru.med.uni-giessen.de (M.L.); Lydia.Anastasopoulou@chiru.med.uni-giessen.de (L.A.); Christoph.Biehl@chiru.med.uni-giessen.de (C.B.); Gabor.Szalay@chiru.med.uni-giessen.de (G.S.); Christian.Heiss@chiru.med.uni-giessen.de (C.H.)

2 Experimental Trauma Surgery, Justus-Liebig-University of Giessen, 35392 Giessen, Germany

3 Department of Anesthesiology, Intensive Care Medicine and Pain Therapy, University Hospital Giessen, 35392 Giessen, Germany; Florian.Brenck@chiru.med.uni-giessen.de

* Correspondence: martin.heinrich@chiru.med.uni-giessen.de; Tel.: +49-641-98544601

Received: 30 June 2020; Accepted: 30 July 2020; Published: 4 August 2020

Abstract: Introductio: Although management of severely injured patients in the Trauma Resuscitation Unit (TRU) follows evidence-based guidelines, algorithms for treatment of the slightly injured are limited. Methods: All trauma patients in a period of eight months in a Level I trauma center were followed. Retrospective analysis was performed only in patients ≥18 years with primary TRU admission, Abbreviated Injury Scale (AIS) ≤ 1, Maximum Abbreviated Injury Scale (MAIS) ≤ 1 and Injury Severity Score (ISS) ≤3 after treatment completion and ≥24 h monitoring in the units. Cochran's Q-test was used for the statistical evaluation of AIS and ISS changes in units. Results: One hundred and twelve patients were enrolled in the study. Twenty-one patients (18.75%) reported new complaints after treatment completion in the TRU. AIS rose from the Intermediate Care Unit (IMC) to Normal Care Unit (NCU) 6.2% and ISS 6.9%. MAIS did not increase >2, and no intervention was necessary for any patient. No correlation was found between computed tomography (CT) diagnostics in TRU and AIS change. Conclusions: The data suggest that AIS, MAIS and ISS did not increase significantly in patients without a severe injury during inpatient treatment, regardless of the type of CT diagnostics performed in the TRU, suggesting that monitoring of these patients may be unnecessary.

Keywords: trauma resuscitation unit; emergency medicine; injury severity; abbreviated injury scale; injury severity score

1. Introduction

Acute care of trauma patients in Germany, Austria, Switzerland, the Netherlands, Belgium and Luxembourg is ensured by local, regional and supraregional trauma centers (level I-III) according to the TraumaNetwork DGU® initiative.

TraumaNetwork DGU® initiative has enabled the German Society for Trauma Surgery (DGU) to establish first-class nationwide care for the severely injured. Clinics and University hospitals in order to provide high-quality patient care in trauma centers in addition to specialized medical requirements, also require specific spatial and material resources [1,2]. According to the guidelines of the DGU and the "Association of the Scientific Medical Societies in Germany" specific criteria must be fulfilled for the activation of the Trauma Resuscitation Unit (TRU). These criteria are divided into three groups: "disturbance of vital signs", "detected injuries" and "mechanism of the accident or accident constellation" [2,3]. However, based on the last criterion, it has been observed that in Germany that many slightly injured patients are admitted to the TRU, yet only one in five are severely injured with an Injury Severity Score (ISS) ≥ 16 [4,5].

In 2019 the German Society for Trauma Surgery published the "Whitebook Medical Care of the Severely Injured" 3rd edition, which provides guidelines for the clinical and diagnostic steps, as well as for the first operative phase of the "Trauma Resuscitation Unit treatment" [2,6,7]. However, until now, there are no recommendations for the duration of treatment and whether further monitoring is necessary for the slightly injured trauma patients, who have suffered a dangerous trauma and who according to the TRU criteria must be treated in the TRU.

In addition, it has been shown that the intake of mind-altering substances (e.g drugs, alcohol or medication) in combination with a dangerous trauma, even if the patient is slightly injured, leads to the monitoring of the patient [8]. In individual and defined cases, if the patient has not suffered a severe injury, after implementation of the standardized Trauma Resuscitation Unit treatment, and if the occurrence of possible further complications is excluded, prolonged monitoring appears not to be necessary [9–11]. However, relevant injuries (such as cerebral contusion, occipital skull fracture or pneumothorax) have been initially overlooked and were only subsequently detected [8].

This might be the reason, that it has been reported in the literature that many patients with minor trauma are admitted to the Intermediate Care Unit (IMC) for monitoring without any comprehensible medical reason [12].

A national or international study that considers the entire cohort of patients that have been treated in the TRU and were initially diagnosed as slightly injured does not exist.

In the present study, it is therefore investigated whether (1) inpatients surveillance after the interdisciplinary TRU diagnostic is necessary so that injuries with an Abbreviated Injury Scale (AIS) ≥2 are not overlooked; and (2) whether the inquired experience of the trauma team along with the improved computed tomography (CT) imaging makes the inpatient monitoring unnecessary.

2. Materials and Methods

2.1. University Hospital of Giessen and Data Acquisition

The University Hospital of Giessen, located in the middle of Germany, is a National Trauma Center (Level I) of the DGU. In 2018, 370 patients were admitted with moderate to severe injuries, which was the greatest number of patients registered by the TraumaRegister DGU® in a single hospital throughout Germany at that time. In addition, a total of about 1000 trauma patients are treated annually in the TRU [13].

When treating trauma patients, the procedures of the TRU-algorithm at the University Hospital of Giessen strictly adhere to the Advanced Trauma Life Support (ATLS) protocol. More specifically, patient care is carried out by a defined TRU team, which consists of five attending physicians from the fields of trauma surgery, visceral surgery, anesthesia, neurosurgery and radiology. While the diagnostic steps of the primary survey are strictly defined in the treatment protocol and are identical for all patients, diagnostic imaging in the TRU is individually adapted to each trauma patient by the trauma team.

After admission in the TRU, regardless of the type of injuries, trauma patients are monitored for 24 h, initially in the Intermediate Care Unit (IMC). They are then transferred to the Normal Care Unit (NCU) until their discharge from the hospital. All patient documentation is carried out promptly in the electronic patient file. "MEONA" software from Meona GmbH, Freiburg, Germany is used at NCU and "icudata" from IMESO-IT GmbH, Giessen, Germany is used at IMC, both are used in the TRU.

2.2. Inclusion and Exclusion Criteria

Ethical approval was given by the Justus-Liebig-University Giessen's ethics committee (approval number AZ 67/20). The study included during the eight month observation period between April and

November 2019 data from 112 adult (≥18 years) trauma patients admitted to the TRU at the University Hospital of Giessen, Department of Trauma, Hand and Reconstructive Surgery, who had Maximum Abbreviated Injury Scale (MAIS) ≤1, Injury Severity Score (ISS) ≤3 and had been monitored at IMC or NCU for 24 h.

Children, as well as patients with less than 24-h monitoring or with severe injuries (MAIS ≥2) or patients with incomplete data files, were excluded from the study.

2.3. Definitions

All 112 patients injuries were rated using the AIS (AIS Version 2005/Update 2008, Association for the Advancement of Automotive Medicine, Barrington, IL), using a scale from 0 to 6 according to injury severity (Table 1) [14]. From the AIS the MAIS and ISS were derived [15]. Evaluation of injuries took place retrospectively, based on the electronic patient record at the end of the TRU management, the IMC-observation and at the end of hospitalization at NCU.

Table 1. The severity of the Abbreviated Injury Scale (AIS).

	Injury Severity
1	Minor
2	Moderate
3	Serious
4	Severe
5	Critical
6	Maximum

In the case of changes at the AIS during hospitalization, a consultant evaluated the consequences, and if necessary, advised for a change in therapy. If the patients reported new symptoms, the current location, IMC or NCU, was also noted.

Furthermore, additional parameters as gender, age and the course of the accident ("motor vehicle accident", "motorcycle/bicycle accident", "high and low falls", "pedestrian vs. vehicle crash", "corporal violence", "others") were included. The performance of a head and body trunk CT, only head or body trunk CT or no CT during the initial TRU assessment was noted. The respective medical units extended diagnostics that were performed were also recorded.

2.4. Statistical Analysis

For statistical assessment of the changes in the AIS and ISS a binary form of the two scores was encoded (AIS: =0 as 0 and >0 as 1; ISS: ≤3 as 0 and >3 as 1). Cochran´s Q tests were used for ISS and AIS variables. For the recoded data, the number and percentage of persons with an AIS/ISS = 1 in the respective hospital unit and the percentage of persons for whom the value has changed from TRU to IMC or IMC to NCU were also shown. Risk assessment and risk differences were also calculated. The Chi^2-test was used to determine whether AIS changes depended on CT diagnostics carried out in the TRU.

Statistical analysis was performed using SPSS (Version 23, IBM Inc., Armonk, NY, USA), and the level of significance was 5%.

The total length of stay (LOS, in hours) in relation to different variables was also analyzed. A minimum LOS of 24 h was mandatory for all patients. Thus, this was defined as the null by subtracting 24 from all values. The explanatory variables were changed (three categories: "no change", "new symptoms" and "AIS change"—with the first one used as a reference category for dummy coding to which the others were compared), age (in years), gender (men as reference category), and extended diagnostics (in this sample, people received extended diagnostics once at maximum if at all; thus, not receiving extended diagnostics was simply chosen as the reference category).

A generalized linear regression model was applied due to the right-skewed distribution of the variable "length of stay". A gamma distribution was chosen in combination with the natural logarithm as the link function between mean length of stay and the explanatory variables. Then the regression coefficients were back-transformed using the exponential function. Hence, they represent a multiplicative change in length of stay. For all analyses, a significance level of 5% was chosen. Statistical analysis was carried out using R 3.6.3. [16].

Data are presented as mean ± standard deviation (mean ± SD). In the case of asymmetrical distribution, the median was also calculated.

3. Results

3.1. Demographic Data

The study included 112 (19.55%) out of the 573 trauma patients admitted in the TRU of the University Hospital of Giessen during the eight month observation period between April and November 2019 who fulfilled the inclusion criteria (≥18 years, primary TRU admission, AIS ≤ 1, MAIS ≤ 1 and ISS ≤ 3 after TRU treatment completion, ≥24 h monitoring in the units). Participants' mean age was 41.18 ± 19.63 years; 69 (62%) were males and 43 (38%) females (Table 2).

Table 2. Demographic data.

N = 112		
Age	Mean = 41.18	SD = 19.63
Gender n (%)	69 (62%) male	43 (38%) female

N = Total sample size; n = Group sample size; SD = Standard Deviation.

The car accident was the reason for admission in 62 cases (55.36 %). Other accidents included falls in 20 cases (17.86%), accidents between cars and pedestrians or cyclists in 12 cases (10.71%), falls from motorcycles or bicycles in nine cases (8.04%), physical abuse in five cases (4.46%), and other types of accidents (circular saw and pinch point injuries) in four cases (3.57%) (Table 3).

Table 3. Mechanisms of injuries.

	Total (n)	Total (%)
Motor vehicle accident	62	55.36
Motorcycle/bicycle accident	9	8.04
High and low falls	20	17.86
Pedestrian vs. vehicle crash	12	10.71
Physical abuse	5	4.46
Others	4	3.57

n = Group sample size.

3.2. Average ISS, AIS and MAIS

All patients admitted in the TRU had an average ISS of 1.45 after treatment. The average score increased to 1.47 in the IMC and to 1.55 in the NCU. An overall increase of 6.9% from the TRU to NCU was observed. The average AIS of all regions rose from an initial 1.45 in the TRU to 1.47 in IMC and to 1.54 in NCU, resulting in an overall increase of 6.2%. The MAIS was 1 in the TRU and IMC and 2 in the NCU. Out of the 112 patients, a total of four (3.57%) were completely unharmed, and therefore, had an AIS and ISS of 0. These scores did not change during inpatient hospitalization (Table 4).

Table 4. ISS Average and MAIS.

	ISS Average *	Range **	MAIS *	Range **
TRU	1.45	0–3	1	0–1
IMC	1.47	0–3	1	0–1
NCU	1.55	0–5	2	0–2

TRU = Trauma Resuscitation Unit; IMC = Intermediate Care; NCU = Normal Care Unit; ISS = Injury Severity Score; AIS = Abbreviated Injury Scale; MAIS = Maximum Abbreviated Injury Scale. * Average of the ISS and AIS in the different units; ** Minimum and Maximum of ISS, AIS range.

The frequency distribution of the individual ISS-values throughout the different units showed that ISS in the IMC increased one point in only two patients from the initial ISS in the TRU. In six patients, the ISS change occurred in the NCU, and in one of these patients, the ISS rose to five (Table 5).

Table 5. Frequencies of all observed ISS values in the units.

ISS	TRU	IMC	NCU
0	4	4	4
1	59	57	53
2	43	45	46
3	6	6	8
5	0	0	1

ISS = Injury Severity Score; TRU = Trauma Resuscitation Unit; IMC = Intermediate Care; NCU = Normal Care Unit.

Figure 1 shows, that there was no significant change of the ISS during patients' hospitalization in the different units. Means and medians were almost at the same level, suggesting that ISS values, and thus, the overall severity of injuries did not change significantly in the different units. Only in NCU the ISS mean rose slightly (ISS 1.55) which can be explained by an individual outlier (Figure 1).

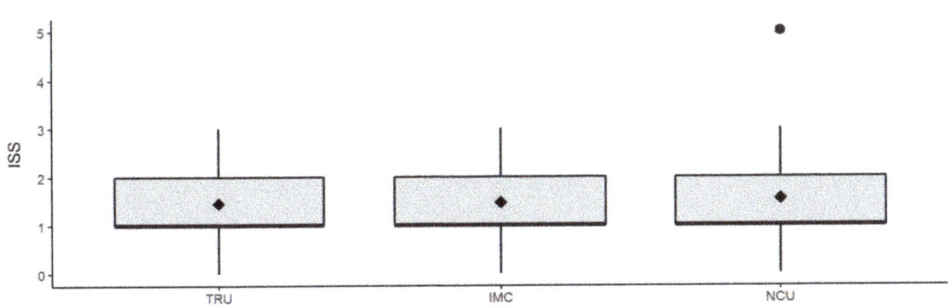

Figure 1. Distribution of ISS in each unit (TRU, IMC, NCU). Rhombuses represent the arithmetic mean. Medians are located at the bottom of the boxes (ISS = 1). The dot indicates outliers. TRU = Trauma Resuscitation Unit; IMC = Intermediate Care Unit; NCU = Normal Care Unit.

3.3. *New Complaints, New Diagnoses and AIS/ISS Changes*

A total of 21 patients (18.75%) after completion of TRU treatment, complained about new symptoms, such as pain, abnormal sensations, and in one case, visual disturbances, during the course of their inpatient stay. Nine of these patients reported new symptoms in the IMC, while 10 only reported new symptoms in the NCU. Two of these patients reported new complaints on both IMC and NCU (Table 6). A new diagnosis was made in 9/112 patients (8.04%) that led to an AIS change. Eight of these patients (7.14%) had an AIS change, as well as an ISS change. In one patient, the MAIS rose from 1 to 2 (0.89%), and thus, the ISS to 5. In all of the rest patients the MAIS remained at 1 and ISS ≤ 3.

A new diagnosis was made in IMC in 2/9 patients (22.2%) and in the other seven (77.8%) patients in the NCU.

Table 6. Frequencies of patients with new symptoms.

	N	% of N = 112
Only IMC *	9	8.036
Only NCU **	10	8.93
Both	2	1.78
Total	21	18.75

* IMC = Intermediate Care; ** NCU = Normal Care Unit; N = Total sample size; n = Group sample size.

Evaluation of the changes in AIS and ISS values during the course of inpatient stay showed no significant change in AIS values for any region of the body (AIS HN: $p = 0.368$; AIS F: $p = 0.223$; AIS C: $p = 0.368$; AIS AbP: $p = 0.368$; AIS ExP $p = 0.135$; AIS E: $p = 0.223$) and also no significant ISS increase ($p = 0.368$) (Table 7). Data analysis showed that the risk difference for an AIS increase by 1 in the extremities during an inpatient stay in NCU was 1.79% ($p = 0.135$). Table 7 shows the distribution of AIS ≥ 1 throughout the different units, as well as the probability of change (RD = Risk Difference).

Table 7. Comparison of patients' frequencies with AIS and ISS ≥1 throughout stations.

				Number of N = 112 with Score > 0			Rate in % with Score > 0			RD in %	
Score	Q	df	p **	TRU	IMC	NCU	TRU	IMC	NCU	TRU to IMC	IMC to NCU
ISS *	2	2	0.368	0	0	1	0.00	0.00	0.89	0.00	0.89
AIS HN	2	2	0.368	51	51	52	45.54	45.54	46.43	0.00	0.89
AIS F	3	2	0.223	14	15	16	12.50	13.39	14.29	0.89	0.89
AIS C	2	2	0.368	1	1	2	0.89	0.89	1.79	0.00	0.89
AIS AbP	2	2	0.368	0	0	1	0.00	0.00	0.89	0.00	0.89
AIS ExP	4	2	0.135	1	1	3	0.89	0.89	2.68	0.00	1.79
AIS E	3	2	0.223	96	97	98	85.71	86,61	87.50	0.89	0.89

* Binary coded (≤3 as 0 and >3 as 1); Q = Test value; df = Degrees of freedom; ** $p = p$ value (Level of Significance = 0.05); RD = Risk difference (proportion in % at which the score changes); TRU = Trauma Resuscitation Unit; IMC = Intermediate Care Unit; NCU = Normal Care Unit; ISS = Injury severity score; AIS = Abbreviate injury scale; HN = Head or Neck; F = Face; C = Chest; Abp = Abdominal or pelvic contents; Exp = Extremities or pelvic girdle; E = External.

3.4. TRU Computed Tomography (CT) and AIS Change

No correlation was found between CT diagnostics performed in the TRU and change in AIS during inpatient's hospitalization ($p = 0.542$). Each of the nine patients, who had an AIS change after completion of TRU treatment, had received a CT diagnostic in the TRU. Eight of them (88.9%) received a trauma CT (head and body-trunk), and one patient only received a CT head. Of all patients who received a CT body trunk (80/112), eight (10%) had an AIS change despite the extensive TRU CT diagnostics. Only head CT diagnostic was performed in the TRU in 25/112 patients and only one of them, received during the hospitalization in the NCU X-rays of the shoulder, which led to an AIS change. The head CT examination that was carried out in the TRU had no influence on this change (Table 8).

Table 8. Correlation between received diagnostic computed tomography (CT) and AIS change.

		AIS Alteration		Total
		No	Yes	
No CT	Number	7	0	7
	Expected number	6.4	0.6	7.0
	% within the category	100.0%	0.0%	100.0%
Only CT body-trunk	Number	4	0	4
	Expected number	3.7	0.3	4.0
	% within the category	100.0%	0.0%	100.0%
Only CT head	Number	24	1	25
	Expected number	23.0	2.0	25.0
	% within the category	96.0%	4.0%	100.0%
CT head and body-trunk	Number	68	8	76
	Expected number	69.9	6.1	76.0
	% within the category	89.5%	10.5%	100.0%
Total	Number	103	9	112
	Expected number	103.0	9.0	112.0
	% within the category	92.0%	8.0%	100.0%
Alteration	Chi^2	df	p *	
AIS	2.15	3	0.542	

Chi^2 = Test Value; df = Degrees of freedom; * p = p value (Level of Significance = 0.05); CT = Computed tomography; AIS = Abbreviated Injury Scale.

3.5. Total Length of Stay (LOS) and Factors Influencing the Length of Stay

The average total LOS (TRU+IMC+NCU) was 53.57 h with a standard deviation of 42.23 h. Most hospitalization time was spent on the NCU, while the time spent on the IMC only accounted for 33.28% of total LOS. As expected, the length of stay at the TRU was short—with an average total of 1.08h (Table 9).

Table 9. The average length of stay (LOS).

	Hours (%)
Overall LOS	53.57 (SD = 42.23; Median = 41.48)
NCU	34.65 (64.68%)
IMC	17.83 (33.28%)
TRU	1.08 (2.01%)
	Number (%)
Patients who stayed >100 h	6 (5.35%)
Patients who stayed >200 h	4 (3.57%)

LOS = Length of stay; NCU = Normal Care Unit; IMC = Intermediate Care Unit; TRU = Trauma Resuscitation Unit; SD = Standard Deviation.

It was also shown, that the average length of stay of patients, who had reported new symptoms without any change in AIS was 65%, and of those who had changes in AIS was 85% of the length of stay of patients who had neither reported new symptoms nor had changes in AIS ($p = 0.350$ and $p = 0.770$) (Table 10, Figure 2).

Table 10. Regression analysis results for length of stay.

Variable	B	SE	t	p *	exp(B)
(Intercept)	2.81	0.30	9.36	<0.001	16.59
Progress (Reference: No change)					
New symptoms	−0.43	0.46	−0.94	0.350	0.65
AIS change	−0.16	0.55	−0.29	0.770	0.85
Age (years)	0.01	0.01	1.87	0.064	1.01
Gender (Reference: male)					
Female	−0.18	0.25	−0.71	0.481	0.84
Extended diagnostics (Reference: none)					
Once	1.28	0.56	2.31	0.023	3.61

* $p = 0.05$; B = Regression coefficient; SE = Standard error; t = Test value; * $p = p$ value (Level of Significance = 0.05); exp(B) = Relative change.

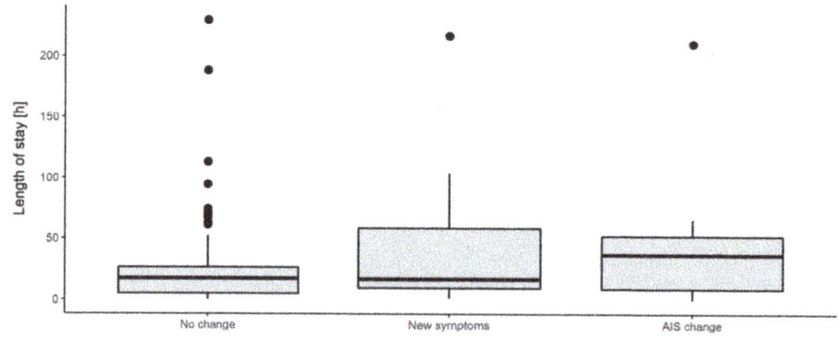

Figure 2. Distribution of length of stay (LOS) in correlation to the variables "No change", "New symptoms", and "AIS Change". Dots represent outliers.

The average total length of stay of female patients was shorter compared to male patients ($p = 0.481$).

The data further showed that for every one year increase in age, there was an increase in the length of stay by a factor of 1.01 ($p = 0.064$) (Figure 3). The necessity of extended diagnostics in the course of inpatients' stay led to a statistically significant increase of the total length of stay by a factor of 3.61 ($p = 0.023$).

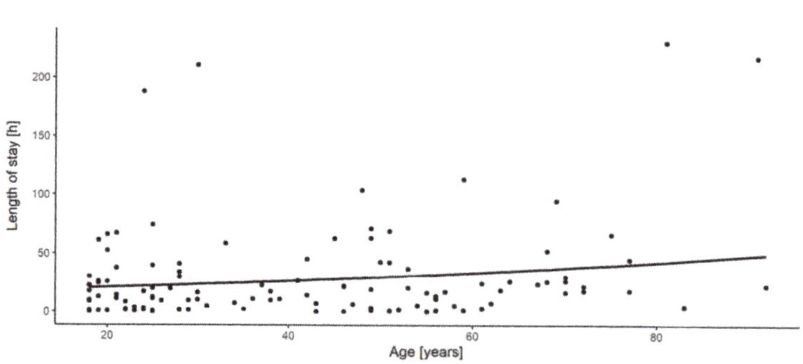

Figure 3. Correlation between length of stay and age of patients. The solid line (regression line) represents the correlation according to the transformed regression coefficient (Table 10).

4. Discussion

The aim of this study was to examine whether monitoring of patients with only minor injuries or no injuries at all after completion of TRU treatment is beneficial in order to identify new relevant injuries during hospitalization. The authors retrospectively analyzed the data of 573 patients that were admitted in the TRU. One hundred and twelve of them had ISS ≤ 3 (MAIS ≤ 1) and were included in the study. This corresponds to 19.55% of all primary TRU patients of Level I trauma center in Giessen, Germany, in the examination period 2019 (April-November). In comparison to the annual report of the Trauma-Register DGU® in 2019, the overall proportion of patients, who were only slightly injured or not injured at all was 13%. Since the slightly injured patients are only being recorded in the Trauma-Register without any further analysis of their data, it can be assumed that most of these patients do not enter the register, and therefore, they are not fully reflected in the statistics [17,18]. Marzi showed an increase of patient admission to TRU of 70 % from 2012 to 2016, although the number of patients with an ISS ≥ 16 or a MAIS ≥ 3 is slightly constant over the years [4]. We made a similar observation in our center and saw this as a reason for the high number of patients with MAIS ≤ 1.

The mean age of these study population was 41 ± 19 years in accordance with the literature (30–50 years). The large fluctuations in mean age can be explained by the differences in the inclusion and exclusion criteria between the various studies [8,11,19]. More specifically in the study of Lansink et al. in 2004 mean age was 30 years, but patients with known coronary artery disease, anticoagulant medication, blood clotting disorder and patients admitted in the ICU were excluded from the study [11]. As these criteria mostly apply to older patients, mean age was therefore smaller. The proportion of male participants in the present study was 62%, which is comparable to other study populations (66–70%) [8,10,11,18–20].

Considering our demographic data, the mechanisms of accidents in this study are comparable with the ones reported in previous studies [8,10,11,19], with the exception of Salim et al., who reported a slightly higher incidence of pedestrian struck-accidents (25.9%) [20].

The severity of the injury was assessed using the internationally recognized Abbreviated Injury Scale (AIS), which was first introduced in 1969. The AIS-Codebook, first published in 1979, has been since then continuously revised. The AIS© 2005 Update 2008 was used for this study [14,21].

The AIS is the basis for calculating the Injury Severity Score (ISS) of a multiply injured patient; a scoring system which was first described in 1974 by Baker et al. [22,23]. In addition to the AIS and ISS, the Maximum Abbreviated Injury Scale (MAIS) was also determined, which gives the maximum AIS value of each patient and estimates the severity of an injury [17].

We observed that after completion of TRU diagnostics, mean AIS for all body regions and ISS were 1.45 and as none of our trauma patients had MAIS > 1 they all belonged to the category of slightly injured patients [14,22–24].

It was shown that AIS, ISS and MAIS did not change significantly during an inpatient hospital stay. Only in one case, AIS increased to 2 and ISS to 5, which led according to Baker et al. (1976) to an insignificant increase in mortality [23]. This delayed diagnosed injury was a sternal fracture, which was already demonstrated in the initial TRU imaging, but was not documented among the diagnoses in the electronic patient's file.

There are only a few studies with a comparable population as this present study, as most clinical studies focus on missed injuries in severely injured patients. In our study, ISS increased by 6.9% during inpatient stay, while AIS increased by 6.2%. New diagnosis in the present study was made in 9/112 patients (8%). Four of the newly diagnosed injuries were classified as relevant but did not lead to a change of further treatment regimen. Zamboni et al. reported 7.6% newly diagnosed injuries in the course of inpatient stay, whereby at this study, the diagnoses were only mentioned without a calculation of AIS or ISS [25]. Moreover, Stephan et al. reported new diagnoses in 35/630 patients (5.56%) during a 23-h patient surveillance period, of which 14 (2.22%) were relevant [8].

Lansink et al. evaluated the necessity of clinical observation of high-energy trauma patients without significant injury. In this study, the patients' ISS was higher than ours (1.37–3.09), and it did not increase during inpatients' hospitalization. The authors attributed their findings, to the high-quality examination in the TRU based on ATLS guidelines [11]. The authors of the present study also believe that the reason for not having many new diagnosed (previously overlooked) injuries in the course of inpatients' stay, is the application of the standardized ATLS-based TRU treatment in Giessen, whereby the comparison between the two studies, due to the extensive exclusion criteria in Lansink et al. study, is restricted [11].

However, it is known, that there is a significant association between the severity of injury and occurrence of overlooked injuries, as in slightly injured patients, who were admitted in the TRU only a few injuries were subsequently detected [26]. In the current study, a large number of delayed diagnoses was not expected. However, relative studies report a widespread of incidence (1.3–39%) of delayed diagnosed injuries, and this can be attributed to the fact that each study has a different design, as well as different definitions for an overlooked injury. Pfeifer et al. 2008 reported that 15–22.3% of the subsequently diagnosed injuries were classified as clinical significant [26]. Regarding our discovered diagnoses we showed that in our study population, 44.44% of them were in extremities. This is in line with relative studies from the literature, in which the proportion of the overlooked extremity injuries is between 33–60% [27–29].

In addition, our finding that 3.57% of the patients had no injuries both in the TRU and in their further hospitalization is consistent with relative German literature [5].

Furthermore, our data showed that AIS and ISS, regardless of TRU diagnostics, did not significantly increase in the course of inpatient stay. It was only after the development of multislice CT that a whole-body CT was possible, and this was first described as a diagnostic tool for seriously injured patients in 1997 [30–32]. Since then, performing a whole-body computed tomography (CT) in the seriously injured patients in the TRU is recommended according to the German guidelines as "Grade of Recommendation A", as among others, it increases the probability of survival of the severely injured patients [3,33–35] While the retrospective data in the literature appear to be clear considering the seriously injured patients, there are no recommendations regarding the indication for performing a whole-body CT or if necessary, a focused CT. Only the parameters "disturbed vital signs", a "relevant mechanism of injury" and the presence of "at least two injured regions" can be used as "Grade of Recommendation B" [3,36,37].

An extensive imaging diagnostic alone does not appear to be required in order to discharge patients after TRU treatment or transferring them to the NCU. Kendall et al. defined some criteria for low risk of overlooking abdominal injuries after blunt abdominal trauma, which would allow the patient to be discharged from the emergency department (ED) without having a CT scan of the abdomen. The authors showed a low risk in the absence of intoxication, prehospital or ED settled hypotension, tachycardia in the ED, abdominal pain or tension, gross hematuria and distracting injury [10]. Similar results demonstrated Nagy et al. and Livingston et al. regarding head trauma patients with a Glasgow Coma Score (GCS) 15 and a negative head CT result. Both authors considered, in this case, an inpatient admission for further monitoring to be unjustified [38,39].

For the isolated high-energy trauma, Lansink et al. suggested that there is no evidence for inpatient monitoring if an ATLS-based TRU treatment has been previously carried out. However, many groups of patients were excluded from this study [11]. This observation by Lansink et al. is also in accordance with our results for all the TRU patients without a significant injury after completion of TRU diagnostics. The insignificant increase ($p = 0.368$) in the ISS, which is presented in the current study is a further indication that the ATLS-based TRU management increases the quality of treatment.

Another reason for a large number of slightly injured patients is the increasing use of the TRU in the last years leading to an increase in overtriage, and thus, to the admission of uninjured or slightly injured patients, whereby an overtriage of 25–35% appears to be necessary [4,40,41]. The high number of TRU activations after a specific mechanism of accident also play a decisive role here [5].

We demonstrated that there were no relevant changes in the AIS and ISS in the course of inpatient stay, regardless of how long the patient was hospitalized for. The average total length of stay in the current study was 2.23 days, which coincides with Stefan et al., who reported a total length of stay of three days (+/−2 days) [8]. The results of the present study were also comparable with other relative studies, in which patients were monitored between 8 and >24 h in an NCU, a clinical decision unit and an IMC [8–11,19].

5. Conclusions

The results of the present study lead to the conclusion that an individualized extended diagnostics using focused CT or whole-body CT combined with a specialized TRU medical team and an ATLS-based TRU treatment in a Level I trauma center is a good algorithm in order not to overlook relevant injuries in the TRU. Hence, an inpatient monitoring in the IMC for patients with an AIS ≤ 1 or an ISS ≤ 3 after completion of the TRU treatment is unnecessary.

In conclusion, our results show that patients who were diagnosed with no injuries or only minimal injuries in the TRU with an ISS ≤ 3 do not need to be monitored in the IMC, regardless of whether they have received in the TRU a trauma CT or only a basic diagnostic procedure according to the ATLS-standards, as clinical examination, extended focused assessment with sonography in trauma (eFAST) and X-rays.

The authors, therefore, suggest that the use of AIS/ISS, which is until now only used retrospectively, could be a good tool for deciding whether the monitoring of a slightly injured patient is necessary, or whether the patient after receiving, for example, a scheduled appointment could be actually discharged. Since monitoring in the IMC requires a highly qualified medical and nursing staff, the latest procedure would relieve the clinical-spatial and personnel-resources and the healthcare system. The aim should be saving resources in order to be able to maintain sufficient TRU and monitoring capacities in the future, which can lead to life-saving treatment.

6. Patents

There are no patents resulting from the work reported in this manuscript.

Author Contributions: Conceptualization, C.H., M.H., M.L.; Methodology, M.H., M.L.; Validation, C.H., M.H.; Formal analysis, M.H., M.L.; Investigation, M.H., M.L., G.S., L.A.; Data curation, M.L., F.B.; Writing—original draft preparation, M.H., M.L., C.B.; Writing—review and editing, C.H., G.S., C.B., F.B.; Visualization, M.L.; Supervision, C.H., M.H.; Project administration, M.H.; All authors have read and agreed to the published version of the manuscript.

Funding: This research received no external funding.

Conflicts of Interest: The authors declare no conflicts of interest.

References

1. Lendemans, S.; Ruchholtz, S. S3-leitlinie polytrauma/schwerverletzten-Behandlung: Schockraumversorgung. *Unfallchirurg* **2012**, *115*, 14–21. [CrossRef]
2. Gesellschaft für Unfallchirurgie, D. Weißbuch Schwerverletztenversorgung, 3. Erweiterte Auflage. Available online: https://www.dgu-online.de/fileadmin/published_content/5.Qualitaet_und_Sicherheit/PDF/2019_DGU_Weissbuch_Schwerverletztenversorgung_Vorabdruck.pdf (accessed on 11 June 2020).
3. Arbeitsgemeinschaft der Wissenschaftlichen Medizinischen Fachgesellschaften: Leitlinie "Polytrauma/Schwerverletzten-Behandlung". Available online: www.awmf.org/leitlinien/detail/ll/012--019.html (accessed on 11 June 2020).
4. Marzi, I.; Lustenberger, T.; Störmann, P.; Mörs, K.; Wagner, N.; Wutzler, S. Increasing overhead ressources of the trauma room. *Unfallchirurg* **2019**, *122*, 53–58. [CrossRef] [PubMed]
5. Schweigkofler, U.; Sauter, M.; Wincheringer, D.; Barzen, S.; Hoffmann, R. Emergency room activation due to trauma mechanism. *Unfallchirurg* **2020**, *123*, 386–394. [CrossRef] [PubMed]
6. Williams, M.J.; Lockey, A.S.; Culshaw, M.C. Improved trauma management with advanced trauma life support (ATLS) training. *Emerg. Med. J.* **1997**, *14*, 81–83. [CrossRef]

7. Sturm, J.A.; Lackner, C.K.; Bouillon, B.; Seekamp, A.; Mutschler, W.E. "Advanced Trauma Life Support ®" (ATLS ®) und "Systematic Prehospital Life Support ®" (SPLS ®). *Unfallchirurg* **2002**, *105*, 1027–1032. [CrossRef] [PubMed]
8. Stephan, P.J.; McCarley, C.M.; O'Keefe, G.E.; Minei, J.P. 23-Hour Observation Solely for Identification of Missed Injuries After Trauma: Is It Justified? *J. Trauma* **2002**, *53*, 895–900. [CrossRef] [PubMed]
9. Livingston, D.H.; Lavery, R.F.; Passannante, M.R.; Skurnick, J.H.; Fabian, T.C.; Fry, D.E.; Malangoni, M.A. Admission or observation is not necessary after a negative abdominal computed tomographic scan in patients with suspected blunt abdominal trauma: Results of a prospective, multi-institutional trial. *J. Trauma Inj. Infect. Crit. Care* **1998**, *44*, 273–282. [CrossRef]
10. Kendall, J.L.; Kestler, A.M.; Whitaker, K.T.; Adkisson, M.M.; Haukoos, J.S. Blunt abdominal trauma Patients are at very low risk for intra-abdominal injury after emergency department observation. *West. J. Emerg. Med.* **2011**, *12*, 496–504. [CrossRef]
11. Lansink, K.W.W.; Cornejo, C.J.; Boeije, T.; Kok, M.F.; Jurkovich, G.J.; Ponsen, K.J. Evaluation of the necessity of clinical ohservation of high-energy trauma patients without significant injury after standardized emergency room stabilization. *J. Trauma Inj. Infect. Crit. Care* **2004**, *57*, 1256–1259. [CrossRef]
12. Crenshaw, L.A.; Lindsell, C.J.; Storrow, A.B.; Lyons, M.S. An evaluation of emergency physician selection of observation unit patients. *Am. J. Emerg. Med.* **2006**, *24*, 271–279. [CrossRef]
13. Sektion Intensiv- & Notfallmedizin, S. der D.G. für U. e. V.A.– A. der U.G. *Jahresbericht 2019 Sektion Notfall- & Intensivmedizin & Schwerverletztenversorgung der Deutschen Gesellschaft für Unfallchirurgie e.V. AUC-Akademie der Unfallchirurgie GmbH*, 2019.
14. Haasper, C.; Junge, M.; Ernstberger, A.; Brehme, H.; Hannawald, L.; Langer, C.; Nehmzow, J.; Otte, D.; Sander, U.; Krettek, C.; et al. Die Abbreviated Injury Scale (AIS): Potenzial und probleme bei der anwendung. *Unfallchirurg* **2010**, *113*, 366–372. [CrossRef] [PubMed]
15. Garthe, E.; States, J.D.; Mango, N.K. Abbreviated injury scale unification: The case for a unified injury system for global use. *J. Trauma Inj. Infect. Crit. Care* **1999**, *47*, 309–323. [CrossRef] [PubMed]
16. R Core Team. *R: A Language and Environment for Statistical Computing*; R Core Team: Vienna, Austria, 2020.
17. Lefering, R.; Nienaber, U.; Paffrath, T. Was ist ein Schwerverletzter? Differenzierte Betrachtung der Fallschwere eines Traumapatienten. *Unfallchirurg* **2017**, *120*, 898–901. [CrossRef]
18. Lefering, R.; Höfer, C. Annual Report 2019 TraumaRegister DGU, Committee on Emergency Medicine, Intensive Care and Trauma Management of the German Trauma Society (DGU), AUC - Academy for Trauma Surgery, 2019, 1–68. Available online: http://www.traumaregister-dgu.de/fileadmin/user_upload/traumaregister-dgu.de/docs/Downloads/Annual_report_2019.pdf (accessed on 11 June 2020).
19. Cowell, V.L.; Ciraulo, D.; Gabram, S.; Lawrence, D.; Cortes, V.; Edwards, T.; Jacobs, L. Trauma 24-h observation critical path. *J. Trauma Inj. Infect. Crit. Care* **1998**, *45*, 147–150. [CrossRef] [PubMed]
20. Salim, A.; Sangthong, B.; Martin, M.; Brown, C.; Plurad, D.; Demetriades, D. Whole Body Imaging in Blunt Multisystem Trauma Patients Without Obvious Signs of Injury. *Arch. Surg.* **2015**, *141*. [CrossRef] [PubMed]
21. AAAM International Injury Scaling Committee (IISC) Abbreviated Injury Scale, Association for the Advancement of Automotive Medicine. Available online: https://www.aaam.org/abbreviated-injury-scale-ais/ (accessed on 10 June 2020).
22. Baker, S.P.; O'Neill, B.; Haddon, W.; Long, W.B. The injury severity score: A method for describing patients with multiple injuries and evaluating emergency care. *J. Trauma* **1974**, *14*, 187–196. [CrossRef] [PubMed]
23. Baker, S.P.; O'Neill, B. The injury severity score: An update. *J. Trauma Inj. Infect. Crit. Care* **1976**, *16*, 882–885. [CrossRef]
24. Greenspan, L.; McLellan, B.A.; Greig, H. Abbreviated injury scale and injury severity score: A scoring chart. *J. Trauma Inj. Infect. Crit. Care* **1985**, *25*, 60–64. [CrossRef]
25. Zamboni, C.; Yonamine, A.M.; Faria, C.E.N.; Filho, M.A.M.; Christian, R.W.; Mercadante, M.T. Tertiary survey in trauma patients: Avoiding neglected injuries. *Injury* **2014**, *45*, S14–S17. [CrossRef]
26. Pfeifer, R.; Pape, H.-C. Missed injuries in trauma patients: A literature review. *Patient Saf. Surg.* **2008**, *2*. [CrossRef]
27. Kalemoglu, M.; Demirbas, S.; Akin, M.L.; Yildirim, I.; Kurt, Y.; Uluutku, H.; Yıldız, M. Missed Injuries in Military Patients with Major Trauma: Original Study. *Mil. Med.* **2006**, *171*, 598–602. [CrossRef] [PubMed]
28. Buduhan, G.; McRitchie, D.I. Missed injuries in patients with multiple trauma. *J. Trauma Inj. Infect. Crit. Care* **2000**, *49*, 600–605. [CrossRef] [PubMed]

29. Pehle, B.; Kuehne, C.A.; Block, J.; Waydhas, C.; Taeger, G.; Nast-Kolb, D.; Ruchholtz, S. Die bedeutung von verzögert diagnostizierten läsionen bei polytraumatisierten. Eine studie an 1187 schockraumpatienten. *Unfallchirurg* **2006**, *109*, 964–974. [CrossRef] [PubMed]
30. Löw, R.; Düber, C.; Schweden, F.; Lehmann, L.; Blum, J.; Thelen, M. Ganzkorper-Spiral-CT zur Primardiagnostik polytraumatisierter Patienten unter Notfallbedingungen. *RoFo Fortschr. auf dem Geb. der Rontgenstrahlen und der Neuen Bildgeb. Verfahr.* **1997**, *166*, 382–388. [CrossRef] [PubMed]
31. Klingenbeck-Regn, K.; Schaller, S.; Flohr, T.; Ohnesorge, B.; Kopp, A.F.; Baum, U. Subsecond multi-slice computed tomography: Basics and applications. *Eur. J. Radiol.* **1999**, *31*, 110–124. [CrossRef]
32. Fox, S.H.; Tanenbaum, L.N.; Ackelsberg, S.; He, H.D.; Hsieh, J.; Hu, H. Future directions in CT technology. *Neuroimaging Clin. N. Am.* **1998**, *8*, 497–513.
33. Huber-Wagner, S.; Biberthaler, P.; Häberle, S.; Wierer, M.; Dobritz, M.; Rummeny, E.; van Griensven, M.; Kanz, K.G.; Lefering, R. Whole-Body CT in Haemodynamically Unstable Severely Injured Patients—A Retrospective, Multicentre Study. *PLoS ONE* **2013**, *8*, e68880. [CrossRef]
34. Huber-Wagner, S.; Lefering, R.; Qvick, L.M.; Körner, M.; Kay, M.V.; Pfeifer, K.J.; Reiser, M.; Mutschler, W.; Kanz, K.G. Effect of whole-body CT during trauma resuscitation on survival: A retrospective, multicentre study. *Lancet* **2009**, *373*, 1455–1461. [CrossRef]
35. Kanz, K.-G.; Körner, M.; Linsenmaier, U.; Kay, M.V.; Huber-Wagner, S.M.; Kreimeier, U.; Pfeifer, K.-J.; Reiser, M.; Mutschler, W. Prioritätenorientiertes Schockraummanagement unter Integration des Mehrschichtspiralcomputertomographen. *Unfallchirurg* **2004**, *107*, 937–944. [CrossRef]
36. Davies, R.M.; Scrimshire, A.B.; Sweetman, L.; Anderton, M.J.; Holt, E.M. A decision tool for whole-body CT in major trauma that safely reduces unnecessary scanning and associated radiation risks: An initial exploratory analysis. *Injury* **2016**, *47*, 43–49. [CrossRef]
37. Hsiao, K.H.; Dinh, M.M.; Mcnamara, K.P.; Bein, K.J.; Roncal, S.; Saade, C.; Waugh, R.C.; Chi, K.F. Whole-body computed tomography in the initial assessment of trauma patients: Is there optimal criteria for patient selection? *EMA Emerg. Med. Australas.* **2013**, *25*, 182–191. [CrossRef] [PubMed]
38. Nagy, K.K.; Joseph, K.T.; Krosner, S.M.; Roberts, R.R.; Leslie, C.L.; Dufty, K.; Smith, R.F.; Barrett, J. The utility of head computed tomography after minimal head injury. *J. Trauma Inj. Infect. Crit. Care* **1999**, *46*, 268–270. [CrossRef] [PubMed]
39. Livingston, D.H.; Lavery, R.F.; Passannante, M.R.; Skurnick, J.H.; Baker, S.; Fabian, T.C.; Fry, D.E.; Malangoni, M.A. Emergency department discharge of patients with a negative cranial computed tomography scan after minimal head injury. *Ann. Surg.* **2000**, *232*, 126–132. [CrossRef] [PubMed]
40. Dehli, T.; Fredriksen, K.; Osbakk, S.A.; Bartnes, K. Evaluation of a university hospital trauma team activation protocol. *Scand. J. Trauma. Resusc. Emerg. Med.* **2011**, *19*, 18. [CrossRef] [PubMed]
41. Follin, A.; Jacqmin, S.; Chhor, V.; Bellenfant, F.; Robin, S.; Guinvarc'H, A.; Thomas, F.; Loeb, T.; Mantz, J.; Pirracchio, R. Tree-based algorithm for prehospital triage of polytrauma patients. *Injury* **2016**, *47*, 1555–1561. [CrossRef] [PubMed]

Journal of
Clinical Medicine

MDPI

Article

Isolated Pubic Ramus Fractures Are Serious Adverse Events for Elderly Persons: An Observational Study on 138 Patients with Fragility Fractures of the Pelvis Type I (FFP Type I)

Pol Maria Rommens [1,*], Johannes Christof Hopf [1], Michiel Herteleer [1], Benjamin Devlieger [1], Alexander Hofmann [2] and Daniel Wagner [1]

1 Department of Orthopedics and Traumatology, University Medical Center Mainz, Langenbeckstrasse 1, 55131 Mainz, Germany; johannes.hopf@unimedizin-mainz.de (J.C.H.); michiel.herteleer@unimedizin-mainz.de (M.H.); benjamin.devlieger@unimedizin-mainz.de (B.D.); daniel.wagner@unimedizin-mainz.de (D.W.)

2 Department of Orthopedics and Traumatology, Westpfalz Klinikum Kaiserslautern, Hellmut-Hartert Straße 1, 67655 Kaiserslautern, Germany; Hofmann.trauma-surgery@gmx.net

* Correspondence: pol.rommens@unimedizin-mainz.de; Tel.: +49-6131-177292

Received: 17 June 2020; Accepted: 29 July 2020; Published: 3 August 2020

Abstract: Background: Fractures of the pubic ramus without involvement of the posterior pelvic ring represent a minority of fragility fractures of the pelvis (FFP). The natural history of patients suffering this FFP Type I has not been described so far. Material and methods: All patients, who were admitted with isolated pubic ramus fractures between 2007 and mid-2018, have been reviewed. Epidemiologic data, comorbidities, in-hospital complications, and one-year mortality were recorded. Of all surviving patients, living condition before the fracture and at follow-up was noted. Mobility was scored with the Parker Mobility Score, quality of life with the European Quality of Life 5 Dimensions 3 Level (EQ-5D-3L), subjective sensation of pain with the Numeric Rating Scale (NRS). Results: A consecutive series of 138 patients was included in the study. There were 117 women (84.8%) and 21 men (15.2%). Mean age was 80.6 years (SD 8.6 years). 89.1% of patients presented with comorbidities, 81.2% of them had cardiovascular diseases. Five patients (4%) died during hospital-stay. Median in-hospital stay was eight days (2–45 days). There were in-hospital complications in 16.5%, urinary tract infections, and pneumonia being the most frequent. One-year mortality was 16.7%. Reference values for the normal population of the same age are 5.9% for men and 4.0% for women. One-year mortality rate was 22.2% in the patient group of 80 years or above and 8.8% in the patient group below the age of 80. The rate of surviving patients living at home with or without assistance dropped from 80.5% to 65.3%. The median EQ-5D-Index Value was 0.62 (0.04–1; IQR 0.5–0.78). Reference value for the normal population is 0.78. Average PMS was 4 and NRS 3. Within a two-year period, additional fragility fractures occurred in 21.2% and antiresorptive medication was taken by only 45.2% of patients. Conclusion. Pubic ramus fractures without involvement of the posterior pelvis (FFP Type I) are serious adverse events for elderly persons. During follow-up, there is an excess mortality, a loss of independence, a restricted mobility, and a decreased quality of life. Pubic ramus fractures are indicators for the need to optimize the patient's general condition.

Keywords: pubic ramus fractures; fragility fractures of the pelvis; mortality; living condition; mobility; quality of life

1. Introduction

Pubic ramus fractures are part of complex pelvic injuries in high-energy trauma [1]. They also occur in isolation or in combination with fractures of the posterior pelvis due to low-energy trauma. In communities with a high life expectancy, the incidence of fragility fractures of the pelvis (FFP) surpasses that of high-energy pelvic trauma [2,3]. Of all FFP, isolated pubic rami fractures represent only one fifth [4]. They are described as FFP Type I in the classification of Rommens and Hofmann [4]. A combination of fractures of the pubic ramus with fractures of the posterior pelvic ring is present in more than 80% of FFP. These fracture combinations are described as FFP Types II, III, or IV in the same classification [4]. Pubic ramus fractures are usually diagnosed on a conventional pelvic radiograph, which is the first diagnostic step after a domestic fall with pain in the pelvic region. On this radiograph, crush zones and fissures or non-displaced fractures in the sacrum may be overlooked. The real extent of the pelvic injury is then underestimated. With a pelvic CT, fractures and dislocations of the posterior pelvis can be analyzed in more detail [5]. Consequently, a pelvic CT is indispensable for complete evaluation of an FFP. Multiple publications deal with epidemiology, treatment, and outcome of elderly patients with pubic ramus fractures [6–11]. None of them differentiates between isolated pubic ramus fractures and pubic ramus fractures in combination with posterior pelvis fractures. In this retrospective analysis, we first analyzed the pelvic CT-images of all patients admitted with FFP in an 11.5-year period. We then looked at quality of life, mobility, level of independence, and mortality of patients with FFP Type I (isolated pubic ramus fractures) under exclusion of the FFP Types II, III, and IV. We compared our data with available data on the level of independence of the same patients before the fall and with data on quality of life and mortality of a representative group in the normal population.

2. Patients and Methods

We retrospectively reviewed the medical charts and radiological data (pelvic overviews and pelvic CT-images) of all patients with an FFP, who presented at the Department of Orthopedics and Traumatology of the University Medical Center Mainz, Germany between 1 January 2007 and 30 June 2018 (11.5-years period). We identified 519 patients with this diagnosis. We analyzed the pelvic CT-data of these patients to identify involvement of the posterior pelvic ring and classified all FFP according to the classification of Rommens and Hofmann [4]. We then excluded FFP with a non-displaced or displaced fracture of the posterior pelvic ring (FFP Type II (n = 251), Type III, and Type IV (n = 130)). We also excluded patients with acetabular fractures, patients with pelvic fractures due to high-energy trauma and patients with pelvic fractures due to malignancies. In addition, 138 of 519 (26.6%) of FFP were classified as FFP Type I. A flowchart of selected and excluded patients is presented in Figure 1. They build the patient cohort for this study.

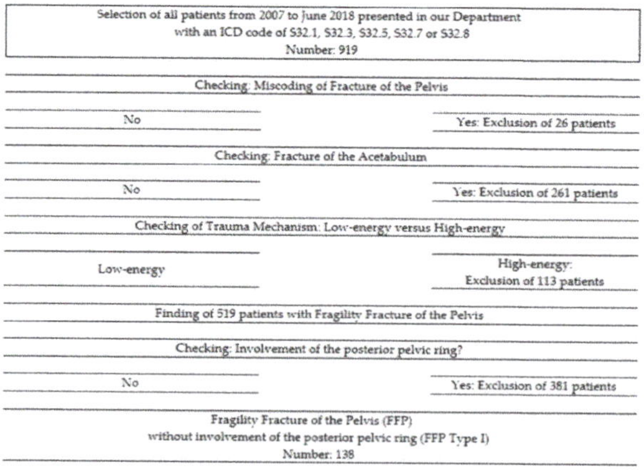

Figure 1. Flowchart of selected and excluded patients.

The following epidemiologic data of these 138 patients were collected: age, sex, trauma mechanism, conservative or operative treatment, duration of hospital stay, in-hospital complications and destination at discharge from hospital. The patient's records were searched for the physical status just before admission, current medication and for the following comorbidities at the time of first presentation: cardiovascular disease, pulmonary disease, osteoporosis, malignancies, diabetes mellitus, rheumatoid arthritis, and dementia. Images were assessed for existing hip replacement or lumbar spine fusion. In-hospital medical complications included cardiovascular events, pneumonia, symptomatic deep venous thrombosis, symptomatic pulmonary embolism, symptomatic urinary tract infection, and skin ulcer.

Patients or their relatives were contacted by phone asking to answer several questionnaires. If this was not possible, their general practitioner or the bureau of vital statistics was contacted to ask about vital status. Quality of life was assessed by a European Quality of Life five dimensions—three level (EQ-5D-3L) questionnaire, and scores range from 0 to 1.0 (higher scores indicating better quality of life) [12–14]. Subjective sensation of pain was rated with the numeric rating scale (NRS), with scores from 0 to 10 (higher scores indicating heavier pain) [15]. The actual place of living and mobility status was asked, the mobility further specified by Parker Mobility Score (PMS), ranging from 0 to 9, higher scores equal to better mobility [16]. Patients were asked for the occurrence of subsequent fragility fractures.

Mean values with standard deviation (SD) were given in case of normal distribution, median values with min and max together with 25–75 inter quartal ranges (IQR) in case of non-normal distribution. Continuous data were compared using the unpaired Mann–Whitney U test for non-normally distributed data. Linear regression was tested with Spearman Rho. The chi-square test was used to compare nominal groups. A p-value of ≤ 0.05 was considered statistically significant. Statistical analysis was performed using SPSS software (IBM SPSS Statistics for Windows, Version 23.0; IBM Corp, Armonk, NY, USA).

3. Results

3.1. Baseline Characteristics

In addition, 138 patients with fragility fractures of the anterior pelvic ring only (FFP Type I) were identified. There were 130 patients with unilateral pubic rami fractures (FFP Type Ia = 94.2%) and eight patients with bilateral fractures (FFP Type Ib = 5.8%). Mean body mass index (BMI) of all patients was 24 (15–42). Sex ratio was 5.6/1 in favor of women. The average age of women was 5.6 years higher than that of men. The vast majority of patients suffered a fall from standing position or recurrent falls. Only 15 patients (10.9%) had no comorbidities at first presentation. Among the patients with comorbidities (89.1%), cardiovascular diseases, osteoporosis, and actual or previous malignancies were the most frequently present. In addition, 107 patients received anticoagulants and/or antithrombotic drugs (77.5%). Median time delay between trauma and primary presentation was 0 days (0–264, IQR 0–2). More than 84% of patients presented within one week after trauma. Patients with a presentation of seven or more days after trauma were younger (77.7 years ± 8.14 vs. 81.3 years ± 8.64, $p = 0.045$), had shorter stays in hospital (median 4 vs. 8 days, $p < 0.001$) and they suffered medical complications less often (3.8% vs. 22.3%, $p = 0.030$).

Demographics, trauma mechanism, time of presentation, comorbidities, relevant medication, and previous surgeries at hip joint or lumbar spine of all patients, prior to suffering an FFP Type I, are depicted in Table 1.

Table 1. Baseline characteristics of all patients before suffering an FFP Type I.

	Number	%	Mean Age	SD
Demographics				
All patients	138	100	80.6	8.6
Women	117	84.8	81.5	8.2
Men	21	15.2	75.9	9.2
Patients younger than 80	57	41.3	72.5	6.1
Patients age 80 and older	81	58.7	86.2	4.8
Trauma Mechanism	**Number**	**%**		
Fall from standing position	106	77		
Other trauma mechanism	19	13.8		
Recurrent falls	7	5.1		
No trauma memorable	6	4.2		
Time of Presentation	**Number**	**%**		
Day of trauma	86	62.3		
Within first week	30	21.7		
After one week	22	16.0		
Comorbidities	**Number**	**%**		
Patients without comorbidities	15	10.9		
Patients with comorbidities	123	89.1		
Cardiovascular disease	112	81.2		
Osteoporosis	54	39.1		
Actual/previous malignancies	28	20.3		
Diabetes mellitus	27	19.6		
Pulmonary disease	7	12.3		
Dementia	15	10.9		
Rheumatoid arthritis	5	3.6		
Medication	**Number**	**%**		
Anticoagulants	107	77.5		
Cortisone	20	14.5		
Previous surgeries	**Number**	**%**		
Total hip arthroplasty	20	14.5		
Lumbar spine fusion	5	3.6		

Age and sex of patients with pubic ramus fractures, published in representative original articles of the last decades are listed in Table 2

Table 2. Age and sex of patients with pubic ramus fractures in previous publications.

Author [Reference]	Year	Number of Patients	Age (Range)	Sex (F/M)
Hill et al. [7]	2001	286	74.7 (17–97)	231/55
Taillander et al. [17]	2003	60	83 (65–99)	54/6
Krappinger et al. [8]	2009	534	73.3 (SD 19.8)	448/86
van Dyck et al. [18]	2010	99	80.1 (60–98)	88/11
Maier et al. [19]	2016	93	76.8 (n.a.)	64/29
Banierink et al. [20]	2019	153	79 (65–100)	108/45
Schmitz et al. [21]	2019	196	75.3 (60–94)	138/58
Hamilton et al. [10]	2019	43	78.4 (S.D 9.2)	32/11
Loggers et al. [11]	2019	117	83 (65–97)	101/16
Own series	2020	138	80.6 (52–98)	117/21

3.2. Care Pathways

In total, 136 patients were treated conservatively (98.6%). Conservative treatment consisted of pain therapy, mobilization in bed, sitting and standing at the bedside, followed by short transfers and assisted walking. Weight bearing was allowed at all times, when tolerated. Two patients were treated operatively (1.4%). In one patient, a retrograde transpubic screw was inserted and another patient received a plate and screw osteosynthesis of the anterior pelvic ring.

Fourteen patients (10.1%) received an outpatient treatment, and 124 patients were admitted in our trauma unit (89.9%). Five patients died during hospital stay (4.0%). The reasons of death were not directly related to the pubic ramus fractures: pneumonia in two, cardiovascular arrest, cardiac infarction and multiple organ failure in one patient each. Median in-hospital stay of the surviving patients was eight days (2–45 days, IQR 5–10 days). Twenty-two patients (16.5%) suffered complications during hospital stay of which urinary tract infection and pneumonia were the most frequent. Thrombosis and pulmonary embolism were not noticed. Complications occurred more often with a longer stay in hospital (median 11 days vs. 7 days, p <0.001) and in patients with more comorbidities (median 2 vs. 1, $p = 0.085$). They did not differ with age (median 83.5 years vs. 81 years, $p = 0.201$). At discharge, almost three quarters of the patients were mobile on the ward or in the room. Nearly two thirds of patients could be discharged at home, and the remaining were discharged in different caring institutes. More data on in-hospital complications, on mobility, and destination at discharge are depicted in Table 3.

Table 3. In-hospital complications, mobility, and destination at discharge.

	Number	%
In-Hospital Complications		
All in-hospital patients	124	100
In-hospital death	5	4.0
Number of patients with in-hospital complications	22	17.7
Type of In-Hospital Complication		
Urinary tract infection	17	13.7
Pneumonia	7	5.6
Skin ulcer	6	4.8
Cardiovascular accident	3	2.4
Mobility at Discharge		
All surviving in-hospital patients	119	100
Type		
Mobile on the ward	68	57.1
Mobile in the room	18	15.2
Need help for out-of-bed mobilization	15	12.6
Immobilized in bed	0	0
Unknown	18	15.2
Destination of Discharge		
All surviving in-hospital patients	119	100
Type		
Discharge at home	74	62.2
Geriatric rehabilitation center	13	11.0
Geriatric clinic	10	8.4
Nursing home	10	8.4
Short-time nursing care	6	5.0
Assisted living environment	3	2.5
Other hospital	1	0.8
Unknown	16	13.4

3.3. Follow-Ups

Forty-five patients had died at follow-up (32.6%). Median delay between primary presentation and death was 50 weeks (0–345 weeks, IQR 22–112 weeks). Twenty-three patients died within the first year after primary presentation (16.7%), 41 within 5 years (29.7%). None of the patients died due to a direct complication of the pubic ramus fractures. One-year mortality of patients below and above 80 years was 8.8% resp. 22.2%. Five-year mortality of patients below and above 80 years was 17.5% resp. 39.5%. Figure 2 shows the Kaplan–Meier curve of the cumulative survival of both age groups.

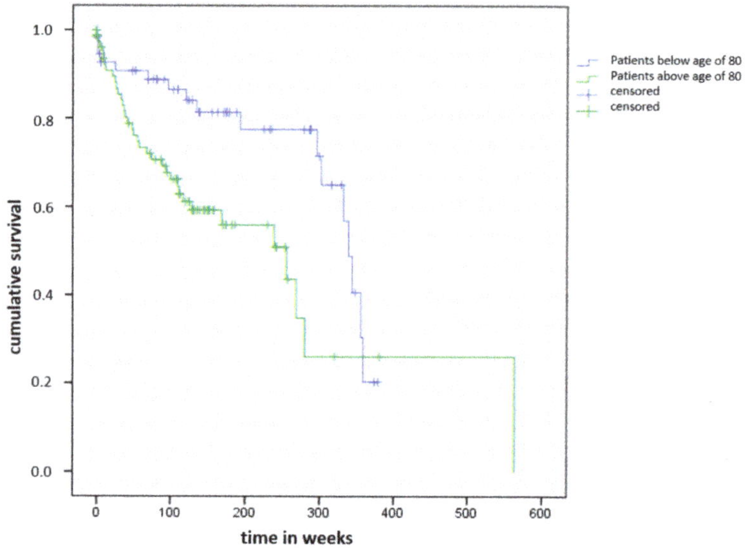

Figure 2. Kaplan–Meier curve of the cumulative survival of patient groups below and above age of 80.

One-year mortality rates of reference populations and of published series of patients with FFP are listed in Table 4.

Table 4. One-year mortality rates of reference populations and of published series of patients with FFP.

Author (Reference)	Year	Number	Mean Age of Patients	One-Year Mortality Rate, in %	Reference Group in %
Hill et al. [7]	2001	286	74.7	13.3	4.7 ***
Leung et al. [22]	2001	60	78	11.7	
Krappinger et al. [8]	2009	534	73.3	11.2	
Krappinger et al. [8]	2009	270 *	n.a.	3.7	
Krappinger et al. [8]	2009	264 **	n.a.	18.9	12.5 ****
van Dyck et al. [18]	2010	99	80.1	24.7	7.5 *****
Maier et al. [19]	2016	93	76.8		
Andrich et al. [23]	2017	5685	80	21	11
Banierink et al. [20]	2019	153	79	26.8	
Banierink et al. [20]	2019	65	76–8531	5 *****	
Banierink et al. [20]	2019	34	>85	35	15 *****
Loggers et al. [11]	2019	117	83	23	
Loggers et al. [11]	2019	94	n.a.	20 ‡	
Own series	2020	138	80.6	16.7	5.9 ¥/4.0 ¥¥
Own series	2020	57 *	74	8.8	
Own series	2020	81 **	86	22.2	
Own series	2020	21 ŧ	75	19.1	5.5
Own series	2020	117 ŧ	82	16.2	4.0

* Patients below age of 80, ** Patients with age of 80 and above, *** Data from the Scottish Institute for Statistics, **** Data from Austrian Institute for Statistics, ***** Data from the Dutch Institute for Statistics, ‡ Patients with isolated anterior pelvic ring fractures, ¥ Male population [24], ¥¥ Female population [24].

Seventeen patients were lost to follow-up (12.3%) and 4 refused participation in our retrospective study (2.9%). In addition, 72 of 93 surviving patients completed the questionnaires (77.4%). Median time delay between presentation and follow-up of the responding 72 patients was 149 weeks (53–382 weeks, IQR 113–237 weeks). All patients had a minimum follow-up of one year. At follow-up, the vast majority of patients was able to walk independently or with walking aids. The rate of surviving patients living at home with or without assistance dropped from 80.5% to 65.3%. Detailed data on mortality, mobility, and living conditions before trauma and at follow-up is depicted in Table 5.

Table 5. Mortality, mobility and living condition before trauma and at follow-up.

	Number		%	
All patients	138		100	
Death at follow-up	45		32.6	
Lost to follow-up	17		12.3	
Refused participation	4		2.9	
Remaining patients	72		52.2	
	Mobility at Follow-Up			
All patients	72		100	
	Type			
Independent walking	20		27.8	
Walking with walking aid	36		50	
Walking inside home	12		16.7	
Immobilized in bed	4		5.6	
	Living Condition at Primary Presentation and at Follow-Up			
	Primary Presentation		**Follow-Up**	
	Number	**%**	**Number**	**%**
Number of patients	72	100	72	100
Independent at home	44	61.1	27	37.5
At home with assistance	14	19.4	20	27.8
Nursing home	6	8.3	14	19.4
Hospitalized	3	4.2	1	1.4
Assisted living environment	2	2.8	4	5.6
Unknown	3	4.2	6	8.3

The median Parker Mobility Score was 4 (0–9; IQR 3–7). The median EQ-5D-Index Value of 72 patients, who answered this questionnaire, was 0.62 (0.04–1; IQR 0.5–0.78). The median value of NRS was 3 (0–10, IQR 0–5). The EQ-5D-Index Value correlated with the PMS ($p < 0.001$), inversely with age ($p < 0.001$) and with NRS ($p = 0.011$). The number of comorbidities correlated inversely with the EQ-5D-Index Value ($p = 0.022$) and with the PMS ($p = 0.010$). The occurrence of a medical complication did not influence the quality of life (EQ-5D-Index Value) at follow-up ($p = 0.107$). Nevertheless, the PMS was higher in patients without medical complication (median 4 vs. 3, $p = 0.072$). There was no correlation of the EQ-5D-Index Value with delayed presentation ($p = 0.529$).

Fourteen out of 66 patients (21.2%), who answered this question, expressed having suffered an additional fragility fracture after the pubic ramus fractures: five times a progression of the FFP Type I to another FFP Type, three times an osteoporotic vertebral fracture, three times a fracture of the lower extremities, two times rib fractures, and once a fracture of the upper extremities. The median time delay between the index injury and the new fracture was 123 weeks (46–413, IQR 58–167).

Of 66 patients, who answered this question, only 28 (45.2%) expressed taking an anti-resorptive medication.

4. Discussion

This is the first and unique study on mobility, level of independency, quality of life, and survival rate of elderly patients with isolated pubic ramus fractures. Isolated pubic ramus fractures are the least unstable fracture types in FFP [4]. Stability of the pelvic ring with pubic ramus fractures and intact peri-pelvic soft tissues is only reduced by 7% [25]. It seems reasonable to hypothesize that isolated pubic ramus fractures have limited impact on the patient's outcome and can be treated with "careful neglect". The results of this study show the opposite: isolated pubic ramus fractures are serious adverse events for elderly persons as they have a distinct influence on their mobility, level of independence, and survival rate.

Age and sex ratio of our patient cohort was similar to that of the populations of previous publications, although all types of FFP were included in previously published studies.

The mean age of the patients in the presented papers ranges from 75.3 to 83 years, sex ratio was always in favor of women and ranged from 2.2/1 to 8/1. The variation in sex ratio can be explained by the different inclusion criteria used (e.g., minimum age). Demographic data of our 138 patients—mean age of 80.6 years and female to male ratio of 5.6/1—are situated in the middle of this spectrum of data.

Unilateral pubic ramus fractures were diagnosed in 94.2% and bilateral in 5.8%. These findings are in accordance with data from other publications: Hill et al. found bilateral fractures in 3.5% in a series of 286 consecutive patients [7], and Krappinger et al. in 6.6% in a series of 534 patients [8].

Only 10.9% of our patients presented without comorbidities. The very high rate of comorbidities is a direct sign for the vulnerability of this patient population. Hypotensive drugs, impaired vision, vertigo, walking impairment and intake of analgesics may be at the origin of their falls [26–28]. In a multidisciplinary approach, the reasons for the falls must be explored and treated, if possible. Multidisciplinary co-management prevents recurrent falls and further deterioration of the patient's condition [29].

Complication rate within hospital-stay was 16.5%, urinary tract infection and pneumonia being the most frequent complications. For comparison, van Dyck et al. registered 20.2% of in-hospital complications, of which urinary tract infection and pneumonia also were the most frequent [18]. Banierink et al. calculated a complication rate of 23% within 30 days after injury, in which delirium was included, whereas the last was not represented in other studies [20]. In-hospital complications occurred more often in patients with a longer hospital stay and with more comorbidities. It is therefore most important for reducing the length of hospital stay while providing uninterrupted medical care and continuous support for mobilization.

One-year mortality of our patients was three times higher than in the reference population. One-year mortality rate of our male patients was 19.1%, of our female patients 16.2%. The one-year mortality rates in the reference population are 5.9% for males and 4% for females [24].

In the studies listed in Table 4, there always is an excess mortality in FFP patients when compared with the general population of the same age, be it in Scotland, the Netherlands, Austria, or Germany. As in the publications of Krappinger [8] and Banierink [20], we found a strong dependence of the one-year mortality on age: the rates of our patients below and above the age of 80 were 8.8% resp. 22.2%. In both groups below and above the age of 80, mortality rates exceeded the rates of the general population. We did not find a remarkable difference in the one-year mortality between our study population without involvement of the posterior pelvic ring and other study populations, in which at least a part had involvement in the posterior pelvic ring. The one-year mortality rate of 16.7% in our patient cohort is situated at the lower end of data given in the published series in Table 4, ranging from 11.2% [8] to 26.8% [20].

More than three quarters of surviving patients could be reached for follow-up. We registered a clear reduction of the level of independence at follow-up. The percentage of patients living independent at home dropped from 61.1% to 37.5%, and the rate of patients living in a nursing home increased from 8.3% to 19.4%. The median PMS of our patients was 4. PMS rates mobility at home (3 points), mobility out of home (3 points), and shopping (3 points). The score has a minimum of 0 (immobility) and a maximum of 9 (independent mobility). Our patients scored low, which means that most of them needed help in their activities of daily life. These data are also supported by the EQ-5D-Index Value of our patients being 0.62. This value is 0.78 for a previously described German patient population older than 75 years of age [30]. Unsurprisingly, there was a significant positive correlation between quality of life (EQ-5D-Index Value) and mobility (PMS). Patients with more comorbidities had a lower quality of life and were less mobile. With these data, it becomes clear that isolated pubic ramus fractures cannot be regarded merely as "tissue damage". The results of our study show a similarity instead between the natural course of patients with an FFP Type I and patients with more unstable types of FFP, as shown in Table 4. As the origin of the fragility fractures can be multifactorial, a multidisciplinary co-management is needed for the treatment of existing comorbidities [29].

Patients scored on average 3 points in their subjective sensation of pain, depicted in the NRS. NRS scores range from 0 (no pain) to 10 (unbearable pain) [15]. A value of three points means that patients suffer from a lower degree of continuous burden in their daily life, even after a follow-up of at least one year.

One fifth of our patients suffered an additional fragility fracture during follow-up, whereas only 45.2% took anti-resorptive medication. The additional fractures do not occur immediately but rather later during follow-up, in our series after a median of 123 weeks. van Dyck published a rate of 24.1% additional fractures of which the majority occurred in the first 24 months [18]. Maier et al. found that only 50% of their 93 patients received anti-osteoporotic therapy [19]. Suhm et al. stated that only 46% of their 50 follow-up patients received any form of anti-resorptive therapy and additional fractures occurred in 22% [31]. Although the occurrence of isolated pubic rami fractures is a serious adverse event for elderly persons, prevention of further fractures with anti-resorptive drugs seems not to be widely accepted. One important part of geriatric co-management is exploration of bone metabolism and treatment of osteoporosis for the prevention of the occurrence of additional fragility fractures [29,31].

This study has several limitations. It concerns a retrospective study, in which patients were recruited over a time of more than 10 years. The follow-up time varied from one to more than seven years. The influence of pubic ramus fractures on mobility, level of independency, and quality of life may become less important with greater time interval. We could not compare our data with other series of patients with FFP Type I, as they are not available in literature. We compared our results with those of patient series, which also involved fractures of the posterior pelvic ring and found several similarities. The published series so far are not completely comparable with our patient group, but—to the best of our knowledge—represent the most comparable data available. From our data, we cannot give recommendations for a different, more specific type of conservative treatment of the fractures themselves. Our data rather show that pubic ramus fractures arise as the consequence of co-existing problems of different origin. These problems should be explored and treated by multidisciplinary geriatric co-management [29].

5. Conclusions

Pubic ramus fractures without involvement of the posterior pelvic ring are serious adverse events for elderly persons. They are much more than merely a tissue damage, which can be treated with careful neglect. They have a direct influence on level of independence, mobility, and quality of life of these patients. One-year mortality is three times as high as in a reference population. Pubic ramus fractures are a warning signal of the patient to his/her medical caretakers and simultaneously a demand for exploration and treatment of comorbidities, which may lead to recurrent falls, additional fragility fractures, and further deterioration of his/her general condition.

Author Contributions: Conceptualization and methodology: P.M.R. and D.W.; investigation: J.C.H., M.H., and B.D.; writing—original draft preparation, P.M.R.; writing—review and editing, D.W., M.H., and B.D.; supervision: A.H.; funding acquisition, P.M.R. All authors have read and agreed to the published version of the manuscript.

Funding: This research was funded by the Zimmer-Biomet Company. Sulzerallee 6, PO Box CH-9404 Winterthur, Switzerland, Grant No. IRE 2017-56CH.

Acknowledgments: We sincerely thank Kirsten Schuelke for meticulous data collection.

Conflicts of Interest: The authors declare no conflict of interest. The funders had no role in the design of the study; in the collection, analyses, or interpretation of data; in the writing of the manuscript, or in the decision to publish the results.

References

1. Scheyerer, M.J.; Osterhoff, G.; Wehrle, S.; Wanner, G.A.; Simmen, H.P.; Werner, C.M. Detection of posterior pelvic injuries in fractures of the pubic rami. *Injury* **2012**, *43*, 1326–1329. [CrossRef] [PubMed]
2. Kannus, P.; Parkkari, J.; Niemi, S.; Sievänen, H. Low-Trauma Pelvic Fractures in Elderly Finns in 1970–2013. *Calcif. Tissue Int.* **2015**, *97*, 577–580. [CrossRef] [PubMed]
3. Holstein, J.H.; Stuby, F.M.; Herath, S.C.; Culemann, U.; Aghayev, E.; Pohlemann, T. Einfluss des Beckenregisters der DGU auf die Versorgung von Beckenringfrakturen [Influence of the pelvic trauma registry of the DGU on treatment of pelvic ring fractures]. *Unfallchirurg* **2016**, *119*, 475–481. [CrossRef] [PubMed]
4. Rommens, P.M.; Hofmann, A. Comprehensive classification of fragility fractures of the pelvic ring: Recommendations for surgical treatment. *Injury* **2013**, *44*, 1733–1744. [CrossRef]
5. Rommens, P.; Wissing, H.; Serdarevic, M. Significance of computerized tomography in the diagnosis and therapy of fractures of the posterior pelvic ring and hip joint. *Unfallchirurgie* **1987**, *13*, 32–37. [CrossRef]
6. Koval, K.J.; Aharonoff, G.B.; Schwartz, M.C.; Alpert, S.; Cohen, G.; McShinawy, A.; Zuckerman, J.D. Pubic rami fracture: A benign pelvic injury? *J. Orthop. Trauma* **1997**, *11*, 7–9. [CrossRef]
7. Hill, R.M.; Robinson, C.M.; Keating, J.F. Fractures of the pubic rami. Epidemiology and five-year survival. *J. Bone Joint Surg. Br.* **2001**, *83*, 1141–1144. [CrossRef]
8. Krappinger, D.; Struve, P.; Schmid, R.; Kroesslhuber, J.; Blauth, M. Fractures of the pubic rami: A retrospective review of 534 cases. *Arch. Orthop. Trauma Surg.* **2009**, *129*, 1685–1690. [CrossRef]
9. Lau, T.W.; Leung, F. Occult posterior pelvic ring fractures in elderly patients with osteoporotic pubic rami fractures. *J. Orthop. Surg.* **2010**, *18*, 153–157. [CrossRef]
10. Hamilton, C.B.; Harnett, J.D.; Stone, N.C.; Furey, A.J. Morbidity and mortality following pelvic ramus fractures in an older Atlantic Canadian cohort. *Can. J. Surg.* **2019**, *62*, 270–274. [CrossRef]
11. Loggers, S.A.I.; Joosse, P.; Jan Ponsen, K. Outcome of pubic rami fractures with or without concomitant involvement of the posterior ring in elderly patients. *Eur. J. Trauma Emerg. Surg.* **2019**, *45*, 1021–1029. [CrossRef]
12. Group, T.E. EuroQoL—A new facility for the measurement of health-related quality of life. *Health Policy* **1990**, *16*, 199–208.
13. Brooks, L. EuroQoL: The current state of the play. *Health Policy* **1996**, *37*, 53–72. [CrossRef]
14. Hinz, A.; Klaiberg, A.; Brähler, E.; König, H.H. The Quality of Life Questionnaire EQ-5D: Modelling and norm values for the general population. *Psychother. Psychosom. Med. Psychol.* **2006**, *56*, 42–48. [CrossRef] [PubMed]
15. Rodriguez, C.S. Pain measurement in the elderly: A review. *Pain Manag. Nurs.* **2001**, *2*, 38–46. [CrossRef] [PubMed]
16. Parker, M.; Palmer, C. A new mobility score for predicting mortality after hip fracture. *J. Bone Joint Surg. Br.* **1993**, *75*, 797–798. [CrossRef]
17. Taillandier, J.; Langue, F.; Alemanni, M.; Taillandier-Heriche, E. Mortality and functional outcomes of pelvic insufficiency fractures in older patients. *Joint Bone Spine* **2003**, *70*, 287–289. [CrossRef]
18. Van Dijk, W.A.; Poeze, M.; van Helden, S.H.; Brink, P.R.; Verbruggen, J.P. Ten-year mortality among hospitalised patients with fractures of the pubic rami. *Injury* **2010**, *41*, 411–414. [CrossRef]
19. Maier, G.S.; Kolbow, K.; Lazovic, D.; Horas, K.; Roth, K.E.; Seeger, J.B.; Maus, U. Risk factors for pelvic insufficiency fractures and outcome after conservative therapy. *Arch. Gerontol. Geriatr.* **2016**, *67*, 80–85. [CrossRef]

20. Banierink, H.; Ten Duis, K.; de Vries, R.; Wendt, K.; Heineman, E.; Reininga, I.; IJpma, F. Pelvic ring injury in the elderly: Fragile patients with substantial mortality rates and long-term physical impairment. *PLoS ONE* **2019**, *14*, e0216809. [CrossRef]
21. Schmitz, P.; Lüdeck, S.; Baumann, F.; Kretschmer, R.; Nerlich, M.; Kerschbaum, M. Patient-related quality of life after pelvic ring fractures in elderly. *Int. Orthop.* **2019**, *43*, 261–267. [CrossRef] [PubMed]
22. Leung, W.Y.; Ban, C.M.; Lam, J.J.; Ip, F.K.; Ko, P.S. Prognosis of acute pelvic fractures in elderly patients: Retrospective study. *HKMJ* **2001**, *7*, 139–145. [PubMed]
23. Andrich, S.; Haastert, B.; Neuhaus, E.; Neidert, K.; Arend, W.; Ohmann, C.; Grebe, J.; Vogt, A.; Jungbluth, P.; Thelen, S.; et al. Excess Mortality After Pelvic Fractures Among Older People. *J. Bone Miner. Res.* **2017**, *32*, 1789–1801. [CrossRef] [PubMed]
24. Rheinland_Pfalz. Statistisches Landesamt. Statistische Berichte 2018. Available online: https://www.statistik.rlp.de/fileadmin/dokumente/berichte/A/2033/A2033_201600_1j_L.pdf (accessed on 14 May 2020).
25. Fensky, F.; Weiser, L.; Sellenschloh, K.; Vollmer, M.; Hartel, M.J.; Morlock, M.M.; Püschel, K.; Rueger, J.M.; Lehmann, W. Biomechanical analysis of anterior pelvic ring fractures with intact peripelvic soft tissues: A cadaveric study. *Eur. J. Trauma Emerg. Surg.* **2019**, 1–7. [CrossRef] [PubMed]
26. Bradley, S.M. Falls in older adults. *Mt. Sinai J. Med.* **2011**, *78*, 590–595. [CrossRef] [PubMed]
27. Enderlin, C.; Rooker, J.; Ball, S.; Hippensteel, D.; Alderman, J.; Fisher, S.J.; McLeskey, N.; Jordan, K. Summary of Factors Contributing to Falls in Older Adults and Nursing Implications. *Geriatr. Nurs.* **2015**, *36*, 397–406. [CrossRef]
28. While, A.E. Falls and older people: Understanding why people fall. *Br. J. Community Nurs.* **2020**, *25*, 173–177. [CrossRef]
29. Bukata, S.V.; Digiovanni, B.F.; Friedman, S.M.; Hoyen, H.; Kates, A.; Kates, S.L.; Mears, S.C.; Mendelson, D.A.; Serna, F.H., Jr.; Sieber, F.E.; et al. A guide to improving the care of patients with fragility fractures. *Geriatr. Orthop. Surg. Rehabil.* **2011**, *2*, 5–37. [CrossRef]
30. Janssen, M.F.; Szende, A.; Cabases, J.; Ramos-Goñi, J.M.; Vilagut, G.; König, H.H. Population norms for the EQ-5D-3L: A cross-country analysis of population surveys for 20 countries. *Eur. J. Health Econ.* **2019**, *20*, 205–216. [CrossRef]
31. Suhm, N.; Egger, A.; Zech, C.; Eckhardt, H.; Morgenstern, M.; Gratza, S. Low acceptance of osteoanabolic therapy with parathyroid hormone in patients with fragility fracture of the pelvis in routine clinical practice: A retrospective observational cohort study. *Arch. Orthop. Trauma Surg.* **2020**, *140*, 321–329. [CrossRef]

Journal of
Clinical Medicine

MDPI

Article

Retrospective Analysis of the Clinical Outcome in a Matched Case-Control Cohort of Polytrauma Patients Following an Osteosynthetic Flail Chest Stabilization

Marcel Niemann *,†, Frank Graef †, Serafeim Tsitsilonis, Ulrich Stöckle and Sven Märdian

Center for Musculoskeletal Surgery, Charité–University Medicine Berlin, Augustenburger Platz 1, 13353 Berlin, Germany; frank.graef@charite.de (F.G.); serafeim.tsitsilonis@charite.de (S.T.); ulrich.stoeckle@charite.de (U.S.); sven.maerdian@charite.de (S.M.)

* Correspondence: marcel.niemann@charite.de; Tel.: +49-30-450-652-256; Fax: +49-30-450-552-901

† These authors contributed equally to this work.

Received: 30 June 2020; Accepted: 24 July 2020; Published: 26 July 2020

Abstract: Background: In polytrauma (PT) patients, osseous thoracic injuries are commonly observed. One of the most severe injuries is the flail chest where the rib cage is broken in such a way that leads to a partial functional detachment of the thoracic wall. Especially in PT patients, the integrity of the respiratory system and especially, of the respiratory muscles is essential to prevent respiratory failure. Besides conservative treatment options, flail chest injuries may be surgically stabilized. However, this treatment option is rarely carried out and evidence on the outcome of surgically treated flail chest patients is rare. Objective: This study intends to investigate the clinical outcome of PT patients with the diagnosis of a flail chest who received an osteosynthetic stabilization for that compared to the same group of patients without an operative treatment. The between-groups outcome was compared regarding the duration of the total hospital and the intensive care unit (ICU) stay, the total of the invasive ventilation days, the incidence of pneumonia, and the dosage of the pain medication at the hospital discharge. Methods: A retrospective analysis was conducted including all PT patients who received an osteosynthetic stabilization of a flail chest. Furthermore, another cohort of PT patients and the diagnosis of a flail chest but without operative treatment was determined. Both groups were case-control matched for the Injury Severity Score (ISS) and age. Further statistical analysis was performed using the Wilcoxon signed-rank test and the McNemar's test. Results: Out of eleven operatively and 59 conservatively treated patients, eleven patients per group were matched. Further analysis revealed no significant differences in the normal ward treatment duration (5.64 ± 6.62 and 6.20 ± 5.85 days), the invasive ventilation duration (was 6.25 ± 7.17 and 7.10 ± 6.14 days), the morphine equivalent dosage of the oral analgesia (61.36 ± 67.23 mg and 39.67 ± 65.65 mg), and the pneumonia incidence (36.4 and 54.5%) when conservatively and operatively treated patients were compared, respectively. However, surgically treated patients had a longer ICU (25.18 ± 14.48 and 15.27 ± 12.10 days, $Z = -2.308$, $p = 0.021$) and a longer total hospital treatment duration (30.10 ± 13.01 and 20.91 ± 10.34 days, $Z = -2.807$, $p = 0.005$) when compared to conservatively treated patients. Conclusion: In the present study cohort, there was no outcome difference between conservatively and operatively treated patients with the diagnosis of a flail chest regarding the normal ward treatment duration, the invasive ventilation duration, the morphine equivalent dosage of the oral analgesia, and the pneumonia incidence while ICU treatment duration and hospital treatment duration was longer in operatively treated patients.

Keywords: Polytrauma; flail chest; thoracic injury

1. Introduction

In 2018, the TraumaRegister® DGU counted 17,664 severely injured trauma patients, who were admitted to a hospital in Germany. Out of these, 4735 patients met the criteria of a polytrauma (PT) [1].

In PT patients, severe injuries of the thorax are regularly observed. At least 53.2% of the PT patients after a fall from a height [2], 42.8% of the pedestrians, and 60.1% of the motor vehicle occupants with a blunt trauma [3] presented with a severe injury of the thorax with an Abbreviated Injury Scale (AIS) [4] ≥ 3. Osseous injuries of the thorax are associated with a high level of pain [5] and, potentially, with a longer hospital stay and a prolonged invasive ventilation, especially when associated with sternal fractures [6]. Accordingly, a surgical stabilization of flail chest injuries might entail avoiding such issues. Yet, evidence of the benefits on patient outcome following surgical flail chest treatment is rare.

There is one meta-analysis comparing three randomized controlled trials (RCTs) of traumatic flail chests which concludes that surgical stabilization of a flail chest leads to a lower incidence of pneumonia, a shorter duration of mechanical ventilation, and a shorter length of intensive care unit (ICU) stay [7]. The authors of the primary studies used heterogenous inclusion criteria, surgical indications, and surgical methods [8–10] which might be the reason for the data heterogeneity observed by the authors of the meta-analysis [7].

Therefore, we conducted a retrospective study with a case-control matched cohort of PT patients and the diagnosis of a flail chest. Uniquely, there was no exclusion of patients because of any associated injury. Patients who received a surgical stabilization of the rib cage were compared to a conservative treatment group. The between-groups outcome was compared regarding the length of the hospital and the ICU stay, the invasive ventilation days, the incidence of pneumonia, and the dosage of the pain medication at the hospital discharge.

2. Methods

A retrospective analysis was conducted between January 2012 and December 2019 concerning all patients transmitted to the Campus Virchow clinic of the Center for Musculoskeletal Surgery of the Charité–University Medicine Berlin, a German level 1 trauma center. The electronic medical data system used at this clinic, SAP (SAP ERP 6.0 EHP4, SAP AG, Walldorf, Germany), was searched for PT patients in the aforementioned time span. PT patients were defined as patients whose clinically and radiographically objectified injuries counted up to an ISS ≥ 16. Therefore, the recorded diagnoses codes of the 10th version of the International Classification of Diseases (ICD-10) and the injuries described in the radiology reports were manually translated to their specific AIS codes in the version of 2005. The Injury Severity Score (ISS) was calculated by adding up the squares of the AIS codes of the three most injured body regions [11]. Furthermore, regarding the already described limitations of such scoring systems in patients with injuries of one region, solely [12], it was decided to include patients as previously described only when matching to the 'Berlin Definition' [13], as well. Patients who preclinically died or passed away after hospital but before ICU admittance were excluded from any further analysis.

Out of these patients, those with a flail chest according to the documented clinical and radiographic findings were included in the subsequent analysis. Flail chest was defined as either at least three contiguous ribs with segmental fractures or more than five adjacent rib fractures. All patients meeting the described criteria were included in the definite analyses. Demographic data were assessed, such as sex, age, the dates of hospital admittance, ICU discharge, and hospital discharge and morphine equivalent dosage at hospital discharge.

During the hospital stay, some of the included patients required secondary osteosynthetic stabilization of their rib cage. The indication for that intervention was made in a multidisciplinary approach both with trauma surgeons and intensive care physicians. Surgery was planned only if both disciplines agreed on the necessity of a surgical chest wall stabilization. At our clinic, PT patients with the radiographic diagnosis of a flail chest were selected for surgery when they presented a clinically observed paradoxical breathing pattern that lead to a prolonged weaning process. A paradoxical breathing pattern was defined as a flail segment moving inward due to the negative pleural pressure during regular inspiration while the rest of the thoracic wall physiologically moved outward [14]. A prolonged weaning process was defined as a futile extubation attempt ≥48 h or the necessity of a re-intubation within 48 h and, in the meantime, an observed paradoxical breathing pattern.

At our clinic, the MatrixRib™ system (DePuy Synthes, Raynham, MA, USA) was used for such operations. Commonly, this intervention was performed by an anterolateral thoracotomy. Following an exploration of the thoracic cavity and, depending on the injuries found, appropriate interventions such as evacuation of a hemothorax, coagulation of an active intrathoracic bleeding or overhaul of injured lung parenchyma, the rib cage was reconstructed. Therefore, the ribs beyond and above the thoracotomy as well as another more cranial rib were reduced and stabilized using plates out of the aforementioned osteosynthetic system. Furthermore, a thoracic drainage was inserted and the operation site was closed in a usual manner using non-resorbable sutures.

In order to avoid confounding when comparing conservatively and operatively treated patients with a flail chest, a case-control matching in the mentioned subgroups was performed. Tolerance limits were set as ± four and ± five and, correspondingly, patients were matched for ISS [15] and for age [16], respectively, in a ratio of 1:1.

The statistical analysis was performed using SPSS (SPSS Statistics for Mac OS, Version 25, IBM Corp., Armonk, NY, USA). Initially, the implemented case-control matching was used to create a matched case-control cohort of conservatively and operatively treated flail chest cases in the aforementioned manner. The resulting data were analyzed for normal distribution using histograms, Q-Q plots, and the Shapiro–Wilk test. Accordingly, the Wilcoxon signed-rank test and the McNemar's test were used for dependent samples. Unless stated otherwise, values are represented as mean ± SD. All p-values are two-tailed and p-values ≤ 0.05 were considered statistically significant.

3. Results

3.1. Demographic Data of the Study Cohort

Regarding the described inclusion criteria, a total of 70 PT patients (17 females, 53 males) with a flail chest were included in the analysis. The entire demographic data of the study cohort are displayed in Table 1.

Table 1. Demographic overview of the study cohort.

	Total Sample (N = 70)	Conservative Treatment (N = 59)	Operative Treatment (N = 11)
sex (female/male)	17/53	17/42	0/11
age [years]	50.69 ± 16.18 (range 16–82)	51.46 ± 16.25 (range 16–81)	46.55 ± 15.85 (range 29–82)
ISS	33.24 ± 12.17 (range 16.0–75.0)	33.97 ± 12.07 (range 16–75)	29.36 ± 12.55 (range 16–57)
Flail chest (unilateral/bilateral)	50/20	48/11	2/9
Pneumonia (no/yes)	39/31	34/25	5/6
Morphine equivalent dosage [mg p. o.]	100.65 ± 236.95 (range 0–1200.0)	111.0 ± 253.87 (range 0–1200.0)	39.67 ± 65.65 (range 0–180.0)
Hospital treatment [days]	23.90 ± 13.69 (range 1.0–68.0)	22.85 ± 13.63 (range 1.0–68.0)	30.10 ± 13.01 (range 12.0–54.0)
Intensive care unit treatment [days]	17.91 ± 14.59 (range 1.0–68.0)	16.56 ± 14.33 (range 1.0–68.0)	25.18 ± 14.48 (range 5.0–48.0)
Normal ward treatment [days]	6.28 ± 7.61 (range 0–35.0)	6.29 ± 7.91 (range 0–35.0)	6.20 ± 5.85 (range 0–15.0)
Invasive ventilation [days]	7.93 ± 9.10 (range 0–42.0)	8.17 ± 9.85 (range 0–42.0)	7.10 ± 6.14 (range 0–19.0)

ISS injury severity score, p. o. per os.

In the conservative treatment group, 13 (22.0%) patients were regularly sent home, twelve (20.3%) patients were discharged to an intensive care rehabilitation program, and 28 (47.5%) patients were discharged to a regular care rehabilitation program. In the operative treatment group, three (27.3%) patients were regularly sent home, three (27.3%) patients were discharged to an intensive care rehabilitation program, and four (36.4%) patients were discharged to a regular care rehabilitation program.

In the conservative treatment group, six patients (10.2%) died during the primary hospital stay. One patient (1.7%) died of a pulmonary embolism, three patients (5.1%) of a post-hypoxic cerebral edema >24 h after hospital admittance, and in two patients (3.4%), a palliative therapy was multidisciplinarily chosen after the primary computed tomography scan. In the operative treatment group, one patient (9.1%) died of a pulmonary embolism.

3.2. Demographic Data of the Case-Control Matched Cohort

Following the case-control matching, eleven patients (3 females, 19 males) remained in the conservative treatment group. Those were matched with the operative treatment group. None of the conservatively treated patients died during the primary hospital stay, but one surgically treated patient (male, 52 years old, ISS 20) died of a pulmonary embolism at day 18 after the primary hospital admission. The demographic data of the case-control matched cohort are represented in Table 2. There were no surgical site complications noted during the hospital stay.

Table 2. Demographic overview of the case-control matched cohort.

	Conservative Treatment (N = 11)	Operative Treatment (N = 11)
sex (female/male)	3/8	0/11
age [years]	46.18 ± 13.78 (range 25–77)	46.55 ± 15.85 (range 29–82)
ISS	29.27 ± 11.58 (range 20–57)	29.36 ± 12.55 (range 16–57)
Flail chest (unilateral/bilateral)	11/0	2/9
Pneumonia (no/yes)	7/4	5/6

ISS injury severity score, p. o. per os.

In the conservative and in the operative treatment group, four (36.36%) and three (27.27%) patients were regularly sent home, two (18.18%) and three (27.27%) patients were discharged to an intensive care rehabilitation program, and five (45.45%) and four (36.36%) patients were discharged to a regular care rehabilitation program, respectively.

3.3. Outcome Analysis of the Case-Control Matched Cohort

While patients of the conservative treatment group stayed at the hospital for 20.91 ± 10.34 days (range 7.0–36.0 days), patients of the operative treatment group stayed for 30.10 ± 13.01 days (range 12.0–54.0 days). This difference was statistically significant ($Z = -2.807$, $p = 0.005$).

During that time, conservatively treated patients stayed at the ICU for 15.27 ± 12.10 days (range 1.0–36.0 days) and at the normal ward for 5.64 ± 6.62 days (range 0–17.0 days). Operatively treated patients stayed at the ICU for 25.18 ± 14.48 days (range 5.0–48.0 days) and at the normal ward for 6.20 ± 5.85 days (range 0–15.0 days). The difference in the ICU treatment duration significantly differed between groups ($Z = -2.308$, $p = 0.021$), while the difference of the normal ward treatment duration did not reach significance between groups ($Z = -1.054$, $p = 0.292$).

During the ICU stay, patients conservatively treated stayed for 6.25 ± 7.17 days (range 0–20.0 days) and patients operatively treated stayed for 7.10 ± 6.14 days (range 0–19.0 days). The differences between groups did not significantly differ ($Z = -1.192$, $p = 0.233$).

At the time of hospital discharge, conservatively treated patients needed an equivalence of 61.36 ± 67.23 mg (range 0–195.0 mg), while operatively treated patients needed an equivalence of 39.67 ± 65.65 mg (range 0–180.0 mg) oral morphine as a pain medication. The differences between groups did not reach significance ($Z = -0.845$, $p = 0.398$).

A total of four patients (36.4%) out of the conservatively treated and six patients (54.5%) out of the operatively treated group received antibiotic treated due to the clinical and radiographic diagnosis of a pneumonia. This difference did not reach significance ($p = 0.687$).

Figure 1 displays the outcome of the case-control matched cohort regarding the intensive care unit treatment duration, the regular ward treatment duration, the total hospital treatment duration, the invasive ventilation treatment duration, and the morphine equivalent dosage at hospital discharge.

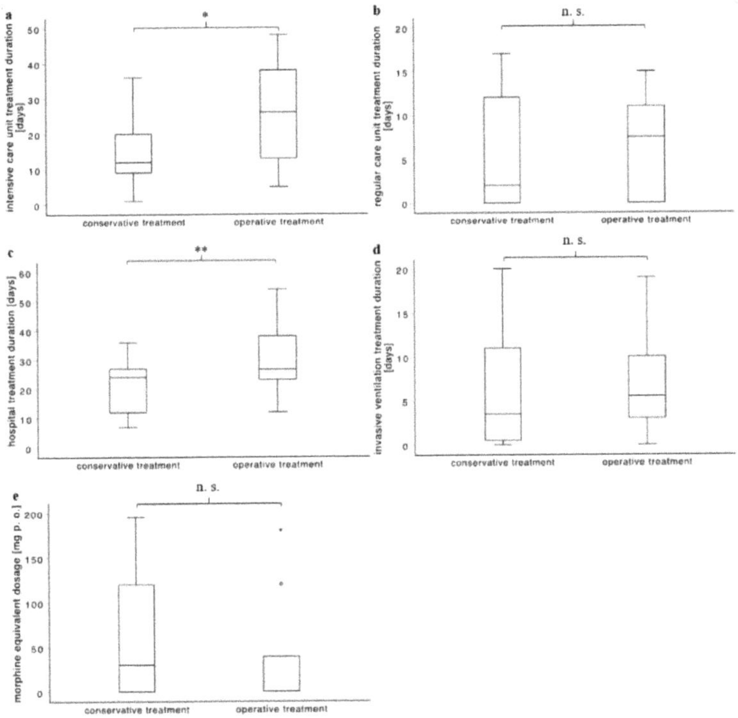

Figure 1. Overview of the outcome of the case-control matched cohort. (**a**) depicts the duration of the intensive care unit treatment duration which was 15.27 ± 12.10 and 25.18 ± 14.48 days in conservatively and operatively treated patients, respectively ($Z = -2.308$, $p = 0.021$). (**b**) depicts the duration of the normal ward treatment duration which was 5.64 ± 6.62 and 6.20 ± 5.85 days in conservatively and operatively treated patients, respectively ($Z = -1.054$, $p = 0.292$). (**c**) depicts the total hospital treatment duration which was 20.91 ± 10.34 and 30.10 ± 13.01 days in conservatively and operatively treated patients, respectively ($Z = -2.807$, $p = 0.005$). (**d**) depicts the duration of the invasive ventilation which was 6.25 ± 7.17 and 7.10 ± 6.14 days in conservatively and operatively treated patients, respectively ($Z = -1.192$, $p = 0.233$). (**e**) depicts the pain medication at the time of hospital discharge as morphine equivalent dosage. This was 61.36 ± 67.23 mg and 39.67 ± 65.65 mg in conservatively and operatively treated patients, respectively ($Z = -0.845$, $p = 0.398$). * $p \leq 0.05$, ** $p \leq 0.01$, n. s. *not significant*.

4. Discussion

The presented study investigated clinical outcome differences in a matched case-control cohort of PT patients with the diagnosis of a flail chest. While the normal ward treatment duration, the invasive ventilation duration, the morphine equivalent dosage of the oral analgesia at the time of hospital discharge, and the pneumonia incidence did not significantly differ between groups, the ICU and the total hospital treatment duration were significantly longer when the flail chests were surgically stabilized.

Granhed and Pazooki provided a prospective cohort study including 60 patients who received a chest wall stabilization due to a flail chest. The definition of the flail chest as an indication for surgery and the surgical procedure were very similar to the ones mentioned above. The authors compared that cohort with historical controls who did not receive surgery and found a significantly shorter invasive ventilation duration for operated patients [15]. This is supported by some authors who had similar results [8], while others did not find any significant difference between groups [10]. However, Granhed and Pazooki did not match for the ISS which was 30.9 ± 13.3 in the historical cohort compared to 21.7 + 10.7 in the primary analyzed cohort. The authors claimed that the ISS did not significantly differ between groups. Regardless of that, they found a linear correlation between the ISS and the invasive ventilation duration [15]. Therefore, the different ISS, although not reaching significance, should be discussed as a potential confounder of the published results.

Nevertheless, the different results of previous authors [8,15] when compared to our results might be a result of the point of time when surgery took place. While other authors reported an early intervention, at our department the indication for a surgical intervention in flail chest patients is made when other conservative treatment options repeatedly failed. This decision is made in the manner of a last treatment option. This needs to be taken into account when comparing our results to previously published data.

Farquhar et al. provided a retrospective cohort of 19 patients with a mean ISS of 31 who received surgery for a flail chest injury. The included patients were matched for the AIS of the thoracic injury, their age, and the AIS of the other injured regions with a historical cohort of conservatively treated patients with a mean ISS of 29. The authors found significantly less invasive ventilation days, a shorter ICU and hospital stay, and lower rates of pneumonia in the control group when compared to the surgically treated group [17]. Other authors, on the other hand, found a lower pneumonia incidence and a shorter ICU treatment duration [8,10] as well as a shorter total hospital treatment duration [10] in surgically treated when compared to conservatively treated patients.

Another recent study by Caragounis et al. analyzed a prospective consecutive series of 49 patients surgically treated due to a flail chest. The authors found a decreasing pain level as well as an improving forced vital capacity (FVC) during the observation period of one year. However, the authors excluded patients with severe head injury or any spinal cord injury which, as already described above, might confound the cohort when PT patients are considered [18]. In the presented study, the morphine equivalent dosage of the oral analgesia at the time of hospital discharge appeared to be lower following surgery but the difference between groups did not reach significance. This might be a result of the small study cohort. Olsén et al. provided a cohort of 31 prospectively acquired patients with a mean ISS of 22 and the diagnosis of a flail chest who received surgical stabilization. These were compared to 30 unmatched historical patients with a mean ISS of 18.5 who were treated conservatively for the same diagnosis. The authors did not find any significant differences regarding pain and FVC in the follow-up [19].

The currently available literature about the surgical stabilization of a flail chest is heterogenous regarding the indication, the material used, the patient groups themselves, and the type of statistical analysis. Concurrently more data in a RCT-design needs to be published in order to derive general recommendations regarding the aforementioned intervention. Especially, the timing of a surgical intervention for a flail chest in PT patients needs to be investigated. When used as a last treatment option after conservative treatment failure, surgical flail chest stabilization cannot facilitate any benefits regarding the outcomes observed in this study.

Perchance, algorithms such as the one provided by Bemelmann et al. [20] need to be taken into account when such future studies are planned in order to generate some kind of standard operating procedure.

Up until now, previous studies proved that several biomarkers are associated with infectious complications as well as general outcome after polytrauma [21,22]. Moreover, authors were able to show that fracture healing is connected with individual's immune reaction [23–25]. Correspondingly, the interactions between the immunoinflammatory mechanisms in polytrauma patient with associated osseous thoracic injuries should be addressed in future study designs as well.

This study has both strengths and limitations. Firstly, the study was designed in a matched-case control design including a matching for commonly known confounders. This effectively reduces selection bias. However, both groups are not totally identical. Patients of the operatively treated cohort had a bilateral flail chest more often than patients of the conservatively treated group. Although not adequately represented in the ISS, a bilateral flail chest might potentially compromise the physiological breathing mechanisms even more. Secondly, there was no patient exclusion because of any related injuries. In such fashion, the general cohort of PT patients is adequately represented in this study. On the other hand, the overall study population was low considering a total of 22 patients that could matched. Future studies need to be designed to investigate a larger population in order to generate more evidence for recommendations. Also, the severity of the thoracic injuries differed between groups. In the conservative treatment group, all patients solely had a unilateral flail chest. In the operative treatment group, only two patients had a unilateral flail chest, while nine patients had a bilateral flail chest. This might compromise the patients' outcomes and, therefore, needs to be taken into account when comparing this study results to previously published data. Even though case-control matched, the groups might not be completely identical. Lastly, a surgical chest wall stabilization was chosen as a last treatment option. Correspondingly, operatively treated patients already stayed longer at the ICU when the definite treatment procedure was chosen. This needs to be taken into account when interpreting the presented data.

5. Conclusions

In the present study, there were no significant differences between flail chest patients who were operatively treated when compared to conservatively treated patients regarding the length of the regular ward stay, the invasive ventilation days, the morphine equivalent dosage at the time of hospital discharge, and the pneumonia incidence. The ICU and the general hospital treatment duration were longer in the surgically treated group.

However, neither from the presented nor from the already published data can a general recommendation be derived. Especially in PT patients, data are lacking. There is a high need for RCTs in order to generate such data. Until then, the indication for surgical stabilization of flail chest injuries might remain as a last treatment option.

Author Contributions: Writing—original draft, M.N. and F.G.; Writing—review & editing, S.T.; U.S. and S.M. All authors have read and agreed to the published version of the manuscript.

Funding: This research received no external funding.

Acknowledgments: We acknowledge support from the German Research Foundation (DFG) and the Open Access Publication Fund of Charité – Universitätsmedizin Berlin.

Conflicts of Interest: The authors declare no conflict of interest.

References

1. Jahresbericht 2019—TraumaRegister DGU®. Sektion Notfall- & Intensivmedizin & Schwerverletztenversorgung der Deutschen Gesellschaft für Unfallchirurgie e.V. 2019. Available online: http://www.traumaregister-dgu.de/fileadmin/user_upload/traumaregister-dgu.de/docs/Downloads/Jahresbericht_2019.pdf (accessed on 23 June 2020).
2. Topp, T.; Müller, T.; Kiriazidis, I.; Lefering, R.; Ruchholtz, S. Trauma Registry of the German Trauma Society, et al. Multiple blunt trauma after suicidal attempt: An analysis of 4754 multiple severely injured patients. *Eur. J. Trauma Emerg. Surg.* **2012**, *38*, 19–24. [CrossRef] [PubMed]
3. Reith, G.; Lefering, R.; Wafaisade, A.; Hensel, K.O.; Paffrath, T.; Bouillon, B.; Probst, C.; TraumaRegister DGU. Injury pattern, outcome and characteristics of severely injured pedestrian. *Scand. J. Trauma Resusc. Emerg. Med.* **2015**, *23*, 56. [CrossRef] [PubMed]
4. Gennarelli, T.A.; Wodzin, E. AIS 2005: A contemporary injury scale. *Injury* **2006**, *37*, 1083–1091. [CrossRef]
5. Kerr-Valentic, M.A.; Arthur, M.; Mullins, R.J.; Pearson, T.E.; Mayberry, J.C. Rib fracture pain and disability: Can we do better? *J. Trauma Acute Care Surg.* **2003**, *54*, 1058–1064. [CrossRef]
6. Schulz-Drost, S.; Krinner, S.; Langenbach, A.; Oppel, P.; Lefering, R.; Taylor, D.; Hennig, F.F.; Mauerer, A.; TraumaRegister DGU. Concomitant Sternal Fracture in Flail Chest: An Analysis of 21,741 Polytrauma Patients from the TraumaRegister DGU®. *Thorac. Cardiovasc. Surg.* **2017**, *65*, 551–559.
7. Coughlin, T.A.; Ng, J.W.G.; Rollins, K.E.; Forward, D.P.; Ollivere, B.J. Management of rib fractures in traumatic flail chest: A meta-analysis of randomised controlled trials. *Bone Jt. J.* **2016**, *98*, 1119–1125. [CrossRef]
8. Tanaka, H.; Yukioka, T.; Yamaguti, Y.; Shimizu, S.; Goto, H.; Matsuda, H.; Shimazaki, S. Surgical stabilization of internal pneumatic stabilization? A prospective randomized study of management of severe flail chest patients. *J. Trauma* **2002**, *52*, 727–732. [CrossRef]
9. Granetzny, A.; Abd El-Aal, M.; Emam, E.; Shalaby, A.; Boseila, A. Surgical versus conservative treatment of flail chest. Evaluation of the pulmonary status. *Interact. Cardiovasc. Thorac. Surg.* **2005**, *4*, 583–587. [CrossRef]
10. Marasco, S.F.; Davies, A.R.; Cooper, J.; Varma, D.; Bennett, V.; Nevill, R.; Lee, G.; Bailey, M.; Fitzgerald, M. Prospective randomized controlled trial of operative rib fixation in traumatic flail chest. *J. Am. Coll. Surg.* **2013**, *216*, 924–932. [CrossRef] [PubMed]
11. Baker, S.P.; O'Neill, B.; Haddon, W.; Long, W.B. The injury severity score: A method for describing patients with multiple injuries and evaluating emergency care. *J. Trauma* **1974**, *14*, 187–196. [CrossRef] [PubMed]
12. Paffrath, T.; Lefering, R.; Flohé, S.; TraumaRegister DGU. How to define severely injured patients?—An Injury Severity Score (ISS) based approach alone is not sufficient. *Injury* **2014**, *45*, S64–S69. [CrossRef] [PubMed]
13. Pape, H.-C.; Lefering, R.; Butcher, N.; Peitzman, A.; Leenen, L.; Marzi, I.; Lichte, P.; Josten, C.; Bouillon, B.; Schmucker, U.; et al. The definition of polytrauma revisited: An international consensus process and proposal of the new "Berlin definition". *J. Trauma Acute Care Surg.* **2014**, *77*, 780–786. [CrossRef] [PubMed]
14. Hess, D.R. Respiratory Mechanics in Mechanically Ventilated Patients. *Respir. Care* **2014**, *59*, 1773–1794. [CrossRef] [PubMed]
15. Granhed, H.P.; Pazooki, D. A Feasibility Study of 60 Consecutive Patients Operated for Unstable Thoracic Cage. *J. Trauma Manag. Outcomes* **2014**, *8*, 20. Available online: https://www.ncbi.nlm.nih.gov/pmc/articles/PMC4311414/ (accessed on 24 June 2020). [CrossRef] [PubMed]
16. Holcomb, J.B.; McMullin, N.R.; Kozar, R.A.; Lygas, M.H.; Moore, F.A. Morbidity from rib fractures increases after age 45. *J. Am. Coll Surg.* **2003**, *196*, 549–555. [CrossRef]
17. Farquhar, J.; Almarhabi, Y.; Slobogean, G.; Slobogean, B.; Garraway, N.; Simons, R.K.; Hameed, S.M. No benefit to surgical fixation of flail chest injuries compared with modern comprehensive management: Results of a retrospective cohort study. *Can. J. Surg.* **2016**, *59*, 299–303. [CrossRef] [PubMed]
18. Caragounis, E.-C.; Fagevik Olsén, M.; Pazooki, D.; Granhed, H. Surgical treatment of multiple rib fractures and flail chest in trauma: A one-year follow-up study. *World J. Emerg. Surg.* **2016**, *11*, 1–7. [CrossRef]
19. Olsén, M.F.; Slobo, M.; Klarin, L.; Caragounis, E.-C.; Pazooki, D.; Granhed, H. Physical function and pain after surgical or conservative management of multiple rib fractures—A follow-up study. *Scand. J. Trauma Resusc. Emerg. Med.* **2016**, *24*, 128. [CrossRef]
20. Bemelman, M.; De Kruijf, M.W.; Van Baal, M.; Leenen, L. Rib Fractures: To Fix or Not to Fix? An Evidence-Based Algorithm. *Korean J. Thorac. Cardiovasc. Surg.* **2017**, *50*, 229–234. [CrossRef]

21. Papurica, M.; Rogobete, A.F.; Sandesc, D.; Dumache, R.; Cradigati, C.A.; Sarandan, M.; Nartita, R.; Popovici, S.E.; Bedreag, O.H. Advances in Biomarkers in Critical Ill Polytrauma Patients. *Clin. Lab.* **2016**, *62*, 977–986. [CrossRef]
22. Ciriello, V.; Gudipati, S.; Stavrou, P.Z.; Kanakaris, N.K.; Bellamy, M.C.; Giannoudis, P.V. Biomarkers predicting sepsis in polytrauma patients: Current evidence. *Injury* **2013**, *44*, 1680–1692. [CrossRef] [PubMed]
23. Reinke, S.; Geissler, S.; Taylor, W.R.; Schmidt-Bleek, K.; Juelke, K.; Schwachmeyer, V.; Dahne, M.; Hartwig, T.; Akyüz, L.; Meisel, C.; et al. Terminally differentiated $CD8^+$ T cells negatively affect bone regeneration in humans. *Sci. Transl. Med.* **2013**, *5*, 177ra36. [CrossRef] [PubMed]
24. Sass, F.A.; Schmidt-Bleek, K.; Ellinghaus, A.; Filter, S.; Rose, A.; Preininger, B.; Reinke, S.; Geissler, S.; Volk, H.; Duda, G.N.; et al. $CD31^+$ Cells From Peripheral Blood Facilitate Bone Regeneration in Biologically Impaired Conditions Through Combined Effects on Immunomodulation and Angiogenesis. *J. Bone Miner. Res.* **2017**, *32*, 902–912. [CrossRef] [PubMed]
25. Schlundt, C.; Reinke, S.; Geissler, S.; Bucher, C.H.; Giannini, C.; Märdian, S.; Dahne, M.; Kleber, C.; Samans, B.; Baronet, U.; et al. Individual Effector/Regulator T Cell Ratios Impact Bone Regeneration. *Front. Immunol.* **2019**, *10*, 1954. [CrossRef]

Journal of
Clinical Medicine

MDPI

Article

Reduced Recovery Capacity After Major Trauma in the Elderly: Results of a Prospective Multicenter Registry-Based Cohort Study

Viola Freigang [1,*], Karolina Müller [2], Antonio Ernstberger [1], Marlene Kaltenstadler [3], Lisa Bode [4], Christian Pfeifer [1], Volker Alt [1] and Florian Baumann [1]

1 Department of Trauma, Regensburg University Medical Center, 93053 Regensburg, Germany; antonio.ernstberger@ukr.de (A.E.); christian.pfeifer@ukr.de (C.P.); volker.alt@ukr.de (V.A.); florian.baumann@ukr.de (F.B.)
2 Center for Clinical Studies, Regensburg University Medical Center, 93053 Regensburg, Germany; karolina.mueller@ukr.de
3 Department of Surgery, Regensburg University Medical Center, 93053 Regensburg, Germany; marlene.kaltenstadler@ukr.de
4 Department of Orthopaedics and Trauma Surgery, Faculty of Medicine, Medical Center—Albert-Ludwigs-University of Freiburg, 79085 Freiburg im Breisgau, Germany; lisa.bode@uniklinik-freiburg.de
* Correspondence: viola.freigang@ukr.de; Tel.: +49-094-1944-6805

Received: 11 May 2020; Accepted: 21 July 2020; Published: 23 July 2020

Abstract: Aims: Considering the worldwide trend of an increased lifetime, geriatric trauma is moving into focus. Trauma is a leading cause of hospitalization, leading to disability and mortality. The purpose of this study was to compare the global health-related quality of life (HRQoL) of geriatric patients with adult patients after major trauma. Methods: This multicenter prospective registry-based observational study compares HRQoL of patients aged ≥65 years who sustained major trauma (Injury Severity Score (ISS) ≥ 16) with patients <65 years of age within the trauma registry of the German Trauma Society (DGU). The global HRQoL was measured at 6, 12, and 24 months post trauma using the EQ-5D-3L score. Results: We identified 405 patients meeting the inclusion criteria with a mean ISS of 25.6. Even though the geriatric patients group (≥65 years, $n = 77$) had a lower ISS (m = 24, SD = 8) than patients aged <65 years ($n = 328$), they reported more difficulties in each EQ dimension compared to patients <65 years. Contrary to patients <65, the EQ-5D Index of the geriatric patients did not improve at 12 and 24 months after trauma. Conclusions: We found a limited HRQoL in both groups after major trauma. The group of patients ≥65 showed no improvement in HRQoL from 6 to 24 months after trauma.

Keywords: health service research; management of major trauma; geriatric major trauma; outcome research; patient-reported outcome

1. Introduction

Since the geriatric population is forecasted to further increase, tremendous challenges are coming our way. The number of persons over 65 years of age in industrial societies is already over 20% and will reach over 35% by 2060 [1]. It is likely that the number of severely injured geriatric patients will rise in line with demographic trends. In 2017, a total of 26% of the patients included in the Trauma Register DGU® of the German Trauma Society (DGU) were over 70 years old [2]. Physiological changes and comorbidities of the elderly population are challenging factors in treatment. The likelihood of severe impact on the quality of life even after minor injury increases with age, leading to hospitalization and impairment [3]. A generally decreased ability to tolerate stress imposed by traumatic incidents leads to a significant increase in social costs and risk of mortality [4,5].

In general, major trauma research applies mortality for the measurement of initial trauma severity and outcome [6]. Using patient-centered analysis methods like the multidimensional EQ-5D (European Quality of Life 5 Dimensions) score requires a more demanding longitudinal follow up [7]. However, the personal consequences of major trauma are generally severe, which makes investigating health-related quality of life (HRQoL) fundamentally necessary, especially in the vulnerable elderly patient population.

The purpose of this study is to compare the progress of HRQoL in patients equal or over 65 years of age to patients under 65 years of age after major trauma. We hypothesized that there is an impairment in evolution of HRQoL after major trauma in the elderly.

2. Methods

In a multicenter prospective registry-based observational cohort study within the East Bavarian trauma network (TNO), we monitored the development of health-related quality of life of adult patients after major trauma (ISS ≥ 16). The TNO is part of the trauma registry of the German Trauma Society (DGU), and consists of 25 hospitals. Two hospitals are maximum care facilities, 15 hospitals provide basic care and 8 hospitals provide standard care [8]. We assured excellent quality of the recorded data. As described in the methodical paper of this study by Koller et al. [9], substantial effort has been made, to exclude confounding factors and bias. The study was approved by the Ethics Committee of the University of Regensburg (reference number 10-101-0077). The study was funded by a grant from the German Federal Ministry of Education and Research (reference number 01GY1153), and was registered in the database of the German Network of Health Services Research (reference number VfD_Polyqualy_12_001978), as well as in the German Clinical Trials Register (reference number DRKS00010039).

Between March 2012 and February 2014, 2596 patients were treated for severe trauma and were documented in the TNO data base. Overall, 56% of these patients (n = 1453 patients) had to be excluded due to an Injury Severity Score (ISS) below 16. EQ 5D data were collected from 508 patients between September 2012 and February 2016. For 456 patients, a match in both databases (TNO and EQ 5D) was complete. For the present analyses, patients below the age of 18 years were excluded, resulting in 405 patients with an age ≥ 18 years, ISS ≥ 16, and a HRQoL assessment (Figure 1). For the maintenance of a representative sample and the evaluation of bias, we compared the baseline data of included patients and patients lost to follow up. We found no clinically significant differences between participants and the excluded patient population.

We used the web-based registry of the German Trauma Society (DGU) for data acquisition. It contains 130 single items per patient. For the present study, the following baseline data were used: sociodemographic data including age and sex, clinical data including level of care of the trauma center, mechanism of injury, intensive care, intubation and duration of intubation, ISS, Glasgow Coma Scale (GCS), ASA physical status (American Society of Anesthesiologists Score), Revised Injury Severity Classification II (RISC II) and Functional Capacity Index (FCI).

Additionally, we assessed the global HRQoL, which was measured using the EQ-5D-3L at 6, 12, and 24 months after trauma. The first part of the EQ-5D evaluates the health status regarding mobility, self-care, usual activities, pain/discomfort, and anxiety/depression. The responses were dichotomized into no problems versus problems. Additionally, five dimensions were converted into EQ index ranging from −0.21 (worst health) to 1.00 (best health) [10]. The second part of the EQ-5D-3L measures the patient's assessment of their current global health status and contains a 100 mm global health visual analog scale (EQ VAS) ranging from 0 points (worst health) to 100 points (best health) concerning the patient's assessment of their current global health status. The EQ-5D is available in German and validated [11].

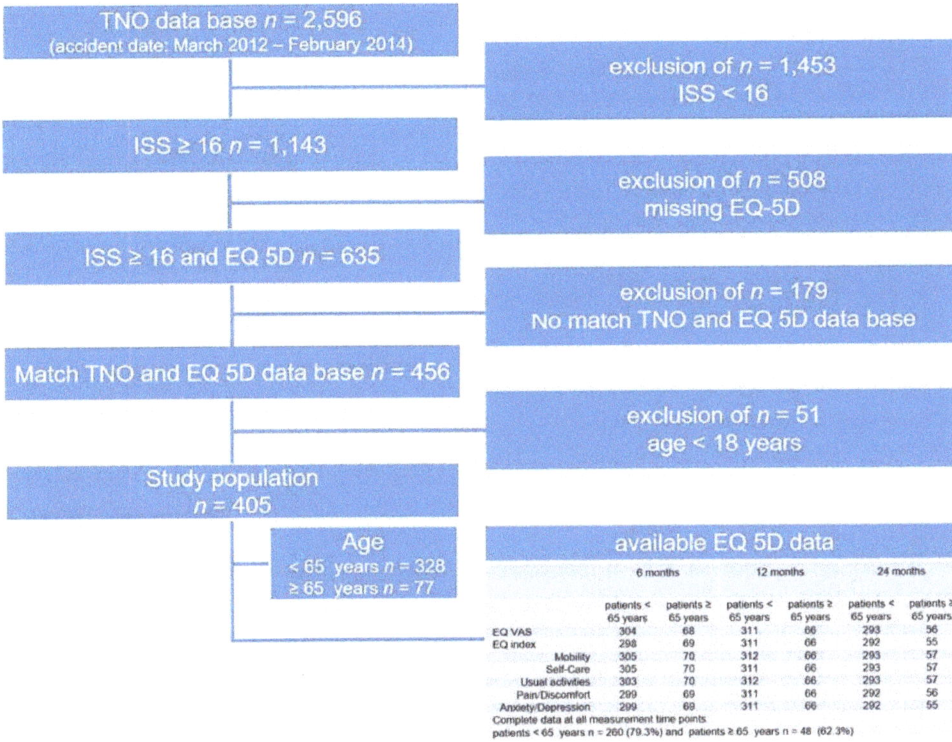

Figure 1. Selection procedure of the study population.

The ISS assess the severity trauma based on the Abbreviated Injury Scale (AIS). Each injury of the three most affected body regions is rated. The square of each score is then summed up to an ISS. A major trauma is defined as an ISS ≥ 16 [12].

The RISC II is a prognostic score evaluating different factors at initial evaluation of trauma patients. It comprises ten items of clinical and laboratory parameters to evaluate early mortality of the patient [13].

The FCI is a score used to estimate the patient's level of functional impairment within the following year after trauma. It is based on ten physical functions which are evaluated and transformed into a numerical score on a scale of 0–100. An index of 100 represents no functional limitation [14].

3. Statistics

Statistical analysis was performed using the software package SPSS (Version 25, SPSS Inc, Chicago, IL, USA). The level of significance was set at $p \leq 0.05$ for all tests. Data analyses were of an exploratory manner. Thus, no adjustments for multiple testing were conducted. Missing values were not imputed. The study was conducted in the context of health services research. No sample size calculation was conducted, as all patients were treated for major trauma between March 2012 and February 2014 with EQ 5D data, and at least at one of the three measurement time points were included.

Descriptive analyses were done using frequency (n), percentage (%), mean (m), standard deviation (sd), 95% confidence interval (95% CI), median (med), and interquartile range (IQR). Chi-square tests were used for categorial data and U-tests were used for metric data, in order to compare baseline characteristics of geriatric patients (≥65 years) and patients under the age of 65 years. Fisher-exact tests were used to compare five EQ dimensions (no problem versus any problem) between both patient groups.

Linear mixed models (maximum likelihood method, unstructured repeated covariance type) were used to evaluate repeated measures of HRQoL (i.e., EQ index and EQ VAS) 6, 12, and 24 months after trauma within and between patient groups (interaction effect time * patient group). Additionally, covariates RISC II (main effect) and FCI (main effect) and AIS for the body regions head, face, thorax, abdomen, extremities, and soft tissue (main effects) were included in the linear mixed linear models to adjust for injury severity. The mixed linear models use the full data set, and thus will give unbiased estimates.

4. Results

4.1. Baseline Characteristics

Four hundred and five patients met the inclusion criteria (Figure 1). There were 328 (81%) patients under 65 years of age and 77 (19%) patients aged 65 years or older. Overall, 72% of the patients were male. The majority (57%) of the patients were treated in a level II trauma center. Most patients sustained a high-velocity trauma in a traffic accident (32%). Most patients had to be treated in the intensive care unit (91%) and 52% of the patients had to be intubated. The mean time of intubation was 9 days (sd = 10). The mean ISS was 26 (sd = 10), the mean RISC II was 7 (sd = 15), and the mean FCI was 4 (sd = 1). Table 1 presents the baseline characteristics for the total sample and separately for geriatric patients and for patients under the age of 65 years and the mechanism of injury.

Table 1. Baseline characteristics of the study population.

		Patients < 65 years n = 328		Patients ≥ 65 years n = 77		p Value
Age (in years)		43.0	(24.3/53.0)	73.0	(70.0/78.0)	<0.001
Sex						
	male	245	(74.7%)	45	(58.4%)	0.007
	female	83	(25.3%)	32	(41.6%)	
Level of Trauma Center Facility						
	Level I	131	(39.9%)	21	(27.3%)	
	Level II	186	(56.7%)	46	(59.7%)	0.001
	Level III	11	(3.4%)	10	(13.0%)	
ISS		22.0	(18.0/30.0)	20.0	(17.0/27.5)	0.018
	AIS head	2.0	(0/3.0)	2.0	(0/4.0)	0.513
	AIS face	0	(0/0)	0	(0/0)	0.251
	AIS thorax	3.0	(2.0/4.0)	3.0	(0/4.0)	0.937
	AIS abdomen	0	(0/2.00)	0	(0/2.0)	0.186
	AIS extremities	2.0	(0/3.0)	2.0	(0/2.5)	0.020
	AIS soft tissue	0	(0/1.0)	0	(0/1.0)	0.995
RISC II [1]		1.2	(0.7/3.9)	6.3	(2.2/16.5)	<0.001
FCI [2]		4.0	(2.0/5.0)	5.0	(3.0/5.0)	0.073
ASA physical status [3]		1.0	(1.0/1.0)	2.0	(2.0/3.0)	<0.001
GCS [4]		15.0	(12.0/15.0)	15.0	(13.8/15.0)	0.266
Type of injury						
	blunt	309	(96.3%)	73	(97.3%)	1.000
	penetrating	12	(3.7%)	2	(2.7%)	
In hospital stay (in days)		15.6	(9.8/24.5)	17.0	(11.1/26.9)	0.215

Table 1. *Cont.*

	Patients < 65 years n = 328	Patients ≥ 65 years n = 77	p Value
Emergency surgery			
no	215 (70.0%)	55 (80.9%)	0.075
yes	92 (30.0%)	13 (19.1%)	
Time between accident and emergency surgery (in hours) [5]	3.0 (2.4/4.5)	3.6 (1.9/6.4)	0.599
	33.8%	27.0%	
	22.8%	4.1%	
	6.5%	9.5%	
	4.0%	10.8%	
stabbing	16%	13.5%	
	8.6%	20.3%	
	1.2%	0.0%	
	3.2%	5.4%	
	0.6%	0.0%	

Data show median (IQR) for metric variables or number of patients (%, column percentage of all patients without missing values) for categorical variables; Level of Trauma Center Facility; Injury Severity Score (ISS); Revised Injury Severity Classification Score II (RISC II); Functional Capacity Index (FCI); ASA physical status (American Society of Anesthesiologists Score); Glasgow Coma Scale (GCS); p-value (comparison of patient age groups): U-test or Chi-squared test. [1] $n = 300/n = 68$; [2] $n = 327/n = 77$; [3] $n = 309/n = 70$; [4] $n = 292/n = 62$; [5] $n = 85/n = 12$.

4.2. Quality of Life

The EQ-5D dimensions at 6, 12, and 24 months after trauma are presented for geriatric patients (≥65 years) and patients under 65 years of age (Figures 2–4). In general, severe trauma patients reported more difficulties in all five HRQoL dimensions than the German general population. Geriatric patients reported significantly more impairment than patients under the age of 65 years of age. Significant differences between geriatric patients (≥65 years) and patients under 65 years of age were found for self-care at 6 months (p = 0.046), 12 months (p = 0.003), and 24 months post-trauma (p = 0.036). Significant differences between age groups were also found in mobility 12 months after trauma (p = 0.014).

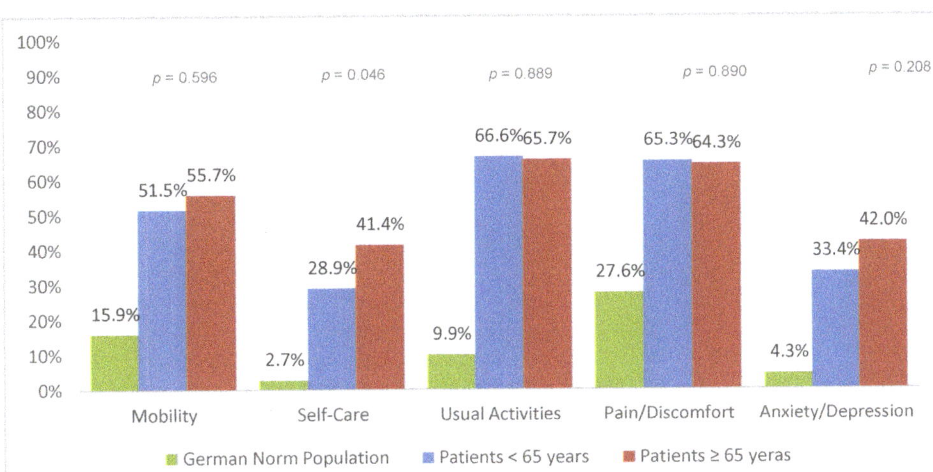

Figure 2. Reported problems in EQ-5D-3L dimension 6 months after trauma (European Quality of Life 5 Dimensions 3 Level Version).

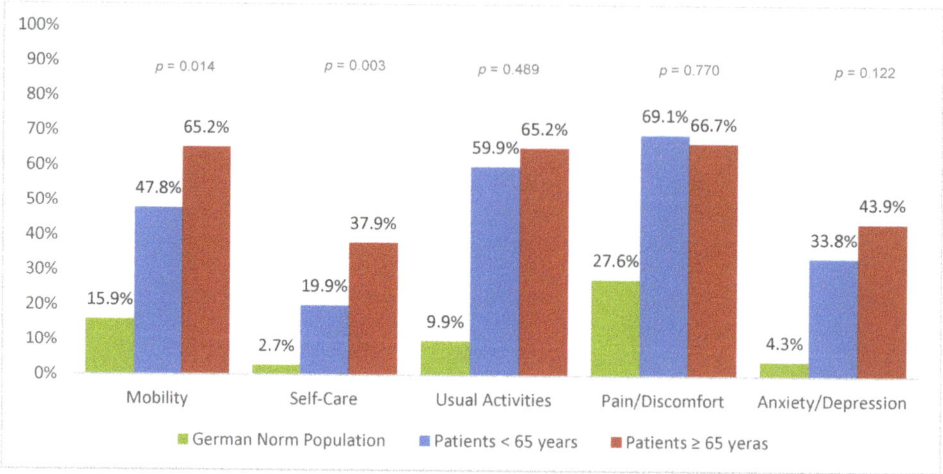

Figure 3. Reported problems in EQ-5D-3L dimensions 12 months after trauma (European Quality of Life 5 Dimensions 3 Level Version).

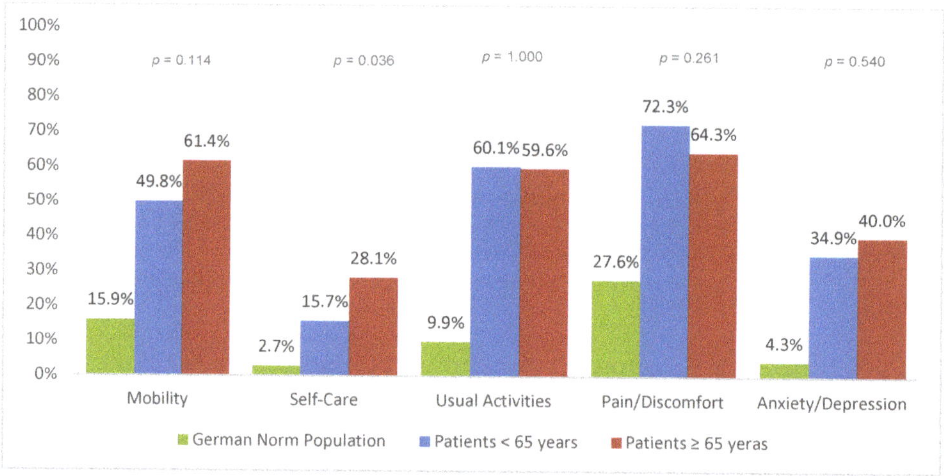

Figure 4. Reported problems in EQ-5D-3L dimension 24 months after trauma (European Quality of Life 5 Dimensions 3 Level Version).

The results of the mixed linear models support the notion that FCI, RISC II, AIS face, as well as AIS extremities, and ASA physical status have an impact on quality of life (Table 2). The EQ index and EQ VAS decreased with increasing RISC II as well as increasing ASA physical status, and increased with increasing FCI. With increasing AIS extremities, the EQ index and EQ VAS decreased.

Table 2 presents results of the main effects of AIS indices on quality of life.

Table 2. Impact of injury severity on quality of life.

		Estimate	95% CI		p Value
EQ index					
	FCI	0.04	0.02	0.06	<0.001
	RISC II	−0.003	−0.005	−0.001	0.001
	AIS head	−0.01	−0.02	0.01	0.315
	AIS face	0.03	0.00	0.06	0.026
	AIS thorax	−0.01	−0.03	0.01	0.198
	AIS abdomen	0.01	−0.01	0.03	0.178
	AIS extremities	−0.02	−0.04	0.00	0.016
	AIS soft tissue	−0.01	−0.04	0.03	0.742
	ASA physical status	−0.08	−0.12	−0.03	<0.001
EQ VAS					
	FCI	2.50	0.98	4.02	0.001
	RISC II	−0.23	−0.38	−0.09	0.001
	AIS head	−0.25	−1.60	1.09	0.712
	AIS face	1.86	−0.46	4.18	0.116
	AIS thorax	0.18	−1.16	1.52	0.789
	AIS abdomen	1.20	−0.24	2.64	0.101
	AIS extremities	−2.01	−3.49	−0.53	0.008
	AIS soft tissue	0.26	−2.41	2.93	0.847
	ASA physical status	−7.20	−10.63	−3.77	<0.001

Mixed linear models were used to assess the course of quality of life between patients aged <65 years and aged ≥65 years. These models were adjusted for injury severity measured by RISC II, FCI, AIS for each body region, and ASA physical status. Estimates of these injury severity parameters are presented.

Geriatric patients (≥65 years) reported a lower EQ index and EQ VAS 12 months and 24 months after trauma than patients under the age of 65 years (p-values < 0.012, (Table 3, Figures 5 and 6). The EQ index as well as the EQ VAS of geriatric patients (≥65 years) did not significantly change from 6 to 24 months after trauma (Table 3, Figures 5 and 6). The EQ index as well as the EQ VAS of patients under 65 years of age increased significantly from 6 to 12 to 24 months after trauma (Table 3, Figures 5 and 6). Post hoc tests showed that the EQ index of patients under the age of 65 years increased significantly from 6 to 12 months post trauma ($p = 0.037$), and from 12 to 24 months post trauma ($p = 0.028$). Moreover, EQ VAS was significantly lower 6 months post trauma than 12 as well as 24 months post trauma (p values < 0.001), but did not differ between 12 and 24 months post trauma ($p = 0.664$).

Table 3. Course of quality of life data depending on age.

	6 Months Post Trauma				12 Months Post Trauma				24 Months Post Trauma				p Value [2]
	n	m	95% CI		n	m	95% CI		n	m	95% CI		
EQ Index													
<65 years	256	0.70	0.66	0.74	268	0.74	0.70	0.77	247	0.77	0.74	0.81	0.004
≥65 years	55	0.69	0.61	0.77	55	0.69	0.61	0.76	44	0.73	0.64	0.81	0.558
p value [1]			0.755				0.232				0.304		
EQ VAS													
<65 years	262	61.2	58.2	64.2	268	69.3	66.6	72.1	248	68.8	65.9	71.6	<0.001
≥65 years	55	59.4	53.2	65.6	55	62.7	57.0	68.5	45	63.8	57.3	70.3	0.262
p value [1]			0.618				0.051				0.177		

Differences in quality of life between age groups and the course of quality of life within each age group were assessed by mixed linear models. Presented are the means (95% CI) of EQ index and global health visual analog scale (EQ VAS) for patients aged <65 years aged≥ 65 years 6, 12, and 24 months after trauma adjusted for RISC II, FCI, AIS for six body areas, ASA physical status, and sex. AIS, Abbreviated Injury Scale; RISC II, Revised Injury Severity Classification Score II; FCI, Functional Capacity Index; ASA physical status, American Society of Anesthesiologists Score; [1] p-value of differences between age groups; [2] p-value of course of quality of life over time with each age group.

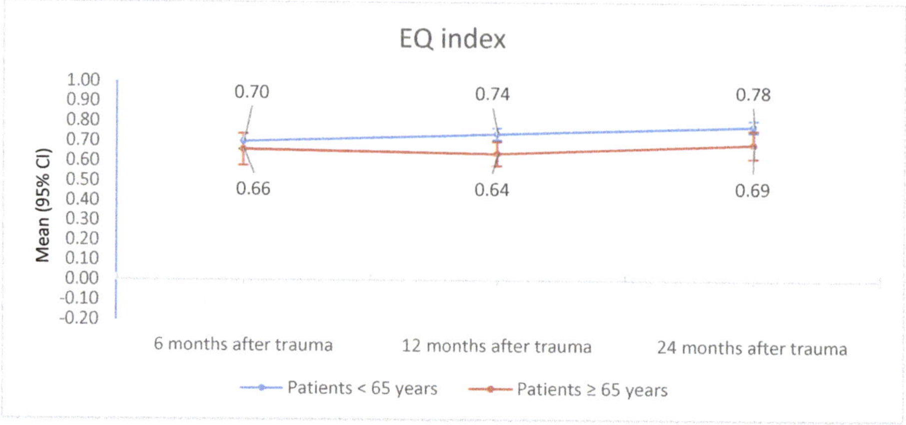

Figure 5. EQ index, adjusted for RISC II and FCI, of patients <65 years and ≥65 years of age 6, 12, and 24 months after trauma.

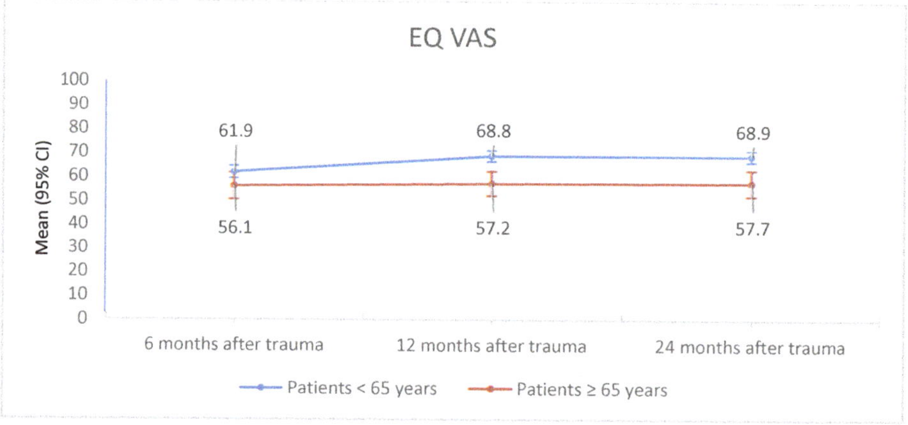

Figure 6. EQ VAS of patients <65 years and ≥65 years of age 6, 12, and 24 months after trauma.

The EQ index after 6, 12, and 24 months did not differ between male and female patients (Table 4). Moreover, the EQ index did not change over time within female and male patients (Table 4). Within male patients, no changes in EQ VAS from 6 to 24 months after trauma were found (Table 4). The EQ VAS of female patients increased significantly from 6 to 12 to 24 months after trauma (Table 4). Post hoc tests showed that EQ VAS was significantly lower 6 months post trauma than 12 as well as 24 months post trauma (p values < 0.001), but did not differ between 12 and 24 months post trauma ($p = 0.736$). However, female patients started with significantly lower EQ VAS than male patients ($p = 0.036$).

Table 4. Course of quality of life data depending on sex.

	6 Months Post Trauma				12 Months Post Trauma				24 Months Post Trauma				p Value [2]
	n	m	95% CI		n	m	95% CI		n	m	95% CI		
EQ Index													
male	220	0.72	0.67	0.78	232	0.72	0.68	0.77	212	0.76	0.72	0.81	0.193
female	91	0.67	0.60	0.74	91	0.70	0.64	0.76	79	0.74	0.67	0.81	0.242
p value [1]			0.209				0.546				0.548		
EQ VAS													
male	226	63.8	59.8	67.8	232	65.8	62.1	69.5	213	65.4	61.6	69.3	0.413
female	91	56.8	51.6	62.1	91	66.3	61.4	71.1	80	67.1	61.5	72.7	<0.001
p value [1]			0.036				0.883				0.614		

Differences in quality of life between male and female patients and the course of quality of life within each sex were assessed by mixed linear models. Presented are the means (95% CI) of EQ index and EQ VAS for male and female patients 6, 12, and 24 months after trauma adjusted for RISC II, FCI, and AIS for six body areas, ASA physical status, and age. AIS, Abbreviated Injury Scale; RISC II, Revised Injury Severity Classification Score II; FCI, Functional Capacity Index; ASA physical status, American Society of Anesthesiologists Score; [1] p-value of differences between age groups; [2] p-value of course of quality of life over time with each age group.

The EQ index as well as the EQ VAS of geriatric patients (≥65 years) did not significantly change from 6 to 24 months after trauma (Table 3, Figures 5 and 6). The EQ index as well as the EQ VAS of patients under 65 years of age increased significantly from 6 to 12 to 24 months after trauma (Table 3, Figures 5 and 6). Post hoc tests showed that the EQ index of patients under the age of 65 years increased significantly from 6 to 12 months post trauma, and from 12 to 24 months post trauma.

Moreover, EQ VAS was significantly lower 6 months post trauma than 12 as well as 24 months post trauma, but did not differ between 12 and 24 months post trauma.

5. Discussion

To our knowledge, this is the first study comparing HRQoL after major trauma in different age groups with a focus on geriatric patients. We found a limited HRQoL in geriatric patients up to 24 months after major trauma. Contrary to patients under the age of 65 years, geriatric patients showed no significant improvement in HRQoL (EQ index and EQ VAS) from 6 to 24 months after trauma.

The influence of age on mortality in severe injuries is a topic of ongoing research. Demetriades et al. found that geriatric trauma patients have a higher mortality in general, compared to younger patients, even after minor injury. Concordant with our results, they found that geriatric patients are also more likely to need intensive care unit (ICU) treatment and operations [15]. Kühne et al. and Morris et al. found that mortality rises with increasing age, regardless of ISS [16]. This is concordant with the findings in our study: The elderly had a lower mean ISS but a greater impairment in HRQoL. Grossman found that elderly trauma patients suffer more significant injuries compared to a younger cohort and have a higher mortality rate [17,18]. Sterling et al. found that death after same-level falls as a cause of death were 10 times more likely in the elderly [19]. The increased comorbidities in the elderly are often the reason for injury and contribute to worse outcome [4]. The unequal distribution of patients in the two groups in our study represents the typical age structure in major trauma. However, with a demographic trend towards the inverted population pyramid, a shift is to be expected. Rising numbers of elderly people will probably lead to an increase in geriatric trauma. Moreover, the baby boomers are starting to grow into the geriatric age group. It is assumed that this generation has a higher risk propensity [20] and a strong desire for optimum care and physical fitness and participation [21]. Therefore, this topic is gaining even more importance.

As life expectancy increases, the probability of comorbidities such as osteoporosis, leading to complex injury patterns even after minor traumatic incidents, also increases [22,23]. A systematic review and meta-analysis of several articles by Sammy et al. investigated contributing reasons for mortality in geriatric trauma patients. The factors affecting mortality included age and gender, comorbidities and medication (especially blood-thinning medication), as well as injury type and severity. Interestingly, mortality after low-level falls in the elderly was shown to be higher than after high velocity injuries [24–27]. In our study, low-level falls were the second most common reason for major trauma in geriatric patients. Falls are a common mechanism for geriatric trauma patients. Even though they present an overall lower ISS, they often sustain severe injuries to the head [28]. Unsteady gait, vision, hearing, and polypharmacy increase the risk of collapse, and anticoagulation medication increases the risk of hemorrhage [29]. Head, chest and proximal femur fractures are also more likely to occur.[17] For the comparison of the evolution of HRQoL over time, we included FCI, RISC II and the AIS of the body regions into the mixed linear model (MLM) to reduce confounding factors. Overall, the MLM revealed a significant impact of AIS face and AIS extremities on HRQoL

The subscale analysis of EQ index revealed larger impairments in geriatric patients for the categories self-care and mobility. An increase in mobility and self-care in the elderly leads to an improved physical and mental quality of life [30]. A lack of mobility is associated with reduced independence, decreased mental function, falls and consequently death [31,32]. Therefore, means of increasing elderly patient's mobility and involvement in self-care should be the main goal of rehabilitation.

Younger adults had lower values for pain/discomfort. Several studies indicated a higher pain threshold in the geriatric population [33]. However, older people are not simply less sensitive to pain. Sofaer et al. suggested that old people see pain as a normal part of aging, and therefore perceive pain as normal and inevitable [34]. Hence, older patients tend to report pain to a lesser extent and demand pain medication less frequently [35]. Nonetheless, pain leads to suffering and disability. This is why multimodal pain management is compulsory, especially in the elderly [36]. Mędrzycka-Dąbrowska et al. found that proper pain management can reduce mortality in geriatric patients [37]. Therefore, evidence-based guidelines for in-hospital treatment and rehabilitation are needed to standardize the care of geriatric trauma patients [38–40].

The paradoxical finding that geriatric patients with low impact trauma are at higher risk than patients who sustained higher velocity trauma should reflect on the triage of geriatric trauma patients [41]. The question remains whether established trauma severity measurement tools are able to reflect the patient's condition and if this is associated with the prognosis. Currently, the ISS is the standard evaluation instrument in the initial management of major trauma [16]. An ISS over 16 indicates major trauma associated with significant mortality. In the present study, only patients with an ISS greater than 16, indicating major trauma, were included. Although many patients with a lower ISS might be facing a comparable impairment of HRQoL, we focused on the high-risk population of geriatric major trauma reflected by an ISS over 16. Even though the ISS is a very effective tool to assess the severity of the injury and predict initial mortality, it has shown weakness in the prediction of prognosis and inclusion of interfering factors, such as comorbidities [24,28]. Therefore, the development of an assessment tool specifically for geriatric trauma for initial triage and further treatment might be valuable. Under-triage of geriatric patients often begins during the pre-hospital assessment. A worse general health status and preexisting conditions complicate clinical examination and the initial grading of injury severity [42]. Advanced age is associated with transport to a lower level of trauma care [43]. We also recorded a trend to a lower level of care of the primary admission facility with advanced patient age. In the literature, initial under-triage is associated with increased mortality [43]. Unconscious age bias occurs in pre-hospital providers, as well as hospitals, and therefore one must maintain a high clinical suspicion for serious injuries, regardless of the mechanism of injury [42,44]. The triage to a high-level trauma center, especially one with a high number of geriatric cases, is linked to better outcomes for the elderly [44]. A team approach with interdisciplinary care involving geriatricians, social workers, and pharmacists supervised by surgeons improves the quality of trauma care to address comorbidities, geriatric syndromes, care planning and rehabilitation, medication and pain management right from the beginning of hospitalization may reduce mortality and improve functional outcome [38,42]. Post-discharge issues are as important as the initial management of severe injuries in the elderly population. Post-acute rehabilitation and the patients' functionality have a relevant impact on outcome [29]. There are few studies focusing on geriatric severe trauma. Measurement of outcome in geriatric trauma is mostly limited to mortality [6].

Facing the socio-economic impact of trauma and a decreasing mortality due to preventive measures and patient-centered outcome tools are increasingly relevant. More than ever, the aspect of HRQoL after severe trauma gains importance [45,46]. The main focus of this study was the assessment of posttraumatic HRQoL in geriatric major trauma patients. HRQoL can be defined as "how well a person functions in their life and his or her perceived wellbeing in physical, mental, and social domains of health" [47]. We used the EQ-5D-3L for HRQoL assessment 6, 12, and 24 months post trauma. Even though HRQoL decreases throughout life [48], we found significant impairment of HRQoL in geriatric patients compared to the general population.

Our study also reveals a significantly worse recovery over time for geriatric patients. The impairment of major trauma on geriatric patient's HRQoL is greater than in patients younger than 65 years. Contrary to geriatric patients, the control group under 65 years experienced a significant improvement in HRQoL within the first year after trauma. Even though PROM tools are gaining importance, HRQoL is under-researched in elderly severe trauma patients. Our study shows that geriatric patients particularly reported a loss of mobility, self-care and an increase in anxiety and depression. Few data exist on recovery for the elderly trauma patients. Undesirable conditions such as delirium, posttraumatic stress disorder, and depression might have a significant impact and lead to persistence in limitations of HRQoL [38]. In the last couple of years, ortho-geriatric trauma centers have been founded aiming for an improvement in the quality of care of elderly after trauma. Since this initiative was started after the closure of recruitment for this study, the question remains whether this has a significant impact on the quality of life after major trauma in the elderly.

The main limitation of our study is the limited number of cases. Even though major trauma in geriatrics is on the rise, there are only a limited number of cases even in a large trauma network like the TNO. Reporting on a specific patient cohort implicates a limitation of generalizability and bias. The low number of penetrating injuries is only one example, such that the data are specific for the reported patient population and the results might not be transferrable to other populations where the majority of patients sustain penetrating injuries due to violence. Another limitation is that due to the design of this large multicenter trial, an extension to clinical follow-up examinations was not possible. Therefore, we cannot present clinical follow-up data for correlation with HRQoL. Since this study was conducted in a heath-service context, there are many potential sources of bias or imprecision. Great efforts have been taken to improve data quality, as published before [9]. Assessment of data quality proved an excellent documentation rate of >95% in all major trauma patients. To reduce the impact of not uniformly distributed confounders between both age groups, the MLM included factors that were assumed to be potentially influencing the results, such as FCI, RISC II, and AIS of each body region. Furthermore, the MLM replaces missing values by using maximum likelihood estimates. Thus, all patients, even those with missing quality of life values at specific points of time, could be used for the analyses.

In general, non-participation is a major issue in longitudinal studies. Our strategy for diminishing this effect was to compare baseline characteristics of participants with non-participants, which showed no significant discrepancy between the two groups. Still, participation dissent can introduce selection bias.

There might be other confounding factors that we did not take into account. However, including all major trauma patients in a specific geographic region and considering all clinically relevant factors, we aimed for unbiased estimates of HRQoL means. The strength of this study lies in its prospective multicenter registry-based design and data quality. Even though the study lacks a sample size calculation, we think it serves its purpose as a reference point when calculating sample sizes for further studies. However, further studies on the evaluation of HRQoL in post-traumatic conditions of the elderly would be valuable to confirm these results.

6. Conclusions

Our study is the largest elaboration on geriatric HRQoL after major trauma. We found a limited HRQoL measured by EQ-5D-3L in geriatric patients after major trauma. HRQoL of geriatric patients stagnated at a low level from 6 to 24 months after trauma. Compared to patients under the age of 65 years and the normal values of the general population, this suggests a relevant impairment of HRQoL after major trauma. Further evolution of ortho-geriatric initiatives is necessary to improve the care of the elderly after major trauma.

Author Contributions: Conceptualization, V.F. and F.B.; Data curation, V.F. and F.B.; Formal analysis, K.M.; Funding acquisition, A.E.; Methodology, A.E.; Project administration, V.A. and F.B.; Supervision, V.A.; Writing–original draft, V.F.; Writing–review & editing, M.K., L.B., C.P., V.A. and F.B. All authors have read and agreed to the published version of the manuscript.

Funding: This research received no external funding.

Conflicts of Interest: The authors declare that they have no conflict of interest.

References

1. Statistisches Bundesamt (Destatis). Bevölkerung im Wandel Annahmen und Ergebnisse der 14. koordinierten Bevölkerungsvorausberechnung. 2019. Available online: https://www.destatis.de/DE/Presse/Pressekonferenzen/2019/Bevoelkerung/pressebroschuere-bevoelkerung.pdf?__blob=publicationFile (accessed on 1 February 2020).
2. Gather, A.; Grützner, P.A.; Münzberg, M. Polytrauma in old Age-Knowledge from the TraumaRegister DGU®. *Chirurg* **2019**, *90*, 791–794. [CrossRef]
3. Shankar, K.N.; Liu, S.W.; Ganz, D.A. Trends and Characteristics of Emergency Department Visits for Fall-Related Injuries in Older Adults, 2003–2010. *West J. Emerg. Med.* **2017**, *18*, 785–793. [CrossRef]
4. Kirshenbom, D.; Ben-Zaken, Z.; Albilya, N.; Niyibizi, E.; Bala, M. Older Age, Comorbid Illnesses, and Injury Severity Affect Immediate Outcome in Elderly Trauma Patients. *J. Emerg. Trauma Shock* **2017**, *10*, 146–150.
5. Bala, M.; Willner, D.; Klauzn, D.; Bdolah-Abram, T.; Rivkind, A.; Abu Gazala, M.; Elazary, R.; Almogy, G. Pre-hospital and admission parameters predict in-hospital mortality among patients 60 years and older following severe trauma. *Scand. J. Trauma Resusc. Emerg. Med.* **2013**, *21*, 91. [CrossRef]
6. Crawford, S.M. Changing the System-Major Trauma Patients and Their Outcomes in the NHS (England) 2008-17. *Eclinicalmedicine* **2018**, *4*, 3. [CrossRef]
7. Wang, M.C.; Bellows, J. Quality of Life and Patient-Centered Outcomes. In *Chronic Illness Care: Principles and Practice*; Daaleman, T.P., Helton, M.R., Eds.; Springer International Publishing: Cham, Switzerland, 2018; pp. 95–107. [CrossRef]
8. Ernstberger, A.; Koller, M.; Nerlich, M. Quality circle in a trauma network of the German Association for Trauma Surgery. Upgrading patient care. *Unfallchirurg* **2011**, *114*, 172–181. [CrossRef]
9. Koller, M.; Ernstberger, A.; Zeman, F.; Loss, J.; Nerlich, M. Trauma Network Eastern Bavaria (TNO). Outcome after polytrauma in a certified trauma network: Comparing standard vs. maximum care facilities concept of the study and study protocol (POLYQUALY). *BMC Health Serv. Res.* **2016**, *16*, 242. [CrossRef]
10. Rabin, R.; de Charro, F. EQ-5D: A measure of health status from the EuroQol Group. *Ann. Med.* **2001**, *33*, 337–343. [CrossRef]
11. Greiner, W.; Claes, C.; Busschbach, J.J.V.; von der Schulenburg, J.-M.G. Validating the EQ-5D with time trade off for the German population. *Eur. J. Health Econ.* **2005**, *6*, 124–130. [CrossRef]
12. Baker, S.P.; O'Neill, B.; Haddon, W.; Long, W.B. The injury severity score: A method for describing patients with multiple injuries and evaluating emergency care. *J. Trauma* **1974**, *14*, 187–196. [CrossRef]
13. Lefering, R.; Huber-Wagner, S.; Nienaber, U.; Maegele, M.; Bouillon, B. Update of the trauma risk adjustment model of the TraumaRegister DGU™: The Revised Injury Severity Classification, version II. *Crit. Care* **2014**, *18*, 476. [CrossRef] [PubMed]
14. MacKenzie, E.J.; Damiano, A.; Miller, T.; Luchter, S. The development of the Functional Capacity Index. *J. Trauma* **1996**, *41*, 799–807. [CrossRef]

15. Demetriades, D.; Sava, J.; Alo, K.; Newton, E.; Velmahos, G.C.; Murray, J.A.; Belzberg, H.; Asensio, J.A.; Berne, T.V. Old age as a criterion for trauma team activation. *J. Trauma* **2001**, *51*, 754–756, discussion 756–757. [CrossRef] [PubMed]
16. Kuhne, C.A.; Ruchholtz, S.; Kaiser, G.M.; Nast-Kolb, D.; Working Group on Multiple Trauma of the German Society of Trauma. Mortality in severely injured elderly trauma patients-when does age become a risk factor? *World J. Surg.* **2005**, *29*, 1476–1482. [CrossRef] [PubMed]
17. Bergeron, E.; Clement, J.; Lavoie, A.; Ratte, S.; Bamvita, J.-M.; Aumont, F.; Clas, D. A simple fall in the elderly: Not so simple. *J. Trauma* **2006**, *60*, 268–273. [CrossRef]
18. Grossman, M.D.; Miller, D.; Scaff, D.W.; Arcona, S. When is an elder old? Effect of preexisting conditions on mortality in geriatric trauma. *J. Trauma* **2002**, *52*, 242–246. [CrossRef] [PubMed]
19. Sterling, D.A.; O'Connor, J.A.; Bonadies, J. Geriatric falls: Injury severity is high and disproportionate to mechanism. *J. Trauma* **2001**, *50*, 116–119. [CrossRef]
20. Puac-Polanco, V.; Keyes, K.M.; Li, G. Mortality from motorcycle crashes: The baby-boomer cohort effect. *Inj. Epidemiol.* **2016**, *3*, 19. [CrossRef]
21. Arendt, E.A.; DiNubile, N.D. Toward optimal health: The experts discuss fitness among baby boomers. Interview by Jodi Godfrey Meisler. *J. Womens Health* **2003**, *12*, 219–225.
22. Skaga, N.O.; Eken, T.; Søvik, S.; Jones, J.M.; Steen, P.A. Pre-injury ASA physical status classification is an independent predictor of mortality after trauma. *J. Trauma* **2007**, *63*, 972–978. [CrossRef]
23. Ringdal, K.G.; Skaga, N.O.; Steen, P.A.; Hestnes, M.; Laake, P.; Jones, J.M.; Lossius, H.M. Classification of comorbidity in trauma: The reliability of pre-injury ASA physical status classification. *Injury* **2013**, *44*, 29–35. [CrossRef]
24. Sammy, I.; Lecky, F.; Sutton, A.; Leaviss, J.; O'Cathain, A. Factors affecting mortality in older trauma patients-A systematic review and meta-analysis. *Injury* **2016**, *47*, 1170–1183. [CrossRef]
25. Zhu, Z.; Shang, X.; Qi, P.; Ma, S. Sex-based differences in outcomes after severe injury: An analysis of blunt trauma patients in China. *Scand. J. Trauma Resusc. Emerg. Med.* **2017**, *25*, 47. [CrossRef] [PubMed]
26. Angele, M.K.; Frantz, M.C.; Chaudry, I.H. Gender and sex hormones influence the response to trauma and sepsis: Potential therapeutic approaches. *Clinics* **2006**, *61*, 479–488. [CrossRef]
27. Sperry, J.L.; Nathens, A.B.; Frankel, H.L.; Vanek, S.L.; Moore, E.E.; Maier, R.V.; Minei, J.P. Characterization of the gender dimorphism after injury and hemorrhagic shock: Are hormonal differences responsible? *Crit. Care Med.* **2008**, *36*, 1838–1845. [CrossRef] [PubMed]
28. Brown, C.V.R.; Rix, K.; Klein, A.L.; Ford, B.; Teixeira, P.G.R.; Aydelotte, J.; Coopwood, B.; Ali, S. A Comprehensive Investigation of Comorbidities, Mechanisms, Injury Patterns, and Outcomes in Geriatric Blunt Trauma Patients. *Am. Surg.* **2016**, *82*, 1055–1062. [CrossRef] [PubMed]
29. DiMaggio, C.; Ayoung-Chee, P.; Shinseki, M.; Wilson, C.; Marshall, G.; Lee, D.C.; Wall, S.; Maulana, S.; Pachter, H.L.; Frangos, S. Traumatic injury in the United States: In-patient epidemiology 2000–2011. *Injury* **2016**, *47*, 1393–1403. [CrossRef] [PubMed]
30. Fagerström, C.; Borglin, G. Mobility, functional ability and health-related quality of life among people of 60 years or older. *Aging Clin. Exp. Res.* **2010**, *22*, 387–394. [CrossRef]
31. Patel, A.V.; Bernstein, L.; Deka, A.; Spencer Feigelson, H.; Campbell, P.T.; Gapstur, S.M.; Colditz, G.A.; Thun, M.J. Leisure time spent sitting in relation to total mortality in a prospective cohort of US adults. *Am. J. Epidemiol.* **2010**, *172*, 419–429. [CrossRef] [PubMed]
32. Hirvensalo, M.; Rantanen, T.; Heikkinen, E. Mobility difficulties and physical activity as predictors of mortality and loss of independence in the community-living older population. *J. Am. Geriatr. Soc.* **2000**, *48*, 493–498. [CrossRef]
33. Kaye, A.D.; Baluch, A.; Scott, J.T. Pain management in the elderly population: A review. *Ochsner J.* **2010**, *10*, 179–187.
34. Sofaer, B.; Moore, A.P.; Holloway, I.; Lamberty, J.M.; Thorp, T.A.; O'Dwyer, J. Chronic pain as perceived by older people: A qualitative study. *Age Ageing.* **2005**, *34*, 462–466. [CrossRef] [PubMed]
35. McCleane, G.; Smith, H. *Clinical Management of the Elderly Patient in Pain*; CRC Press: Boca Raton, FL, USA, 2006.
36. Noroozian, M.; Raeesi, S.; Hashemi, R.; Khedmat, L.; Vahabi, Z. Pain: The Neglect Issue in Old People's Life. *Open Access Maced. J. Med. Sci.* **2018**, *6*, 1773–1778. [CrossRef] [PubMed]

37. Wioletta, M.-D.; Sebastian, D.; Andrzej, B. Perception of barriers to postoperative pain management in elderly patients in Polish hospitals—A multicentre study. *J. Nurs. Manag.* **2016**, *24*, 1049–1059. [CrossRef] [PubMed]
38. Kozar, R.A.; Arbabi, S.; Stein, D.M.; Shackford, S.R.; Barraco, R.D.; Biffl, W.L.; Brasel, K.J.; Cooper, Z.; Fakhry, S.M.; Livingston, D.; et al. Injury in the aged: Geriatric trauma care at the crossroads. *J. Trauma Acute Care Surg.* **2015**, *78*, 1197–1209. [CrossRef]
39. Fares, A. Pharmacological and Non-Pharmacological Means for Prevention of Fractures among Elderly. *Int. J. Prev. Med.* **2018**, *9*, 78. [CrossRef] [PubMed]
40. Verhoeff, K.; Glen, P.; Taheri, A.; Min, B.; Tsang, B.; Fawcett, V.; Widder, S. Implementation and adoption of advanced care planning in the elderly trauma patient. *World J. Emerg. Surg.* **2018**, *13*, 40. [CrossRef]
41. Wong, T.H.; Wong, Y.J.; Lau, Z.Y.; Nadkarni, N.; Lim, G.H.; Seow, D.C.; Ong, M.E.; Tan, K.B.; Nguyen, H.V.; Wong, C.H. Not All Falls Are Equal: Risk Factors for Unplanned Readmission in Older Patients After Moderate and Severe Injury-A National Cohort Study. *J. Am. Med. Dir. Assoc.* **2019**, *20*, 201–207.e3. [CrossRef]
42. Southern, A.P.; Lopez, R.A.; Jwayyed, S. Geriatric Trauma. In *StatPearls*; StatPearls Publishing: Bethesda, MD, USA, 2020. Available online: https://www.ncbi.nlm.nih.gov/books/NBK442020/ (accessed on 1 February 2020).
43. Gage, A.M.; Traven, N.; Rivara, F.P.; Jurkovich, G.J.; Arbabi, S. Compliance with Centers for Disease Control and Prevention field triage guidelines in an established trauma system. *J. Am. Coll. Surg.* **2012**, *215*, 148–154; discussion 154–156. [CrossRef]
44. Chang, D.C.; Bass, R.R.; Cornwell, E.E.; Mackenzie, E.J. Undertriage of elderly trauma patients to state-designated trauma centers. *Arch Surg.* **2008**, *143*, 776–781; discussion 782. [CrossRef]
45. Ruchholtz, S.; Lefering, R.; Paffrath, T.; Oestern, H.J.; Neugebauer, E.; Nast-Kolb, D.; Pape, H.C.; Bouillon, B. Reduction in mortality of severely injured patients in Germany. *Dtsch Arztebl Int.* **2008**, *105*, 225–231. [CrossRef] [PubMed]
46. Von Oelreich, E.; Eriksson, M.; Brattström, O.; Discacciati, A.; Strömmer, L.; Oldner, A.; Larsson, E. Post-trauma morbidity, measured as sick leave, is substantial and influenced by factors unrelated to injury: A retrospective matched observational cohort study. *Scand. J. Trauma Resusc. Emerg. Med.* **2017**, *25*, 100. [CrossRef] [PubMed]
47. Hays, R.D. Measurement and Modeling of Health-Related Quality of Life. In *Epidemiology and Demography in Public Health*; Killewo, J., Heggenhougen, H.K., Quah, S.R., Eds.; Academic Press: Cambridge, MA, USA, 2010; pp. 195–205.
48. Hinz, A.; Klaiberg, A.; Brähler, E.; König, H.-H. The Quality of Life Questionnaire EQ-5D: Modelling and norm values for the general population. *Psychother. Psychosom. Med. Psychol.* **2006**, *56*, 42–48. [CrossRef] [PubMed]

Journal of
Clinical Medicine

MDPI

Article

Is the Additional Effort for an Intraoperative CT Scan Justified for Distal Radius Fracture Fixations? A Comparative Clinical Feasibility Study

Sascha Halvachizadeh [1,2,*], Till Berk [1], Alexander Pieringer [1], Emanuael Ried [1], Florian Hess [3], Roman Pfeifer [1,2], Hans-Christoph Pape [1,2] and Florin Allemann [1]

1 Department of Trauma, University Hospital Zurich, Raemistrasse 100, 8091 Zurich, Switzerland; Till.Berk@usz.ch (T.B.); Alexander.Pieringer@usz.ch (A.P.); Emanuael.Ried@balgrist.ch (E.R.); Roman.Pfeifer@usz.ch (R.P.); Hans-Christoph.Pape@usz.ch (H.-C.P.); Florin.Allemann@usz.ch (F.A.)

2 Harald-Tscherne Research Laboratory, University Hospital Zurich, Sternwartstrasse 14, 8091 Zurich, Switzerland

3 Department of Orthopaedic Surgery and Traumatology, Cantonal Hospital Frauenfeld, Pfaffenholzstrasse 4, 8501 Frauenfeld, Switzerland; florian.hess@stgag.ch

* Correspondence: Sascha.Halvachizadeh@usz.ch; Tel.: +41-794-648-233

Received: 5 May 2020; Accepted: 14 July 2020; Published: 16 July 2020

Abstract: Introduction: It is currently unclear whether the additional effort to perform an intraoperative computed tomography (CT) scan is justified for articular distal radius fractures (DRFs). The purpose of this study was to assess radiological, functional, and clinical outcomes after surgical treatment of distal radius fractures when using conventional fluoroscopy vs. intraoperative CT scans. Methods: Inclusion criteria: Surgical treatment of DRF between 1 January 2011 and 31 December 2011, age 18 and above. Group distribution: intraoperative conventional fluoroscopy (Group Conv) or intraoperative CT scans (Group CT). Exclusion criteria: Use of different image intensifier devices or incomplete data. DRF classification according to the Arbeitsgemeinschaft für Osteosynthesefragen (AO) classification. Outcome variables included requirement of revision surgeries, duration of surgery, absorbed radiation dose, and requirement of additional CT scans during hospitalization. Results: A total of 187 patients were included (Group Conv n = 96 (51.3%), Group CT n = 91 (48.7%)). AO Classification: Type A fractures n = 40 (50%) in Group Conv vs. n = 16 (17.6%) in Group CT, $p < 0.001$; Type B: 10 (10.4%) vs. 11 (12.1%), not significant (n.s.); Type C: 38 (39.6%) vs. 64 (70.3%), $p < 0.001$. In Group Conv, four (4.2%) patients required revision surgeries within 6 months, but in Group CT no revision surgery was required. The CT scan led to an intraoperative screw exchange/reposition in 23 (25.3%) cases. The duration of the initial surgery (81.7 ± 46.4 min vs. 90.1 ± 43.6 min, n.s.) was comparable. The radiation dose was significantly higher in Group CT (6.9 ± 1.3 vs. 2.8 ± 7.8 mGy, $p < 0.001$). In Group Conv, 11 (11.5%) patients required additional CT scans during hospitalization. Conclusion: The usage of intraoperative CT was associated with improved reduction and more adequate positioning of screws postoperatively with comparable durations of surgery. Despite increased efforts by utilizing the intraoperative CT scan, the decrease in reoperations may justify its use.

Keywords: intraoperative CT scan; distal radius fracture; O-arm radius fracture; intraoperative CT scan in trauma

1. Introduction

Distal radius fractures (DRFs) represent the most common fractures of the upper extremity in adults (17.5%) [1]. Exact restoration of the anatomy and correct screw placement in the relevant fragment can be challenging, especially if the posterior articular surface is involved, or in cases of severe impaction [2]. These cases require revision surgery and the outcome is unfavorable (decreased range of motion, later wrist fusion) [3]. With conventional intraoperative imaging, incomplete reduction and inadequate screw placements have been reported [4]. The use of conventional fluoroscopy during surgery provides limited information, especially in complex DRFs [5]. Imaging of DRFs may include computed tomography (CT), especially in complex intra-articular fractures. The CT scan is a well-established imaging method that has proven diagnostic value [6]. To date, the majority of CT studies, however, are obtained for diagnostic reasons and for classification of injuries [7,8]. Advancements in intraoperative imaging, including mobile CT scans, have improved intraoperative image quality and allowed for immediate control of the osteosynthesis [9]. CT-based navigations have been used to increase the accuracy of screw and plate positioning during open reduction internal fixation (ORIF) of DRFs [10].

There continues to be a lack of studies that investigate the effects of intraoperative CT scans on the treatment of DRFs. The objective of this study was to compare surgical, radiological, and functional outcomes after operative treatment of DRFs with and without the use of intraoperative CT scans. We therefore aimed to answer the following questions:

- Is the use of intraoperative CT scans associated with increased surgical time and radiation dosage?
- Does an intraoperative CT scan lead to intraoperative revisions that may prevent reoperations?
- Does the intraoperative CT scan reduce the requirement of secondary CT scans during hospitalization?

2. Methods

This study was conducted with the approval of the cantonal ethical committee (Kantonale Ethikkommission, KEK, Zürich) and the institutional review board (IRB) under the license numbers 2019-01957 and 2018-00146.

2.1. Study Design and Study Population

This retrospective comparative study was performed among patients treated between 1 January 2011 and 31 December 2018, and was conducted in compliance with the Strengthening the Reporting of Observational studies in Epidemiology (STROBE) guidelines [11].

The inclusion criteria were as follows: patients aged 18 years and over who required surgical treatment of a distal radius fracture at one academic Level 1 trauma center.

Exclusion criteria: patients with incomplete data sets, missing radiation values, usage of other imaging techniques/devices, reoperations, open fractures, or more than one surgical intervention during the same session.

All patients were treated by a variable angle-locked compression plate (VA-LCP) and a two-column volar distal radius plate 2.4 (VA-LCP 2.4 mm, DePuy Synthes, 4436 Oberdorf, Switzerland).

The follow-up period was six months after surgery. Our standardized follow-up foresees 2 weeks, 6 weeks, 12 weeks, and 6 months of post-operative clinical and radiological examination.

2.2. Group Distribution and Intraoperative Radiologic Protocol

Intraoperative imaging defined the stratification of patients: conventional fluoroscopy (Group Conv) or additional intraoperative CT scans using the O-arm (O-arm; Medtronic, Minneapolis, MN) with standard configurations for extremity scans (Group CT).

2.3. Protocol for Intraoperative CT Use

According to our in-house protocol, an intraoperative CT scan has been used in all Type C fractures since 2015. After initial reduction, a fluoroscopic assessment of the plate and screw position is performed. The final assessment is then performed by a CT scan. If correction is required, a second CT scan is added after revision.

2.4. Definitions and Outcome Parameters

All DRFs were classified according to the Arbeitsgemeinschaft für Osteosynthesefragen (AO) classification [12]. Surgical factors: fracture classification with associated intraoperative imaging technique, duration of surgery, revision rate intraoperatively, and revision surgeries within six months after initial treatment. These data were retrieved from the radiological statement prior to surgery and the surgical report.

The radiological outcome included intraoperative radiation doses and the requirement of secondary CT scans after surgery during hospitalization. These data are automatically calculated by the imaging intensifier device (conventional fluoroscopy or intraoperative CT scan) and electronically sent to the patient's chart.

During re-examination, the senior author (F.A.) measured the range of motion (ROM) in person to minimize inter-observer variability. The ROM was measured in six degrees of freedom: dorsal extension, palmar flexion, radial abduction, ulnar abduction, pronation, and supination.

A potential confounder was the fracture classification according to AO [13]. Therefore, the analysis included additional stratification according to the AO classification. The study size is based on the maximal available data set, according the inclusion and exclusion criteria.

2.5. Statistical Analysis

Continuous variables are summarized as mean and standard deviation, and categorical variables as number and percentage. Group comparison of two groups was performed using Student's *t*-test for continuous variables, and the Pearson chi-squared test for discrete variables. ANOVA was performed to compare groups of more than two partners. Patients were stratified according to the imaging technique during surgery, and according to the fracture classification to control for confounding. Statistical significance was assumed at an alpha of 5% ($p < 0.05$). All analyses were performed using R (R Core Team (2019). R: a language and environment for statistical computing. R Foundation for Statistical Computing, Vienna, Austria. URL https://www.R-project.org/).

3. Results

We included 187 patients (mean age 55.1 years (±19.4 y)), among which 131 (70.1%) were females. In all patients, an acute fracture was the reason for fixation. The distribution according to the AO classification was as follows: Type A fracture (n = 64, 34.2%), Type B fracture (n = 21, 11.2%), Type C fracture (n = 102, 54.5%).

3.1. Patient Demographics

Group Conv (n = 96, 51.3%) and Group CT (n = 91, 48.7%) were comparable in age, gender distribution, body mass index (BMI), length of stay, and duration until returning to work. The incidence of Type A fractures in the Conv Group was 50% vs. 17.6% in the CT Group ($p < 0.001$). In Group CT, the leading fracture was Type C fractures, with 70.3% vs. 39.6% in the Conv Group ($p < 0.001$) (Table 1).

Table 1. Patient demographics.

	Group Conv	Group CT	p-Value
n	96	91	
Age (years), mean (SD)	54.8 (19.7)	55.4 (19.1)	n.s.
Female gender, n (%)	67 (69.8)	64 (70.3)	n.s.
BMI (kg/m^2), mean (SD)	24.6 (4.4)	26.5 (17.3)	n.s.
AO classification, n (%)			
A	48 (50.0)	16 (17.6)	<0.001
B	10 (10.4)	11 (12.1)	n.s.
C	38 (39.6)	64 (70.3)	<0.001
Length of stay (days), mean (SD)	7.0 (8.8)	7.9 (6.6)	n.s.
Weeks until return to work, mean (SD)	5.9 (4.4)	6.2 (4.5)	n.s.

n = Number of patients; SD = Standard Deviation; n.s. = Not Significant ($p > 0.05$); BMI = Body Mass Index; AO = Arbeitsgemeinschaft für Osteosynthesefragen.

3.2. Intraoperative Revisions and Revision Surgeries

In Group Conv, 11 patients (11.5%) required a secondary CT scan after surgery. Out of these, four patients (36.4%) required revision surgeries: one case required a revision surgery due to intra-articular screw positioning, two cases required revision due to a malreduced fracture, and one case required a secondary stabilization of the distal radio-ulnar joint. None of the patients in Group CT required revision surgeries within six months. However, in 23 cases (25.3%) the CT scan revealed inadequate reduction, or inadequate implant position, that led to intraoperative revision.

3.3. Duration of Surgery and Radiation Dosage

Group Conv and Group CT were comparable in duration of surgery (95%CI 21.4 to 4.6, $p = 0.21$). The intraoperative radiation dose was significantly lower in Group Conv compared with Group CT (2.8 ± 7.8 mGy vs. 6.9 ± 1.3, $p < 0.001$). Group Conv required secondary CT scans after surgery during hospitalization in 11.5% of cases (Table 2). The radiation dosage of a secondary CT scan was significantly higher in Group Conv compared with the total intraoperative radiation dosage of Group CT (8.3 ± 2.5 mGy vs. 6.9 ± 1.3 mGy, 95%CI 0.4 to 3.2, $p = 0.02$).

Table 2. Radiographic and intraoperative data.

	Group Conv	Group CT	p-Value
n	96	91	
Revision Surgeries within 6 months, n (%)	4 (4.2)	0 (0.0)	n.s.
Intraoperative revision based on CT, n (%)	Not documented	23 (25.3%)	NA
Duration of surgery (minutes), mean (SD)	81.7 (46.4)	90.1 (43.6)	n.s.
Intraoperative Radiation Dose (mGy), mean (SD)	2.8 (7.8)	6.9 (1.3)	<0.001
Requirement of secondary CT scan, n (%)	11 (11.5%)	0 (0%)	<0.001
Radiation Dose of secondary CT scan (mGy), mean (SD)	8.3 (2.5)	NA	

AO = Arbeitsgemeinschaft für Osteosynthesefragen; n = Number of patients; SD = Standard Deviation; mGy = milligray; n.s. = Not Significant ($p > 0.05$).

3.4. Range of Motion

In Group Conv: Ulnar abduction Type A 30.4 ± 8.9° vs. Type B 51.0 ± 10.0°, $p = 0.0026$; Pronation Type A 85.7 ± 4.3° vs. Type B 65.0 ± 28.3°, $p < 0.001$ and vs. Type C 82.1 ± 8.2, $p = 0.03$; and Supination Type A 85.6 ± 5.7° vs. Type B 66.0 ± 32.9° $p = 0.001$ and vs. Type C 75.1 ± 26.8, $p = 0.004$. Type A, Type B, and Type C fractures had comparable ROMs in Group CT (Figure 1).

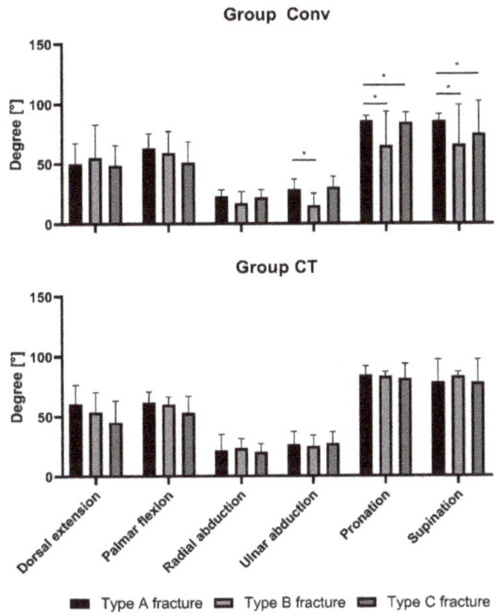

Figure 1. Comparison of Range of Motion (ROM) at six months after initial surgery of Group CT and Group Conv. While there is a significant difference amongst the subgroups in Group Conv, the ROM appears to be independent of the severity of fracture in Group CT. Types of fracture are classified according to the AO classification; * = significant difference ($p < 0.05$).

4. Discussion

Intraoperative anatomic reduction has been known to be a cofactor for good results in intra-articular fractures and those adjacent to joints [12]. Recent advancements in radiological imaging and improvement of CT technologies have led to an increased use of CT scans intraoperatively to guide and facilitate surgical interventions [14–16]. Currently, spine surgeons routinely use intraoperative CT scans [17,18]. Reports about the use for intra-articular fractures of the extremity are sparse [5]. In distal radius fractures, the variable anatomy and limited ability to visualize the dorsal aspect of the fracture's articular surface represents a special challenge during surgical fixation of these fractures [19].

Our study provides the following main results:

1. The use of an intraoperative CT scan did not increase duration of surgery.
2. Intraoperative correction of screw positioning was performed in 25.3% of cases in Group CT. No further revision surgery was required.
3. Secondary CT scans were required in 11.5% of cases where no intraoperative CT was performed, resulting in an increased cumulative radiation dosage and revision surgeries in 36.4% of cases.

According to our data, the use of an intraoperative CT scan did not affect the overall duration of surgery. The time required for an intraoperative CT scan was shown to be 3 to 5 minutes during surgical correction of scoliosis without significant prolongation of the operation time [20]. During surgery of a

DRF, the use of an intraoperative CT scan might take 6.7 ± 1.8 (range 4.3–13.3) minutes [5]. Previous authors have suggested that the duration of surgery may be less dependent on the imaging technique (fluoroscopy, CT scan) and more dependent on the experience of the surgeon, or the indication for surgery [21].

In a laboratory study with cadavers, no significant difference in breach rate between CT scans and fluoroscopy was observed during pedicle screw insertion [22]. Another study concluded that the increased radiation dose after the use of an intraoperative CT scan with an image-guided system was acceptable, given the benefits of CT imaging [23].

The present study indicates that the intraoperative use of CT is associated with higher levels of intraoperative radiation. During the postoperative course, some patients of Group Conv also required CT, which leads to a lesser sustained total radiation exposure. Another study indicates that during surgical treatment of DRFs, radiation exposure from fluoroscopy was 14.1 ± 15.4 $cGycm^2$ compared with 19.3 ± 16.9 $cGycm^2$ in cases where an additional CT scan was used, representing an increase of 36.9% [5]. This increase in radiation after additional usage of intraoperative CT scans is comparable with reported data that might range from 4.8 to 195% [5].

The use of CT scans has been suggested to improve visibility and assessment of intra-articular fractures [24]. Further, the use of postoperative CT scans after ORIF of DRFs provides more information regarding potential intra-articular placements of screws that otherwise would have been missed [25]. Our study revealed that in 11.5% of cases, a secondary CT scan was required that led to revision surgeries in 36.4% of cases. These secondary interventions could be prevented in cases that had an intraoperative CT scan. The quality of conventional fluoroscopy depends on projection and might increase false negative rates of intra-articular screw placement or poorly reduced fractures [26]. The use of intraoperative CT scans has been suggested to improve the assessment of screw placement and the quality of articular reduction independent of the user and projection, potentially decreasing the revision rate.

We are aware of several potential drawbacks. The sample size might introduce a type 2 error. However, based on completeness of data, especially radiologic measures, we believe that this sample size is sufficient. Further, the measurement of ROM might introduce some degree of variability. However, all ROMs were measured by one author (F.A.) to minimize variability. One might argue that the homogeneity of the study population might suffer based on a 7-year inclusion period. Yet, we believe that the inclusion of patients prior to the availability of intraoperative CT scans (2015) reduces confounding and selection bias, and that might increase confidence in our conclusion. The requirements for a secondary CT scan include insufficient information provided by fluoroscopy, pain, and discomfort. Since the intraoperative CT resulted in 25.3% of cases needing revision and the secondary CT scan in 36.4% of cases, we believe that the additional information given by the CT might improve the outcome of the patient. In addition, this is not a prospective study categorized according to severity of fractures. However, we feel that the automatized documentation of radiation dosages and reporting of reoperation rates and intraoperative revisions allows us to draw the following conclusions.

5. Conclusions

In our series, an intraoperative CT scan was not associated with an increased duration of surgery. We observed a decrease in the revision rate and improved screw positioning after the use of an intraoperative CT scan. We feel that these findings support the limited use of intraoperative CT scans in patients with complex fractures of the radius.

Author Contributions: Conceptualization, S.H. and F.A.; methodology, S.H. and H.-C.P.; software, S.H.; validation, T.B, F.H. and R.P.; formal analysis, S.H. and F.A.; investigation, A.P. and E.R.; resources, H.-C.P. and F.A.; data curation, S.H., A.P., E.R. and F.A.; writing—original draft preparation, S.H.; writing—review and editing, T.B., F.H., R.P.; visualization, S.H. and R.P.; supervision, H.-C.P. amd F.A.; project administration, H.-C.P. and F.A.; All authors have read and agreed to the published version of the manuscript.

Funding: No external funding was received for this study.

Conflicts of Interest: None of the authors or their relatives have any conflicts of interest to declare.

References

1. Court-Brown, C.M.; Caesar, B. Epidemiology of adult fractures: A review. *Injury* **2006**, *37*, 691–697. [CrossRef]
2. Kasapinova, K.; Kamiloski, V. Outcomes of surgically treated distal radius fractures associated with triangular fibrocartilage complex injury. *J. Hand Ther.* **2020**. [CrossRef] [PubMed]
3. Kennedy, S.A.; Hanel, D.P. Complex distal radius fractures. *Orthop. Clin. N. Am.* **2013**, *44*, 81–92. [CrossRef]
4. Mauck, B.M.; Swigler, C.W. Evidence-Based Review of Distal Radius Fractures. *Orthop. Clin. N. Am.* **2018**, *49*, 211–222. [CrossRef]
5. Mehling, I.; Rittstieg, P.; Mehling, A.P.; Kuechle, R.; Mueller, L.P.; Rommens, P.M. Intraoperative C-arm CT imaging in angular stable plate osteosynthesis of distal radius fractures. *J. Hand Surg. Eur. Vol.* **2013**, *38*, 751–757. [CrossRef]
6. Huber-Wagner, S.; Kanz, K.G.; Hanschen, M.; van Griensven, M.; Biberthaler, P.; Lefering, R. Whole-body computed tomography in severely injured patients. *Curr. Opin. Crit. Care* **2018**, *24*, 55–61. [CrossRef]
7. Sanders, R.; Fortin, P.; Dipasquale, T.; Walling, A. Operative treatment in 120 displaced intraarticular calcaneal fractures—Results using a prognostic computed-tomography scan classification. *Clin. Orthop. Relat. Res.* **1993**, *290*, 87–95.
8. Chandrabose, R.; Saha, S.; Kumar, H.; Tapadiya, N.; Hd, B. A computed tomography-based classification of Hoffa fracture: Surgical treatment considerations and prognostic outcome with assessment of reproducibility. *J. Orthop.* **2020**, *20*, 21–27. [CrossRef]
9. Richter, P.H.; Gebhard, F.; Eickhoff, A.; Schuetze, K. New advances in intra-operative imaging in trauma. *EFORT Open Rev.* **2018**, *3*, 168–172. [CrossRef]
10. Kaneshiro, Y.; Hidaka, N.; Yano, K.; Kawabata, A.; Fukuda, M.; Sasaoka, R.; Sakanaka, H.; Takamatsu, K. Intraoperative computed tomography with an integrated navigation system versus freehand technique under fluoroscopy in the treatment of intra-articular distal radius fractures. *J. Plast. Surg. Hand Surg.* **2019**, *53*, 255–259. [CrossRef] [PubMed]
11. von Elm, E.; Altman, D.G.; Egger, M.; Pocock, S.J.; Gøtzsche, P.C.; Vandenbroucke, J.P. The Strengthening the Reporting of Observational Studies in Epidemiology (STROBE) statement: Guidelines for reporting observational studies. *Lancet* **2007**, *370*, 1453–1457. [CrossRef]
12. Rüedi, T.P.; Murphy, W.M. *AO Principles of Fracture Management*; AO Publishing: Davos, Switzerland; Georg Thieme Verlag: Stuttgart, Germany; New York, NY, USA, 2000.
13. Marsh, J.L. OTA fracture classification. *J. Orthop. Trauma* **2009**, *23*, 551. [CrossRef] [PubMed]
14. Lavallee, S.; Sautot, P.; Troccaz, J.; Cinquin, P.; Merloz, P. Computer-assisted spine surgery: A technique for accurate transpedicular screw fixation using CT data and a 3-D optical localizer. *J. Image Guided Surg.* **1995**, *1*, 65–73. [CrossRef]
15. Slomczykowski, M.; Roberto, M.; Schneeberger, P.; Ozdoba, C.; Vock, P. Radiation dose for pedicle screw insertion—Fluoroscopic method versus computer-assisted surgery. *Spine* **1999**, *24*, 975–982. [CrossRef] [PubMed]
16. Verhofste, B.P.; Glotzbecker, M.P.; Hresko, M.T.; MacDougall, R.D.; Birch, C.M.; O'Neill, N.P.; Karlin, L.I.; Emans, J.B.; Proctor, M.R.; Hedequist, D.J. Intraoperative Use of O-arm in Pediatric Cervical Spine Surgery. *J. Pediatric Orthop.* **2020**, *40*, e266–e271. [CrossRef]
17. Jentzsch, T.; Sprengel, K.; Peterer, L.; Mica, L.; Werner, C.M.L. 3D navigation of endoscopic rhizotomy at the lumbar spine. *J. Clin. Neurosci.* **2016**, *23*, 101–105. [CrossRef]
18. Sembrano, J.N.; Santos, E.R.G.; Polly, D.W., Jr. New generation intraoperative three-dimensional imaging (O-arm) in 100 spine surgeries: Does it change the surgical procedure? *J. Clin. Neurosci.* **2014**, *21*, 225–231. [CrossRef]
19. Ruedi, T.P.; Buckley, R. *AO Principles of Fracture Management Vol. 2 Specific Fractures*; Thieme: New York, NY, USA, 2007.
20. Skala-Rosenbaum, J.; Jezek, M.; Dzupa, V.; Kaderabek, R.; Dousa, P.; Rusnak, R.; Krbec, M. Surgical Correction of Scoliosis: Does Intraoperative CT Navigation Prolong Operative Time? *Acta Chir. Orthop. Traumatol. Cechoslov.* **2016**, *83*, 344–347.

21. Knafo, S.; Mireau, E.; Bennis, S.; Baussart, B.; Aldea, S.; Gaillard, S. Operative and Perioperative Durations in O-Arm vs C-Arm Fluoroscopy for Lumbar Instrumentation. *Oper. Neurosurg.* **2018**, *14*, 273–278. [CrossRef]
22. Tabaraee, E.; Gibson, A.G.; Karahalios, D.G.; Potts, E.A.; Mobasser, J.-P.; Burch, S. Intraoperative Cone Beam-Computed Tomography With Navigation (O-ARM) Versus Conventional Fluoroscopy (C-ARM). *Spine* **2013**, *38*, 1953–1958. [CrossRef]
23. Costa, F.; Tosi, G.; Attuati, L.; Cardia, A.; Ortolina, A.; Grimaldi, M.; Galbusera, F.; Fornari, M. Radiation exposure in spine surgery using an image-guided system based on intraoperative cone-beam computed tomography: Analysis of 107 consecutive cases. *J. Neurosurg. Spine* **2016**, *25*, 654–659. [CrossRef]
24. Pruitt, D.L.; Gilula, L.A.; Manske, P.R.; Vannier, M.W. Computed-tomography scanning with image-reconstruction in evaluation of distal radius fractures. *J. Hand Surg. Am. Vol.* **1994**, *19A*, 720–727. [CrossRef]
25. Jakubietz, M.G.; Mages, L.; Zahn, R.K.; Kenn, W.; Jakubietz, R.G.; Meffert, R.H. The role of CT scan in postoperative evaluation of distal radius fractures: Retrospective analysis in regard to complications and revision rates. *J. Orthop. Sci.* **2017**, *22*, 434–437. [CrossRef]
26. Kleinlugtenbelt, Y.V.; Hoekstra, M.; Ham, S.J.; Kloen, P.; Haverlag, R.; Simons, M.P.; Bhandari, M.; Goslings, J.C.; Poolman, R.W.; Scholtes, V.A.B. Spectrum bias, a common unrecognised issue in orthopaedic agreement studies: Do CT scans really influence the agreement on treatment plans in fractures of the distal radius? *Bone Jt. Res.* **2015**, *4*, 5. [CrossRef] [PubMed]

Journal of
Clinical Medicine

MDPI

Article

High Prevalence of Sarcopenia in Older Trauma Patients: A Pilot Study

Robert C. Stassen, Kostan W. Reisinger, Moaath Al-Ali, Martijn Poeze, Jan A. Ten Bosch and Taco J. Blokhuis *

Department of Traumatology, Maastricht University Medical Centre+, 6229HX Maastricht, The Netherlands; robert.stassen@mumc.nl (R.C.S.); k.reisinger@zuyderland.nl (K.W.R.); moaath.alali@mumc.nl (M.A.-A.); martijn.poeze@mumc.nl (M.P.); jan.ten.bosch@mumc.nl (J.A.T.B.)

* Correspondence: taco.blokhuis@mumc.nl

Received: 8 June 2020; Accepted: 27 June 2020; Published: 29 June 2020

Abstract: Sarcopenia is related to adverse outcomes in various populations. However, little is known about the prevalence of sarcopenia in polytrauma patients. Identifying the number of patients at risk of adverse outcome will increase awareness to prevent further loss of muscle mass. We utilized data from a regional prospective trauma registry of all polytrauma patients presented between 2015 and 2019 at a single level-I trauma center. Subjects were screened for availability of computed tomography (CT)-abdomen and height in order to calculate skeletal mass index, which was used to estimate sarcopenia. Additional parameters regarding clinical outcome were assessed. Univariate analysis was performed to identify parameters related adverse outcome and, if identified, entered in a multivariate regression analysis. Prevalence of sarcopenia was 33.5% in the total population but was even higher in older age groups (range 60–79 years), reaching 82 % in patients over 80 years old. Sarcopenia was related to 30-day or in-hospital mortality ($p = 0.032$), as well as age ($p < 0.0001$), injury severity score ($p = 0.026$), and Charlson comorbidity index ($p = 0.001$). Log rank analysis identified sarcopenia as an independent predictor of 30-day mortality ($p = 0.032$). In conclusion, we observed a high prevalence of sarcopenia among polytrauma patients, further increasing in older patients. In addition, sarcopenia was identified as a predictor for 30-day mortality, underlining the clinical significance of identification of low muscle mass on a CT scan that is already routinely obtained in most trauma patients.

Keywords: sarcopenia; polytrauma; prevalence; mortality; skeletal mass index; muscle mass

---

1. Introduction

Sarcopenia, a disease characterized by progressive loss of skeletal muscle mass (SMM), muscle strength, and physical performance, is a common condition among senior adults [1]. It is associated with a wide range of adverse outcomes and leads to a decreased quality of life and increased mortality [1–4]. The clinical relevance of sarcopenia has been extensively described in various disorders [5–8]. In addition, the predictive value of skeletal muscle mass measurements for complications has been demonstrated in various areas of surgery, such as general, vascular, colorectal, and liver transplant surgery [7,9,10].

With worldwide increased life expectancy and associated increased incidence in geriatric polytrauma patients, prevalence of sarcopenia in trauma patients is expected to increase as well [11,12]. To date, prevalence of sarcopenia in polytrauma patients is largely unknown. Evidence on adverse outcome related to sarcopenia in polytrauma patients is scarce and quality of available studies is limited [13–15]. One limiting factor is the heterogeneity in polytrauma patients, including all age groups, different trauma mechanisms and a variety in pre-existing medical conditions. In addition, use of different definitions for sarcopenia hampers the comparison of studies in trauma patients [1,16,17]. Nevertheless, on arrival of a trauma patient, a total-body computed tomography (CT) scan is obtained almost routinely, and CT-based measurement of skeletal muscle mass is the gold standard for quantification of SMM. Therefore, the abdominal CT scan offers the opportunity to identify patients with low muscle mass directly.

The aim of this pilot study was to investigate the prevalence of low muscle mass in older polytrauma patients, as well as to explore the relation between low muscle mass and mortality, complications, and inflammatory response. We hypothesize that a low skeletal muscle mass on abdominal CT, as an indicator of sarcopenia, is common in polytrauma patients of increased age and that it could aggravate their clinical outcome by increasing the risk of complications. In addition, we hypothesize that low muscle mass is a predictor of 30-day or in hospital mortality and that it induces an increased early inflammatory response during hospitalization.

2. Patients and Methods

Approval for this study was acknowledged by the local ethics committee of the Maastricht University Medical Centre (MUMC+, Maastricht, the Netherlands). Requirement for informed consent was waived because of the retrospective nature of this study.

2.1. Patients and Determination of Muscle Mass

Data from polytrauma patients (injury severity score (ISS) ≥16) who were admitted to a single level-I trauma center between January 2015 and December 2019 were assessed for study eligibility. Patient records were retrospectively checked for presence of an abdominal CT scan and patient height. Only when both abdominal CT scan on admission and height were available, patient data were included for analysis. Measurement of SMM was performed using abdominal CT images by two independent observers using OsiriX Lite 11.0.2 open software on transverse slides of abdominal CT scan at the level of third lumbar (L3) vertebra as described before [18,19]. All measurements were performed in a semi-automated fashion by setting tissue of interest threshold at −30 to +110 Hounsfield Units (HU) for skeletal muscle [20]. Automatically generated areas of interest were corrected manually. Total muscle mass area was automatically calculated and displayed in square centimeters.

Skeletal mass index (SMI), a derivative of the skeletal muscle mass (SMM) [21], was then calculated using the following equation:

$$\text{Skeletal mass Index} = \text{Skeletal muscle mass (SMM)/height}^2 \quad (1)$$

To estimate prevalence of sarcopenia in the study population, sarcopenia was defined according to cutoff values for SMI as described by Prado et al. [18]. These values were determined at 52.4 cm^2/m^2 and 38.5 cm^2/m^2 for males and females, respectively. Two independent investigators measured the L3 muscle area of all patients and these data were used to calculate the interobserver agreement. Intra-observer agreement was assessed by repeating 50 L3-measurements 6 months after initial analysis.

2.2. Clinical Outcome

Complications were retrieved from patient data by two observers. For this purpose, complications (pneumonia, urinary tract infection, delirium and mortality (both in hospital and 30-day)) and duration of intensive care unit (ICU) admission and hospitalization were all scored. Diagnosis of pneumonia was based on chest radiographs and antibiotic treatment [22]. Urinary tract infection was defined as positive urinary culture and initiation of antibiotic therapy [23]. Delirium was diagnosed by a geriatrician in patients with altered mental status and if they received medical treatment [24]. In addition, inflammatory variables (leukocytes and C-reactive protein (CRP) on admission, after 24 and 48 h) were evaluated. Data from patients with severe head trauma who deceased within 24 h were included in the analysis of prevalence of sarcopenia. However, their data were excluded from analysis of complications.

2.3. Statistical Analysis

Frequencies are presented as absolute numbers and percentages. Continuous data is presented as mean (± standard error of the mean). Normal distribution was tested using Kolmogorov–Smirnov test. Differences between groups were analyzed using Pearson χ^2 test for dichotomous variables. Confidence intervals were calculated using logistic regression analysis. First, univariate analysis was performed to select parameters directly related to adverse outcome. Dependent variables that were identified in univariate analysis were subsequently entered into a multivariate logistic regression analysis. The influence of sarcopenia on 30-day mortality was determined using a log rank test.

The interobserver agreement (R.S., M.A.) of L3 muscle index assessment of sarcopenia was analyzed by the Pearson correlation index. Two-tailed P values less than 0.05 were considered significant. All statistical analyses were performed using SPSS (version 25.0; SPSS Inc. Chicago, IL, USA).

3. Results

3.1. Patients

Data from 846 polytrauma patients were assessed for eligibility. In 428 patients, no abdominal CT-scan was available. Further exclusion was due to missing data regarding patient height (n = 179) and death within 24 hours due to brain injury (n = 1). Therefore, data from 239 polytrauma patients were included in analysis of prevalence and from 238 for complications, excluding the single patient who died of severe brain injury within 24 hours. Patient demographics are listed in Table 1. One-hundred fifty nine of 239 (66.5%) patients were male, and 80 of 239 (33.5%) were female. Average age was 49 years (range 6–89, SD 21.45), with a non-significant distribution among gender (48 (± 20) and 53 (± 24) years for males and females, respectively, p = 0.078). For the total population, the following means were observed: ISS 26.7 (± 9.9), body mass index (BMI) 25.0 kg/m^2 (± 4.3), Charlson Comorbidity Index 1.7 (± 2.1). Patients were hospitalized for an average of 19 days (± 17). Mean L3 SMI for males and females was 57.4 cm^2/m^2 (± 10.24) and 42.7 cm^2/m^2 (± 7.82), respectively.

Table 1. Patient characteristics.

	No. of Patients (%)	Mean (SD)	Sarcopenic	Non-Sarcopenic	Significance
Gender					
Male	159 (66.5%)		51	108	
Female	80 (33.5%)		30	50	
Age					
Male		48 (± 20)	52 (± 21.9)	46 (± 18.7)	p = 0.046
female		53 (± 24)	66 (± 22.7)	46 (± 21.0)	p < 0.0001
>80	20 (8.3%)				
Male		84 (± 3)	5	1	
Female		83 (± 2)	12	2	
BMI					
<18.5	7 (2.9%)		4 (1.7%)	3 (5.1%)	p = 0.174
18.5–24.9	120 (50.5%)		54 (22.7%)	66 (27.7%)	p < 0.0001
25–29.9	88 (36.9%)		20 (8.4%)	68 (28.6%)	p =0.006
>30	23 (9.7%)		2 (0.8%)	21 (8.8%)	p = 0.005
Length of hospital stay (days)		19 (± 17)	17.6 (± 15.9)	20.1 (± 17.3)	p = 0.29
Length of stay ICU (days)		6 (± 8)	5.4 (± 7.5)	6.2 (± 8.6)	p = 0.48
Injury severity score		26.7 (± 9.9)	25.9 (± 9.3)	27.1 (± 10.2)	p = 0.34
Charlson comorbidity index					
0–1	145 (60.9%)		37	108	
>2	94 (39.9%)		44	50	
SMI					
Male <52.4	52 (21.8%)				
Female <38.5	30 (11.8%)				
Complications					
Pneumonia	43 (18.1%)		17 (20.9%)	26 (16.4%)	
Urinary tract infection	11 (5.5%)		2 (2.5%)	9 (5.6%)	
Delirium	51 (21.0%)		22 (27.2%)	29 (18.4%)	
Mortality within 1 month	18 (7.5%)		10 (12.3%)	8 (5.1%)	p = 0.032
Mortality within 1 year	8 (3.4%)		4 (4.9%)	4 (2.5%)	
Mortality after 1 year	5 (2.1%)		3 (3.7%)	2 (1.3%)	
Number of patients requiring emergency (<24 h) surgery	108 (45.4%)		33 (41.3%)	75 (47.5%)	
Number of patients requiring ICU admission	181 (76.1%)		127 (80.4%)	54 (67.5%)	

BMI: body mass index; SD: standard deviation; ICU: intensive care unit; SMI: skeletal mass index.

3.2. Prevalence

Prevalence of sarcopenia using the criteria as defined by Prado et al. was 80 out of 239 patients (33.5%), of whom 52 (65%) were male and 28 out of 80 (35%) were female (see Table 2). Mean SMI in the sarcopenic group was 42.8 (± 6.9) while this was 57.5 (± 10.5) for the non-sarcopenic group. SMI in males was higher compared to females (57.4 cm^2/m^2 (± 10.2) vs 42.7 cm^2/m^2 (± 7.8), respectively). In the older cohort (> 80 years), prevalence increased to 85%, with an even distribution between males and females (83.3% and 85.7%, respectively). Patients defined as sarcopenic were older than non-sarcopenic patients (57 years (± 22.9) and 46 years (± 19.5), respectively, $p < 0.0001$). ISS was comparable in sarcopenic (ISS = 25.9) and non-sarcopenic (ISS = 27.2) patients. The relation between age, ISS, and SMI is represented in Figure 1.

Table 2. Sarcopenia prevalence in polytrauma population.

	General Population (%)	Age 60–79 (%)	Age ≥ 80 (%)
Group			
Females	11.8 (n = 28/239)	13.6 (n = 9/66)	60 (n = 12/20)
Males	21.8 (n = 52/239)	24.2 (n = 16/66)	25 (n = 5/20)

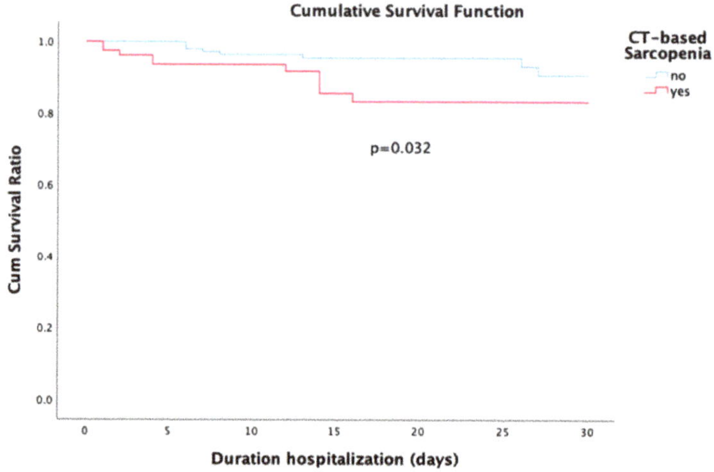

Figure 1. Survival curves for sarcopenia and no sarcopenia.

3.3. In Hospital Mortality

Eighteen (7.6%) patients died within one month or during hospital admission. Log rank analysis identified sarcopenia as an independent predictor of 30-day mortality ($p = 0.032$, Figure 1). In univariate analysis, sarcopenia ($p = 0.045$) was identified as a predictor for 30-day or in-hospital mortality. In addition, age ($p = 0.005$), Charlson Comorbidity Index ($p = 0.001$), ISS ($p = 0.026$), surgical procedures ($p = 0.038$), and hospital length of stay ($p = 0.004$) were significant predictors of mortality within one month. In the binary logistic regression analysis age (OR, 1.08; 95% CI 1.01–1.165; $p = 0.018$), ISS (OR, 1.19; 95% CI 1.04–1.20; $p = 0.003$) and hospital length of stay (OR, 0.83; 95% CI 0.74–0.92; $p < 0.0001$) remained as independent predictors of mortality within one month or during hospital admission. Logistic regression results are summarized in Table 3.

Table 3. Logistic regression analysis of mortality within one month.

		Univariate Analysis		Multivariate Analysis	
	Mortality	Odds Ratio	p-Value	Odds Ratio	p-Value
Gender					
Male	9/150	1			
Female	9/79	2.14 (0.82–5.6)	0.115		
Age		1.05 (1.02–1.08)	0.005		
BMI		0.93 (0.82-1.04)	0.21		
Sarcopenia					
No	8/157	1			
Yes	10/81	2.62 (0.99–6.93)	0.45		
Charlson Comobidity Index		1.46 (1.20–1.77)	0.001		
Injury Severity Score		1.05 (1.00–1.09)	0.026	1.19 (1.00–1.41)	0.05
Surgery during hospitalization					
No		1			
Yes		0.36 (0.14–0.98)	0.38		
Inflammatory parameters					
Plasma CRP at hospitalization		0.97 (0.87–1.07)	0.55		
Plasma Leukocyte at hospitalization		1.01 (0.98–1.03)	0.59		
Plasma CRP after 24 h		0.99 (0.99–1.01)	0.85		
Plasma Leukocytes after 24 h		1.08 (0.95–1.24)	0.25		
Plasma CRP after 48 h		0.99 (0.99–1.00)	0.19		
Plasma leukocytes after 48 h		1.13 (0.94–1.36)	0.20	1.77 (1.06–2.96)	0.029
Complications					
Pneumonia					
No	14/195	1			
Yes	4/43	1.33 (0.41–4.25)	0.63		
Urinary tract infection					
No	18/227				
Yes	0/11		0.33		
Delirium					
No	11/187	1			
Yes	7/51	2.55 (0.93–6.94)	0.06		
ICU length of stay		0.99 (0.93–1.06)	0.84		
Hospital length of stay		0.89 (0.82–9.63)	0.004	0.67 (0.50–0.89)	0.006

CRP: C-reactive protein.

3.4. Complications and Inflammatory Response

The incidence of complications was 68 (45.3%) in non-sarcopenic patients and 41 (52.6%) in sarcopenic patients (p = 0.28). No significant differences were observed between sarcopenic and non-sarcopenic cohorts regarding prevalence of pneumonia (p = 0.25), urinary tract infection (p = 0.34), delirium (p = 0.085) and ICU (p = 0.48) or hospital length of stay (p = 0.29). The inflammatory response in sarcopenic patients showed a significant increase in leukocyte levels at 48 hours compared to non-sarcopenic patients (11.95 (± 3.64) vs 10.08 (± 3.04), respectively, p = 0.002). The other time points (admission and 24 hours after admission) showed no difference for leukocyte levels (p = 0.18 and p = 0.45, respectively).

3.5. Interobserver Agreement of CT Based Muscle Measurement by Osirix

Interobserver agreement analysis of all measurements showed a strong and significant correlation (R^2 = 0.99; $p < 0.0001$). The interclass correlation coefficient (ICC) of sarcopenia assessment by CT image analysis using Osirix was 0.99 ($p < 0.0001$) with a Cronbach alpha of 0.99. The interobserver coefficient of variation (CV) was 10.1%. Intraobserver agreement analysis of 50 L3-measurements showed a significant correlation (0.863; $p < 0.0001$) in the repeated measurements.

4. Discussion

The clinical significance of sarcopenia, defined in this study as a decreased skeletal muscle mass (SMM), is becoming evident in many fields of medicine. The depletion of muscle mass is a risk factor for infection during hospitalization in both non-cancer patients and cancer patients [9,25,26]. Furthermore, it has been revealed that sarcopenia in cancer patients is associated with treatment toxicity, poor functional status, increased length of hospital stay, prolonged rehabilitation care, and increased mortality (Huaiying 2019) [9,18,27–29]. The prevalence of sarcopenia in community-dwelling populations is up to 29%, ranging from 12% to 60% in patients with colorectal cancer [30,31]. However, despite the direct clinical relevance, the prevalence of sarcopenia in polytrauma patients is unclear. This study identified a prevalence of 34% in the overall polytrauma study group, increasing to more than 80% in polytrauma patients aged over 80 years. Furthermore, our data indicate a relationship between sarcopenia and 30-day or in-hospital mortality, regardless of gender, underlining the clinical significance of sarcopenia in polytrauma patients.

Our data are in line with other studies that have described the prevalence of sarcopenia in various populations [32–34]. In general populations, von Haehling and colleagues describe a prevalence of 5–13% in people aged 60–70 years, increasing to 11–50% in those aged 80 or above. These numbers are comparable to the prevalence of sarcopenia in populations suffering from obstructive pulmonary disease (COPD), renal failure and cancer [5,35,36]. The present study shows a higher prevalence of sarcopenia in polytrauma patients compared to other studies using the same age groups. Although the reason for this higher prevalence is beyond the scope of the current analysis, it raises questions on the causal relationship between sarcopenia and accidents. Sarcopenia is associated with an increased risk of falling [37], and in a part of the current population, a fall was registered as mechanism of trauma. Another aspect that has to be taken into account in interpretation of the high prevalence in our population is the applied definition of sarcopenia. In the present study, the criteria for skeletal muscle mass as described by Prado were used. Other definitions of sarcopenia use functional tests in addition to the quantification of muscle mass, such as the EWGSOP-II definition that uses hand-grip strength and gait speed [1]. However, in the polytrauma population these parameters are not readily obtainable. This limitation is mostly due to the extremity injuries frequently present in polytrauma patients, but also admission to the ICU and (prolonged) ventilation makes it impossible to obtain these data. Obtaining data during the admission is not straight forward, as loss of muscle mass and muscle function occurs within days during bedrest [38]. In contrast, a total-body CT scan is performed almost routinely upon arrival of a polytrauma patient, providing detailed imaging of the abdomen. The quantification of skeletal muscle mass is therefore readily available, and our study indicates that this parameter is directly related to survival.

The relation between sarcopenia and mortality, as indicated by many publications, appears in the univariate analysis of our data as well. In addition, a clear prediction of 30-day mortality was found. The identification of sarcopenia in these analyses is in line with available literature, showing increased mortality within one year of diagnosing sarcopenia [39,40]. A recent study by Leeper et al. indicates sarcopenia to be a strong predictor of 6-month post-discharge mortality in elderly trauma patients [41]. However, in the multivariate analysis in our study, we were unable to maintain sarcopenia as an independent risk factor for 30-day or in-hospital mortality. This is likely due to the small sample size in our study, as well as the stronger correlation between mortality and other factors such as age and trauma severity. Notwithstanding this effect, in the study by Leeper et al., an association is described between mortality and a variety of factors including ICU and hospital length of stay and injury scoring systems like Injury Severity Score and Abbreviated Injury Scale. Our data are in accordance with their findings.

Obtaining an abdominal CT scan is becoming a more and more widespread routine in trauma patients [42]. Our data showed the same trend, as the percentage of patients excluded for missing CT data decreased per year. Surprisingly, data from routinely obtained trauma CT scans are only seldom used for muscle mass measurement in clinical practice. We believe that the addition of skeletal mass measurement analysis in trauma patients has a direct beneficial effect, since treatment of low muscle mass can be initiated immediately, and further loss of muscle mass could be prevented. One consideration in using only CT derived data is, however, the mentioned cutoff values for the L3 index, which are used to estimate sarcopenia. As these values are based on obese patients with cancer, caution is advised when translating these values to other populations. Ideally, cutoff values for sarcopenia should be established within each specific patient population and BMI category. A much larger sample size would be required to undertake cutoff values analyses by gender and by Body Mass Index (BMI). It is important to realize that there has been mounting evidence on the clinical importance of BMI in the field of traumatology. An observational prospective study of Childs et al. shows an increased risk of infections, acute renal failure, length of ICU stay, hospital length of stay, and duration of mechanical ventilation in polytrauma patients with a BMI > 30 [43]. In addition, our analyses suggest differences in prevalence of sarcopenia between different BMI ranges, with an increasing portion of sarcopenic trauma patients in higher BMI ranges. However, it is important to acknowledge that BMI does not distinguish between muscle and fat tissues. Increase in routinely obtained CT-scanning gives the opportunity to assess CT-based anthropometric parameters of fat in addition to muscle mass. A recent study of Poros et al. showed that CT-based assessment of abdominal fat is suitable in revealing pathologic body composition in trauma patients [44]. Abdominal fat measurements might add valuable information in relation to complications and mortality in trauma patients in future studies.

The current study was a pilot study, where a retrospective analysis of collected data was performed as a first step to elucidate the clinical impact of sarcopenia in trauma patients. This study has therefore limitations that have to be kept in mind in interpretation of the results. One of the limitations of this study is its retrospective nature. Because only data from patients with an abdominal CT were included in our analysis, there is a potential inclusion bias. Still, all cases were retrieved from a regional prospective trauma registry, thereby limiting the effect of potential selection bias. Another limitation is the heterogeneity of the study population. Traumatic events occur in any age group with different grades of severity. In order to limit the effect of heterogeneity, only patients with an ISS ≥ 16 were included, and age-specific analysis was obtained regarding the prevalence of sarcopenia and its complications. Finally, only CT data were analyzed, and other markers of frailty such as functional and nutritional status were not included in our analysis.

In future studies, functional tests should, if possible, be included in the criteria for sarcopenia. Moreover, the cut-off values for skeletal mass index on CT measurements may require different cut-off points based upon reported outcome in this specific population.

5. Conclusions

The prevalence of sarcopenia in elderly polytrauma patients is high, reaching 85% in people over 80 years old. Our analysis also shows that sarcopenia is an independent predictor for 30-day mortality. Since abdominal CT scans are now almost routinely obtained in trauma patients, we advocate the measurement of skeletal mass measurement to detect decreased muscle mass early. Early identification of people at risk for sarcopenia will lead to early diagnosis and therapy, and more awareness will help to prevent additional loss of muscle mass during the admission after trauma.

Author Contributions: Conceptualization, R.C.S. and T.J.B.; data curation, M.A.-A.; formal analysis, R.C.S., M.P., and T.J.B.; methodology, K.W.R. and J.A.T.B.; supervision, K.W.R., M.P., J.A.T.B., and T.J.B.; writing—original draft, R.C.S., K.W.R., and M.A.-A.; writing—review and editing, M.P., T.J.B. and J.A.T.B. All authors have read and agreed to the published version of the manuscript.

Funding: This research received no external funding.

Acknowledgments: We acknowledge support by the Open Access Publication Funds of the Göttingen University.

Conflicts of Interest: The authors declare no conflicts of interest.

References

1. Cruz-Jentoft, A.J.; Bahat, G.; Bauer, J.; Boirie, Y.; Bruyère, O.; Cederholm, T.; Cooper, C.; Landi, F.; Rolland, Y.; Sayer, A.A.; et al. Sarcopenia: Revised European consensus on definition and diagnosis. *Age Ageing* **2018**, *48*, 16–31. [CrossRef] [PubMed]
2. Cruz-Jentoft, A.J.; Baeyens, J.P.; Bauer, J.M.; Boirie, Y.; Cederholm, T.; Landi, F.; Martin, F.C.; Michel, J.-P.; Rolland, Y.; Schneider, S.M.; et al. Sarcopenia: European consensus on definition and diagnosis: Report

of the European Working Group on Sarcopenia in Older People. *Age Ageing* **2010**, *39*, 412–423. [CrossRef] [PubMed]

3. Dodds, R.M.; Sayer, A.A. Sarcopenia, frailty and mortality: The evidence is growing. *Age Ageing* **2016**, *45*, 570–571. [CrossRef]
4. Marzetti, E.; Calvani, R.; Tosato, M.; Cesari, M.; Di Bari, M.; Cherubini, A.; Collamati, A.; D'Angelo, E.; Pahor, M.; Bernabei, R.; et al. Sarcopenia: An overview. *Aging Clin. Exp. Res.* **2017**, *29*, 11–17. [CrossRef] [PubMed]
5. Jones, S.E.; Maddocks, M.; Kon, S.S.; Canavan, J.L.; Nolan, C.M.; Clark, A.L.; Polkey, M.I.; Man, W.D.-C. Sarcopenia in COPD: Prevalence, clinical correlates and response to pulmonary rehabilitation. *Thorax* **2015**, *70*, 213–218. [CrossRef] [PubMed]
6. Yazar, T.; Yazar, H.O.; Zayimoğlu, E.; Çankaya, S. Incidence of sarcopenia and dynapenia according to stage in patients with idiopathic Parkinson's disease. *Neurol. Sci.* **2018**, *39*, 1415–1421. [CrossRef] [PubMed]
7. Joglekar, S.; Nau, P.N.; Mezhir, J.J. The impact of sarcopenia on survival and complications in surgical oncology: A review of the current literature. *J.Surg.Oncol.* **2015**, *112*, 503–509. [CrossRef]
8. Cruz-Jentoft, A.J.; Landi, F.; Topinková, E.; Michel, J.-P. Understanding sarcopenia as a geriatric syndrome. *Curr. Opin. Clin. Nutr. Metab. Care* **2010**, *13*, 1–7. [CrossRef]
9. Lieffers, J.R.; Bathe, O.F.; Fassbender, K.; Winget, M.; Baracos, V.E. Sarcopenia is associated with postoperative infection and delayed recovery from colorectal cancer resection surgery. *Br. J. Cancer* **2012**, *107*, 931–936. [CrossRef] [PubMed]
10. Friedman, J.; Lussiez, A.; Sullivan, J.; Wang, S.C.; Englesbe, M.J. Implications of Sarcopenia in Major Surgery. *Nutr. Clin. Pr.* **2015**, *30*, 175–179. [CrossRef]
11. Dimitriou, R.; Calori, G.M.; Giannoudis, P.V. Polytrauma in the elderly: Specific considerations and current concepts of management. *Eur. J. Trauma Emerg. Surg.* **2011**, *37*, 539–548. [CrossRef]
12. Braun, B.; Holstein, J.; Fritz, T.; Veith, N.T.; Herath, S.; Mörsdorf, P.; Pohlemann, T. Polytrauma in the elderly: A review. *EFORT Open Rev.* **2016**, *1*, 146–151. [CrossRef] [PubMed]
13. Malekpour, M.; Bridgham, K.; Jaap, K.; Erwin, R.; Widom, K.; Rapp, M.; Leonard, D.; Baro, S.; Dove, J.; Hunsinger, M.; et al. The Effect of Sarcopenia on Outcomes in Geriatric Blunt Trauma. *Am. Surg.* **2017**, *83*, 1203–1208. [CrossRef] [PubMed]
14. Fairchild, B.; Webb, T.P.; Xiang, Q.; Tarima, S.; Brasel, K. Sarcopenia and frailty in elderly trauma patients. *World J. Surg.* **2015**, *39*, 373–379. [CrossRef] [PubMed]
15. DeAndrade, J.; Pedersen, M.; Garcia, L.; Nau, P. Sarcopenia is a risk factor for complications and an independent predictor of hospital length of stay in trauma patients. *J. Surg. Res.* **2018**, *221*, 161–166. [CrossRef] [PubMed]
16. Bhasin, S.; Travison, T.G.; Manini, T.M.; Patel, S.; Pencina, K.M.; Fielding, R.A.; Magaziner, J.M.; Newman, A.B.; Kiel, D.P.; Cooper, C.; et al. Sarcopenia Definition: The Position Statements of the Sarcopenia Definition and Outcomes Consortium. *J. Am. Geriatr. Soc.* **2020**. [CrossRef] [PubMed]
17. Chen, L.-K.; Liu, L.-K.; Woo, J.; Assantachai, P.; Auyeung, T.-W.; Bahyah, K.S.; Chou, M.-Y.; Chen, L.-Y.; Hsu, P.-S.; Krairit, O.; et al. Sarcopenia in Asia: Consensus Report of the Asian Working Group for Sarcopenia. *J. Am. Med Dir. Assoc.* **2014**, *15*, 95–101. [CrossRef]
18. Prado, C.M.; Lieffers, J.R.; McCargar, L.J.; Reiman, T.; Sawyer, M.B.; Martin, L.; Baracos, V.E. Prevalence and clinical implications of sarcopenic obesity in patients with solid tumours of the respiratory and gastrointestinal tracts: A population-based study. *Lancet Oncol.* **2008**, *9*, 629–635. [CrossRef]
19. Reisinger, K.W.; Van Vugt, J.L.A.; Tegels, J.; Snijders, C.; Hulsewé, K.W.E.; Hoofwijk, A.G.; Stoot, J.; Von Meyenfeldt, M.F.; Beets, G.L.; Derikx, J.P.M.; et al. Functional Compromise Reflected by Sarcopenia, Frailty, and Nutritional Depletion Predicts Adverse Postoperative Outcome After Colorectal Cancer Surgery. *Ann. Surg.* **2015**, *261*, 345–352. [CrossRef]
20. Mitsiopoulos, N.; Baumgartner, R.N.; Heymsfield, S.B.; Lyons, W.; Gallagher, D.; Ross, R. Cadaver validation of skeletal muscle measurement by magnetic resonance imaging and computerized tomography. *J. Appl. Physiol.* **1998**, *85*, 115–122. [CrossRef]
21. Mourtzakis, M.; Prado, C.M.; Lieffers, J.R.; Reiman, T.; McCargar, L.J.; Baracos, V.E. A practical and precise approach to quantification of body composition in cancer patients using computed tomography images acquired during routine care. *Appl. Physiol. Nutr. Metab.* **2008**, *33*, 997–1006. [CrossRef]
22. Sattar, S.B.A.; Sharma, S. *Bacterial Pneumonia*; StatPearls Publishing: Tampa/St. Petersburg, FL, USA, 2019.

23. Hooton, T.M.; Stamm, W.E. DIAGNOSIS AND TREATMENT OF UNCOMPLICATED URINARY TRACT INFECTION. *Infect. Dis. Clin. North Am.* **1997**, *11*, 551–581. [CrossRef]
24. Inouye, S.K. Delirium in Older Persons. *N. Engl. J. Med.* **2006**, *354*, 1157–1165. [CrossRef] [PubMed]
25. Pichard, C.; Kyle, U.G.; Morabia, A.; Perrier, A.; Vermeulen, B.; Unger, P. Nutritional assessment: Lean body mass depletion at hospital admission is associated with an increased length of stay. *Am. J. Clin. Nutr.* **2004**, *79*, 613–618. [CrossRef]
26. Cosquéric, G.; Sebag, A.; Ducolombier, C.; Thomas, C.; Piette, F.; Weill-Engerer, S. Sarcopenia is predictive of nosocomial infection in care of the elderly. *Br. J. Nutr.* **2006**, *96*, 895–901. [CrossRef] [PubMed]
27. Prado, C.M.; Baracos, V.E.; McCargar, L.J.; Reiman, T.; Mourtzakis, M.; Tonkin, K.; Mackey, J.R.; Koski, S.; Pituskin, E.; Sawyer, M.B. Sarcopenia as a Determinant of Chemotherapy Toxicity and Time to Tumor Progression in Metastatic Breast Cancer Patients Receiving Capecitabine Treatment. *Clin. Cancer Res.* **2009**, *15*, 2920–2926. [CrossRef]
28. Antoun, S.; Baracos, V.E.; Birdsell, L.; Escudier, B.; Sawyer, M.B. Low body mass index and sarcopenia associated with dose-limiting toxicity of sorafenib in patients with renal cell carcinoma. *Ann. Oncol.* **2010**, *21*, 1594–1598. [CrossRef]
29. Van Vledder, M.G.; Levolger, S.; Ayez, N.; Verhoef, C.; Tran, T.C.K.; Ijzermans, J.N.M. Body composition and outcome in patients undergoing resection of colorectal liver metastases. *BJS* **2012**, *99*, 550–557. [CrossRef]
30. Cruz-Jentoft, A.J.; Landi, F.; Schneider, S.M.; Zúñiga, C.; Arai, H.; Boirie, Y.; Chen, L.-K.; Fielding, R.A.; Martin, F.C.; Michel, J.-P.; et al. Prevalence of and interventions for sarcopenia in ageing adults: A systematic review. Report of the International Sarcopenia Initiative (EWGSOP and IWGS). *Age Ageing* **2014**, *43*, 748–759. [CrossRef]
31. Vergara-Fernandez, O.; Trejo-Avila, M.; Salgado-Nesme, N. Sarcopenia in patients with colorectal cancer: A comprehensive review. *World J. Clin. Cases* **2020**, *8*, 1188–1202. [CrossRef]
32. Morley, J.E. Sarcopenia: Diagnosis and treatment. *J. Nutr. Heal. Aging* **2008**, *12*, 452–456. [CrossRef]
33. Von Haehling, S.; Anker, S.D. Cachexia as a major underestimated and unmet medical need: Facts and numbers. *J. Cachex- Sarcopenia Muscle* **2010**, *1*, 1–5. [CrossRef] [PubMed]
34. Von Haehling, S.; Morley, J.E.; Anker, S.D. An overview of sarcopenia: Facts and numbers on prevalence and clinical impact. *J. Cachex- Sarcopenia Muscle* **2010**, *1*, 129–133. [CrossRef] [PubMed]
35. Kim, J.-K.; Choi, S.R.; Choi, M.J.; Kim, S.G.; Lee, Y.K.; Noh, J.W.; Kim, H.J.; Song, Y.R. Prevalence of and factors associated with sarcopenia in elderly patients with end-stage renal disease. *Clin. Nutr.* **2014**, *33*, 64–68. [CrossRef]
36. Villaseñor, A.; Ballard-Barbash, R.; Baumgartner, K.; Baumgartner, R.; Bernstein, L.; McTiernan, A.; Neuhouser, M.L. Prevalence and prognostic effect of sarcopenia in breast cancer survivors: The HEAL Study. *J. Cancer Surviv.* **2012**, *6*, 398–406. [CrossRef]
37. Yang, M.; Liu, Y.; Zuo, Y.; Tang, H. Sarcopenia for predicting falls and hospitalization in community-dwelling older adults: EWGSOP versus EWGSOP2. *Sci. Rep.* **2019**, *9*, 1–8. [CrossRef]
38. Wall, B.T.; Dirks, M.L.; Van Loon, L. Skeletal muscle atrophy during short-term disuse: Implications for age-related sarcopenia. *Ageing Res. Rev.* **2013**, *12*, 898–906. [CrossRef]
39. Brown, J.C.; Harhay, M.O.; Harhay, M.N. Sarcopenia and mortality among a population-based sample of community-dwelling older adults. *J. Cachex- Sarcopenia Muscle* **2015**, *7*, 290–298. [CrossRef] [PubMed]
40. Liu, P.; Hao, Q.; Hai, S.; Wang, H.; Cao, L.; Dong, B. Sarcopenia as a predictor of all-cause mortality among community-dwelling older people: A systematic review and meta-analysis. *Maturitas* **2017**, *103*, 16–22. [CrossRef]
41. Leeper, C.M.; Lin, E.; Hoffman, M.; Fombona, A.; Zhou, T.; Kutcher, M.; Rosengart, M.; Watson, G.; Billiar, T.; Peitzman, A.; et al. Computed Tomography Abbreviated Assessment of Sarcopenia Following Trauma: The CAAST Measurement Predicts 6-month Mortality in Older Adult Trauma Patients. *J. Trauma Acute Care Surg.* **2016**, *80*, 805–811. [CrossRef]

42. Sierink, J.C.; Treskes, K.; Edwards, M.J.R.; Beuker, B.J.A.; Hartog, D.D.; Hohmann, J.; Dijkgraaf, M.G.W.; Luitse, J.S.K.; Beenen, L.F.M.; Hollmann, M.W.; et al. Immediate total-body CT scanning versus conventional imaging and selective CT scanning in patients with severe trauma (REACT-2): A randomised controlled trial. *Lancet* **2016**, *388*, 673–683. [CrossRef]
43. Childs, B.R.; Nahm, N.J.; Dolenc, A.J.; Vallier, H.A. Obesity Is Associated With More Complications and Longer Hospital Stays After Orthopaedic Trauma. *J. Orthop. Trauma* **2015**, *29*, 504–509. [CrossRef]
44. Poros, B.; Irlbeck, T.; Probst, P.; Volkmann, A.; Paprottka, P.; Böcker, W.; Irlbeck, M.; Weig, T. Impact of pathologic body composition assessed by CT-based anthropometric measurements in adult patients with multiple trauma: A retrospective analysis. *Eur. J. Trauma Emerg. Surg.* **2019**, *2019*, 1–15. [CrossRef]

Journal of
Clinical Medicine

MDPI

Article

Effects of Four-Week Rehabilitation Program on Hemostasis Disorders in Patients with Spinal Cord Injury

Magdalena Mackiewicz-Milewska [1], Małgorzata Cisowska-Adamiak [1], Danuta Rość [2], Iwona Głowacka-Mrotek [1] and Iwona Świątkiewicz [3,4,*]

1 Department of Rehabilitation, Nicolaus Copernicus University in Toruń, Collegium Medicum in Bydgoszcz, 85-094 Bydgoszcz, Poland; magmami@onet.eu (M.M.-M.); malgorzata.cisowska@cm.umk.pl (M.C.-A.); iwona.glowacka@cm.umk.pl (I.G.-M.)

2 Department of Pathophysiology, Nicolaus Copernicus University in Toruń, Collegium Medicum in Bydgoszcz, 85-094 Bydgoszcz, Poland; d.rosc@cm.umk.pl

3 Department of Cardiology and Internal Medicine, Nicolaus Copernicus University in Toruń, Collegium Medicum in Bydgoszcz, 85-094 Bydgoszcz, Poland

4 Division of Cardiovascular Medicine, University of California San Diego, La Jolla, CA 92037, USA

* Correspondence: iwona.swiatkiewicz@gmail.com; Tel.: +1-(858)-246-2510

Received: 10 May 2020; Accepted: 10 June 2020; Published: 12 June 2020

Abstract: Background: Patients with spinal cord injury (SCI) exhibit hemostasis disorders. This study aims at assessing the effects of a 4-week rehabilitation program on hemostasis disorders in patients with SCI. Methods: Seventy-eight in-patients undergoing a 4-week rehabilitation were divided into three groups based on time elapsed since SCI: I (3 weeks–3 months), II (3–6 months), and III (>6 months). Tissue factor (TF), tissue factor pathway inhibitor (TFPI), thrombin–antithrombin complex (TAT) and D-dimer levels, antithrombin activity (AT), and platelet count (PLT) were measured on admission and after rehabilitation. Results: Rehabilitation resulted in an increase in TF in group III ($p < 0.050$), and decrease in TFPI ($p < 0.022$) and PLT ($p < 0.042$) in group II as well as AT in group I ($p < 0.009$). Compared to control group without SCI, TF, TFPI, and TAT were significantly higher in all SCI groups both before and after rehabilitation. All SCI groups had elevated D-dimer, which decreased after rehabilitation in the whole study group ($p < 0.001$) and group I ($p < 0.001$). Conclusion: No decrease in activation of TF-dependent coagulation was observed after a 4-week rehabilitation regardless of time elapsed since SCI. However, D-dimer levels decreased significantly, which may indicate reduction of high fibrinolytic potential, especially when rehabilitation was done <3 months after SCI.

Keywords: spinal cord injury; rehabilitation; exercises; hemostasis; venous thrombosis

1. Introduction

Venous thromboembolism (VTE) is a frequent complication in patients after spinal cord injury (SCI). Deep vein thrombosis (DVT) occurs in 5.4–27% and pulmonary embolism (PE) in 4–5.2% of patients, mainly in the acute period, although these complications have also been described in the chronic phase after SCI [1–7]. The risk of VTE is greatest (up to ~86% of all VTE events) in the first 3 months after injury [1,7]. The occurrence of VTE events drops significantly to about 9% between 3 and 6 months after injury and may still be observed at lower frequency (~5%) in long-term follow-up beyond 6 months [7]. Furthermore, our previous findings indicate that for patients beyond 3 months after SCI and diagnosed with DVT, 80% of DVT was detected during the period up to 6 months after injury [6]. The high risk of thromboembolic complications in SCI patients is associated with several factors including venous stasis resulting from immobilization, paresis or paralysis, decreased muscle contractibility, previous VTE, and infections [1,7,8]. In addition, patients with SCI exhibit hemostasis disorders, which can contribute to the VTE [6,9,10].

Rehabilitation of patients after SCI in the subacute or chronic phase involves regular physical activity of moderate intensity. The effect of a systematic moderate-intensity rehabilitation on hemostasis in the SCI patients has not been definitely assessed. Based on the results of previous studies that were conducted in other populations, it has been proven that exercise, especially of high intensity, has an impact on coagulation and fibrinolysis and may be responsible for the sudden death of persons participating in a marathon or triathlon [11,12]. On the other hand, it is widely known that regular, moderate exercise exerts a positive effect on the cardiovascular system [13].

In clinical practice, D-dimer concentration, platelet (PLT) count, and antithrombin (AT) activity are the most commonly measured parameters in patients with suspected VTE. Tissue factor (TF), tissue factor pathway inhibitor (TFPI) and thrombin–antithrombin (TAT) complex levels are rarely assessed in routine clinical practice. TF, previously known as thromboplastin, is a protein that initiates coagulation through the so-called extrinsic coagulation pathway [14–16]. It serves as a receptor for factor VII with which it forms the TF/VII complex, resulting in thrombin formation as well as deposition of fibrin and platelets in the process of clot formation [16–19]. TPFI is an endogenous physiological inhibitor of the TF/VII complex. Its anticoagulant properties are involved only in the coagulation pathway initiated by TF [20,21]. TAT complex is an indicator of prothrombin to thrombin activation and is one of the principal markers of blood hypercoagulability [22].

The objective of this research was to assess whether a four-week systematic rehabilitation involving moderate-intensity exercises affects selected parameters of coagulation and fibrinolysis in patients with SCI. To the best of our knowledge, our study is the first to investigate these interactions in such a specific population of patients. We measured the concentration of TAT complex, AT activity, D-dimer levels, PLT count, and extrinsic coagulation pathway factors, such as TF and TFPI levels. Our hypothesis was that regular, moderate exercise can reduce the activation of coagulation and fibrinolysis factors and, thus, may mitigate thromboembolic complications in the SCI patients.

2. Material and Methods

2.1. Study Design

This prospective study included patients with SCI who were hospitalized at the Department of Rehabilitation, the University Hospital No. 1 in Bydgoszcz, Poland, from 2011 to 2017. Every patient with SCI admitted to the Department of Rehabilitation in the period from 2011 to 2017 who agreed to participate was included in the study. Based on previous studies on the time course of the occurrence of VTE events post-SCI [1,6,7] as briefly summarized in Section 1, the patients were divided into the following three groups according to time elapsed since injury: group I (>3 weeks to 3 months, subacute phase), group II (>3 months to 6 months, early chronic phase), and group III (>6 months, late chronic phase). The study was approved by the local bioethical committee (KB 295/2011, 5 May 2011) and all patients signed an informed consent form.

All patients underwent clinical examination for assessment of paresis and symptoms of DVT such as edema, increased temperature, and erythema of the upper and lower limbs. They were also subjected to Doppler ultrasound examination of the lower-limb venous system and were graded according to the American Spinal Injury Association Impairment Scale (AIS). The occurrence of post-traumatic complications, such as decubitus ulcers, heterotopic ossifications, or urinary tract infection was also recorded (Table 1). PLT count, TF, TFPI, TAT complex and D-dimer plasma levels, and AT activity were measured in all patients at the time of admission and after four weeks of rehabilitation. Because normal reference ranges for TF, TFPI and TAT plasma concentrations were not available, their levels were also assessed in a control group of 42 individuals without SCI.

Table 1. Study group characteristics: number of patients (*N*) with specific symptoms.

Symptom or Incident	*N* (%)
Tetraplegia	34 (43.6%)
Flaccid paraplegia	18 (23.1%)
Spastic paraplegia	26 (33.3%)
Cervical spine injury	37 (44.4%)
Thoracic spine injury	33 (42.3%)
Lumbosacral spine injury	8 (10.3%)
AIS A	34 (43.6%)
AIS B	30 (36.5%)
AIS C	14 (17.9%)
Decubitus ulcers	11 (14.1%)
Urinary tract infection	26 (33.3%)
Heterotopic ossifications	13 (16.6%)
Administration of LMWH	53 (67.9%)
Deep vein thrombosis	7 (9.0%)
Superficial vein thrombosis of the lower limbs	4 (5.1%)
Pulmonary embolism	0

Data represent the number of patients (*N*) including the percentage of total number (%). Abbreviations: AIS—American Spinal Injury Association Impairment Scale; AIS A—impairment is complete according to AIS; AIS B and C—impairment is incomplete according to AIS; LMWH—low-molecular-weight heparin.

All patients underwent a four-week course of rehabilitation program, which included about two hours of moderate exercise a day with verticalization, wheelchair adaptation if necessary, passive and active exercises of the upper and lower limbs, resistance training, learning to move in a wheelchair, self-service, or learning to walk. The intensity of exercise was estimated as moderate but the maximal oxygen consumption (VO_2 max) parameter that qualifies exercise as low, moderate, or high intensity was not assessed.

The plasma concentrations of TF, TFPI, and TAT complex were determined by enzyme-linked immunosorbent assay (ELISA) using specific IMUBIND® kits (Sekisui Diagnostics). Plasma levels of D-dimer were determined by INNOVANCE® D-Dimer (Siemens Healthcare Diagnostic Products GmbH), which is a particle-enhanced immunoturbidimetric assay for the quantitative determination of cross-linked fibrin degradation products (D-dimers). AT activity was measured by a chromogenic test, INNOVANCE Antithrombin (Siemens Healthcare). Platelets were counted with a Sysmex hematology analyzer.

There was no control group of patients with SCI who did not receive rehabilitation after injury due to the difficulty in accessing such patients, especially in the subacute stage up to three months after injury. If patients are not receiving rehabilitation during this period, it is usually because of severe complications of the trauma that preclude rehabilitation.

2.2. Statistical Analysis

Statistical analyses were conducted using Statistica 13.1 software (StatSoft Europe GmbH, Hamburg, Germany). Analyzed parameters were characterized by non-normal distribution. Hence, the non-parametric tests, Mann–Whitney U and Wilcoxon signed-rank, were used to evaluate the differences between groups for hemostasis parameters. For demographic and clinical characteristics, the differences between the groups were analyzed using the Kruskal–Wallis and post hoc Fisher's Least Significant Difference tests. A probability level of $p < 0.05$ was considered statistically significant. Median (Me) and quartiles (lower Q25 and upper Q75) were used to describe the variables.

3. Results

Initially, 88 patients with SCI were enrolled in the study, but 10 patients discontinued rehabilitation prematurely, so 78 patients were included in the final analyses. Reasons for not completing the rehabilitation program included transfer to another hospital or a rehabilitation time of less than four weeks. The final group comprised 66 men (84.6% of total) and 12 women (15.4%). The average age of the patients in the study group was 37.7 years (±15.7 years); the women were older (42 ± 20.8 years) compared to men (37 ± 14.6 years). The minimum age was the same in the women and the men (18 years), while the maximum age varied; it was higher in men at 80 years. The mean time elapsed since injury was 7.9 months (±13.3 months). There were 34 patients in group I, 22 patients in group II, and 22 patients in group III.

The clinical characteristics of the study group are shown in Table 1.

No significant differences were found between groups I, II, and III for age, gender, body mass index, urinary tract infections, decubitus ulcers, the AIS grades, as well as thoracic and lumbosacral spine injuries. There were more patients with cervical spine injury in group III (77.3% of patients) compared to group II (40.9%) and group I (32.3%) ($p = 0.012$ for group II vs. III, $p = 0.001$ for group I vs. III). This result is expected because the patients with cervical spine injury often undergo rehabilitation in the chronic phase of SCI due to significant neurologic deficits. Heterotopic ossifications occurred at higher rate in groups II and III (27.3% of patients in each group) compared to group I (2.9%) ($p = 0.016$ for group I vs. II and I vs. III). Low-molecular-weight heparin (LWMH) was used more frequently in group I (94.1% of patients) compared to group II (63.6%) and group III (31.8%) ($p = 0.006$ for group I vs. II, $p = 0.009$ for II vs. III, and $p = 0.001$ for I vs. III). It is clinically justifiable that LMWH is administered most frequently for VTE prophylaxis and treatment in patients with most recent SCI and higher thromboembolic risk.

In the entire study group, seven patients (9% of all patients) were diagnosed with DVT and four patients (5.1%) with superficial vein thrombosis, and all these patients were from group I. No cases of PE were observed in the studied population during hospitalization when the rehabilitation program was conducted. No significant correlations were found between DVT occurrence and the following clinical factors: urinary tract infections, heterotopic ossifications, decubitus ulcers, AIS score, level of spinal injury, or type of paresis. The majority of patients (67.9% of total) received LMWH. No bleeding complications were observed. In addition, we note that patients enrolled in this study had no underlying bleeding disorders. The control group consisted of 42 subjects without SCI including 31 men and 11 women, with an average age of 41.2 years (±15.4 years).

The results of TF, TFPI, and TAT complex assays, which were performed in the study group and in the control group before rehabilitation program, are presented in Table 2. In the study group, the concentration of TF was over threefold higher, the TFPI almost twofold higher, and the TAT complex 4.5-fold higher than in the control group. These differences were statistically significant.

Table 2. Plasma concentrations of TF, TFPI, and TAT complex in the study group vs. the control group before four-week rehabilitation program.

	Study Group $N = 78$		**Control Group** $N = 42$		***p*-Value between Groups**
Parameter	Median	Q25/Q75	Median	Q25/Q75	
TF (pg/mL)	453.84	327.30/567.66	128.26	90.44/183.40	0.000
TFPI (ng/mL)	103.26	59.36/131.50	59.90	43.30/96.76	0.001
TAT (ng/mL)	8.75	5.29/17.54	2.20	1.98/3.36	0.000

Abbreviations: TAT—thrombin–antithrombin complex; TF—tissue factor; TFPI—tissue factor pathway inhibitor; Q25—lower quartile; Q75—upper quartile.

Evaluation of hemostatic parameters in the study group before and after a four-week rehabilitation program is displayed in the Table 3. Before rehabilitation, high TF, TAT complex, and D-dimer concentrations were observed. After rehabilitation, we observed a significant reduction in D-dimer level. TFPI concentrations and AT activity also decreased after the rehabilitation and the differences before and after rehabilitation reached approximately the level of significance. The median values of AT activity and PLT count in SCI patients were within normal limits both before and after rehabilitation.

Table 3. Parameters of hemostasis in the study subjects before and after a four-week rehabilitation program.

Test ($N = 78$)		Before Rehabilitation		After Rehabilitation		p-Value between Groups
Parameter	Units	Median	Q25/Q75	Median	Q25/Q75	
PLT count	g/L	252.00	204.00/352.00	249.00	211.00/317.00	0.116
TF	pg/mL	453.84	327.30/567.66	459.76	348.20/546.84	0.371
TFPI	ng/mL	103.26	59.36/131.50	92.34	52.84/132.04	0.075
AT	%	101.95	94.80/112.00	101.05	91.40/106.70	0.071
TAT	ng/mL	8.75	5.29/17.54	6.70	4.50/10.88	0.48
D-dimer	ng/mL	1249.50	600.00/2540.00	903.50	430.00/1743/00	0.001

Abbreviations: AT—antithrombin activity; PLT—platelet; TAT—thrombin–antithrombin complex; TF—tissue factor; TFPI—tissue factor pathway inhibitor; Q25—lower quartile; Q75—upper quartile.

The results of the measurements of hemostatic parameters in the groups of patients based on time elapsed since SCI are presented in the Table 4 (group I), Table 5 (group II), and Table 6 (group III). Elevated levels of TF, TFPI, and TAT complex, as well as very high D-dimer concentrations were found on admission in patients from group I (3 weeks to 3 months from injury) (Table 4). After four weeks of rehabilitation, in group I we observed a significant reduction in D-dimer levels from a median of 2387 to 1252 ng/mL. There was also a significant reduction in AT activity after rehabilitation in group I, although it stayed within reference ranges both before and after rehabilitation.

Table 4. Parameters of hemostasis before and after a four-week rehabilitation program in patients from group I (three weeks to three months after injury).

Test ($N = 34$)		Before Rehabilitation		After Rehabilitation		p-Value between Groups
Parameter	Units	Median	Q25/Q75	Median	Q25/Q75	
PLT count	g/L	262.0	242.0/352.0	255.0	218.0/348.0	0.180
TF	pg/mL	482.1	338.9/572.6	492.2	366.6/582.4	0.447
TFPI	ng/mL	90.5	52.8/155.9	93.3	47.7/139.9	0.301
AT	%	102.5	97.4/114.9	100.2	91.1/105.0	0.009
TAT	ng/mL	10.3	5.9/18.9	7.5	5.8/12.6	0.326
D-dimer	ng/mL	2387.5	1250.0/5190.0	1252.0	580.0/2240.0	0.000

Abbreviations: AT—antithrombin activity; TAT—thrombin–antithrombin complex; TF—tissue factor; TFPI—tissue factor pathway inhibitor; Q25—lower quartile; Q75—upper quartile.

Table 5. Parameters of hemostasis before and after a four-week rehabilitation program in patients from group II (three months to six months after injury).

Test ($N = 22$)		Before Rehabilitation		After Rehabilitation		p-Value between Groups
Parameter	Units	Median	Q25/Q75	Median	Q25/Q75	
PLT count	g/L	322.00	229.00/363.00	262.50	216.00/322.00	0.042
TF	pg/mL	453.84	337.59/617.60	451.31	333.12/506.50	0.485
TFPI	ng/mL	111.34	72.20/143.44	88.32	60.96/139.70	0.022
AT	%	97.65	90.30/111.00	99.10	87.00/107.80	0.126
TAT	ng/mL	10.40	7.18/23.48	9.66	4.50/15.22	0.906
D-dimer	ng/mL	1033.50	515.00/1800.00	935.50	430.00/1475.00	0.733

Abbreviations: AT—antithrombin activity; TAT—thrombin–antithrombin complex; TF—tissue factor; TFPI—tissue factor pathway inhibitor; Q25—lower quartile; Q75—upper quartile.

Table 6. Parameters of hemostasis before and after a four-week rehabilitation program in patients from group III (more than six months after injury).

Test ($N = 22$)		Before Rehabilitation		After Rehabilitation		p-Value between Groups
Parameter	Units	Median	Q25/Q75	Median	Q25/Q75	
PLT count	g/L	205.50	181.00/265.00	221.00	204.00/262.00	0.372
TF	ng/mL	388.90	290.25/532.81	442.09	357.50/498.14	0.050
TFPI	ng/mL	93.75	59.36/118.12	104.46	58.36/126.60	0.808
AT	%	102.55	94.00/109.20	104.05	100.50/112.00	0.095
TAT	ng/mL	5.40	3.65/11.52	5.15	3.06/6.26	0.091
D-dimer	ng/mL	522.00	284.00/1057.00	420.00	262.00/711.00	0.768

Abbreviations: AT—antithrombin activity; TAT—thrombin–antithrombin complex; TF—tissue factor; TFPI—tissue factor pathway inhibitor; Q25—lower quartile; Q75—upper quartile.

Among patients from group II (3 to 6 months after injury) high TF, TFPI, TAT complex, and D-dimer levels were noted on admission (Table 5). A significant decrease in PLT count and TFPI level was observed after rehabilitation in group II.

The patients from group III (>6 months after SCI) demonstrated on admission high concentrations of TF, TFPI, and TAT complex compared to the control group, as well as slightly elevated D-dimer levels (Table 6). A significant increase in TF concentrations was observed after rehabilitation in group III. A decrease in D-dimer levels after rehabilitation was not statistically significant in group III; however, the median value of D-dimer concentration was within normal limits after rehabilitation (Table 6).

The analysis of the measurements of hemostasis parameters in all three groups of SCI patients indicated that D-dimer levels decreased gradually with increasing time elapsed since SCI both at hospital admission (i.e., before rehabilitation) and after rehabilitation, from the highest values in group I before rehabilitation to almost normal levels in group III after rehabilitation (Tables 4–6). It should be emphasized that TF, TFPI, and TAT levels were significantly higher in all SCI groups both before and after rehabilitation compared to the control group (Tables 2 and 4–6). However, we did observe a gradual reduction in TF and TAT complex concentrations as time progressed.

4. Discussion

To our knowledge, this is the first study to examine the effect of a systematic rehabilitation program on hemostasis in patients with SCI. We found that patients after SCI showed a continued activation of coagulation and fibrinolytic system long term after injury despite participation in a four-week rehabilitation program. Importantly, no decrease in activation of TF-dependent coagulation was observed after rehabilitation, as evidenced by persistently high TF, TFPI, and TAT, regardless of time period within which rehabilitation was carried out. Significant increase in TF level after rehabilitation that was conducted beyond six months after injury suggests that rehabilitation may even induce prothrombotic potential in patients leading a sedentary lifestyle in the chronic phase of SCI. However, D-dimer levels decreased significantly after rehabilitation, the most within 3 months after SCI, which may indicate a reduction of high fibrinolytic potential, especially when rehabilitation was done in the subacute phase of SCI.

Our findings consistently demonstrate the presence of pronounced activation of coagulation in patients hospitalized in both the subacute and chronic phase of SCI, which was manifested by significantly elevated concentrations of TF and to a lesser extent TFPI, in all examined groups of patients regardless of time elapsed since SCI. In addition, we observed that TF level remained elevated after a four-week course of rehabilitation, or even increased significantly in patients undergoing rehabilitation beyond six months after SCI. Moreover, TFPI levels remained high after rehabilitation, although a significant drop in TFPI was observed after rehabilitation that was carried out between three to six months after SCI. Similarly, a high concentration of the TAT complex was observed both before and after rehabilitation in all SCI groups regardless of time elapsed since injury, but particularly in patients up to six months after injury. Beyond six months after SCI, the TAT complex concentrations both before and after rehabilitation were found to be lower, although they still exceeded the values found in the control group more than twofold.

Additionally, we observed a significant contribution of fibrinolysis in the process of hemostasis among patients after SCI. Increased concentrations of D-dimer in SCI patients suggest activation of fibrinolysis, which is secondary to excessive blood coagulation. Activation of fibrinolysis was noted especially in patients who were up to six months after SCI. Fibrinolysis is a natural compensation mechanism in the presence of blood hypercoagulability. Endothelial cells lining the circulatory system produce and secrete tissue plasminogen activator (tPA) into the blood, which degrades micro-clots forming in the endothelium by transforming plasminogen to plasmin [23]. However, our study demonstrated that systematic exercise of moderate intensity led to a reduction of blood D-dimer levels in SCI patients. The greatest reduction of D-dimer levels following rehabilitation was observed in the group of patients undergoing a four-week program of rehabilitation in the subacute phase (up to three months) after SCI, while a smaller effect of rehabilitation was found with increasing time elapsed since injury.

Detailed analysis of study parameters showed varying results depending on the time after SCI when rehabilitation took place. In a group of 34 patients undergoing rehabilitation within the first three months after injury, we observed a decrease of D-dimer level, as well as a reduction in AT activity. In a group of 22 patients who were subject to rehabilitation between three and six months after SCI, exercise led to a decrease of PLT count and TFPI concentration. Rehabilitation that was conducted in 22 patients who were after six months from injury caused a significant increase in TF concentration.

Several publications have reported elevated D-dimer levels in patients after SCI in both the acute and chronic phase [6,24,25]. It should be emphasized that increased D-dimer is often observed in patients after SCI without a diagnosis of VTE [24–26]. D-dimer is formed by the degradation of fibrin, the main component of a clot, by plasmin. Boudaoud et al. [24] and Roussi et al. [25] stated that persistently elevated D-dimer levels in the chronic phase after injury were associated with persistent prothrombotic processes and absence of proper fibrinolytic potential. This is consistent with our results, which indicated a persistent activation of coagulation in patients admitted to hospital in the period from three weeks to over six months after injury. The patients after SCI exhibited significantly elevated concentrations of TF, TFPI, and TAT compared to the control group, while increased D-dimer levels, especially within the first three months, indicated persistently increased fibrinolytic potential.

The influence of physical activity on coagulation and fibrinolysis was investigated in various populations and, while some studies reported increased coagulation and fibrinolysis after exertion, others found a reduction [27–31]. In our study, we observed a decrease in D-dimer formation in patients after four weeks of rehabilitation, which was most pronounced in the group of patients who had rehabilitation within the first three months after injury. In addition, the D-dimer levels decreased with time since injury. The decrease in D-dimer after rehabilitation may be related to the rehabilitation itself or to reduced number of complications in the subacute and chronic phase after SCI such as infections, decubitus ulcers, or acute heterotopic ossifications, which may affect activation of coagulation and fibrinolysis [32].

In a study of 4000 elderly men, Wannamethee et al. [27] concluded that physical activity had an inversely proportional effect on many components of hemostasis including PLT count, factors VII and XI, tPA, activated partial thromboplastin time (APTT), D-dimer, as well as inflammatory factors such as C-reactive protein (CRP) and leukocyte count. Their study confirmed that systematic physical activity produced changes in factors involved in coagulation as well as fibrinolysis. In our study, after a four-week rehabilitation program, we observed a reduction in fibrinolysis and persistently high values of the coagulation parameters such as TF and TAT. In contrast, Molz et al. [28] observed an increase in factors involved in fibrinolysis such as D-dimer, plasminogen activator inhibitor (PAI) concentration, and PAI activity immediately after moderate-to-intense exercise as well as during the 30-minute recovery time. These authors suggested that elevated D-dimer levels after exercise and in the first 30 min of recovery indirectly indicate an increase in fibrin formation. They also observed shortening of APTT which could reflect simultaneous activation of coagulation and fibrinolysis during moderate-to-intensive exercise. Other researchers, including van den Burg et al. [33], also observed an increase in D-dimer concentration after physical exercise. Lippi et al. [30] measured D-dimer levels and concentrations of coagulation factors such as VIIa, VIIIa, and von Willebrand Factor (vWF) in professional cyclists and cross-country skiers and compared them to individuals leading sedentary lifestyle, but did not find significant differences between the two groups. Similarly, Clark et al. [31], who evaluated the hemostatic parameters such as D-dimer, tPA, and fibrinogen as well as CRP in volunteers after four weeks of endurance training, did not observe significant changes other than a sudden increase in tPA levels immediately after exercise.

Dimitriadou et al. [34] reported an increased number of PLTs and augmented platelet aggregation in Finish runners after a marathon. Increased PLT counts were also found in sedentary children after moderate exercise, and the elevated PLT levels persisted for 24 h [35]. In our study, however, we did not observe an increased number of PLT after four weeks of rehabilitation but the opposite, i.e., PLT level decreased in group of patients undergoing rehabilitation between three to six months after SCI. Lippi et al. [29] claimed that intense physical activity led to transient hypercoagulability, especially in normally sedentary patients, which might result in thrombotic complications and sudden death. In our study, we observed significant increase in TF concentration after rehabilitation when it was conducted beyond six months after SCI. Such patients are usually wheelchair-bound for many months and their ability to exercise is limited. However, no complications such as DVT were observed in our study in this group of patients.

A review of the literature reveals that changes in hemostasis depend on the intensity of exertion and on when the clotting and fibrinolysis parameters are measured, i.e., whether they are analyzed immediately after single exercise or, as in our study, after a rehabilitation program consisting of several weeks of exercise. Lippi et al. [29] postulated that intense exertion led only to short-lasting, transient changes in coagulation. Van den Burg et al. [33] observed after exercises in healthy subjects with different ages increased concentrations of selected parameters of the intrinsic coagulation pathway in the absence of changes in the extrinsic and common coagulation pathways. They reported increases in concentrations of coagulation factors of the intrinsic pathway and TAT complex, which reflected thrombin formation (common pathway). Further augmentation of components of the intrinsic coagulation pathway occurred immediately after exercise. These authors also demonstrated increased fibrinolysis as reflected by increased D-dimer formation during submaximal and maximal exercise, as well as immediately afterward [33]. Collins et al. [36], on the other hand, examined parameters of hemostasis immediately after physical activity among patients with intermittent claudication vs. healthy subjects. They noted increased TAT and D-dimer levels after exertion in both groups. A review of available studies on the effects of various types of physical activity on hemostasis reveals some disparities with regard to the involvement of extrinsic (TF, TFPI, fVII, PT) or intrinsic (fV, VIII, IX, APTT) coagulation pathways in the processes of hemostasis.

In our study, after four weeks of rehabilitation, we observed no changes in TF (except for elevated levels in patients undergoing rehabilitation during a period that begins more than six months after SCI), TFPI (except for a decrease in patients between three to six months after SCI), and TAT levels. The lack of activation of the extrinsic coagulation pathway after exertion in our study is consistent with results of Weiss et al. [37] and Lund et al. [38], who also observed no increase in TF expression following intensive exercise. Weiss et al. [37] postulated that the extrinsic coagulation pathway was not responsible for the formation of thrombin and fibrin after exercise. Menzel et al. [39], however, studied the influence of maximal and submaximal exertion in a group of young (24 years old) and middle-aged (48 years old) people and observed an increase in the levels of selected components of the extrinsic and intrinsic pathways after exercise.

The incidence of VTE in the general population averages 0.5% among individuals less than 50 years of age and increases with age, reaching 3.8% in patients above the age of 80 [40]. Patients after SCI are usually young and at a very high risk of VTE, especially in the acute phase after injury, as evidenced by the frequency of DVT of 5.4 to 27% and PE of 4 to 5.2% [1–7]. In our study that included patients in the subacute and chronic phase after SCI, with an average age of 37.7 years, VTE was observed in 9% of patients. The significant disturbances of hemostasis following SCI have been reported to contribute to higher incidence of VTE in the SCI patients [6,9,10,41,42]. Our findings indicate that systematic moderate exercise can affect the hemostasis disorders in patients with SCI and these effects vary depending on time elapsed since injury. The SCI patients participating in an exercised-based rehabilitation program showed a continued activation of coagulation and fibrinolytic system with accompanying depletion of fibrinolysis. In general, these results imply the persisting risk of VTE events in patients participating in the rehabilitation program after SCI. These findings have clinical implications for post-SCI management, especially with regard to the modalities and timing of rehabilitation programs. However, further studies are needed with longer-term follow-up and larger groups of SCI patients, including those at a higher risk of VTE complications in the acute phase of SCI, to identify the prognostic markers for VTE events and address the mechanisms of hemostasis disorders.

5. Limitations of the Study

There was no control group that included SCI patients who did not undergo rehabilitation due to the difficulty of accessing such patients, especially in the subacute phase of SCI, up to three months after injury. If patients are not subject to rehabilitation during this period, it is usually because they have severe complications that preclude exercising.

6. Conclusions

No decrease in activation of TF-dependent coagulation, as evidenced by persistently high TF, TFPI, and TAT complex levels, was observed in patients with SCI after a four-week rehabilitation program of moderate-intensity exercises regardless of time elapsed since injury. Significant increase in TF levels after rehabilitation that was carried out beyond six-month after SCI implies that exercise may induce additional prothrombotic potential in individuals leading sedentary lifestyle in the chronic phase of SCI. Persistently elevated concentrations of TF, TFPI, and TAT complex were not associated with the occurrence of VTE incidents during the observation period. Significant decrease in D-dimer levels after rehabilitation was observed which may indicate a reduction of high fibrinolytic potential, especially when rehabilitation was carried out in the subacute phase of SCI.

Author Contributions: Conceptualization, M.M.-M., D.R., and I.Ś.; data curation, M.M.-M. and M.C.-A.; formal analysis, M.M.-M., D.R., and I.Ś.; investigation, M.M.-M.; methodology, M.M.-M. and D.R.; project administration, M.M.-M.; resources, I.G.-M. and M.C.-A.; software, M.C.-A.; supervision, M.M.-M. and D.R., validation M.M.-M. and I.Ś., visualization, M.M.-M., writing—original draft, M.M.-M. and I.Ś.; writing—review and editing, M.M.-M., I.Ś., and M.C.-A. All authors have read and approved the submitted version of the manuscript.

Funding: This research received no external funding.

Acknowledgments: We wish to thank the patients and professional personnel in the Department of Rehabilitation, University Hospital No. 1, Bydgoszcz, Poland, for their assistance in this study.

Conflicts of Interest: The authors declare no conflict of interest.

References

1. Jones, T.; Ugalde, V.; Franks, P.; Zhou, H.; White, R.H. Venous Thromboembolism after Spinal Cord Injury: Incidence, Time Course, and Associated Risk Factors in 16,240 Adults and Children. *Arch. Phys. Med. Rehabil.* **2005**, *86*, 2240–2247. [CrossRef] [PubMed]
2. Aito, S.; Pieri, A.; D'Andrea, M.; Marcelli, F.; Cominelli, E. Primary prevention of deep venous thrombosis and pulmonary emboliom in acute spinal cord injured patients. *Spinal Cord* **2002**, *40*, 300–303. [CrossRef] [PubMed]

3. Riklin, C.; Baumberger, M.; Wick, L.; Michel, D.; Sauter, B.; Knecht, H. Deep vein thrombosis and heterotopic ossification in spinal cord injury: A 3 year experience at the Swiss Paraplegic Centre Nottwil. *Spinal Cord* **2003**, *41*, 192–198. [CrossRef] [PubMed]
4. Waring, W.P.; Karunas, R.S. Acute spinal cord injuries and the incidence of clinically occurring thromboembolic disease. *Paraplegia* **1991**, *29*, 8–16. [CrossRef] [PubMed]
5. Furlan, J.C.; Fehlings, M.G. Role of screening tests for deep venous thrombosis in asymptomatic adults with acute spinal cord injury: An evidence-based analysis. *Spine* **2007**, *32*, 1908–1916. [CrossRef] [PubMed]
6. Mackiewicz-Milewska, M.; Jung, S.; Kroszczyński, A.C.; Mackiewicz-Nartowicz, H.; Serafin, Z.; Cisowska-Adamiak, M.; Pyskir, J.; Szymkuć-Bukowska, I.; Hagner, W.; Rość, D. Deep venous thrombosis in patients with chronic spinal cord injury. *J. Spinal Cord Med.* **2016**, *39*, 400–404. [CrossRef] [PubMed]
7. Giorgi-Pierfranceschi, M.; Donadini, M.P.; Dentali, F.; Ageno, W.; Marazzi, M.; Bocchi, R.; Imberti, D. The Short- And Long-Term Risk of Venous Thromboembolism in Patients with Acute Spinal Cord Injury: A Prospective Cohort Study. *Thromb. Haemost.* **2013**, *109*, 34–38.
8. Teasell, R.W.; Hsieh, T.J.; Aubut, J.A.L.; Eng, J.J.; Krassioukov, A.; Tu, L.; The SCIRE Research Team. Venous Thromboembolism Following Spinal Cord Injury. *Arch. Phys. Med. Rehabil.* **2009**, *90*, 232–245.
9. Miranda, A.R.; Hassouna, H.I. Mechanisms of thrombosis in spinal cord injury. *Hematol. Oncol. Clin. N. Am.* **2000**, *14*, 401–416. [CrossRef]
10. Myllynen, P.; Kammonen, M.; Rokkanen, P.; Böstman, O.; Lalla, M.; Laasonen, E.; Vahtera, E. The blood F VIII:Ag/F VIII:C ratio as an early indicator of deep venous thrombosis during post-traumatic immobilization. *J. Trauma* **1987**, *27*, 287–290. [CrossRef]
11. Ikarugi, H.; Yamamoto, J. The exercise paradox may be solved by measuring the overall thrombotic state using native blood. *Drug Discov. Ther.* **2017**, *11*, 15–19. [CrossRef] [PubMed]
12. O'Keefe, J.H.; Patil, H.R.; Lavie, C.J.; Magalski, A.; Vogel, R.A.; McCullough, P.A. Potential Adverse Cardiovascular Effects from Excessive Endurance Exercise. *Mayo Clin. Proc.* **2012**, *87*, 587–595. [CrossRef] [PubMed]
13. Fiuza-Luces, C.; Santos-Lozano, A.; Joyner, M.; Carrera-Bastos, P.; Picazo, O.; Zugaza, J.L.; Izquierdo, M.; Ruilope, L.M.; Lucia, A. Exercise benefits in cardiovascular disease: Beyond attenuation of traditional risk factors. *Nat. Rev. Cardiol.* **2018**, *15*, 731–743. [CrossRef] [PubMed]
14. Steffel, J.; Lüscher, T.F.; Tanner, F.C. Tissue factor in cardiovascular diseases: Molecular mechanisms and clinical implications. *Circulation* **2006**, *113*, 722–731. [CrossRef]
15. Price, C.; Thompson, A.; Kam, C.A. Tissue factor and tissue factor pathway inhibitor. *Anesthesia* **2004**, *59*, 483–492. [CrossRef]
16. Mackman, N. Role of Tissue Factor in Hemostasis, Thrombosis, and Vascular Development. *Arterioscler. Thromb. Vasc. Biol.* **2004**, *24*, 1015–1022. [CrossRef] [PubMed]
17. Hobbs, S.D.; Haggart, P.; Fegan, C.; Bradbury, A.W.; Adam, D.J. The Role of Tissue Factor in Patients Undergoing Open Repair of Ruptured and Nonruptured Abdominal Aortic Aneurysms. *J. Vasc. Surg.* **2007**, *46*, 682–686. [CrossRef]
18. Nemerson, Y. Tissue factor and hemostasis. *Blood* **1988**, *71*, 1–8. [CrossRef]
19. Mackman, N.; Tilley, R.E.; Key, N.S. Role of the Extrinsic Pathway of Blood Coagulation in Hemostasis and Thrombosis. *Arterioscler. Thromb. Vasc. Biol.* **2007**, *27*, 1687–1693. [CrossRef]
20. Kasthuri, R.S.; Glover, S.L.; Boles, J.; Mackman, N. Tissue Factor and Tissue Factor Pathway Inhibitor as Key Regulators of Global Hemostasis: Measurement of Their Levels in Coagulation Assays. *Semin. Thromb. Hemost.* **2010**, *36*, 764–771. [CrossRef]
21. Lwaleed, B.A.; Bass, P.S. Tissue factor pathway inhibitor: Structure, biology and involvement in disease. *J. Pathol.* **2006**, *208*, 327–339. [CrossRef] [PubMed]
22. Fidan, S.; Erkut, M.; Cosar, A.M.; Yogun, Y.; Örem, A.; Sönmez, M.; Arslan, M. Higher Thrombin-Antithrombin III Complex Levels May Indicate Severe Acute Pancreatitis. *Dig. Dis.* **2018**, *36*, 244–251. [CrossRef] [PubMed]
23. Collen, D. Molecular mechanisms of fibrinolysis and their application to fibrin-specific thrombolytic therapy. *J. Cell Biochem.* **1987**, *33*, 77–86. [CrossRef] [PubMed]
24. Boudaoud, L.; Roussi, J.; Lortat-Jacob, S.; Bussel, B.; Dizien, O.; Drouet, L. Endothelial fibrinolytic reactivity and the risk of deep venous thrombosis after spinal cord injury. *Spinal Cord* **1997**, *35*, 151–157. [CrossRef]

25. Roussi, J.; Bentolila, S.; Boudaoud, L.; Casadevall, N.; Vallée, C.; Carlier, R.; Lortat-Jacob, S.; Dizien, O.; Bussel, B. Contribution of D-Dimer determination in the exclusion of deep venous thrombosis in spinal cord injury patients. *Spinal Cord* **1999**, *37*, 548–552. [CrossRef]
26. Matsumoto, S.; Suda, K.; Iimoto, S.; Yasui, K.; Komatsu, M.; Ushiku, C.; Takahata, M.; Kobayashi, Y.; Tojo, Y.; Fujita, K.; et al. Prospective study of deep vein thrombosis in patients with spinal cord injury not receiving anticoagulant therapy. *Spinal Cord* **2015**, *53*, 306–309. [CrossRef]
27. Wannamethee, S.G.; Lowe, G.D.; Whincup, P.H.; Rumley, A.; Walker, M.; Lennon, L. Physical activity and hemostatic and inflammatory variables in elderly men. *Circulation* **2002**, *105*, 1785–1790. [CrossRef]
28. Molz, A.B.; Heyduck, B.; Lill, H.; Spanuth, E.; Röcker, L. The effect of different exercise intensities on the fibrinolytic system. *Eur. J. Appl. Physiol. Occup. Physiol.* **1993**, *67*, 298–304. [CrossRef]
29. Lippi, G.; Maffulli, N. Biological influence of physical exercise on hemostasis. *Semin. Thromb. Hemost.* **2009**, *35*, 269–276. [CrossRef]
30. Lippi, G.; Salvagno, G.L.; Montagana, M.; Guidi, G.C. Chronic influence of vigorous aerobic training on hemostasis. *Blood Coagul. Fibrinolysis* **2005**, *16*, 533–534. [CrossRef]
31. Clark, B.C.; Manini, T.M.; Hoffman, R.L.; Williams, P.S.; Guiler, M.K.; Knutson, M.J.; McGlynn, M.L.; Kushnick, M.R. Relative safety of 4 weeks of blood flow-restricted resistance exercise in young, healthy adults. *Scand. J. Med. Sci. Sports* **2011**, *21*, 653–662. [CrossRef]
32. Perkash, A.; Sullivan, G.; Toth, L.; Bradleigh, L.H.; Linder, S.H.; Perkash, I. Persistent hypercoagulation associated with heterotopic ossification in patients with spinal cord injury long after injury has occurred. *Paraplegia* **1993**, *31*, 653–659. [CrossRef] [PubMed]
33. Van den Burg, P.J.; Hospers, J.E.; Van Vliet, M.; Mosterd, W.L.; Bouma, B.N.; Huisveld, I.A. Changes in haemostatic factors and activation products after exercise in healthy subjects with different ages. *Thromb. Haemost.* **1995**, *74*, 1457–1464. [CrossRef]
34. Dimitriadou, C.; Dessypris, A.; Louizou, C.; Mandalaki, T. Marathon run II: Effects on platelet aggregation. *Thromb. Haemost.* **1977**, *37*, 451–455. [CrossRef] [PubMed]
35. Ribeiro, J.; Almeida-Dias, A.; Ascensão, A.; Magalhães, J.; Oliveira, A.R.; Carlson, J.; Mota, J.; Appell, H.J.; Duarte, J. Hemostatic response to acute physical exercise in healthy adolescents. *J. Sci. Med. Sport* **2007**, *10*, 164–169. [CrossRef]
36. Collins, P.; Ford, I.; Croal, B.; Ball, D.; Greaves, M.; Macaulay, E.; Brittenden, J. Haemostasis, inflammation and renal function following exercise in patients with intermittent claudication on statin and aspirin therapy. *Thromb. J.* **2006**, *4*, 9. [CrossRef] [PubMed]
37. Weiss, C.; Bierhaus, A.; Kinscherf, R.; Hack, V.; Luther, T.; Nawroth, P.P.; Bärtsch, P. Tissue factor-dependent pathway is not involved in exercise-induced formation of thrombin and fibrin. *J. Appl. Physiol.* **2002**, *92*, 211–218. [CrossRef] [PubMed]
38. Lund, T.; Kvernmo, H.D.; Osterud, B. Cellular activation in response to physical exercise: The effect of platelets and granulocytes on monocyte reactivity. *Blood Coagul. Fibrinolysis* **1998**, *9*, 63–69. [CrossRef]
39. Menzel, K.; Hilberg, T. Coagulation and fibrinolysis are in balance after moderate exercise in middle-aged participants. *Clin. Appl. Thromb. Hemost.* **2009**, *15*, 348–355. [CrossRef]
40. Hansson, P.O.; Welin, L.; Tibblin, G.; Eriksson, H. Deep Vein Thrombosis and Pulmonary Embolism in the General Population. 'The Study of Men Born in 1913'. *Arch. Intern. Med.* **1997**, *157*, 1665–1670. [CrossRef]
41. Fujii, Y.; Mammen, E.F.; Farag, A.; Muz, J.; Salciccioli, G.G.; Weingarden, S.T. Thrombosis in spinal cord injury. *Thromb. Res.* **1992**, *68*, 357–368. [CrossRef]
42. Sugimoto, Y.; Ito, Y.; Tomioka, M.; Tanaka, M.; Hasegawa, Y.; Nakago, K.; Yagata, Y. Deep venous thrombosis in patients with acute cervical spinal cord injury in a Japanese population: Assessment with Doppler ultrasonography. *J. Orthop. Sci.* **2009**, *14*, 374–376. [CrossRef] [PubMed]

Journal of
Clinical Medicine

MDPI

Article

Early Spinal Injury Stabilization in Multiple-Injured Patients: Do All Patients Benefit?

Philipp Kobbe [1,*], Patrick Krug [2], Hagen Andruszkow [1], Miguel Pishnamaz [1], Martijn Hofman [1], Klemens Horst [1], Carolin Meyer [3], Max Joseph Scheyerer [3], Christoph Faymonville [3,4], Gregor Stein [5], Frank Hildebrand [1] and Christian Herren [1]

1 Department for Trauma and Reconstructive Surgery, RWTH Aachen University Hospital, Pauwelsstraße 30, 52074 Aachen, Germany; handruszkow@ukaachen.de (H.A.); mpishnamaz@ukaachen.de (M.P.); mhofman@ukaachen.de (M.H.); khorst@ukaachen.de (K.H.); fhildebrand@ukaachen.de (F.H.); cherren@ukaachen.de (C.H.)
2 Department of Orthopedics and Trauma Surgery, Rhein-Maas Klinikum GmbH, Mauerfeldchen 25, 52146 Wuerselen, Germany; patrick.krug@gmx.net
3 Department of Medicine, University of Cologne, Joseph-Stelzmann-Str. 24, 50931 Cologne, Germany; carolin.meyer@uk-koeln.de (C.M.); max.scheyerer@uk-koeln.de (M.J.S.); christoph.faymonville@uk-koeln.de (C.F.)
4 Department of Orthopedics and Trauma Surgery, Evangelic Hospital Cologne-Weyertal, Weyertal 76, 50931 Cologne, Germany
5 Department of Orthopedics, Trauma and Spine Surgery, Helios Hospital Siegburg, Ringstraße 49, 53721 Siegburg, Germany; gregor.stein@helios-gesundheit.de
* Correspondence: pkobbe@ukaachen.de

Received: 14 March 2020; Accepted: 3 June 2020; Published: 5 June 2020

Abstract: Background: Thoracolumbar spine fractures in multiple-injured patients are a common injury pattern. The appropriate timing for the surgical stabilization of vertebral fractures is still controversial. The purpose of this study was to analyse the impact of the timing of spinal surgery in multiple-injured patients both in general and in respect to spinal injury severity. Methods: A retrospective analysis of multiple-injured patients with an associated spinal trauma within the thoracic or lumbar spine (injury severity score (ISS) >16, age >16 years) was performed from January 2012 to December 2016 in two Level I trauma centres. Demographic data, circumstances of the accident, and ISS, as well as time to spinal surgery were documented. The evaluated outcome parameters were length of stay in the intensive care unit (ICU) (iLOS) and length of stay (LOS) in the hospital, duration of mechanical ventilation, onset of sepsis, and multiple organ dysfunction syndrome (MODS), as well as mortality. Statistical analysis was performed using SPSS. Results: A total of 113 multiple-injured patients with spinal stabilization and a complete dataset were included in the study. Of these, 71 multiple-injured patients (63%) presented with an AOSpine A-type spinal injury, whereas 42 (37%) had an AOSpine B-/C-type spinal injury. Forty-nine multiple-injured patients (43.4%) were surgically treated for their spinal injury within 24 h after trauma, and showed a significantly reduced length of stay in the ICU (7.31 vs. 14.56 days; $p < 0.001$) and hospital stay (23.85 vs. 33.95 days; $p = 0.048$), as well as a significantly reduced prevalence of sepsis compared to those surgically treated later than 24 h (3 vs. 7; $p = 0.023$). These adverse effects were even more pronounced in the case where cutoffs were increased to either 72 h or 96 h. Independent risk factors for a delay in spinal surgery were a higher ISS ($p = 0.036$), a thoracic spine injury ($p = 0.001$), an AOSpine A-type spinal injury ($p = 0.048$), and an intact neurological status ($p < 0.001$). In multiple-injured patients with AOSpine A-type spinal injuries, an increased time to spinal surgery was only an independent risk factor for an increased LOS; however, in multiple-injured patients with B-/C-type spinal injuries, an increased time to spinal surgery was an independent risk factor for increased iLOS, LOS, and the development of sepsis. Conclusion: Our data support the concept of early spinal stabilization in multiple-injured patients with AOSpine B-/C-type injuries, especially of the thoracic spine. However, in multiple-injured patients with AOSpine A-type injuries, the beneficial impact of early spinal stabilization has been overemphasized in former studies, and the benefit should be weighed out against the risk of patients' deterioration during early spinal stabilization.

Keywords: multiple-injured patient; spine injury; AOSpine classification; time to surgery; sepsis

---

1. Introduction

The patient with multiple injuries is a unique challenge for the trauma care team, even more so in association with spinal fractures. Traumatic spinal injuries in multiple-injured patients are less common in comparison to extremity injuries but present with an increasing incidence over the last decades [1,2]. Most of these injuries are located within the thoracic and lumbar spine and are accompanied by lung contusion and/or abdominal trauma [3,4]. Beside worse outcomes, a cost analysis showed that apart from injuries of the head, associated spinal lesions in multiple-injured patients result in higher hospitalisation costs and prolonged length of stay (LOS) [5].

Controversy still arises concerning the optimal timing for spinal surgery in the multiple-injured patient. In the literature, the discussion has ultimately focused on the question of early versus late surgical treatment and its consequences on mortality and the patients' outcome [6,7]. Recent register studies generally advocate that early spinal stabilization is beneficial for multiple-injured patients, mainly due to the increased possibility of early patient mobilisation in the ICU [8]; however, these register studies do not differentiate the wide variety of different spinal injuries. For example, although AOSpine A-type fractures are managed surgically in some countries to maintain sagittal spinal balance, they are—from a biomechanical viewpoint—stable enough to tolerate early mobilisation in the ICU without the risk of neurological compromise. Therefore, a general recommendation to perform early spinal stabilization, which is definitely a surgical burden and second hit in this scenario, may not be justified, and may even jeopardize multiple-injured patients with biomechanically stable spinal injuries.

For this reason, the aim of the present study is to analyse the impact of the timing of spinal surgery in multiple-injured patients both in general and in respect to spinal injury severity.

2. Methods

This retrospective two-centre study was conducted on all multiple-injured patients with spinal injuries who were admitted to one of the two level I trauma hospitals between January 2012 and December 2016. Patients were eligible for further analysis if they met the following inclusion criteria: age >16 years; injury severity score (ISS) >16; associated spinal injury within the thoracic or lumbar spine; and a fully available computed tomography scan for spinal injury classification, according to the established AOSpine Classification [9]. Demographic data, circumstances of the accident, overall injury severity score (ISS), and time to spinal surgery (24, 72, and 96 h) were documented. Measured outcome parameters were duration of mechanical ventilation, intensive care unit (ICU) length of stay (iLOS), length of hospital stay (LOS), development of sepsis or multiple organ dysfunction syndrome (MODS), and death. Organ failure was defined according to the sequential organ failure assessment (SOFA) score: a value in one or more organ systems of ≥3 points was defined as single or multiple organ failure. Sepsis was defined as systemic inflammatory response syndrome (SIRS) combined with bacteraemia.

Data were collected from the inhouse clinical documentation system. Counts and frequencies were used to describe the sample. Correlation analysis (Spearman) was used to determine any dependence between the variables. For evaluation of influencing factors on the timing of surgery, a chi-square test and a one-way ANOVA was performed. Fisher's exact test was used for categorical variables. Multivariable logistic regression analysis was performed using time to surgery, LOS, iLOS, and sepsis as dependent variables. Results are presented as odds ratios (ORs) with 95% confidence intervals. Significance was set at $p < 0.05$ for all statistical tests. A power analysis was carried out with G *

Power (3.1.9.3, IBM) and resulted in the following statistical power for each statistical test: 0.998 for the ANOVA, 0.963 for the *t*-test, and 0.999 for both the correlation analysis and the regression analysis.

All testing procedures were performed exploratively, so no adjustment for multiple testing has been made. Statistical analyses were performed with IBM SPSS software (version 23; IBM Corp., Armonk, New York, NY, USA). The study complies with the principles of the Declaration of Helsinki (2013) and was approved by the local ethical committee (#EK056/17).

3. Results

3.1. Demographics

A total of 250 multiple-injured patients with vertebral fractures within the thoracolumbar spine were identified (Table 1). The population consisted of 72 (29%) female and 178 male (71%) patients with a mean age of 46 ± 19 years. The mean ISS was 24.8 ± 12.6 points. The most common injury pattern was a fall of >3 m (n = 102, 41%), followed by car accident (n = 39, 16%) and motorcycle accident (n = 38, 15%). In 153 patients (61%) the lumbar spine and in 97 patients (38%) the thoracic spine was involved. In 127 patients (51%) spinal stabilization was performed, of whom 14 patients had to be excluded due to missing data (Figure 1). Thus, 113 patients were included for further statistical analysis.

Table 1. Baseline demographics for spinal fractures in multiple-injured patients.

Demographics	
mean age (SD, years)	46.4 (18.9)
female (%)	72 (28.8%)
male (%)	178 (71.2%)
mean ISS (SD)	24.8 (12.6)
Mechanism of Injury (*n*)	
high fall (>3 m)	102
car accident	39
motorcycle accident	38
low fall (<3 m)	26
other	19
bicycle accident	15
pedestrian	11
AIS ≥3 (*n*)	
Head and Face	84
Thorax	124
Abdomen	35
Pelvis	54
Extremities	139
Spine Level (*n*)	
thoracic	97
lumbar	153

ISS: injury severity score; AIS: abbreviated injury scale.

3.2. Spinal Injury Severity According to the AOSpine Classification

Within the group of the operatively treated patients, 71 fractures (63%) were classified as AOSpine A-type injuries, whereas 42 fractures (37%) were classified as AOSpine B-/C-type injuries (Figure 2). Seventeen thoracic and 18 lumbar spinal injuries were associated with neurological impairment.

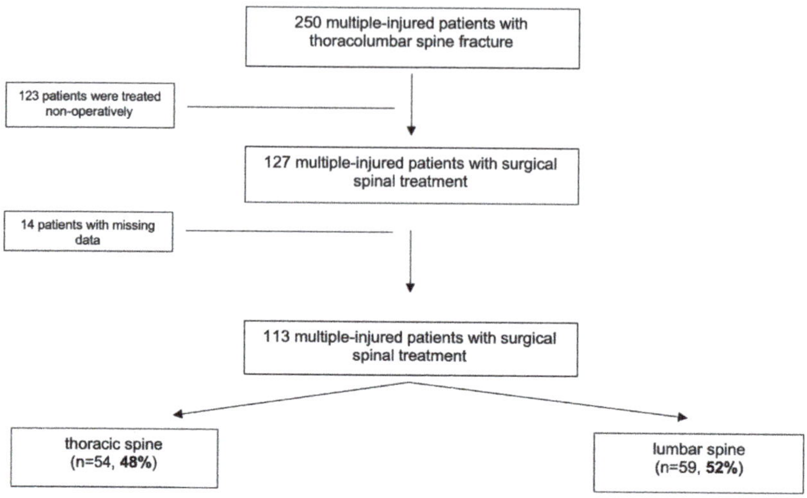

Figure 1. Flowsheet of the included population.

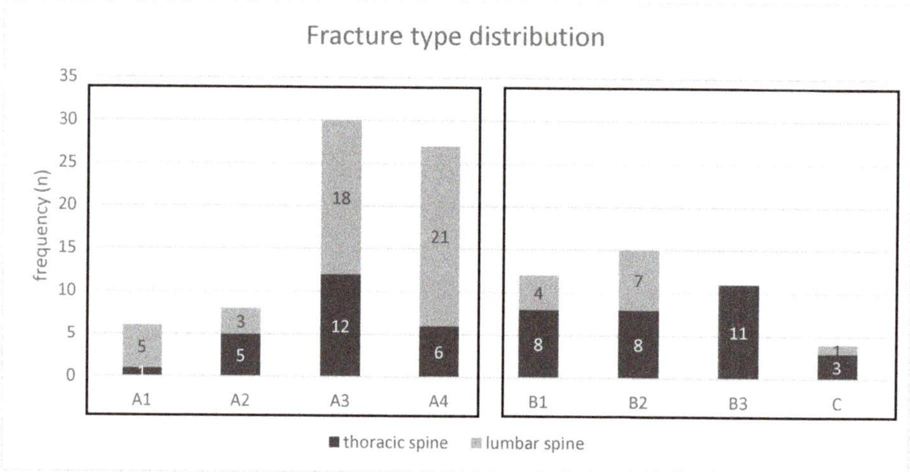

Figure 2. Distribution of the fracture type within the thoracic and lumbar spine of the surgically treated patients.

3.3. Time to Spinal Surgery

Time to spinal surgery for the 113 multiple-injured patients included in the study is presented in Figure 3. Setting a cutoff of 24 h for spinal surgery, 49 patients (43.4%) were treated within 24 h after trauma. Twenty-one of these patients presented with an AOSpine B-/C-type injury. Increasing the cutoff to 72 h for spinal surgery, 75 patients (66.4%) were treated within 72 h after trauma, of whom 32 patients presented with an AOSpine B-/C-type injury. Further increasing the cutoff to 96 h, 81 patients (71.7%) were treated within 96 h after trauma, of whom 33 patients presented with an AOSpine B-/C-type injury. Regression analysis identified a higher ISS, the thoracic spine injury location, A-type injuries, and the absence of an evident neurological deficit as independent risk factors for a delay in spinal surgery (Table 2).

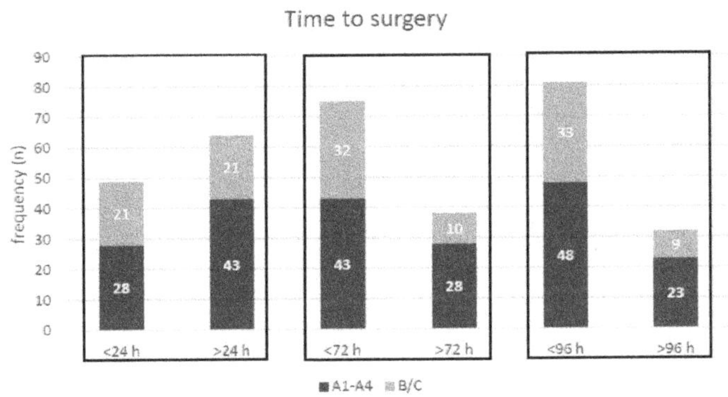

Figure 3. Distribution of the time to surgery related to three defined time points: 24, 72, and 96 h.

Table 2. Regression analysis for time to surgery (dependent variable: >24 h).

	Regression Coefficient	p-Value	OR	95% CI
Age	−0.007	0.604	0.993	0.97–1.02
ISS	0.041	**0.036**	1.042	1.00–1.08
Thoracic spine	1.889	**0.001**	0.151	0.05–0.46
A-type injuries	1.129	**0.048**	3.094	1.01–9.48
No neurological deficit	2.205	**<0.001**	9.069	2.82–29.20

Bold marked values indicate significant parameters. OR: odds ratio.

3.4. *Impact of Time to Spinal Surgery on Patients´ Outcome*

Comparison of multiple-injured patients surgically treated for their spinal injury within 24 h as compared to those surgically treated later than 24 h is shown in Table 3. Multiple-injured patients with their spinal injuries surgically treated within 24 h showed a significantly reduced length of ICU stay by 7 days (7.31 days vs. 14.56 days; $p < 0.001$) as compared to those were operated on later than 24 h while having a comparable overall injury severity (ISS: 23.69 vs. 24.80; $p = 0.672$). Furthermore, the length of hospital stay was significantly reduced by 10 days (23.85 days vs. 33.95 days; $p = 0.048$). The prevalence of sepsis was significantly higher in multiple-injured patients surgically treated for their spinal injury later than 24 h (9 vs. 1, respectively; $p = 0.023$). Mechanical ventilation time was higher in patients surgically treated for their spinal injury later than 24 h, although this did not reach statistical significance (150.94 h vs. 184.05 h, respectively; $p = 0.525$). The prevalence of MODS or death showed no statistical difference between both groups.

Table 3. Stratification analysis (ANOVA and chi-square test) for the time to surgery (<24 vs. >24 h).

Parameter / Time	≤24 h	>24 h	p-Value
n	49	64	
Age (years)	44.07 ± 18.79	47.91 ± 18.40	0.267
ISS	23.69 ± 14.76	24.80 ± 11.29	0.672
LOS (days)	23.85 ± 19.14	33.95 ± 30.63	**0.048**
ICU (days)	7.31 ± 7.19	14.56 ± 13.93	**<0.001**
mechanical ventilation (h)	150.94 ± 266.86	184.05 ± 279.64	0.525
sepsis (n)	1	9	**0.023**
MODS (n)	2	4	0.690
death (n)	2	1	0.592

Significant p-values are marked in bold. LOS: length of stay in the hospital; ICU: intensive care unit; MODS: multiple organ dysfunction syndrome.

Comparison of multiple-injured patients surgically treated for their spinal injury within 72 h as compared to those surgically treated later than 72 h is shown in Table 4. Multiple-injured patients with their spinal injuries surgically addressed later than 72 h showed a significant and twofold longer stay in the ICU (17.5 days vs. 8.46 days, respectively; $p < 0.001$) and in the hospital (44.34 days vs. 22.49 days, respectively; $p < 0.001$). Mechanical ventilation time was higher in patients surgically treated for their spinal injury later than 72 h, although this did not reach statistical significance (229.94 h vs. 141.56 h, respectively; $p = 0.114$). However, patients surgically treated for their spinal injury later than 72 h had a significantly higher ISS as compared to those patients treated within 72 h (28.05 vs. 22.49, respectively; $p = 0.03$). The prevalence of sepsis, MODS, or death showed no statistical difference between both groups.

Table 4. Stratification analysis (ANOVA and chi square test) for the time to surgery (<72 vs. >72 h).

Parameter / Time	≤72 h	>72 h	*p*-Value
n	75	38	
Age (years)	45.70 ± 18.65	47.14 ± 18.70	0.700
ISS	22.49 ± 12.80	28.05 ± 12.60	**0.03**
LOS (days)	22.49 ± 16.99	44.34 ± 35.90	**<0.001**
ICU (days)	8.46 ± 9.13	17.50 ± 14.79	**<0.001**
mechanical ventilation (h)	141.56 ± 258.44	229.94 ± 297.85	0.114
sepsis (*n*)	4	6	0.070
MODS (*n*)	4	2	1.00
death (*n*)	3	0	0.551

Significant *p*-values are marked in bold.

Comparison of multiple-injured patients surgically treated for their spinal injury within 96 h as compared to those surgically treated later than 96 h is shown in Table 5. Multiple-injured patients for whom surgical treatment of their spinal injuries was postponed for more than 96 h showed a significant and twofold longer stay in the ICU (8.55 days vs. 18.41 days respectively; $p < 0.001$) and in the hospital (23.01 days vs. 45.84 days, respectively; $p < 0.001$). Although the overall injury severity was higher in the group surgically treated for their spinal injuries after 96 h, it did not reach statistical significance (27.72 vs. 22.94; $p = 0.075$). Furthermore, mechanical ventilation time was significantly and almost twofold increased from 137.24 h to 250.81 h ($p = 0.046$). The prevalence of sepsis was also significantly higher in the group surgically treated for their spinal injuries later than 96 h (7 vs. 3, respectively; $p < 0.005$). However, the prevalence of MODS or death was not higher in the group of multiple-injured patients treated for their spinal injuries later than 96 h.

Table 5. Stratification analysis (ANOVA and chi-square test) for the time to surgery (<96 vs. >96 h).

Parameter / Time	≤96 h	>96 h	*p*-Value
n	81	32	
Age (years)	45.15 ± 18.71	48.84 ± 18.31	0.340
ISS	22.94 ± 12.50	27.72 ± 13.68	0.075
LOS (days)	23.01 ± 16.81	45.84 ± 37.83	**<0.001**
ICU (days)	8.55 ± 9.94	18.41 ± 15.43	**<0.001**
Mechanical ventilation (hours)	137.24 ± 252.88	250.81 ± 308.83	**0.046**
Sepsis (*n*)	3	7	**<0.005**
MODS (*n*)	4	2	0.673
Death (*n*)	3	0	0.562

Significant *p*-values are marked in bold.

Correlation analysis revealed that there was a significant correlation between time to spinal surgery and outcome parameters (Table 6). Lengths of ICU and hospital stays showed a significant correlation with increasing the time to spinal surgery. The development of sepsis further showed a significant correlation with increasing time to spinal surgery. However, there was no correlation between an increased time to spinal surgery and the development of MODS or death. Regression analysis revealed that increased time to spinal surgery is an independent risk factor for an increased ICU and hospital stay, and spinal stabilization later than 72 h an independent risk factor for the development of sepsis (Table 7).

Table 6. Correlation analysis (Spearman) for time to surgery.

Parameter	Time to Surgery
Age	0.31
ISS	0.25
LOS	**<0.001**
ICU	**<0.001**
Mechanical ventilation	0.08
MODS (n = 6)	0.49
Sepsis (n = 10)	**0.01**
Death (n = 3)	0.28

Significant p-values are marked in bold.

Table 7. Regression analysis with the dependent variables: LOS (days), length of stay in intensive care (iLOS; days), and sepsis.

	p-Value	Regression Coefficient	95% CI
	ICU Stay (iLOS)		
Age	0.878	0.008	−0.10–0.12
ISS	**<0.001**	0.447	0.27–0.62
Localisation	**0.040**	−4.526	−8.85–−0.20
Fracture type	0.330	2.249	−2.31–6.81
Neurological deficit	0.096	−4.197	−9.15–0.76
Time to surgery (h)	**0.020**	0.015	0.02–0.03
	Hospital Stay (LOS)		
Age	0.876	0.017	−0.20–0.23
ISS	0.094	0.293	−0.05–0.64
Localisation	0.158	6.170	−2.43–14.77
Fracture type	0.639	2.114	−6.81–11.04
Neurological deficit	0.100	7.987	−1.55–17.53
Time to surgery (h)	**<0.001**	0.045	0.02–0.07
	Sepsis		
	p-value	**OR**	**95% CI**
Age	0.888	0.997	0.96–1.04
ISS	0.575	0.982	0.92–1.05
Localisation	0.058	0.121	0.01–1.07
Fracture type	0.198	2.974	0.57–15.65
Time to surgery (72 h)	**0.046**	5.543	1.03–29.86

Bold marked values indicate significant parameters.

Subgroup analysis showed that the adverse effect of delayed spinal stabilization is mainly attributable to multiple-injured patients with AOSpine B-/C-type injuries. Regression analysis revealed that in patients with AOSpine A-type spinal injuries, an increased time to spinal surgery was only an independent risk factor for an increased LOS; however, in multiple-injured patients with B-/C-type spinal injuries, an increased time to spinal surgery is an independent risk factor for increased iLOS, LOS, and the development of sepsis (Table 8).

Table 8. Regression analysis for A and B-/C-type fractures with the dependent variables: LOS (days), iLOS (days), and sepsis.

	A-Type Fractures (n = 71)			B/C-Type Fractures (n = 42)		
	p-Value	Regression Coefficient	95% CI	p-Value	Regression Coefficient	95% CI
ICU Stay (iLOS)						
Age	0.59	0.041	−0.11–0.19	0.392	0.067	−0.09–0.23
ISS	**0.003**	0.393	0.14–0.64	**0.002**	−0.4	0.16–0.64
Localisation	**0.028**	−5.889	−11.14–−0.64	0.867	−0.602	−7.83–6.63
Neurological deficit	0.862	−0.593	−7.37–6.19	0.472	−2.661	−10.10–4.78
Time to surgery (h)	0.444	0.005	−0.01–0.02	**<0.001**	0.059	0.03–0.09
Hospital Stay (LOS)						
Age	0.922	0.016	−0.31–0.34	0.378	0.132	−0.17–0.43
ISS	0.823	0.058	−0.46–0.58	0.069	0.42	−0.04–0.88
Localisation	0.758	1.699	−9.26–12.66	**0.024**	16.891	2.32–31.46
Neurological deficit	0.08	12.155	−1.49–25.80	0.237	8.455	−5.84–22.75
Time to surgery (h)	**0.009**	0.039	0.01–0.07	**0.004**	0.081	0.03–0.14
Sepsis						
	p-Value	Odds Ratio (OR)	95% CI	p-Value	Odds Ratio (OR)	95% CI
Age	0.362	0.972	0.91–1.03	0.204	1.074	0.96–1.20
ISS	0.501	0.501	0.93–1.20	0.297	0.914	0.77–1.08
Localisation	0.091	0.091	0.01–1.40	0.999	0	0.01–1.00
Time to surgery (h)	0.857	0.999	0.99–1.01	**0.023**	1.017	1.02–1.03

Bold marked values indicate significant parameters.

3.5. Impact of Spinal Injury Severity on Patients' Outcome

Comparison of multiple-injured patients with AOSpine A-type injuries compared to those multiple-injured patients with AOSpine B-/C-type injuries is shown in Table 9.

Table 9. Stratification analysis (ANOVA and chi-square test) of the fracture type (A-type vs. B-/C-type fractures).

Parameter / Fracture Type	A-Type Fractures	B-/C-Type Fractures	p-Value
n	71	42	
Age (years)	46.04 ± 17.68	47.24 ± 20.82	0.746
ISS (points)	22.75 ± 10.72	26.36 ± 14.85	0.138
LOS (days)	29.12 ± 25.02	27.11 ± 21.40	0.678
ICU (days)	10.05 ± 10.94	14.60 ± 15.56	0.076
Mechanical ventilation (hours)	137.69 ± 242.36	227.85 ± 325.54	0.104
Time to surgery (hours)	113.33 ± 186.62	70.90 ± 130.33	0.206
Sepsis (n)	4	6	0.071
MODS (n)	2	4	0.076
Death (n)	1	2	0.310

Multiple-injured patients with A-type spinal injuries showed a trend towards a lower overall injury severity compared to multiple-injured patients with B-/C-type spinal injuries (ISS: 22.75 vs. 26.36, respectively; $p = 0.138$). Length of ICU stay was on average 4 days shorter, and time of mechanical ventilation roughly 90 h shorter in multiple-injured patients with A-type spinal injuries compared to those with B-/C-type spinal injuries; however, neither observations reached statistical significance (iLOS: 10.05 days vs. 14.60 days, respectively; $p = 0.076$; mechanical ventilation: 137.69 h vs. 227.85 h, respectively; $p = 0.104$). Time to spinal surgery was non-significantly prolonged in multiple-injured patients with A-type spinal injuries as compared to those multiple-injured patients with B-/C-type injuries (113.33 h vs. 70.90 h, respectively; $p = 0.206$). Multiple-injured patients with B-/C-type spinal injuries, compared to multiple-injured patients with A-type spinal injuries, showed a non-significant, higher prevalence of MODS (4 vs. 2, respectively; $p = 0.076$), sepsis (6 vs. 4, respectively; $p = 0.071$), and death (2 vs. 1, respectively; $p = 0.310$).

Correlation analysis showed a significant correlation between higher spinal injury severity and thoracic spinal injury location; however, there was no correlation between spinal injury severity and any measured outcome parameters, and consequently, regression analysis identified that spinal injury severity was not an independent risk factor for adverse outcome.

3.6. Impact of Spinal Injury Location on Patients' Outcomes

A comparison of multiple-injured patients with thoracic spinal injury location compared to those with lumbar spinal injury location is shown in Table 10.

Table 10. Stratification analysis (ANOVA and chi-square test) of the fracture localisation.

Parameter / Localisation	Thoracic Spine	Lumbar Spine	p-Value
n	54	59	
Age (years)	49.79 ± 19.24	42.76 ± 17.65	**0.039**
ISS (points)	25.04 ± 11.69	24.19 ± 14.20	0.728
LOS (days)	25.92 ± 18.05	32.77 ± 32.28	0.180
iLOS (days)	14.58 ± 13.86	9.48 ± 11.41	**0.032**
Mechanical ventilation (hours)	223.41 ± 298.96	136.92 ± 264.55	0.103
Time to surgery (hours)	119.24 ± 190.50	74.24 ± 140.52	0.152
Sepsis (*n*)	8	2	**0.011**
MODS (*n*)	3	3	0.385
Death (*n*)	2	1	0.412

Significant *p*-values are marked bold.

Multiple-injured patients with a thoracic spine injury showed a similar overall injury severity compared to multiple-injured patients with a lumbar spine injury (ISS: 25.04 vs. 24.19, respectively; $p = 0.728$). Length of ICU stay was significantly increased by an average of 5 days in multiple-injured patients with a thoracic spine injury compared to multiple-injured patients with a lumbar spine injury (14.58 days vs. 9.48 days, respectively; $p = 0.032$), whereas length of hospital stay showed no significant difference—although it was shorter in multiple-injured patients with a thoracic spine injury (25.92 days vs. 32.77 days, respectively; $p = 0.180$). Mechanical ventilation time was increased by an average of almost 90 h in multiple-injured patients with a thoracic spine injury compared to multiple-injured patients with a lumbar spine injury; however, this did not reach statistical significance (223.41 h vs. 136.92 h; $p = 0.103$). Time to spinal surgery was prolonged in multiple-injured patients with thoracic spine injury compared to multiple-injured patients with a lumbar spine surgery (119.24 h vs. 74.24 h; $p = 0.152$). The prevalence of MODS and death was comparable in both groups, whereas the prevalence of sepsis was significantly higher in multiple-injured patients with a thoracic spine injury compared to multiple-injured patients with a lumbar spine injury (8 vs. 2; $p = 0.011$).

Correlation analysis revealed that spinal injury location significantly correlated with patients' age, the prevalence of sepsis, the time to spinal surgery, and the spinal injury severity. Regression analysis identified spinal injury location to be an independent risk factor for an increased length of ICU stay ($p = 0.04$, Table 7).

4. Discussion

The clinical course for multiple-injured patients is determined by the initial trauma (first hit), the initial surgical burden (second hit), and the resulting systemic inflammatory response [10]. In contrast to the established damage control orthopedics (DCO) concept for long-bone fractures, which recommends performing a definite long-bone fracture stabilization later in the course of treatment, early definite spinal stabilization in multiple-injured patients is gaining increasing popularity in recent years [11,12]. This "spine damage control" concept advocates immediate posterior spinal stabilization in multiple-injured patients, with delayed anterior spinal stabilization, if required, later in the course [11,13]. Support of this concept is provided by several studies showing that early spinal stabilization in multiple-injured patients appears to be associated with a beneficial medical and socioeconomic outcome [5,8,14,15].

In general, our data support the concept of early posterior spinal stabilization in multiple-injured patients. Our data show that increasing time to spinal surgery in multiple-injured patients is an independent risk factor for an increased ICU and hospital stay, and that spinal stabilization later than 72 h is an independent risk factor for the development of sepsis. We consider immediate spinal stabilization, as advocated above, as spinal surgery within 24 h after trauma. Applying a 24 h cutoff to our patient population, we are able to show that multiple-injured patients with their spinal stabilization later than 24 h had, on average, a significantly longer stay of 7 days in the ICU, and a significantly longer length of hospital stay of 10 days, while having a comparable overall injury severity, as defined by the ISS, compared to those multiple-injured patients with spinal surgery within 24 h. Furthermore, the duration of mechanical ventilation was increased by approximately 30 h, and the prevalence of sepsis was significantly increased in the case of spinal stabilization later than 24 h. These adverse effects were even more pronounced for 72 h or 96 h as time cutoffs for spinal surgery. Several studies have attributed the beneficial effect of early spinal stabilization mainly to a better patient handling in the ICU, which allows, for example, for prone positioning for the improvement of pulmonary function, or even earlier in- or out-of-bed mobilization [8]. Most of these studies, however, do not consider spinal injury severity from a biomechanical point of view. Thus, the above-mentioned reasons for a beneficial effect of early spinal stabilization may only be true for instable spinal injuries (AOSpine B-/C-type), because stable spinal injuries (AOSpine A-type) may be considered for early mobilization anyway.

Therefore, the "spine damage control" concept has to be interpreted with caution and should not result in the recommendation that in multiple-injured patients, every spinal injury requiring surgery should be stabilized as early as possible at almost any cost. Further subgroup analyzation of our patient population supports a more individualized treatment concept, taking into account the degree of spinal injury stability, as described with the AOSpine classification. In multiple-injured patients with AOSpine B-/C-type spinal injuries, which from a biomechanical view are unstable spinal injuries, stabilization as early as possible appears to be beneficial. In these patients, prolonged time to spinal surgery is an independent risk factor for increased length of stay in the ICU and in hospital, as well as for the development of sepsis. In contrast to these findings, the benefit of an early spinal stabilization for multiple-injured patients with AOSpine A-type spinal injuries appears to be less pronounced. In these biomechanically stable spinal injuries, a prolonged time to spinal stabilization is only an independent risk factor for an increased length of hospital stay. Although we could not observe an adverse effect of the stabilization of AOSpine A-type spinal injuries in our multiple-injured patients, this observation reduces the pressure on the trauma team to deal with AOSpine A-type spinal injuries in the acute phase. Since AOSpine A-type injuries are the predominant spinal injury pattern in our multiple-injured patient population, this may have an important impact on trauma care in the future. Although a differentiation of the spinal injury, according to the AOSpine classification, is important for decisions with regard to surgical timing, the injury type in and of itself is not an independent risk factor for adverse outcomes.

Thoracic spinal injury location has been identified by other studies to adversely influence patients' outcome [16,17]. Our data reveals that thoracic spinal injury location is an independent risk factor for prolonged ICU stay. This may be explained by two considerations. First, thoracic spinal injury location in our population is associated with delayed spinal stabilization, probably due to a higher grade of required surgical expertise. Secondly, thoracic spinal injuries are probably associated with a higher rate of thoracic injury (for example, lung contusions). In our population, multiple-injured patients with thoracic spinal injuries on average required 90 h more of mechanical ventilation than those multiple-injured patients with lumbar spinal injuries.

Our data show that in our patient population, almost half of the patients (47.8%) were surgically treated for their spinal injury within 24 h, and almost $\frac{3}{4}$ of the patients (71.7%) within 72 h. Within 24 h, 50% (21/42 patients) of the total AOSpine B-/C-type spinal injuries and 39% (28/71) of the total AOSpine A-type spinal injuries were surgically addressed; thus, the surgeons already recognized the higher surgical urgency of AOSpine B-/C-type injuries. Reasons for a delayed spinal stabilization appear to be multifactorial. Regression analysis identified, in particular, a higher ISS, thoracic spine injury location, A-type injuries, and the absence of an evident neurological deficit as independent risk factors for a delay in spinal surgery.

In our population, 31% of the multiple-injured patients (n = 35) presented with neurological impairment due to their spinal trauma. In the literature, urgent surgical spinal treatment is widely accepted in the event of any neurological impairment focusing on isolated spine trauma. The main target is the decompression of the affected nerve structures and the restoration of the correct spinal alignment. The analysis of the STASCI (Surgical Timing in Acute Spinal Cord Injury) study showed that a general improvement of at least two ASIA (American Spinal Injury Association) grades is observable after early decompression within 24 h [18,19]. Our data show that even in multiple-injured patients with different priority surgeries, neurological impairment resulted in an earlier spinal surgery; however, we were not able to assess whether this had a beneficial impact on neurological outcome.

There are some limitations of our study, which merit further comments. Endpoint selection may not be meticulous enough to identify further differences between the treatment groups, and no in-depth information concerning patients' comorbidities were available for analysis. The clinical course and outcome of multiple-injured patients are influenced by several factors, which might not all be included in our analysis. In particular, spinal trauma with neurological compromise might have a severe impact on outcome parameters of these multiple-injured patients, which might not be valued enough in our data due to early out-of-hospital transfer to neurological rehabilitation units.

Furthermore, the population size is limited as compared to register studies. However, this is the first study to consider spinal injury severity, according to the AOSpine classification, and to correlate this to the impact of surgical timing of spinal injuries. There are several existing fracture classification systems to evaluate the fracture pattern of spinal fractures. Advantages of the AOSpine fracture classification are better reliability and feasibility in clinical practice, in comparison to the thoracolumbar injury classification and severity score (TLICS). Several studies confirmed that the AOSpine classification is superior to the TLICS with regard to reliability for the identification of fracture morphology [20,21].

In conclusion, our data support the concept of early spinal stabilization within 24 h in multiple-injured patients with AOSpine B-/C-type injuries, especially of the thoracic spine. However, in multiple-injured patients with AOSpine A-type injuries, the beneficial impact of early spinal stabilization has been overemphasized in former studies, and the benefit should be weighed against the risk of patients' deterioration, due to the unneglectable surgical burden of spinal surgery.

Author Contributions: Conceptualization, P.K. (Philipp Kobbe) and C.H.; Data curation, P.K. (Patrick Krug), H.A., M.H., K.H., C.M., M.J.S., C.F. and G.S.; Formal analysis, H.A., K.H., M.J.S., C.F., G.S. and C.H.; Investigation, M.P., M.H., C.M., M.J.S. and C.H.; Methodology, P.K. (Patrick Krug) and M.P.; Project administration, P.K. (Philipp Kobbe); Supervision, P.K. (Philipp Kobbe), F.H. and C.H.; Validation, F.H. and C.H.; Writing—original draft, P.K. (Philipp Kobbe); Writing—review & editing, C.H. All authors have read and agreed to the published version of the manuscript.

Funding: This research received no external funding.

Conflicts of Interest: The authors declare no conflicts of interest.

References

1. Harris, M.B.; Sethi, R.K. The Initial Assessment and Management of the Multiple-Trauma Patient With an Associated Spine Injury. *Spine* **2006**, *31*, S9–S15. [CrossRef]
2. Hasler, R.M.; Exadaktylos, A.K.; Bouamra, O.; Benneker, L.M.; Clancy, M.; Sieber, R.; Zimmermann, H.; Lecky, F. Epidemiology and predictors of spinal injury in adult major trauma patients: European cohort study. *Eur. Spine J.* **2011**, *20*, 2174–2180. [CrossRef]
3. Stephan, K.; Huber-Wagner, S.; Häberle, S.; Kanz, K.-G.; Bühren, V.; Van Griensven, M.; Meyer, B.; Biberthaler, P.; Lefering, R.; Huber-Wagner, S. Spinal cord injury—Incidence, prognosis, and outcome: An analysis of the TraumaRegister DGU. *Spine J.* **2015**, *15*, 1994–2001. [CrossRef]
4. McHenry, T.P.; Mirza, S.K.; Wang, J.; Wade, C.E.; O'keefe, G.E.; Dailey, A.T.; Schreiber, M.A.; Chapman, J.R. Risk Factors for Respiratory Failure Following Operative Stabilization of Thoracic and Lumbar Spine Fractures. *J. Bone Jt. Surg.-Am. Vol.* **2006**, *88*, 997–1005. [CrossRef]
5. McKinley, W.; Meade, M.A.; Kirshblum, S.; Barnard, B. Outcomes of early surgical management versus late or no surgical intervention after acute spinal cord injury. *Arch. Phys. Med. Rehabilit.* **2004**, *85*, 1818–1825. [CrossRef]
6. Kerwin, A.J.; Frykberg, E.R.; Schinco, M.A.; Griffen, M.M.; Arce, C.A.; Nguyen, T.Q.; Tepas, J.J. The Effect of Early Surgical Treatment of Traumatic Spine Injuries on Patient Mortality. *J. Trauma* **2007**, *63*, 1308–1313. [CrossRef]
7. Schinkel, C.; Frangen, T.M.; Kmetic, A.; Andress, H.-J.; Muhr, G. Timing of Thoracic Spine Stabilization in Trauma Patients: Impact on Clinical Course and Outcome. *J. Trauma* **2006**, *61*, 156–160. [CrossRef]
8. Bliemel, C.; Lefering, R.; Bücking, B.; Frink, M.; Struewer, J.; Krueger, A.; Ruchholtz, S.; Frangen, T.M. Early or delayed stabilization in severely injured patients with spinal fractures? Current surgical objectivity according to the Trauma Registry of DGU: Treatment of spine injuries in polytrauma patients. *J. Trauma Acute Care Surg.* **2014**, *76*, 366–373. [CrossRef]
9. Vaccaro, A.R.; Öner, F.; Kepler, C.K.; Dvorak, M.; Schnake, K.; Bellabarba, C.; Reinhold, M.; Aarabi, B.; Kandziora, F.; Chapman, J.; et al. AOSpine Thoracolumbar Spine Injury Classification System: Fracture description, neurological status, and key modifiers. *Spine* **2013**, *38*, 2028–2037. [CrossRef]
10. Hildebrand, F.; Giannoudis, P.; Kretteck, C.; Pape, H.-C. Damage control: Extremities. *Injury* **2004**, *35*, 678–689. [CrossRef]
11. Stahel, P.; A Flierl, M.; Moore, E.; Smith, W.R.; Beauchamp, K.; Dwyer, A. Advocating "spine damage control" as a safe and effective treatment modality for unstable thoracolumbar fractures in polytrauma patients: A hypothesis. *J. Trauma Manag. Outcomes* **2009**, *3*, 6. [CrossRef] [PubMed]
12. Stahel, P.; Vanderheiden, T.; A Flierl, M.; Matava, B.; Gerhardt, D.; Bolles, G.; Beauchamp, K.; Burlew, C.C.; Johnson, J.L.; Moore, E.E. The impact of a standardized "spine damage-control" protocol for unstable thoracic and lumbar spine fractures in severely injured patients: A prospective cohort study. *J. Trauma Acute Care Surg.* **2013**, *74*, 590–596. [CrossRef] [PubMed]
13. Kossmann, T.; Trease, L.; Freedman, I.; Malham, G. Damage control surgery for spine trauma. *Injury* **2004**, *35*, 661–670. [CrossRef] [PubMed]
14. Schlegel, J.; Bayley, J.; Yuan, H.; Fredricksen, B. Timing of Surgical Decompression and Fixation of Acute Spinal Fractures. *J. Orthop. Trauma* **1996**, *10*, 323–330. [CrossRef]
15. McLain, R.F.; Benson, D.R. Urgent Surgical Stabilization of Spinal Fractures in Polytrauma Patients. *Spine* **1999**, *24*, 1646. [CrossRef]
16. Chipman, J.G.; Deuser, W.E.; Beilman, G.J. Early Surgery for Thoracolumbar Spine Injuries Decreases Complications. *J. Trauma* **2004**, *56*, 52–57. [CrossRef]
17. Lubelski, D.; Tharin, S.; Como, J.J.; Steinmetz, M.P.; A Vallier, H.; Moore, T. Surgical timing for cervical and upper thoracic injuries in patients with polytrauma. *J. Neurosurg. Spine* **2017**, *27*, 633–637. [CrossRef]
18. Fehlings, M.G.; Vaccaro, A.; Wilson, J.R.; Singh, A.; Cadotte, D.W.; Harrop, J.S.; Aarabi, B.; Shaffrey, C.; Dvorak, M.; Fisher, C.; et al. Early versus Delayed Decompression for Traumatic Cervical Spinal Cord Injury: Results of the Surgical Timing in Acute Spinal Cord Injury Study (STASCIS). *PLoS ONE* **2012**, *7*, e32037. [CrossRef]

19. Fehlings, M.; Tetreault, L.A.; Wilson, J.R.; Aarabi, B.; Anderson, P.; Arnold, P.M.; Brodke, D.S.; Burns, A.S.; Chiba, K.; Dettori, J.R.; et al. A Clinical Practice Guideline for the Management of Patients With Acute Spinal Cord Injury and Central Cord Syndrome: Recommendations on the Timing (≤24 Hours Versus >24 Hours) of Decompressive Surgery. *Glob. Spine J.* **2017**, *7*, 195S–202S. [CrossRef]
20. Kaul, R.; Chhabra, H.; Vaccaro, A.R.; Abel, R.F.; Tuli, S.; Shetty, A.P.; Das, K.D.; Mohapatra, B.; Nanda, A.; Sangondimath, G.M.; et al. Reliability assessment of AOSpine thoracolumbar spine injury classification system and Thoracolumbar Injury Classification and Severity Score (TLICS) for thoracolumbar spine injuries: Results of a multicentre study. *Eur. Spine J.* **2016**, *26*, 1470–1476. [CrossRef]
21. Pishnamaz, M.; Balosu, S.; Curfs, I.; Uhing, D.; Laubach, M.; Herren, C.; Weber, C.; Hildebrand, F.; Willems, P.; Kobbe, P. Reliability and Agreement of Different Spine Fracture Classification Systems: An Independent Intraobserver and Interobserver Study. *World Neurosurg.* **2018**, *115*, e695–e702. [CrossRef] [PubMed]

Journal of
Clinical Medicine

MDPI

Article

Severe Traumatic Brain Injury (TBI) Modulates the Kinetic Profile of the Inflammatory Response of Markers for Neuronal Damage

Cora Rebecca Schindler [1,*], Thomas Lustenberger [1], Mathias Woschek [1], Philipp Störmann [1], Dirk Henrich [1], Peter Radermacher [2] and Ingo Marzi [1]

1 Department of Trauma, Hand and Reconstructive Surgery, University Hospital Frankfurt, 60596 Frankfurt, Germany; tom.lustenberg@gmail.com (T.L.); mathias.woschek@kgu.de (M.W.); philipp.stoermann@kgu.de (P.S.); d.henrich@trauma.uni-frankfurt.de (D.H.); marzi@trauma.uni-frankfurt.de (I.M.)

2 Institute of Anesthesiological Pathophysiology and Process Engineering, University Medical School, 89070 Ulm, Germany; peter.radermacher@uni-ulm.de

* Correspondence: cora.schindler@kgu.de; Tel./Fax: +49-69-6301-83304

Received: 1 May 2020; Accepted: 26 May 2020; Published: 1 June 2020

Abstract: The inflammatory response plays an important role in the pathophysiology of multiple injuries. This study examines the effects of severe trauma and inflammatory response on markers of neuronal damage. A retrospective analysis of prospectively collected data in 445 trauma patients (Injury Severity Score (ISS) ≥ 16) is provided. Levels of neuronal biomarkers (calcium-binding Protein B (S100b), Enolase2 (NSE), glial fibrillary acidic protein (GFAP)) and Interleukins (IL-6, IL-10) in severely injured patients (with polytrauma (PT)) without traumatic brain injury (TBI) or with severe TBI (PT+TBI) and patients with isolated TBI (isTBI) were measured upon arrival until day 5. S100b, NSE, GFAP levels showed a time-dependent decrease in all cohorts. Their expression was higher after multiple injuries ($p = 0.038$) comparing isTBI. Positive correlation of marker level after concomitant TBI and isTBI ($p = 0.001$) was noted, while marker expression after PT appears to be independent. Highest levels of IL-6 and -10 were associated to PT und lowest to isTBI ($p < 0.001$). In all groups pro-inflammatory response (IL-6/-10 ratio) peaked on day 2 and at a lower level on day 4. Severe TBI modulates kinetic profile of inflammatory response by reducing interleukin expression following trauma. Potential markers for neuronal damage have a limited diagnostic value after severe trauma because undifferentiated increase.

Keywords: multiple trauma; traumatic brain injury (TBI); risk prediction; biomarker; IL-6; IL-10; posttraumatic inflammation; S100b; NSE; GFAP

1. Introduction

Polytrauma (PT) and severe traumatic brain injury (TBI) caused by road traffic accidents and falls are the main causes of death and disability in young patients under 45 years with immense socioeconomic impact through loss of productivity, medical and rehabilitation costs [1,2]. The treatment of patients with multiple organ injuries poses a particular challenge due to different injury patterns and severity, but also due to the complex immune response [3]. Post-traumatic exaggerated immunomodulation often leads to postinjury complications, multiple organ failure (MOF) or death and are predictors of mortality in trauma [4,5]. The brain is vulnerable to damage and failure due to its high metabolic rate and limited intrinsic energy reserve. The (neuro-)inflammatory environment subsequently leads to cell death and neurodegeneration in secondary brain damage but also to neuro reparative mechanisms in later stages. Secondary brain injury due to inflammatory processes is one of the main reasons for worsening of outcome [6–8]. Detecting the severity of injuries at an early stage, predicting their development and preventing secondary damage is of highest clinical interest, with biomarkers playing an important role [9]. One of the most studied serum biomarkers in TBI is the calcium binding protein B (S100B). The oligomeric cytoplasmic protein is predominantly found in astrocytes and involved in cellular processes and signal transduction [10]. Neuron-specific enolase 2 (NSE) is mainly found in the cytoplasm of neurons and neuroendocrine tissue and is involved in glycolysis in both neuronal cells and erythrocytes. Its detection in blood is considered as marker for neuronal damage [11,12]. The gliafibrillary acidic protein (GFAP) is a monomeric intermediate filament concentrated in the astroglial cytoskeleton. GFAP is brain-specific and is released into the peripheral blood circulation after death of astrocytes [13]. After multiple injuries and/or TBI, both the membrane integrity of brain cells and the integrity of the blood–brain barrier (BBB) is disturbed [14]. S100B, NSE and GFAP are released into the blood, with kinetic profile being related to injury pattern and (neuro-)inflammatory process [15,16]. Pro- and anti-inflammatory cytokines such as interleukin-6 and -10 (IL-6, IL-10) are released in response to tissue injury and lead to both reactive and restorative inflammatory processes [17]. Although interleukins are clear markers for immune activation, further investigation is needed to determine the extent to which they reflect brain damage as diagnostic factors [18]. In the acute phase reaction, IL-6 is known to regulate inflammation, immunity and neural development. An acute local and systemic release in brain tissue, blood and cerebrospinal fluid can be observed as a reaction to injury [19,20]. IL-10 is commonly known as an anti-inflammatory cytokine that performs immunomodulatory functions and is particularly important in the resorption phase. Its expression increases with the pathology of the Central Nervous System (CNS), promoting survival of nerve and glial cells and attenuating inflammatory responses [21]. Understanding the (neuro)immunological effect of TBI on the systemic inflammatory response is a key factor in the development of early targeted therapies [8]. Although several studies have investigated systemic cytokine levels in severely injured trauma patients [22,23] the specific influence of severe trauma or TBI on the neuronal and inflammatory response and expression of brain-specific biomarkers has not been described.

The aim of the present study was to characterize the systemic profiles of neuronal biomarkers S100b, NSE, GFAP and the pro- and anti-inflammatory markers IL-6 and Il-10 in severely injured patients and to assess the influence of severe TBI on the state of acute inflammation in these patients. Furthermore, it will be shown to what extent neuronal biomarkers used in TBI have sufficient significance to assess the influence of initial or indirect secondary intracranial damage in polytrauma.

2. Experimental Section

The study was performed at the University Hospital Frankfurt, Goethe University after approval by the Institutional Review Board (89/19) in accordance with the Declaration of Helsinki and following STROBE guidelines [24]. Written informed consent was obtained for enrolled patients or their legally authorized representatives in accordance with ethical standards.

We retrospectively reviewed a cohort of severely injured trauma patients admitted to the emergency department (ED) of the University Hospital of the Goethe University Frankfurt from 2012 to 2016. All clinical data were prospectively taken during the quality documentation of the TraumaRegister der Deutschen Gesellschaft für Unfallchirurgie (DGU)®, Berlin, Germany. All trauma patients in the ED were treated according to the Advanced Trauma Life Support (ATLS® American College of Surgeons, Chicago, IL, USA) standard and the polytrauma guidelines [25]. Injury severity from trauma was calculated using the Injury Severity Score (ISS) based on the Abbreviated Injury Scale (AIS) score which assigns each injury a severity level between 1 (mild) and 6 (maximum) in different regions (head, face, thorax, abdomen, extremities and external injuries) [26,27]. The New Injury Severity Score (NISS) was calculated to better correlate the assessment measure with the polytrauma of the patients [28]. We evaluated 445 trauma patients with an ISS $\geq$ 16 between 18 and 80 years of age. Patients who met inclusion criteria were stratified into 3 groups: isolated severe TBI ((isTBI); $AIS_{head} \geq 4$, all other body areas AIS ≤ 1, polytraumatized patients with severe TBI ((PT + TBI); AIS_{head} and AIS of other body area ≥3;) and polytraumatized patients without relevant brain injury ((PT); $AIS_{head} \leq 1$;). Patients with known pre-existing immunological disorders, immunosuppressive medication, burns, concomitant acute myocardial infarction, thromboembolic events and patients who died within 5 days of hospital admission (incomplete serial blood samples) were excluded. Documentation containing further information on demography (age and sex) and injury.

Serial venous blood samples were obtained from traumatized patients on admittance to the ED through day 1–5 daily after trauma. Following baseline sample, subsequent blood was collected following the standard hospital procedures in pre-chilled ethylenediaminetetraacetic acid (EDTA) tubes (BD vacutainer, Becton Dickinson Diagnostics, Aalst, Belgium) and stored on ice. Blood was centrifuged at 2000× *g* for 15 min at 4 °C and the supernatant (serum) was stored at −80 °C until analysis. IL-6 and IL-10 concentrations were measured by IL-6/IL-10 Eli-pair Enzyme-linked Immunosorbent Assay ((ELISA); Diaclone, Hoelzel Diagnostica, Cologne, Germany) according to the manufacturer's instructions. The following markers of brain injury were assessed using commercially available ELISA assays (Bio-Techne GmbH (R & D Systems GmbH, Wiesbaden, Germany): S100B (DY1820-05 Human S100B; assay range: 47–3000 pg/mL)), glial fibrillary acidic protein (DY2594-05 GFAP; assay range: 0.3–20 ng/mL) and neuron-specific enolase 2 (DY5169-05 Human Enolase 2/Neuron-specific Enolase; assay range: 78–5000 pg/mL), after sample dilution as needed.

Continuous normally distributed variables were summarized using means ± standard error of the mean (*SEM*), while categorical or continuous variables with skewed distributions were summarized using means ± standard deviation (*SD*). The *p*-values for categorical variables were derived from the two-sided Fisher's exact test, and for continuous variables from the Mann–Whitney U test or the Kruskal–Wallis test. Significant values were adjusted by the Bonferroni post hoc test. Spearman's rank correlation coefficients were calculated to determine correlations between inflammatory and neuronal biomarkers and injury characteristics. A p-value < 0.05 was considered to be statistically significant. Values are reported as means for continuous variables and as percentages for categorical variables. All analyses were performed using the Statistical Package for Social Sciences (SPSS for Mac©), version 26 (SPSS Inc., Chicago, IL, USA).

3. Results

3.1. Demographics and Clinical Injury Characteristics

Table 1 shows the demographic and clinical characteristics stratified by injury pattern. During the 5-year study period a total of 445 severely injured patients (ISS ≥ 16) was evaluated. A total of 104 patients met the inclusion criteria. Of these, 43 patients were severely injured without TBI (PT), 35 patients were polytrauma patients with severe TBI (PT+TBI) and 26 patients suffered from isolated severe TBI (isTBI). A total of 76.0% of the trauma patients were men. Patients with isolated TBI were significantly older (61 ± 3 years, $p < 0.001$) than those in other groups, about 70% of them were older than 55 years. Mean ISS of the patients with isolated TBI was significantly lower (24 ± 1, $p < 0.01$) but in NISS ($p = 0.135$) no significant difference was found. Computed tomographic findings of patients with PT severe TBI or isolated severe TBI usually suffered not only from one type of intracranial hemorrhage but from several entities simultaneously.

3.2. Systemic Profiles of Neuro Markers in Relation to Injury Pattern

Figure 1 displays neuronal serum marker levels over the time course from ED admission to hospital day 5 stratified by injury pattern.

Table 1. Demographic and clinical injury characteristics stratified by injury pattern.

	PT (n = 43)	PT + TBI (n = 35)	isTBI (n = 26)	p-Value
Male	69.8%	80.0%	80.8%	
Age (y, ± SEM)	46 (±2)	43 (±3)	61 (±3)	<0.001
Age ≥ 55 years	32.6%	25.7%	69.2%	<0.001
ISS (±SEM)	30 (±2)	37 (±2)	24 (±1)	<0.01
ISS ≥ 25	74.4%	77.1%	53.9%	<0.01
NISS (±SEM)	37 (±2)	44 (±2)	38 (±2)	0.135
AIS_{head} (±SEM)	0.3 (±0.1)	4.1 (±0.2)	4.5 (±0.1)	<0.001
AIS_{chest} ≥ 3	81.4%	68.6%	0.0%	<0.001
$AIS_{abdomen}$ ≥ 3	46.5%	11.1%	0.0%	<0.001
$AIS_{extremity}$ ≥ 3	51.2%	37.1%	0.0%	<0.001
ICH (%)		57.1%	61.5%	0.730
SDH (%)		37.1%	61.5%	0.059
SAH (%)		34.3%	57.7%	0.069
EDH (%)		20.0%	11.5%	0.377

Abbreviations: PT = Polytrauma, isTBI = isolated Traumatic Brain Injury, SEM = Standard Error of Mean, y = years, ISS = Injury Severity Score, NISS = New Injury Severity Score, AIS = Abbreviated Injury Score, ICH = intracerebral hemorrhage, SDH = subdural hematoma, SAH = subarachnoid hemorrhage, EDH = epidural hematoma.

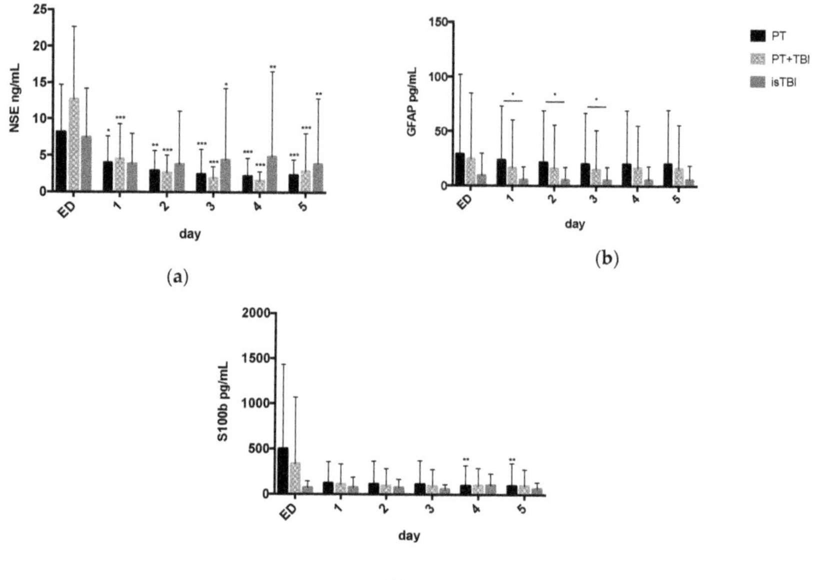

Figure 1. Neuronal serum marker levels (mean ± Standard Deviation) over the time course from admission to Emergency Department (ED) through to hospital day 5 stratified by injury pattern. * $p < 0.05$, ** $p < 0.01$, *** $p < 0.001$. (**a**) Neuron-specific enolase 2 (NSE) (**b**); glial fibrillary acidic protein (GFAP); (**c**) calcium-binding Protein B (S100b).

After trauma, the NSE expression is highest on the day of admission with maximum serum level of 8 ± 1 ng/mL (PT), 13 ± 2 ng/mL (PT + TBI) and 7 ± 1 ng/mL (isTBI) and steadily decreases over time.

Significantly higher GFAP expression was found in the PT cohort (day 1: 23.80 ± 7.94 pg/mL) comparing to isTBI (day 1: 5.82 ± 2.33 pg/mL, p = 0.038) 24 to 72 h after trauma.

For S100b highest marker expression was found in PT patients (495 ± 150 pg/mL) on time of admission, followed by the PT + TBI group (333 ± 128 pg/mL). After isolated TBI the S100b expression was over all lower (71 ± 15 pg/mL) comparing PT and PT + TBI.

3.3. Systemic Profiles of Inflammatory Markers in Relation to Injury Pattern

Figure 2 shows inflammatory serum marker levels over the time course from ED admission through to hospital day 5 stratified by injury pattern.

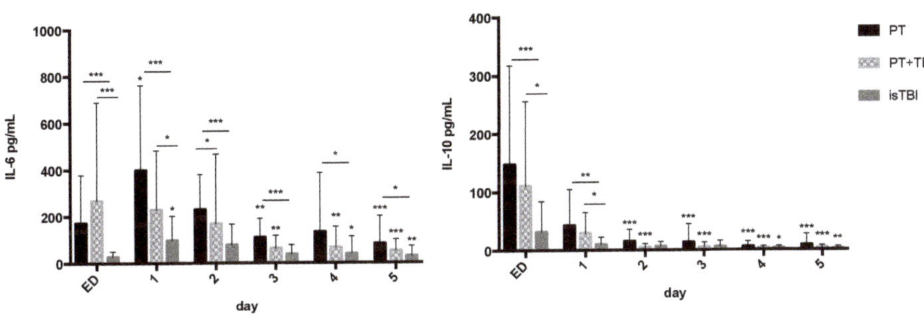

(a) (b)

Figure 2. Inflammatory serum marker levels (mean ± Standard Deviation) over the time course from emergency department (ED) admission through to hospital day 5 stratified by injury pattern. * $p < 0.05$, ** $p < 0.01$, *** $p < 0.001$. (**a**) Interleukin (IL)-6 (**b**); Interleukin (IL)-10.

In PT (day 1: 400 ± 71 pg/mL) and isTBI (day 1: 98 ± 22 pg/mL) group IL-6 peaked on hospital day 1 while in PT + TBI group highest IL-6 level was detected on admission (267 ± 86 pg/mL). All groups showed significant cytokine drop over time course. Over the entire time course, IL-6 levels were significantly higher in the PT cohort ($p < 0.001$) as well within the first 24 h in PT + TBI group ($p < 0.001$) compared to the isTBI group.

All groups showed highest IL-10 expression on admission (PT 148 ± 33 > PT + TBI 111 ± 30 > isTBI 31 ± 11 pg/mL) with significant decline from day 2 in the PT (− 71.2%) and PT + TBI (− 73.6%) groups and from day 4 in isTBI (− 9.5%) group. Within 24 h after trauma, IL-10-level was significantly higher in the PT ($p < 0.001$) and PT + TBI ($p < 0.05$) cohorts according to isolated TBI.

3.4. Relation between Marker Expression and Injury Severity

On admission we found significant positive correlation of increased IL-10 expression and injury severity (Spearman correlation (*rho*), ISS $r = 0.4$, $p = 0.04$; NISS $r = 0.5$, $p = 0.01$) as well as and positive correlation between increased cytokine expression (IL-10 $r = 0.6$, $p = 0.001$; IL-6 $r = 0.5$, $p = 0.01$) and higher risk of mortality (Revised Injury Severity Classification Score (RISC II)) in severely injured patients (PT) within 24 h after severe trauma (PT).

In PT + TBI group the S100b expression showed significant positive correlation with injury severity (ISS $r = 0.4$, $p = 0.02$), mortality risk (RISC II $r = 0.4$, $p = 0.02$) and severity of TBI (AIS_{head} $r = 0.4$, $p = 0.05$) up to 72 h after trauma.

In isTBI cohort we found negative correlation between GFAP expression and age ($r = -0.4$, $p = 0.03$). After isolated TBI the inflammatory response correlated 24 h after trauma with the ISS (IL-6 $r = 0.6$, $p = 0.01$), NISS (IL-6 $r = 0.6$, $p = 0.003$; IL-10 $r = 0.5$, $p = 0.04$) and severity of head injury (AIS_{head}/IL-10 $r = 0.6$, $p = 0.002$) as well as with risk of mortality (IL-10 $r = 0.6$, $p = 0.004$).

3.5. Inflammatory Status (IL-6/IL-10 Ratio) and Kinetic Profile of Neuro Markers

Table 2 displays the relation between inflammatory response and neuronal markers expression stratified by injury pattern. Figure 3 shows inflammatory status (IL-6/IL-10 ratio) together with the kinetics of neuro marker expression during the time course. The comparison of the marker levels within a group in percentage ratio serves to illustrate the proportionality.

Table 2. Relation between inflammatory response and neuronal marker expression.

Day		PT					PT + TBI					isTBI				
		GFAP	**S100ß**	**IL6**	**IL10**	**Ratio**	**GFAP**	**S100ß**	**IL6**	**IL10**	**Ratio**	**GFAP**	**S100ß**	**IL6**	**IL10**	**Ratio**
ED	NSE	0.21	0.06	0.024	0.00	0.12	0.13	−0.05	0.37	0.46 *	− 0.12	0.55 **	0.44 *	−0.17	−0.00	−0.30
	GFAP		0.08	0.18	0.06	0.04		0.30	−0.11	−0.14	−0.06		0.27	−0.03	0.25	−0.58 *
	S100ß			−0.06	0.01	−0.08			−0.14	0.06	−0.31			0.05	0.09	−0.23
	IL6				0.78 ***	0.39				0.64 **	0.31				0.76 ***	−0.19
	IL10					−0.21					−0.50 *					−0.80 ***
1	NSE	−0.14	0.32 *	0.09	0.29	−0.15	0.17	0.07	0.12	−0.35	−0.29	0.44 *	0.12	0.23	0.39	−0.30
	GFAP		0.17	0.18	−0.08	−0.09		0.52 **	0.08	0.27	−0.28		0.54 *	−0.03	0.03	−0.31
	S100ß			−0.12	−0.7	−0.06			0.13	0.27	−0.28			0.18	−0.10	0.00
	IL6				0.41 *	0.34				0.48 *	0.33				0.66 **	0.28
	IL10					−0.64 ***					0.61 **					−0.66 **
2	NSE	−0.16	0.23	0.33	0.00	0.07	0.29	0.23	0.06	0.17	0.11	0.63 *	0.22	0.18	0.08	0.06
	GFAP		0.30	−0.12	0.38	−0.53 *		0.46 *	0.23	0.20	−0.20		0.48 *	−0.05	−0.14	−0.07
	S100ß			−0.25	0.10	0.15			0.06	0.27	0.42			0.25	0.24	−0.18
	IL6				0.08	0.31				0.28	0.61 *				0.33	0.56 *
	IL10					−0.85 ***					−0.22					−0.69 **
3	NSE	0.02	0.21	0.20	−0.08	−0.02	0.24	0.23	0.15	0.18	0.04	0.54 *	0.48 *	0.03	−0.05	−0.17
	GFAP		0.26	−0.20	0.24	0.17		0.43 *	0.36	0.27	−0.10		0.50 *	−0.24	−0.17	−0.25
	S100ß			−0.05	−0.15	0.44			0.03	0.42 *	−0.28			−0.05	−0.87	−0.08
	IL6				0.49 *	0.26				0.74	0.46				0.34	0.38
	IL10					−0.7 ***					−0.78 ***					−0.44
4	NSE	−0.02	0.27	0.07	0.01	−0.08	0.24	0.17	0.15	−0.74	−0.00	0.55 *	−0.10	−0.04	−0.06	0.48
	GFAP		0.26	−0.06	0.22	−0.32		0.44 *	0.36	0.16	0.21		0.17	−0.10	−0.01	0.25
	S100ß			0.4 *	0.03	0.22			0.10	0.28	0.17			0.08	0.03	0.06
	IL6				0.38	0.76 ***				0.01	0.75 **				0.53 *	0.84 **
	IL10					0.21					−0.23					0.04
5	NSE	0.00	0.31	0.07	0.12	−0.20	0.03	0.25	−0.03	−0.02	0.10	0.56 *	0.22	−0.07	−0.16	0.73 **
	GFAP		0.27	−0.20	0.00	−0.02		0.49 *	0.04	0.27	−0.36		0.30	−0.17	−0.30	0.54
	S100ß			0.42 *	0.31	0.21			−0.11	0.42	−0.35			0.21	−0.22	0.31
	IL6				0.65 ***	0.52 *				0.42	0.72 **				0.68 ***	0.21
	IL10					0.34					−0.71 **					0.24

Spearman correlation (*rho*), * $p < 0.05$, ** $p < 0.01$, *** $p < 0.001$. Abbreviations: PT = Polytrauma, isTBI = isolated Traumatic Brain Injury, ED = Admission to Emergency Department, NSE = Neuron-specific enolase 2, GFAP = glial fibrillary acidic protein, S100b = calcium-binding Protein B.

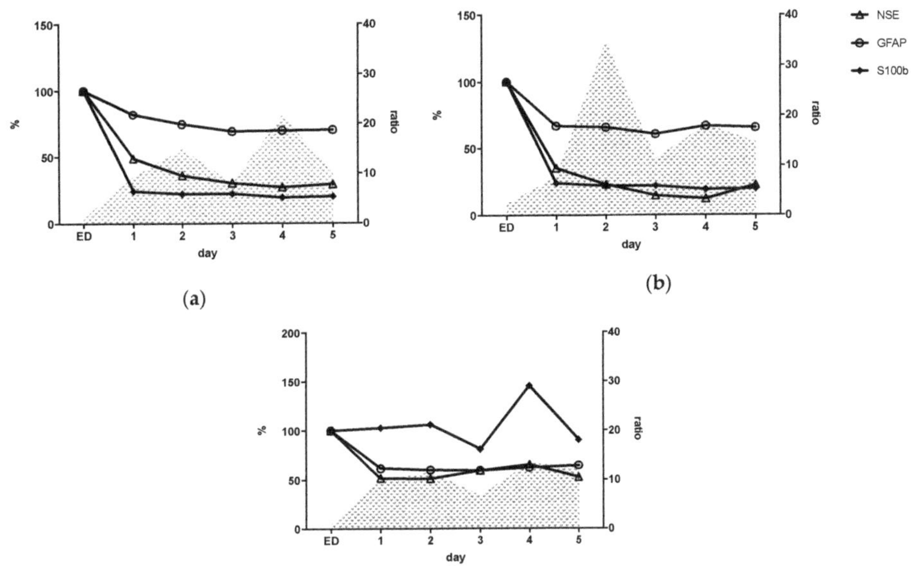

(a)

(b)

(c)

Figure 3. Pro-inflammatory response (Interleukin (IL)-6/Interleukin (IL)-10 ratio, grey-hatched) and neuronal marker expression (Neuron-specific enolase 2 (NSE), glial fibrillary acidic protein (GFAP), calcium-binding Protein B (S100b)) after (**a**) polytrauma (PT); (**b**) polytrauma + traumatic brain injury (TBI); (**c**) isolated TBI (isTBI). ED = Admission to Emergency Department.

Kinetic profiles of PT and PT-TBI groups showed similar course from ED admission through to hospital day 5. While the PT and PT+TBI groups continued to decrease over time until 29.3% (PT) and 22.9% (PT + TBI), the TBI group showed constantly elevated NSE expression (52.3%) 5 days following trauma. All groups showed synchronous decline over time with a maximum reduction of GFAP expression to 64.2–70.0%. For S100b we found a drop down to 24.1% in PT and 33.9% in PT + TBI group within 24 h. After isolated TBI consistent S100b expression over time course (min. 80.9%, day 3) with a secondary peak on day 4 (145.0%) was found.

Based on the IL-6/IL-10 ratio we identified two phases of pro-inflammation for all groups: increase from admission to day 3 with peak after 48 h and secondary from day 3 to day 5 with peak on day 4. The pro-inflammatory quotient after 48 h was higher in the PT + TBI group (ratio = 34.8) than after PT (ratio = 15.0) and isTBI (ratio = 11.6). The lowest pro-inflammatory reaction was found for isTBI.

3.6. Relation between Inflammatory Response and Neuronal Markers

After severe PT a significant correlation was found between IL-6 and IL-10 level ($r = 0.8$, $p < 0.001$) on admission and day 1 to day 5. Over the entire time course, a positive correlation was observed between S100b and NSE and IL-6 expression with statistical significance from day 4 (NSE $r = 0.04$, $p = 0.01$, IL-6 $r = 0.4$, $p = 0.04$) and GFAP.

After PT with severe TBI, GFAP and S100b expression showed statistically significant synchronous decrease ($r = 0.3$, $p = 0.04$) over the entire time course. Positive correlation was found as well between NSE and S100b ($r = 0.3$, $p = 0.04$) from day 3.

A positive relation of GFAP with NSE (admission: $r = 0.3$, $p = 0.05$) and with S100b ($r = 0.5$, $p = 0.001$) levels over the entire time course and between NSE ($r = 0.4$, $p = 0.01$) and with S100b on admission, day 2, 3 and 5 was measured in patients with isTBI.

4. Discussion

Of 104 patients included, 75% were male and the cohort with isolated TBI was significantly older than the PT and PT+TBI group. Polytrauma is the leading cause of death in Western countries for people up to 45 years of age, in a male-to-female ratio of 2.6:1. Older patients cause most TBI-related hospitalizations and deaths [1,29]. In this study it was shown that the application of both the already used and the more recent biomarkers S100b, NSE and GFAP have limited value in the assessment of TBI in polytraumatized patients. Nevertheless, biomarkers are certainly the optimal complement to clinical and radiological findings to assess the course and outcome of the injury sufficiently. Biomarkers can reveal the extent of cell death, provide early indications of occult or later visible organ damage, and thus have an immense clinical value.

4.1. S100b Missing Diagnostic Value after Severe Trauma

One of the most often studied serum biomarkers in TBI is S100b [7]. Due to its high molecular weight, the protein is only able to pass through the BBB, if it has an increased permeability caused by injury [14]. Therefore, this marker was used to detect (sensitivity 81–100%) and predict the outcome of a severe TBI. The potential pitfalls of S100b in the different areas are usually related to its specificity (20–67%) and sensitivity in the detection and assessment of intracranial injury. Consistent cut-off levels (51 pg/mL to 210 ng/mL at admission) are difficult to find in the literature [10,12,15]. In this study, the highest serum levels for S100b were measured in polytrauma patients (495 ± 150 pg/mL) at admission, followed by the PT + TBI group (333 ± 128 pg/mL) and isolated TBI (71 ± 15 pg/mL). S100b is thus expressed lowest after isTBI, although not significantly. S100b is also expressed in peripheral nervous tissue in addition to the CNS. Furthermore, muscle tissue, chondrocytes and adipocytes were identified to release S100b after injury [3]. TBI could only be detected with a predictive power of 67% in pediatric polytrauma patients with TBI and fracture of long bones [30]. Orth-Nissen et al. found higher serum levels of S100b in patients with multiple injuries than in patients with isolated TBI or without TBI. This suggests that elevated serum concentration of S100b after trauma seems to be significantly influenced by an extra-cerebral injury and is an indicator for a global tissue and organ damage [31]. It was shown that pro-inflammatory cytokines such as IL-6 induce an increase of S100b and GFAP secretion via the mitogen-activated protein kinase (MAPK) pathway [32]. Furthermore, a positive correlation between neuro marker expression over time was found after PT + TBI and isolated TBI. Possibly this is an indicator of congruent marker expression after neuronal damage in TBI.

4.2. Non-Specific Increase of NSE Expression by Cofounding Effect after Severe Trauma

NSE is localized in the cytoplasm of neurons, erythrocytes, platelets and neuroendocrine cells. It has been discussed as a biomarker for neuronal damage and has been associated with the severity of injury and clinical outcome after severe TBI. In the literature, serum levels after trauma ranged between 6.5–21.2 ng/mL [9,12,30]. In this study it was shown that after polytrauma with TBI, the NSE expression is highest on the day of admission with a maximum serum level of 13 ± 2 ng/mL (PT + TBI) > 8 ± 1 ng/mL (PT) > 7 ± 1 ng/mL (isTBI) and decreases steadily until day 5. A possible explanation for this finding could be an NSE release due to hemolysis after polytrauma. Another possibility might be the release of neuronal NSE due to reperfusion damage in the course of polytrauma with subsequent BBB disruption by immune reaction. Serum protein S100b and NSE increased temporarily as a result of multiple trauma associated with hemorrhagic shock might lead to cerebral hypoperfusion and brain damage in porcine model [33,34]. Due to its expression in neuroendocrine cells NSE is also studied in association with malignant and inflammatory lung diseases and first studies analyzing NSE release after lung injury have been published [35,36]. Methodological and technical problems such as slow elimination and potential artifacts in trauma patients call into question their diagnostic value as a screening tool [33]. It is striking that the isTBI group still shows an increased NSE expression (isTBI

52.3% > PT + TBI 22.9%, PT 29.3%) 5 days after the trauma, which may be an expression of severe neuronal damage during the secondary brain swelling and injury.

4.3. GFAP Expression Is Induced by Multiple Injuries

GFAP was largely considered brain-specific and is released into the peripheral bloodstream after death of astrocytes [11]. Meanwhile GFAP expression is also described in Schwann cells, myoepithelial cells, chondrocytes and fibroblasts [37]. An acute intracerebral hemorrhage leads to an immediate mechanical destruction of the astroglia with subsequent release of GFAP into the bloodstream [38]. According to Lei et al., human GFAP serum levels are elevated from admission and during the first 5 days after severe TBI and are predictive of the neurological outcome after 6 months. In the literature, different GFAP cut off levels from 6.8 pg/mL to 0.7 ng/mL are described after TBI for unfavorable outcome [13,39]. In the present study, significantly higher GFAP levels in the PT group (day 1: 24 ± 8 pg/mL) compared to isTBI (day 1: 6 ± 2 pg/mL, $p < 0.05$) were measured 24 to 72 h after trauma. Hsieh et al. demonstrated that over a 6 h period of reperfusion after intestinal ischemia, microglial cells and astrocytes were significantly activated in the brain [40]. Polytrauma increases GFAP and neutrophil expression and leads to secondary brain damage in the presence of exacerbated neuroinflammation, edema and disruption of the BBB [41]. In the isTBI cohort, a negative correlation between GFAP expression and age ($r = -0.4$, $p = 0.03$) was found. It is possible that GFAP is less expressed by the significantly older isTBI patients.

4.4. Severe Traumatic Brain Injury (TBI) Modulates Kinetic Profile of Inflammatory Response

The acute inflammatory reaction plays an important role in immune defense, but can also exert serious adverse consequences, if the excessive immune response leads to systemic inflammation, secondary organ damage and subsequent MOF [3,21]. After TBI, activation of glial cells, microglia and astrocytes as well as infiltration of blood leukocytes takes place within minutes, releasing pro- and anti-inflammatory mediators and various growth factors and triggering a local neuroinflammation as well as a systemic inflammatory response. In this case, the brain functions as both target and effector organ [42]. Among these mediators, interleukins play a particularly prominent role in the development of posttraumatic complications [18,21]. IL-6 is secreted in increased amounts early after trauma. Serum concentrations in available studies range from 47 to 245 pg/mL [8,19,43]. Following TBI, IL-6 levels increase with peak concentrations of 93 to 269 pg/mL in human serum and IL-6 levels greater than 100 pg/mL in the first 24 h after trauma have been associated with severe brain injury [8,18,44]. In this study, IL-6 expression in polytraumatized patients with and without concomitant head injury was significantly higher compared to isTBI (day 1: PT 400 ± 71, PT + TBI 230 ± 53 pg/mL, > isTBI 98 ± 22 pg/mL, $p < 0.001$); all groups showed a relevant cytokine decrease ($p < 0.001$) over time.

IL-10 is an anti-inflammatory cytokine that regulates and limits acute inflammation in response to trauma to prevent tissue damage, such as secondary brain damage after TBI [21,45]. IL-10 plays a crucial role in inflammatory and autoimmune diseases of the intestine, chronic infections, tumor development, neuroinflammation, -degeneration as well as multiple organ dysfunction syndrome (MODS) and MOF after polytrauma, where IL-10 levels from 21.0 to 340.7 pg/mL were shown [42,46]. In this study, the highest IL-10 levels were measured on admission and a continuous decrease until day 5 was shown. The overall increase within the first 24 h was significantly higher in PT (148 ± 33 pg/mL, $p < 0.001$) and PT+TBI (111 ± 30 pg/mL, $p < 0.05$) than after isTBI (31 ± 11 pg/mL). Previous studies described a correlation of IL-6 with the severity of injury (ISS) or insult and mortality, especially during the first post-traumatic hours. IL-6 is associated with the occurrence of MODS and sepsis together with IL-10 within 24 h after trauma [23]. In the present study, IL-10 was positively correlated with ISS and NISS on the day of admission and day 1.

In addition, a positive correlation between IL-6 and IL-10 expression with the mortality risk (RISC II) was shown. Thus, the inflammatory reactions are most likely associated with the severity of injury (ISS: PT + TBI 37 > PT 30 > isTBI 24, $p < 0.01$) and the extent of tissue trauma itself.

Interestingly, polytraumatized patients with severe head trauma showed—although not statistically significant—lower IL-6 values than severely injured patients without TBI despite a higher ISS. This corresponds to already published results from 2016, which raised the question of an immunosuppressive role of TBI [8]. With increasing severity of TBI (AIS_{head} isTBI 4.5 > + TBI 4.1 > PT 0.3), an overall lower cytokine expression was observed. Based on the IL-6/IL-10 ratio, two phases of pro-inflammation can be identified for all three groups from hospital admission to day 3 with a first peak after 48 h and from day 3 to day 5 with a second peak on day 4. Overall, the pro-inflammatory quotient was higher after PT and PT + TBI than after isTBI, with the first phase being strongest after PT + TBI. It is possible that the limited cytokine expression and depressed pro-inflammatory ratio indicates an immunomodulatory effect after severe TBI, but the pro-inflammatory immune response was ultimately relatively strongest after PT + TBI. Data on the predictive ability of IL-6 serum and the neurological outcome are limited and contradictory. While in the pediatric TBI serum IL-6 showed no association with the neurological outcome [47], others showed that high IL-6 correlates with a poor neurological outcome [44]. The determination of cytokine levels can serve not only as a prognostic value for the development of complications, but also for the early identification of patients who are at risk of suffering a "second hit" by renewed immune stimulus in the form of a secondary intervention.

An important pathophysiological factor in the development of posttraumatic complications is the dysfunction of the external (skin) and internal paracellular blood and organ barriers, including the brain (BBB), air and gut blood barriers, resulting in tissue flooding with immune cells and microbial invasion [48]. IL-6 modulates the expression of tight junction proteins in cerebral microvasculature of sheep, and the release of adhesion molecules in plasma of polytrauma patients (ISS ≥ 18) correlates with disease severity and organ dysfunction [49]. Furthermore, the hemorrhagic shock is associated with barrier dysfunction of the gut and development of MODS after the trauma and can lead to a traumatic endotheliopathy by glycocalyx degradation, like in the CNS [50]. Studies have shown that paracellular hyperpermeability due to inflammatory reactions and abnormal release of neurotransmitters is the basis for intestinal barrier dysfunction after TBI [51]. The increased permeability of the organ barriers allows metabolites to enter the bloodstream and to detect specific biomarkers [14]. Identifying the severity of injuries at an early stage, predicting their development in order to prevent secondary damage is of paramount interest in trauma treatment, with the detection of biomarkers playing an important role [43].

4.5. Limitations of the Study

The most important limitation is the retrospective nature of the data analysis; however, all clinical data were acquired in a prospective manner, and only the cytokines and the neuro-specific markers were measured later-on. Furthermore, patients with isolated TBI were significantly older than the comparison groups. In a recently published multicenter study, older patients with blunt trauma showed significantly lower plasma cytokine and chemokine concentrations, including IL-6 levels, than patients <55 years of age [52]. The patients included in the isTBI cohort also suffered from several types of intracranial bleeding simultaneously, which does not allow differentiation between bleeding entities and marker expression. In the present study we found a difference between patient's age of the PT and PT+TBI vs. isTBI group and in their interleukin expression. Ultimately, no conclusions can be drawn as to how age may have altered the inflammatory response. The variance of the individual values is large, specifically of neuronal markers, which is due to potential confounders such as volume administration, blood products, shock, which are difficult to standardize.

5. Conclusions

Although no significant correlation between cytokine expression and release of neuronal markers after trauma could be shown, it is clear that the application of the biomarkers NSE, GFAP and S100b have limited value in the assessment of TBI in polytrauma patients, the levels are not substantially elevated. Possible cause could be a modulation of the kinetic profile of the inflammatory response following severe traumatic brain injury (TBI). IL-6 and IL-10 levels were lower in patients with multiple injuries and concomitant TBI compared to those without severe TBI, suggesting a reduced visible systemic inflammatory response due to traumatic brain injury. In addition, significant correlations were shown between IL-6 and IL-10 levels and injury severity after TBI, indicating the general posttraumatic inflammatory course.

Author Contributions: Conceptualization, I.M., D.H. and T.L.; methodology, D.H. and T.L.; validation, T.L.; formal analysis, C.R.S.; investigation, P.R. and C.R.S.; resources, I.M. and P.R.; data curation, C.R.S.; writing—original draft preparation, C.R.S.; writing—review and editing, P.R., P.S., D.H. and I.M.; visualization, M.W.; supervision, I.M. and D.H.; project administration, I.M. and D.H. All authors have read and agreed to the published version of the manuscript.

Acknowledgments: P.R. was funded by the CRC 1149.

Conflicts of Interest: C. R. Schindler, T. Lustenberger, M. Woschek, P. Störmann, D. Henrich, P. Radermacher, I. Marzi declare that the research was conducted in the absence of any commercial or financial relationships that could be construed as a potential conflict of interest.

References

1. Bäckström, D.; Larsen, R.; Steinvall, I.; Fredrikson, M.; Gedeborg, R.; Sjöberg, F. Deaths caused by injury among people of working age (18–64) are decreasing, while those among older people (64+) are increasing. *Eur. J. Trauma Emerg. Surg.* **2018**, *44*, 589–596. [CrossRef] [PubMed]
2. Verboket, R.; Verboket, C.; Schöffski, O.; Tlatlik, J.; Marzi, I.; Nau, C. Costs and proceeds from patients admitted via the emergency room with mild craniocerebral trauma. *Unfallchirurg* **2018**. [CrossRef]
3. Störmann, P.; Wagner, N.; Köhler, K.; Auner, B.; Simon, T.-P.; Pfeifer, R.; Horst, K.; Pape, H.-C.; Hildebrand, F.; Wutzler, S.; et al. Monotrauma is associated with enhanced remote inflammatory response and organ damage, while polytrauma intensifies both in porcine trauma model. *Eur. J. Trauma Emerg. Surg.* **2020**, *46*, 31–42. [CrossRef]
4. Van Wessem, K.J.P.; Leenen, L.P.H. Reduction in Mortality Rates of Postinjury Multiple Organ Dysfunction Syndrome: A Shifting Paradigm? A Prospective Population-Based Cohort Study. *Shock* **2018**, *49*, 33–38. [CrossRef] [PubMed]
5. Balogh, Z.J.; Marzi, I. Novel concepts related to inflammatory complications in polytrauma. *Eur. J. Trauma Emerg. Surg.* **2018**, *44*, 299–300. [CrossRef] [PubMed]
6. Lenzlinger, P.M.; Morganti-Kossmann, M.C.; Laurer, H.L.; McIntosh, T.K. The duality of the inflammatory response to traumatic brain injury. *Mol. Neurobiol.* **2001**, *24*, 169–181. [CrossRef] [PubMed]
7. Makinde, H.M.; Just, T.B.; Cuda, C.M.; Perlman, H.; Schwulst, S.J. The Role of Microglia in the Etiology and Evolution of Chronic Traumatic Encephalopathy. *Shock* **2017**, *48*, 276–283. [CrossRef]
8. Lustenberger, T.; Kern, M.; Relja, B.; Wutzler, S.; Störmann, P.; Marzi, I. The effect of brain injury on the inflammatory response following severe trauma. *Immunobiology* **2016**, *221*, 427–431. [CrossRef]
9. Vos, P.E.; Lamers, K.J.B.; Hendriks, J.C.M.; Van Haaren, M.; Beems, T.; Zimmerman, C.; Van Geel, W.; De Reus, H.; Biert, J.; Verbeek, M.M. Glial and neuronal proteins in serum predict outcome after severe traumatic brain injury. *Neurology* **2004**, *62*, 1303–1310. [CrossRef]
10. Thelin, E.P.; Nelson, D.W.; Bellander, B.M. A review of the clinical utility of serum S100B protein levels in the assessment of traumatic brain injury. *Acta Neurochir.* **2017**, *159*, 209–225. [CrossRef]
11. Yamazaki, Y.; Yada, K.; Morii, S.; Kitahara, T.; Ohwada, T. Diagnostic significance of serum neuron-specific enolase and myelin basic protein assay in patients with acute head injury. *Surg. Neurol.* **1995**, *43*, 267–271. [CrossRef]
12. Park, D.W.; Park, S.H.; Hwang, S.K. Serial measurement of S100B and NSE in pediatric traumatic brain injury. *Child's Nerv. Syst.* **2019**, *35*, 343–348. [CrossRef] [PubMed]
13. Lei, J.; Gao, G.; Feng, J.; Jin, Y.; Wang, C.; Mao, Q.; Jiang, J. Glial fibrillary acidic protein as a biomarker in severe traumatic brain injury patients: A prospective cohort study. *Crit. Care* **2015**, *19*, 1–12. [CrossRef] [PubMed]
14. Kapural, M.; Krizanac-Bengez, L.; Barnett, G.; Perl, J.; Masaryk, T.; Apollo, D.; Rasmussen, P.; Mayberg, M.R.; Janigro, D. Serum S-100β as a possible marker of blood-brain barrier disruption. *Brain Res.* **2002**, *940*, 102–104. [CrossRef]

15. Ercole, A.; Thelin, E.P.; Holst, A.; Bellander, B.M.; Nelson, D.W. Kinetic modelling of serum S100b after traumatic brain injury. *BMC Neurol.* **2016**, *16*, 1–8. [CrossRef] [PubMed]
16. Dadas, A.; Washington, J.; Diaz-Arrastia, R.; Janigro, D. Biomarkers in traumatic brain injury (TBI): A review. *Neuropsychiatr. Dis. Treat.* **2018**, *14*, 2989–3000. [CrossRef]
17. Nomellini, V.; Kaplan, L.J.; Sims, C.A.; Caldwell, C.C. Chronic Critical Illness and Persistent Inflammation: What can we Learn from the Elderly, Injured, Septic, and Malnourished? *Shock* **2018**, *49*, 4–14. [CrossRef]
18. Woodcock, T.; Morganti-Kossmann, M.C. The role of markers of inflammation in traumatic brain injury. *Front. Neurol.* **2013**, *4*, 1–18. [CrossRef]
19. Maier, B.; Lefering, R.; Lehnert, M.; Laurer, H.L.; Steudel, W.I.; Neugebauer, E.A.; Marzi, I. Early versus late onset of multiple organ failure is associated with differing patterns of plasma cytokine biomarker expression and outcome after severe trauma. *Shock* **2007**, *28*, 668–674. [CrossRef]
20. Swartz, K.R.; Liu, F.; Sewell, D.; Schochet, T.; Campbell, I.; Sandor, M.; Fabry, Z. Interleukin-6 promotes post-traumatic healing in the central nervous system. *Brain Res.* **2001**, *896*, 86–95. [CrossRef]
21. Burmeister, A.R.; Marriott, I. The interleukin-10 family of cytokines and their role in the CNS. *Front. Cell. Neurosci.* **2018**, *12*, 1–13. [CrossRef] [PubMed]
22. Frink, M.; Van Griensven, M.; Kobbe, P.; Brin, T.; Zeckey, C.; Vaske, B.; Krettek, C.; Hildebrand, F. IL-6 predicts organ dysfunction and mortality in patients with multiple injuries. *Scand. J. Trauma. Resusc. Emerg. Med.* **2009**, *17*, 1–7. [CrossRef] [PubMed]
23. Stensballe, J.; Christiansen, M.; TØnnesen, E.; Espersen, K.; Lippert, F.K.; Rasmussen, L.S. The early IL-6 and IL-10 response in trauma is correlated with injury severity and mortality. *Acta Anaesthesiol. Scand.* **2009**, *53*, 515–521. [CrossRef] [PubMed]
24. Von Elm, E.; Altmann, D.G.; Egger, M.; Pocock, S.C.; Gøtzsche, P.C.; Vandenbroucke, J.P. Das Strengthening the Reporting of Observational Studies in Epidemiology (STROBE-) Statement. *Internist (Berl)* **2008**, *49*, 688–693. [CrossRef] [PubMed]
25. Bouillon, B.; Kanz, K.G.; Lackner, C.K.; Mutschler, W.; Sturm, J. Die bedeutung des Advanced Trauma Life Support®(ATLS®) im schockraum. *Unfallchirurg* **2004**, *107*, 844–850. [CrossRef]
26. Haasper, C.; Junge, M.; Ernstberger, A.; Brehme, H.; Hannawald, L.; Langer, C.; Nehmzow, J.; Otte, D.; Sander, U.; Krettek, C.; et al. Die Abbreviated Injury Scale (AIS). *Unfallchirurg* **2010**, *113*, 366–372. [CrossRef]
27. Baker, S.P.; O'Neill, B.; Haddon, W. The Injury Severity Score. *J. Trauma-Inj. Infect. Crit. Care* **1974**, *14*, 187–196. [CrossRef]
28. Stevenson, M.; Segui-Gomez, M.; Lescohier, I.; Di Scala, C.; McDonald-Smith, G. An overview of the injury severity score and the new injury severity score. *Inj. Prev.* **2001**, *7*, 10–13. [CrossRef]
29. Fröhlich, M.; Caspers, M.; Lefering, R.; Driessen, A.; Bouillon, B.; Maegele, M.; Wafaisade, A. Do elderly trauma patients receive the required treatment? Epidemiology and outcome of geriatric trauma patients treated at different levels of trauma care. *Eur. J. Trauma Emerg. Surg.* **2019**, 1–7. [CrossRef]
30. Bechtel, K.; Frasure, S.; Marshall, C.; Dziura, J.; Simpson, C. Relationship of serum S100B levels and intracranial injury in children with closed head trauma. *Pediatrics* **2009**, *124*. [CrossRef]
31. Ohrt-Nissen, S.; Friis-Hansen, L.; Dahl, B.; Stensballe, J.; Romner, B.; Rasmussen, L.S. How does extracerebral trauma affect the clinical value of S100B measurements? *Emerg. Med. J.* **2011**, *28*, 941–944. [CrossRef] [PubMed]
32. De Souza, D.F.; Wartchow, K.; Hansen, F.; Lunardi, P.; Guerra, M.C.; Nardin, P.; Gonçalves, C.A. Interleukin-6-induced S100B secretion is inhibited by haloperidol and risperidone. *Prog. Neuro-Psychopharmacol. Biol. Psychiatry* **2013**, *43*, 14–22. [CrossRef] [PubMed]
33. Pelinka, L.E.; Hertz, H.; Mauritz, W.; Harada, N.; Jafarmadar, M.; Albrecht, M.; Redl, H.; Bahrami, S. Nonspecific increase of systemic neuron-specific enolase after trauma: Clinical and experimental findings. *Shock* **2005**, *24*, 119–123. [CrossRef] [PubMed]
34. Vogt, N.; Herden, C.; Roeb, E.; Roderfeld, M.; Eschbach, D.; Steinfeldt, T.; Wulf, H.; Ruchholtz, S.; Uhl, E.; Schöller, K. Cerebral Alterations Following Experimental Multiple Trauma and Hemorrhagic Shock. *Shock* **2018**, *49*, 164–173. [CrossRef]
35. Xu, C.M.; Luo, Y.L.; Li, S.; Li, Z.X.; Jiang, L.; Zhang, G.X.; Owusu, L.; Chen, H.L. Multifunctional neuron-specific enolase: ITS role in lung diseases. *Biosci. Rep.* **2019**, *39*, 1–16. [CrossRef]

36. Crawford, A.M.; Yang, S.; Hu, P.; Li, Y.; Lozanova, P.; Scalea, T.M.; Stein, D.M. Concomitant chest trauma and traumatic brain injury, biomarkers correlate with worse outcomes. *J. Trauma Acute Care Surg.* **2019**, *87*, S146–S151. [CrossRef]
37. Hainfellner, J.A.; Voigtländer, T.; Ströbel, T.; Mazal, P.R.; Maddalena, A.S.; Aguzzi, A.; Budka, H. Fibroblasts can express glial fibrillary acidic protein (GFAP) in vivo. *J. Neuropathol. Exp. Neurol.* **2001**, *60*, 449–461. [CrossRef]
38. Foerch, C.; Pfeilschifter, W.; Zeiner, P.; Brunkhorst, R. Saures gliafaserprotein beim patienten mit akuten schlaganfallsymptomen: Diagnostischer marker einer hirnblutung. *Nervenarzt* **2014**, *85*, 982–989. [CrossRef]
39. Lumpkins, K.M.; Bochicchio, G.V.; Keledjian, K.; Simard, J.M.; McCunn, M.; Scalea, T. Glial fibrillary acidic protein is highly correlated with brain injury. *J. Trauma* **2008**, *65*, 778–782. [CrossRef]
40. Hsieh, Y.H.; McCartney, K.; Moore, T.A.; Thundyil, J.; Gelderblom, M.; Manzanero, S.; Arumugam, T.V. Intestinal ischemia-reperfusion injury leads to inflammatory changes in the brain. *Shock* **2011**, *36*, 424–430. [CrossRef]
41. Shultz, S.R.; Sun, M.; Wright, D.K.; Brady, R.D.; Liu, S.; Beynon, S.; Schmidt, S.F.; Kaye, A.H.; Hamilton, J.A.; O'Brien, T.J.; et al. Tibial fracture exacerbates traumatic brain injury outcomes and neuroinflammation in a novel mouse model of multitrauma. *J. Cereb. Blood Flow Metab.* **2015**, *35*, 1339–1347. [CrossRef] [PubMed]
42. Morganti-Kossmann, M.C.; Satgunaseelan, L.; Bye, N.; Kossmann, T. Modulation of immune response by head injury. *Injury* **2007**, *38*, 1392–1400. [CrossRef] [PubMed]
43. Maier, B.; Schwerdtfeger, K.; Mautes, A.; Holanda, M.; Müller, M.; Steudel, W.I. Differential release of interleukines 6, 8, and 10 in cerebrospinal fluid and plasma after traumatic brain injury. *Shock* **2001**, *15*, 421–426. [CrossRef] [PubMed]
44. Woiciechowsky, C.; Schöning, B.; Cobanov, J.; Lanksch, W.R.; Volk, H.D.; Döcke, W.D. Early il-6 plasma concentrations correlate with severity of brain injury and pneumonia in brain-injured patients. *J. Trauma* **2002**, *52*, 339–345. [CrossRef] [PubMed]
45. Garcia, J.M.; Stillings, S.A.; Leclerc, J.L.; Phillips, H.; Edwards, N.J.; Robicsek, S.A.; Hoh, B.L.; Blackburn, S.; Doré, S. Role of interleukin-10 in acute brain injuries. *Front. Neurol.* **2017**, *8*, 1–17. [CrossRef]
46. Sapan, H.B.; Paturusi, I.; Islam, A.A.; Yusuf, I.; Patellongi, I.; Massi, M.N.; Pusponegoro, A.D.; Arief, S.K.; Labeda, I.; Rendy, L.; et al. Interleukin-6 and interleukin-10 plasma levels and mRNA expression in polytrauma patients. *Chin. J. Traumatol.* **2017**, *20*, 318–322. [CrossRef]
47. Kalabalikis, P.; Papazoglou, K.; Gouriotis, D.; Papadopoulos, N.; Kardara, M.; Papageorgiou, F.; Papadatos, J. Correlation between serum IL-6 and CRP levels and severity of head injury in children. *Intensive Care Med.* **1999**, *25*, 288–292. [CrossRef]
48. Wrba, L.; Ohmann, J.J.; Eisele, P.; Chakraborty, S.; Braumüller, S.; Braun, C.K.; Klohs, B.; Schultze, A.; Von Baum, H.; Palmer, A.; et al. Remote intestinal injury early after experimental polytrauma and hemorrhagic shock. *Shock* **2019**, *52*, e45–e51. [CrossRef]
49. Cohen, S.S.; Min, M.; Cummings, E.E.; Chen, X.; Sadowska, G.B.; Sharma, S.; Stonestreet, B.S. Effects of Interleukin-6 on the Expression of Tight Junction Proteins in Isolated Cerebral Microvessels from Yearling and Adult Sheep. *Neuroimmunomodulation* **2013**, *20*, 264–273. [CrossRef]
50. Halbgebauer, R.; Braun, C.K.; Denk, S.; Mayer, B.; Cinelli, P.; Radermacher, P.; Wanner, G.A.; Simmen, H.P.; Gebhard, F.; Rittirsch, D.; et al. Hemorrhagic shock drives glycocalyx, barrier and organ dysfunction early after polytrauma. *J. Crit. Care* **2018**, *44*, 229–237. [CrossRef]
51. Pan, P.; Song, Y.; Du, X.; Bai, L.; Hua, X.; Xiao, Y.; Yu, X. Intestinal barrier dysfunction following traumatic brain injury. *Neurol. Sci.* **2019**, *40*, 1105–1110. [CrossRef] [PubMed]
52. Vanzant, E.L.; Hilton, R.E.; Lopez, C.M.; Zhang, J.; Ungaro, R.F.; Gentile, L.F.; Szpila, B.E.; Maier, R.V.; Cuschieri, J.; Bihorac, A.; et al. Advanced age is associated with worsened outcomes and a unique genomic response in severely injured patients with hemorrhagic shock. *Crit. Care* **2015**, *19*, 1–15. [CrossRef] [PubMed]

Journal of
Clinical Medicine

MDPI

Article

Which Risk Factors Predict Knee Ligament Injuries in Severely Injured Patients?—Results from an International Multicenter Analysis

Christian D. Weber [1,*], Lucian B. Solomon [2], Rolf Lefering [3], Klemens Horst [1], Philipp Kobbe [1], Frank Hildebrand [1] and TraumaRegister DGU [4]

1 Department of Orthopaedics and Trauma Surgery, RWTH Aachen University, 52074 Aachen, Germany; khorst@ukaachen.de (K.H.); pkobbe@ukaachen.de (P.K.); fhildebrand@ukaachen.de (F.H.)
2 Orthopaedic and Trauma Service, Royal Adelaide Hospital and Centre for Orthopaedic and Trauma Research, The University of Adelaide, SA 5005, Adelaide, Australia; bogdansolomon@me.com
3 Institute for Research in Operative Medicine (IFOM), Witten/Herdecke University, 51109 Cologne, Germany; rolf.lefering@uni-wh.de
4 Committee on Emergency Medicine, Intensive Care and Trauma Management (Sektion NIS) of the German Trauma Society (DGU), 10623 Berlin, Germany; traumaregister@auc-online.de
* Correspondence: chrweber@ukaachen.de; Tel.: +49-241-8036161

Received: 4 April 2020; Accepted: 7 May 2020; Published: 12 May 2020

Abstract: *Introduction:* Ligament injuries around the knee joint and knee dislocations are rare but potentially complex injuries associated with high-energy trauma. Concomitant neurovascular injuries further affect their long-term clinical outcomes. In contrast to isolated ligamentous knee injuries, epidemiologic data and knowledge on predicting knee injuries in severely injured patients is still limited. *Methods:* The TraumaRegister DGU® (TR-DGU) was queried (01/2009–12/2016). Inclusion criteria for selection from the database: maximum abbreviated injury severity ≥ 3 points (MAIS 3+). Participating countries: Germany, Austria, and Switzerland. The two main groups included a "control" and a "knee injury" group. The injury severity score (ISS) and new ISS (NISS) were used for injury severity classification, and the abbreviated injury scale (AIS) was used to classify the severity of the knee injury. Logistic regression analysis was performed to evaluate various risk factors for knee injuries. *Results:* The study cohort included 139,462 severely injured trauma patients. We identified 4411 individuals (3.2%) with a ligament injury around the knee joint ("knee injury" group) and 1153 patients with a knee dislocation (0.8%). The risk for associated injuries of the peroneal nerve and popliteal artery were significantly increased in dislocated knees when compared to controls (peroneal nerve from 0.4% to 6.7%, popliteal artery from 0.3% to 6.9%, respectively). Among the predictors for knee injuries were specific mechanisms of injury: e.g., pedestrian struck (Odds ratio [OR] 3.2, 95% confidence interval [CI]: 2.69–3.74 $p \leq 0.001$), motorcycle (OR 3.0, 95% CI: 2.58–3.48, $p \leq 0.001$), and motor vehicle accidents (OR 2.2, 95% CI: 1.86–2.51, $p \leq 0.001$) and associated skeletal injuries, e.g., patella (OR 2.3, 95% CI: 1.99–2.62, $p \leq 0.001$), tibia (OR 1.9, 95% CI: 1.75–2.05, $p \leq 0.001$), and femur (OR 1.8, 95% CI: 1.64–1.89, $p \leq 0.001$), but neither male sex nor general injury severity (ISS). *Conclusion:* Ligament injuries and knee dislocations are associated with high-risk mechanisms and concomitant skeletal injuries of the lower extremity, but are not predicted by general injury severity or sex. Despite comparable ISS, knee injuries prolong the hospital length of stay. Delayed or missed diagnosis of knee injuries can be prevented by comprehensive clinical evaluation after fracture fixation and a high index of suspicion is advised, especially in the presence of the above mentioned risk factors.

Keywords: risk factors; knee joint injuries; knee dislocation; ligament injuries

1. Introduction

High-energy trauma, in particular, can result in multisystem injuries, which may involve both isolated or multi-ligamentous knee injuries [1,2]. The acute traumatic dislocation of the knee is considered the most severe ligament injury of the lower extremity and may be associated with devastating and limb-threatening complications [3–6]. The incidence for knee dislocations is very low and has been estimated to be 1.2 per million person-years, mainly from high-energy trauma [7]. However, recent publications also reported knee dislocations as a result of low-energy mechanisms, including ground level falls in obese individuals [8–10]. The prompt identification, dedicated evaluation, and a comprehensive management of knee injuries have a high impact on long-term functional outcomes [11–14].

In fact, ligament injuries around the knee and dislocations of the knee joint have been poorly described in the context of multiple trauma [15]. Previous studies have suggested anatomic risk factors for knee injuries, including femoral shaft fractures [16,17], combined femur and tibia fractures [18], patella fractures [19], and acetabular fractures [20]. According to Byun et al. around 30% of concomitant knee injuries after femoral shaft fracture are not detected in time [17] and frequently become symptomatic within the first posttraumatic year [20]. The mean time for diagnosis of associated knee ligament injury in neglected cases after fixation of a femoral shaft fracture was around 10.6 weeks (range, 1–32) [17].

While a meta-analysis suggested improved outcomes for the early reconstruction of complex knee injuries [21], this concept would be jeopardized by a delayed diagnosis of injuries to the knee. Therefore, the identification of risk factors based on anatomical injury patterns or injury mechanisms might be helpful to guide the diagnostic and surgical strategy, to improve the early detection of knee injuries, and to prevent long-term complications.

In this context, this study was designed as a multi-center registry analysis to increase the knowledge about ligament injuries around the knee and knee dislocations in severely injured trauma patients. We attempted to answer the following questions:

1. What is the incidence for knee ligament injuries and knee dislocations?
2. What are the predominant injury mechanisms leading to knee injuries?
3. What are independent predictors for knee injuries in severely injured trauma patients?

2. Patients and Methods

2.1. TraumaRegister DGU® and Data Acquisition

The TraumaRegister DGU® of the German Trauma Society (Deutsche Gesellschaft für Unfallchirurgie, DGU) was founded in 1993 [22,23]. The aim of this multi-center database is a pseudonymized and standardized documentation of severely injured patients. Data are collected prospectively in four consecutive time phases from the site of the accident until discharge from hospital: (A) Pre-hospital phase, (B) emergency room and initial surgery, (C) intensive care unit (ICU), and (D) discharge.

The documentation includes detailed information on demographics, injury pattern, comorbidities, pre- and in-hospital management, a course in ICU, relevant laboratory findings including data on transfusion, and the outcome of each individual. The inclusion criterion is admission via the emergency room with subsequent intensive or intermediate care or death before admission to ICU. The infrastructure for documentation, data management, and data analysis are provided by the Academy for Trauma Surgery (AUC—Akademie der Unfallchirurgie GmbH), a company affiliated with the German Trauma Society. The scientific leadership is provided by the Committee on Emergency Medicine, Intensive Care and Trauma Management (Sektion NIS) of the German Trauma Society. The participating hospitals submit their data pseudonymized into a central database via a web-based application. Scientific data analysis is approved according to a peer review procedure established by Sektion NIS. The participating hospitals are primarily located in Germany (90%), but a rising number of hospitals of other countries contribute data as well (at the moment Austria, Switzerland, Belgium, Finland, Luxemburg, Slovenia, The Netherlands, and the United Arab Emirates). Currently, approx. 35,000 cases from almost 700 hospitals are entered into the database per year. Participation in TraumaRegister DGU® is voluntary. For hospitals associated with the TraumaNetzwerk DGU®, however, the entry of at least a basic dataset is obligatory for reasons of quality assurance. The present study is in line with the publication guidelines of the TraumaRegister DGU® and registered as TR-DGU project ID 2014-057.

2.2. Inclusion and Exclusion Criteria

This study included data from all patients included in the TraumaRegister DGU® with severe injuries (MAIS 3+) after admission to a participating trauma center in Germany, Austria, or Switzerland between January 2009 and December 2016.

Patients transferred *out* to another center within 48 h after admission were excluded because of missing outcome data and to exclude the risk of a double counting from the receiving hospital. However, all cases transferred *in* were included to prevent bias in prevalence rates.

2.3. Definitions

2.3.1. Mechanism of Injury

According to the TR-DGU dataset, the following injury mechanisms were considered: (1) Motor vehicle accident (MVA), (2) motorcycle accident (MCA), (3) bicycle accident, (4) pedestrian struck by vehicle, (5) high fall (≥ 3 m), and (6) low fall (< 3 m); further (combined) categories include (7) suicide attempt, (8) other (not shown), (9) blunt/penetrating trauma (not shown), and (10) traffic-related (overall value presented).

2.3.2. Injury Severity

Since 2009, coding follows a uniform protocol, and the data management has been previously described [23]. All injuries were coded according to the Abbreviated Injury Scale (AIS Version 2005/Update 2008, Association for the Advancement of Automotive Medicine, Barrington, IL) [24,25]. According to the AIS, the severity of injuries was documented as follows [26]: 1 (minor), 2 (moderate), 3 (severe, not life-threatening), 4 (serious, life-threatening), 5 (critical, survival uncertain), or 6 (maximum, currently untreatable). The injury severity score (ISS) and the new ISS (NISS) were derived from documented AIS values [26,27].

2.3.3. Identification of Knee Injuries and Group Distribution

Identification of ligament injuries according to AIS codes: (1) AIS 8740**.1: knee ligament injury (including subluxation); (2) AIS 87403*.2: (multi-)ligament injury with knee dislocation; and (3) AIS 84080*.2: partial or complete ligament rupture. Neurovascular injuries around the knee were identified independently from ligamentous injuries either as a popliteal artery injury (AIS 8206**.2) and/or a peroneal nerve injury (AIS 8305**.2).

Patients with one of the aforementioned AIS codes were assigned to the "knee injury" group, whereas patients without these injuries were included in the "control" group.

3. Statistical Analysis

Categorical data were presented as frequencies and percentages. Metric variables were reported as means and standard deviations (SD). For skew distributed data, the median is also reported. Severe trauma patients without a ligament injury of the knee served as a control group. Formal statistical testing was avoided because of the very large sample size. Multivariate logistic regression analysis was performed to evaluate the impact of various risk factors for knee injuries. Results are presented as odds ratios (OR) with 95% confidence intervals. The analysis was performed with SPSS (Version 25, IBM Inc., Armonk, NY, USA).

4. Results

4.1. Demographic Data and Mechanism of Injury

During the study period, 139,462 severely injured patients fulfilled the inclusion criteria. Of these, 4411 patients sustained a knee injury (3.2% overall incidence), and 1152 patients (0.8%) suffered from a multi-ligament injury related to a knee dislocation. Ligamentous knee injuries in polytraumatized patients were most commonly caused by road traffic accidents (84.8%, Table 1). MVA and MCA were equally responsible for 62% of these (1375 patients or 31.7% for MVA and 1305 or 30.1% for MCA), while pedestrians struck by vehicles were responsible for 13.3% of these injuries (578 patients).

Table 1. Mechanisms of injury.

	Control Group n = 131,483	Knee Injury n = 4340	Total
Motor vehicle collision % (n)	20.6% (27,054)	31.7% (1374)	20.9% (28,428)
Motorcycle accident % (n)	12.5% (16,391)	30.1% (1305)	13% (17,696)
Bicycle accident % (n)	8.5% (11,177)	6.1% (263)	8.4% (11,440)
Pedestrian struck % (n)	6.6% (8618)	13.3% (578)	6.8% (9196)
High Fall ≥3 m % (n)	17.6% (21,938)	8.5% (367)	16.4% (22,305)
Low Fall <3 m % (n)	24.1% (31,667)	4.9% (212)	23.5% (31,879)
Traffic-related (all) % (n)	51.7% (64,859)	84.8% (3580)	52.7% (68,439)
Suicide attempt (any) % (n)	4.8% (6221)	3.0% (128)	4.7% (6349)

Of the patients, 98,252 (70.7%) were male (Table 2). The "knee injury" group had a mean age of 43 years (±19), and the control group had a mean age of 52 years (±22). The vast majority of patients with knee ligament injuries were between 16 and 59 years of age (n = 3447, 78.1%). Pediatric and elderly patients infrequently sustained ligamentous knee injuries. The age distribution was found bimodal; we observed two peaks: 20–30 years and 40–50 years (Figure 1).

Table 2. Demographic and outcome data.

	Control Group	Knee Injury
Male sex % (n)	70.5% (94,981)	74.3% (3271)
Mean age (SD), years	52 (22)	43 (19)
Pediatric age (≤ 15 years)	3.3% (4420)	2.3% (102)
ISS: mean (SD), points	21.7 (12)	21.4 (11)
New ISS: mean (SD), points	27.5 (14)	26.0 (12)
ICU LOS: days †	7.4 / 3 (11)	8.4 / 3 (12)
Hospital LOS: days †	19 / 14 (19)	26 / 21 (22)
Delayed injury identification β	8.3% (108)	14.7% (120)

LOS = length of stay; ICU = intensive care unit. (†) mean / median (SD). (β) Injury diagnosed at ICU or later; available for cases with standard documentation only.

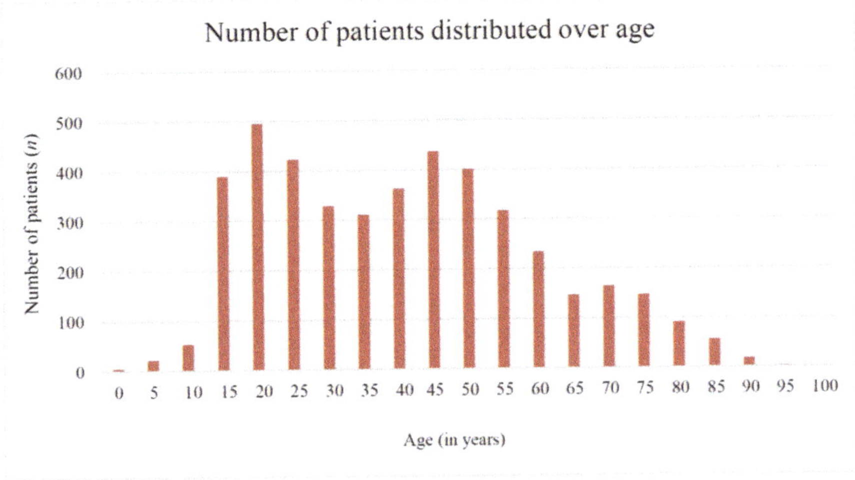

Figure 1. Age distribution of patients with knee ligament injuries (each column represents a 5-year interval).

4.2. Injury Pattern

Mean ISS (21.7 vs. 21.4 points) and NISS (27.5 vs. 26.0 points) values were comparable for both groups. In terms of associated injuries, the control group had a higher rate of head injuries (45.0%) compared to the knee injury group (25.9%).

No clinically relevant variance for facial, chest, and abdominal or spinal injuries was observed (Table 3) between the two groups. However, upper and lower extremity injuries and pelvic fractures were more frequently diagnosed in patients with ligamentous knee injuries. The rate of associated neurovascular injuries was increased in patients with ligamentous knee injuries and even more pronounced in case of knee dislocation (peroneal nerve: 6.7% and popliteal artery: 6.9%).

Table 3. Patterns of injury.

	Control Group	Knee Injury	*Total*
Head injury (AIS ≥3)	45.0% (60,755)	25.9% (1141)	44.4% (61,896)
Facial injury (AIS ≥2)	11.6% (15,634)	10.9% (483)	11.6% (16,117)
Chest injury (AIS ≥3)	47.7% (64,458)	50.7% (2238)	47.8% (66,696)
Abdominal injury (AIS ≥3)	12.4% (16,800)	12.1% (532)	12.4% (17,332)
Extremity injury (AIS ≥3)	30.1% (40,674)	56.9% (2508)	31.0% (43,182)
Spinal injury (AIS ≥2)	29.6% (39,926)	29.1% (1283)	29.5% (41,208)
UE injury (AIS ≥2)	30.0% (40,563)	39.9% (1758)	30.3% (42,321)
LE injury (AIS ≥2)	26.3% (35,542)	76.5% (3375)	27.9% (38,917)
Pelvic injury (AIS ≥2)	17.9% (24,139)	27.1% (1195)	18.2% (25,334)
Femur fracture % (*n*)	13.9% (18,826)	31.6% (1394)	14.5% (20,220)
Tibia fracture % (*n*)	10.3% (13,853)	31.7% (1399)	10.9% (15,252)
Patella fracture % (*n*)	4.5% (6084)	16.6% (731)	4.9% (6815)
Peroneal nerve injury % (*n*)	0.4% (489)	3.9% (63)	0.4% (552)
Popliteal artery injury % (*n*)	0.2% (228)	2.2% (99)	0.2% (327)

UE = upper extremity; LE = lower extremity.

4.3. Length of Hospital Stay and Delayed Diagnosis

The hospital stay was prolonged by seven days in patients with associated ligamentous knee injuries, and 228 patients had a delay longer than 48 h in the diagnosis of a ligamentous knee injury.

4.4. Multivariate Logistic Regression Analysis

The multivariate logistic regression analysis model (Table 4) identified various variables associated with an increased risk for knee ligament injury: (1) Pedestrian struck by vehicle (OR 3.2, 95% CI: 2.69–3.74 $p \leq 0.001$); (2) MCA (OR 3.0, 95% CI: 2.58–3.48, $p \leq 0.001$); (3) patella fracture (OR 2.3, 95% CI: 1.99–2.62, $p \leq 0.001$); (4) MVA (OR 2.2, 95% CI: 1.86–2.51, $p \leq 0.001$); (5) tibia fracture (OR 1.9, 95% CI: 1.75–2.05, $p \leq 0.001$); (6) femur fracture (OR 1.8, 95% CI: 1.64–1.89, $p \leq 0.001$); (7) fibula fracture (OR 1.8, 95% CI: 1.62–1.98, $p \leq 0.001$); (8) bicycle accident (OR 1.5, 95% CI: 1.21–1.74, $p \leq 0.001$); (9) pelvic fracture (OR 1.3, 95% CI: 1.24–1.44, $p \leq 0.001$); and (10) upper extremity fracture (OR 1.1, 95% CI: 1.03–1.18, $p = 0.004$).

Table 4. Logistic regression analysis: predictors for ligamentous knee injuries.

Risk Factors	Odds Ratio (OR)	95% Confidence Interval (CI)	p-Value
Mechanisms of Injury			
Motor vehicle accident	2.2	1.86–2.51	≤ 0.001
Motorcycle accident	3.0	2.58–3.48	≤ 0.001
Pedestrian struck	3.2	2.69–3.74	≤ 0.001
Bicycle accident	1.5	1.21–1.74	≤ 0.001
Skeletal Injuries			
Pelvic fracture	1.3	1.24–1.44	≤ 0.001
Femur fracture	1.8	1.64–1.89	≤ 0.001
Patella fracture	2.3	1.99–2.62	≤ 0.001
Tibia fracture	1.9	1.75–2.05	≤ 0.001
Fibula fracture	1.8	1.62–1.98	≤ 0.001
Upper extremity fracture	1.1	1.03–1.18	0.004
Demographic Data			
Male sex	1.0	0.96–1.12	0.29

5. Discussion

This study interrogated a large registry database to investigate the mechanisms of injury that cause associated ligamentous knee injuries in severely injured patients. Furthermore, demographics and associated injuries in severely injured patients with knee ligament injuries were characterized. Such information is likely to support the development of diagnostic protocols and thereby to increase the early diagnosis of ligamentous knee injuries in this patient cohort. This is of upmost importance because it is known that such injuries are missed in up to 30% of patients [17], and a delayed diagnosis of these injuries can have devastating effects on their outcomes [28]. In a long-term study after multiple trauma, knee injuries were most often responsible for preventing individuals to return to sports [13].

5.1. Incidence and Demographic Data

The incidence of ligamentous knee injuries in our study population was 3.2%, and 0.8% of the included patients suffered a dislocated knee. These findings are in line with recent publications, since ligamentous knee injuries, especially knee dislocations, are rare injuries. Particularly, traumatic knee dislocations are very rare and have been described to account for only 0.02% of orthopedic injuries [29].

We observed a bimodal age distribution for ligamentous knee injuries, with one peak in the third decade of life and a second peak in the fifth decade of life. The highest incidence of ligamentous knee injuries in the severely injured patient was previously identified in men aged between 18 and 29 years (incidence, 29 per 1 million person-years in 2011) [30]. The observed bimodal distribution with a second peak in the fifth life decade may be caused by the current demographic situation in the participating countries [31,32], and therefore might also reflect the reality of social and behavioral changes in people's lives at certain time points.

5.2. Mechanisms and Patterns of Injury

Recently, a number of publications highlighted low-velocity mechanisms in obese individuals as novel and separate mechanism causing ligamentous knee injuries [7–10]. According to our data, low energy falls contributed to only 4.9% of all ligamentous knee injuries, and the vast majority of complex knee injuries were associated with high-energy trauma. Predominant injury mechanisms leading to knee injuries were MVAs, MCAs, and pedestrian struck by a car. Multiple previous studies also reported motor vehicle collisions as the major cause of these injuries [33–36].

5.3. Associated Injuries and Outcome

While we report ligamentous and neurovascular injuries of the knee in dichotomous fashion, we are unable to comment on exact intra-articular pathologies. Krych et al. evaluated 122 dislocated knees in 121 patients and found associated intra-articular injuries in addition to ligament injuries in 76% of patients [37].

We identified a high incidence of concomitant injuries particularly of the lower extremity (i.e., patella fractures) and the chest in our population with ligamentous knee injuries. This finding should prompt a comprehensive assessment of ligamentous knee injuries in all these situations, especially when the knee injury is not obvious. Accordingly, Darcy et al. [29] reported in a group of 80 patients with knee dislocation that 57.1% of the cases were associated with another injury. Also other reports described a number of injuries associated with ligamentous knee injuries. In this context it was found, that 25% of patellar fractures were associated with a posterior cruciate ligament injury [19]. A retrospective analysis of 114 femoral shaft fractures in 110 patients, at an average of 3.9 years post-injury, showed that 27% of patients had some form of knee ligament insufficiency, while 11% complained of knee instability [18]. The same study found that knee instability was even more prevalent, with 54% in cases of combined ipsilateral femur and tibial shaft fractures [18]. As a conclusion, the authors advocated examination of the knee under anesthesia in all patients with a femoral shaft fracture. Accordingly, another study found a 20% risk of ipsilateral ligamentous knee injuries after femoral shaft fractures (87 of 429 cases, 32 of which were multi ligamentous injuries) [17]. Most importantly, 30% of these injuries were only detected at an average of 11 weeks (range 1–32 weeks) after the surgical treatment of the femoral shaft fracture. At 14.7%, the delayed diagnosis of ligamentous knee injuries in our study was half of that.

5.4. Associated Neurovascular Injuries

This study found that the incidence of popliteal artery injuries associated with ligamentous injuries to the knee is bigger than previously reported by large cohort series. Notably, popliteal artery injuries can also be associated with isolated ligamentous injuries of the knee, as our study identified 99 popliteal artery injuries (2.2%) in patients with isolated knee ligamentous injuries. The incidence of popliteal artery injury in patients with knee dislocations at 6.9% (79 cases) in our study was higher than in other studies with large cohorts based on either an analysis of a large insurance database [38] or a prospective review of 303 cases of knee dislocations [39]. This might be explained by a higher proportion of high energy trauma cases in our study. However, the incidences of our and the other aforementioned studies are markedly lower compared to results from smaller cohort series investigating knee dislocations. For example, a review of 67 patients at a multicenter study found the incidence of popliteal artery injury in 12% (9 patients) of patients with knee dislocations in which both cruciate ligaments are injured [40], while a systematic review of 23 studies with rather small study populations with knee dislocation found the incidence of popliteal artery injury to be 18% [3]. Excluding the questions related to relatively small retrospective studies and the associated selection bias, it is possible that such differences are also related to the mechanism of injury and patient-specific factors. In this context, the exact role of the injury mechanism for the development of popliteal injuries is not fully clarified. While this and other studies [3,10,30,41–43] mainly observed vascular injuries associated with knee dislocations in high-energy trauma cases, some authors suggest that knee dislocation-associated vascular injuries preferably appear secondary to low energy injuries (21% in ultra-low energy injuries) when compared with high energy injuries mechanisms (13%) [41]. Also patient- and injury-specific risk factors (increased body mass index and open injuries, OR 3.366; 95% CI, 1.008–11.420; $p = 0.048$) for vascular injuries in case of knee dislocation were identified [42]. This study also found that the incidence of peroneal nerve injuries was smaller than previously reported. We identified 148 (3.9%) peroneal nerve injuries in patients with isolated knee ligamentous injuries and 77 peroneal nerve injuries (6.7%) in patients with knee dislocations. By comparison, a prospective review of 303 patients with knee dislocations found the incidence of peroneal nerve injuries to be 19.2% [39], and a systematic review identified the risk of common peroneal nerve injuries in knee dislocations to be as high as 25% [3]. As with the vascular injuries, injury mechanism and patient-specific factors might again explain these differences. In this context, some literature has suggested that lower energy injuries are more likely to be associated with nerve damage compared with higher energy injuries [41].

5.5. Limitations

This study has several limitations. Owing to the nature of the TraumaRegister DGU® and the well-known inclusion criteria, our data concerning injury mechanisms were biased toward high-energy injuries rather than low-energy injuries. Therefore, our findings are not generalizable to isolated injuries such as ultra-low-energy knee dislocations, e.g., from low-level falls. Furthermore, as the number and anatomic sites of ligament injuries around the knee are not consistently documented within the TraumaRegister DGU®, we are unable to report the exact anatomic injury patterns. Additionally, in severely injured patients, there is a risk of underreporting of knee injuries related to early mortality or limb-loss. The TraumaRegister DGU® is also not designed to capture occult knee injuries that were diagnosed after hospital discharge or transfer to a rehabilitation facility. Especially in patients with limited mobility, knee instability, and associated pain might be clinically unapparent prior to weight-bearing mobilization during rehabilitation. However, the current study also has several strengths to be recognized. First, to our knowledge, this is the largest study analyzing knee injuries in severely injured patients. Therefore, the epidemiologic data, description of injury mechanisms, general injury severity, and concomitant injuries seem to be valid and clinically relevant. Second, the logistic regression analysis involved a wide range of risk factors including injury mechanisms and skeletal injuries. The analysis identified various independent predictors for knee injuries that are also applicable in sedated and ventilated trauma patients.

6. Conclusions

Ligamentous knee injuries caused by high-energy trauma are associated with concomitant injuries of the pelvis, femur, patella, and lower leg, but are not predicted by general injury severity or sex. Despite comparable injury severity, ligamentous knee injuries prolong the hospital length of stay and could therefore be considered a surrogate for increased treatment complexity and costs.

Author Contributions: Conceptualization, C.D.W. and F.H.; data curation, R.L and C.D.W.; formal analysis, L.B.S., K.H., C.D.W. P.K., and F.H.; investigation, C.D.W. and R.L.; methodology, R.L., K.H., C.D.W. P.K., and F.H.; project administration, C.D.W. and F.H.; resources, P.K. and F.H.; supervision, L.B.S., P.K., and F.H.; validation, C.D.W.,

L.B.S., R.L., K.H., P.K., and F.H.; visualization, C.D.W. and F.H.; writing—original draft, C.D.W., R.L., and L.B.S.; writing—review and editing, K.H., P.K., and F.H. All authors have read and agreed to the published version of the manuscript.

Funding: This research received no external funding.

Acknowledgments: Preliminary results of this study (DOI: 10.3205/18dkou778) were presented in October 2018 at the German Congress of Orthopaedics and Traumatology in Berlin (Deutscher Kongress für Orthopädie und Unfallchirurgie). The authors would like to thank the internal review board of the TraumaRegister DGU® for their substantial contribution. Furthermore, we thank all participating trauma centers (complete list at www.traumaregister-dgu.de). The manuscript was proofread by Scribendi Proofreading Services (405 Riverview Drive, Chatham, Canada).

Conflicts of Interest: The authors declare no conflict of interest with respect to the research, authorship, and/or publication of this article.

References

1. Burrus, M.T.; Werner, B.C.; Cancienne, J.M.; Miller, M.D. Simultaneous bilateral multiligamentous knee injuries are associated with more severe multisystem trauma compared to unilateral injuries. *Knee Surg. Sports Traumatol. Arthrosc.* **2015**, *23*, 3038–3043. [CrossRef] [PubMed]
2. Fanelli, G.C. Multiple Ligament Injured Knee: Initial Assessment and Treatment. *Clin. Sports Med.* **2019**, *38*, 193–198. [CrossRef] [PubMed]
3. Medina, O.; Arom, G.A.; Yeranosian, M.G.; Petrigliano, F.A.; McAllister, D.R. Vascular and nerve injury after knee dislocation: A systematic review. *Clin. Orthop. Relat. Res.* **2014**, *472*, 2621–2629. [CrossRef] [PubMed]
4. Teissier, V.; Tresson, P.; Gaudric, J.; Davaine, J.M.; Scemama, C.; Raux, M.; Chiche, L.; Koskas, F. Importance of Early Diagnosis and Care in Knee Dislocations Associated with Vascular Injuries. *Ann. Vasc. Surg.* **2019**, *61*, 238–245. [CrossRef] [PubMed]
5. Matthewson, G.; Kwapisz, A.; Sasyniuk, T.; MacDonald, P. Vascular Injury in the Multiligament Injured Knee. *Clin. Sports Med.* **2019**, *38*, 199–213. [CrossRef] [PubMed]
6. Stannard, J.P.; Schreiner, A.J. Vascular Injuries following Knee Dislocation. *J. Knee Surg.* **2020**, *33*, 351–356. [CrossRef]
7. Peltola, E.K.; Lindahl, J.; Hietaranta, H.; Koskinen, S.K. Knee dislocation in overweight patients. *AJR Am. J. Roentgenol.* **2009**, *192*, 101–106. [CrossRef]
8. Werner, B.C.; Gwathmey, F.W., Jr.; Higgins, S.T.; Hart, J.M.; Miller, M.D. Ultra-low velocity knee dislocations: Patient characteristics, complications, and outcomes. *Am. J. Sports Med.* **2014**, *42*, 358–363. [CrossRef]
9. Carr, J.B.; Werner, B.C.; Miller, M.D.; Gwathmey, F.W. Knee Dislocation in the Morbidly Obese Patient. *J. Knee Surg.* **2016**, *29*, 278–286. [CrossRef]
10. Georgiadis, A.G.; Mohammad, F.H.; Mizerik, K.T.; Nypaver, T.J.; Shepard, A.D. Changing presentation of knee dislocation and vascular injury from high-energy trauma to low-energy falls in the morbidly obese. *J. Vasc. Surg.* **2013**, *57*, 1196–1203. [CrossRef]
11. Engebretsen, L.; Risberg, M.A.; Robertson, B.; Ludvigsen, T.C.; Johansen, S. Outcome after knee dislocations: A 2–9 years follow-up of 85 consecutive patients. *Knee Surg. Sports Traumatol. Arthrosc.* **2009**, *17*, 1013–1026. [CrossRef] [PubMed]
12. Woodmass, J.M.; Johnson, N.R.; Mohan, R.; Krych, A.J.; Levy, B.A.; Stuart, M.J. Poly-traumatic multi-ligament knee injuries: Is the knee the limiting factor? *Knee Surg. Sports Traumatol. Arthrosc.* **2018**, *26*, 2865–2871. [CrossRef] [PubMed]
13. Weber, C.D.; Horst, K.; Nguyen, A.R.; Bader, M.J.; Probst, C.; Zelle, B.; Pape, H.C.; Dienstknecht, T. Return to Sports After Multiple Trauma: Which Factors Are Responsible?-Results From a 17-Year Follow-up. *Clin. J. Sport Med.* **2017**, *27*, 481–486. [CrossRef] [PubMed]
14. Schenck, R.C., Jr.; Richter, D.L.; Wascher, D.C. Knee Dislocations: Lessons Learned From 20-Year Follow-up. *Orthop. J. Sports Med.* **2014**, *2*, 2325967114534387. [CrossRef] [PubMed]
15. Fanelli, G.C.; Fanelli, D.G. Multiple Ligament Knee Injuries. *J. Knee Surg.* **2018**, *31*, 399–409. [CrossRef]
16. Auffarth, A.; Bogner, R.; Koller, H.; Tauber, M.; Mayer, M.; Resch, H.; Lederer, S. How severe are initially undetected injuries to the knee accompanying a femoral shaft fracture? *J. Trauma* **2009**, *66*, 1398–1401. [CrossRef]

17. Byun, S.E.; Shon, H.C.; Park, J.H.; Oh, H.K.; Cho, Y.H.; Kim, J.W.; Sim, J.A. Incidence and risk factors of knee injuries associated with ipsilateral femoral shaft fractures: A multicentre retrospective analysis of 429 femoral shaft injuries. *Injury* **2018**, *49*, 1602–1606. [CrossRef]
18. Szalay, M.J.; Hosking, O.R.; Annear, P. Injury of knee ligament associated with ipsilateral femoral shaft fractures and with ipsilateral femoral and tibial shaft fractures. *Injury* **1990**, *21*, 398–400. [CrossRef]
19. Yoon, Y.C.; Jeon, S.S.; Sim, J.A.; Kim, B.K.; Lee, B.K. Concomitant posterior cruciate ligament injuries with direct injury-related patellar fractures. *Arch. Orthop. Trauma Surg.* **2016**, *136*, 779–784. [CrossRef]
20. Kempegowda, H.; Maniar, H.H.; Tawari, A.A.; Fanelli, G.C.; Jones, C.B.; Sietsema, D.L.; Bogdan, Y.; Tornetta, P., 3rd; Marcantonio, A.J.; Horwitz, D.S. Knee Injury Associated With Acetabular Fractures: A Multicenter Study of 1273 Patients. *J. Orthop. Trauma* **2016**, *30*, 48–51. [CrossRef]
21. Hohmann, E.; Glatt, V.; Tetsworth, K. Early or delayed reconstruction in multi-ligament knee injuries: A systematic review and meta-analysis. *Knee* **2017**, *24*, 909–916. [CrossRef]
22. Ruchholtz, S.; Lefering, R.; Debus, F.; Mand, C.; Kuhne, C.; Siebert, H. TraumaregisterTraumaNetwork DGU(R) und TraumaRegister DGU(R). Success by cooperation and documentation. *Chirurg* **2013**, *84*, 730–738. [CrossRef] [PubMed]
23. DGU, T. 20 years TraumaRegister DGU((R)): Development, aims and structure. *Injury* **2014**, *45* (Suppl. 3), S6–S13. [CrossRef]
24. Greenspan, L.; McLellan, B.A.; Greig, H. Abbreviated Injury Scale and Injury Severity Score: A scoring chart. *J. Trauma* **1985**, *25*, 60–64. [CrossRef] [PubMed]
25. Garthe, E.; States, J.D.; Mango, N.K. Abbreviated injury scale unification: The case for a unified injury system for global use. *J. Trauma* **1999**, *47*, 309–323. [CrossRef] [PubMed]
26. Baker, S.P.; O'Neill, B.; Haddon, W., Jr.; Long, W.B. The injury severity score: A method for describing patients with multiple injuries and evaluating emergency care. *J. Trauma* **1974**, *14*, 187–196. [CrossRef] [PubMed]
27. Osler, T.; Baker, S.P.; Long, W. A modification of the injury severity score that both improves accuracy and simplifies scoring. *J. Trauma* **1997**, *43*, 922–925, discussion 925–926. [CrossRef]
28. McKee, L.; Ibrahim, M.S.; Lawrence, T.; Pengas, I.P.; Khan, W.S. Current concepts in acute knee dislocation: The missed diagnosis? *Open Orthop. J.* **2014**, *8*, 162–167. [CrossRef]
29. Darcy, G.; Edwards, E.; Hau, R. Epidemiology and outcomes of traumatic knee dislocations: Isolated vs multi-trauma injuries. *Injury* **2018**, *49*, 1183–1187. [CrossRef]
30. Sillanpaa, P.J.; Kannus, P.; Niemi, S.T.; Rolf, C.; Fellander-Tsai, L.; Mattila, V.M. Incidence of knee dislocation and concomitant vascular injury requiring surgery: A nationwide study. *J. Trauma Acute Care Surg.* **2014**, *76*, 715–719. [CrossRef]
31. Herbermann, J.D.; Miranda, D. Defusing the demographic "time-bomb" in Germany. *Bull. World Health Organ.* **2012**, *90*, 6–7. [CrossRef] [PubMed]
32. Statistisches Bundesamt. Altersstruktur der Bevölkerung in Deutschland zum 31 Dezember 2017. In Statista—Das Statistik-Portal. 8. February 2019. Available online: https://de.statista.com/statistik/daten/studie/1351/umfrage/altersstruktur-der-bevoelkerung-deutschlands/ (accessed on 27 April 2020).
33. Levy, N.M.; Krych, A.J.; Hevesi, M.; Reardon, P.J.; Pareek, A.; Stuart, M.J.; Levy, B.A. Does age predict outcome after multiligament knee reconstruction for the dislocated knee? 2- to 22-year follow-up. *Knee Surg. Sports Traumatol. Arthrosc.* **2015**, *23*, 3003–3007. [CrossRef] [PubMed]
34. Brautigan, B.; Johnson, D.L. The epidemiology of knee dislocations. *Clin. Sports Med.* **2000**, *19*, 387–397. [CrossRef]
35. Seroyer, S.T.; Musahl, V.; Harner, C.D. Management of the acute knee dislocation: The Pittsburgh experience. *Injury* **2008**, *39*, 710–718. [CrossRef]
36. Twaddle, B.C.; Bidwell, T.A.; Chapman, J.R. Knee dislocations: Where are the lesions? A prospective evaluation of surgical findings in 63 cases. *J. Orthop. Trauma* **2003**, *17*, 198–202. [CrossRef]
37. Krych, A.J.; Sousa, P.L.; King, A.H.; Engasser, W.M.; Stuart, M.J.; Levy, B.A. Meniscal tears and articular cartilage damage in the dislocated knee. *Knee Surg. Sports Traumatol. Arthrosc.* **2015**, *23*, 3019–3025. [CrossRef]
38. Natsuhara, K.M.; Yeranosian, M.G.; Cohen, J.R.; Wang, J.C.; McAllister, D.R.; Petrigliano, F.A. What is the frequency of vascular injury after knee dislocation? *Clin. Orthop. Relat. Res.* **2014**, *472*, 2615–2620. [CrossRef]
39. Moatshe, G.; Dornan, G.J.; Loken, S.; Ludvigsen, T.C.; LaPrade, R.F.; Engebretsen, L. Demographics and Injuries Associated With Knee Dislocation: A Prospective Review of 303 Patients. *Orthop. J. Sports Med.* **2017**, *5*, 2325967117706521. [CrossRef]

40. Boisrenoult, P.; Lustig, S.; Bonneviale, P.; Leray, E.; Versier, G.; Neyret, P.; Rosset, P.; Saragaglia, D. Vascular lesions associated with bicruciate and knee dislocation ligamentous injury. *Orthop. Traumatol. Surg. Res.* **2009**, *95*, 621–626. [CrossRef]
41. Stewart, R.J.; Landy, D.C.; Khazai, R.S.; Cohen, J.B.; Ho, S.S.; Dirschl, D.R. Association of Injury Energy Level and Neurovascular Injury Following Knee Dislocation. *J. Orthop. Trauma* **2018**, *32*, 579–584. [CrossRef]
42. Weinberg, D.S.; Scarcella, N.R.; Napora, J.K.; Vallier, H.A. Can Vascular Injury be Appropriately Assessed With Physical Examination After Knee Dislocation? *Clin. Orthop. Relat. Res.* **2016**, *474*, 1453–1458. [CrossRef] [PubMed]
43. Parker, S.; Handa, A.; Deakin, M.; Sideso, E. Knee dislocation and vascular injury: 4 year experience at a UK Major Trauma Centre and vascular hub. *Injury* **2016**, *47*, 752–756. [CrossRef] [PubMed]

Journal of
Clinical Medicine

MDPI

Article

Clinical Utility of Extracorporeal Shock Wave Therapy on Hypertrophic Scars of the Hand Caused by Burn Injury: A Prospective, Randomized, Double-Blinded Study

So Young Joo [1,†], Seung Yeol Lee [2,†], Yoon Soo Cho [1] and Cheong Hoon Seo [1,*]

1 Department of Rehabilitation Medicine, Hangang Sacred Heart Hospital, College of Medicine Hallym University, Seoul 07247, Korea; anyany98@naver.com (S.Y.J.); hamays@hanmail.net (Y.S.C.)
2 Department of Physical Medicine and Rehabilitation, College of Medicine, Soonchunhyang University Hospital, Bucheon 14584, Korea; shouletz@gmail.com
* Correspondence: chseomd@gmail.com; Tel.: +82-2-2639-5738; Fax: +82-2-2635-7820
† These authors contributed equally to this work.

Received: 8 April 2020; Accepted: 5 May 2020; Published: 7 May 2020

Abstract: Postburn hypertrophic scarring is a common complication in burn injuries to the hands, often associated with impaired hand function. We evaluated the effects of extracorporeal shock wave therapy (ESWT), compared to a sham stimulation therapy, on hypertrophic scars of the hand caused by burn injury and investigated its effects on hand function. This was a double-blinded, randomized, controlled trial of 48 patients with a burn to their dominant right hand. The parameters of ESWT were as follows: energy flux density, 0.05–0.30 mJ/mm^2; frequency, 4 Hz; 1000 to 2000 impulses per treatment; four treatments, once a week for four weeks. The outcomes measured were as follows: a 10-point visual analogue scale pain score; Vancouver scar scale for scar vascularity, height, pliability and pigmentation; ultrasound measurement of scar thickness; Jebsen–Taylor hand function test; grip strength; Perdue pegboard test; and the Michigan hand outcomes questionnaire. The change in the score from baseline to post-treatment was compared between the two groups. ESWT improved the pain score (p = 0.001), scar thickness (p = 0.018), scar vascularity (p = 0.0015), and improved hand function (simulated card-turning, p = 0.02; picking up small objects, p = 0.004). The other measured outcomes were not different between the two groups. ESWT is effective in decreasing pain, suppressing hypertrophic scarring, and improving hand function.

Keywords: extracorporeal shock wave therapy; hypertrophic scar; burn; hand function

1. Introduction

Hypertrophic scarring is a common complication after a burn. Hypertrophic scars result from excessive tissue formation during the wound healing process [1]. The mechanisms underlying hypertrophic scar formation include exaggerated inflammation, prolonged re-epithelialization, excessive extracellular matrix production, and reduced apoptosis [2]. Both types of hypertrophic scars, those which are raised and inflexible [3] and those which are characterized by traction on surrounding tissues, can result in functional limitations [4]. Common complications after burn injuries to the hands include decreased hand performance, sensory impairment, and scar contracture [5]. Hand complications such as these may impair performance of the activities of daily life. Nonsurgical treatments of postburn hypertrophic scars include intralesional corticosteroid injection, laser therapy, compression therapy, and silicone therapy. The outcomes of these nonsurgical treatments of hypertrophic scars on the hands, however, have not yielded satisfactory outcomes. Recently, there has been increased focus on shortening the healing time and improving hand function to reduce the risk of hypertrophic scarring.

Extracorporeal shock wave therapy (ESWT) is effective in the treatment of orthopedic diseases and neuropathic pain and has also been used in regenerative medicine of the skin [6], with neoangiogenesis and anti-inflammatory effects having been reported [7]. The regeneration effects of ESWT have been demonstrated in improving the healing of burn wounds [8,9] as well as in decreasing hypertrophic scarring after a burn [10]. ESWT may also improve the pliability and the subjectively evaluated appearance of postburn scar contracture [11]. Studies in our own institution found ESWT to be useful for burn-associated pain and pruritus and demonstrated that ESWT can suppress the hypertrophic scarring. The anti-fibrotic effects of ESWT can likely be attributed to its molecular effect on hypertrophic scars [1,12,13]. However, the effects of ESWT on hypertrophic scarring of the hand and on hand function have not been evaluated to date. Therefore, this research aimed to evaluate the effectiveness of ESWT on hypertrophic scars and on the hand functions affected by such scarring.

2. Experimental Section

2.1. Methods

Study Design and Statement of Ethics

This was a double-blinded, randomized, controlled trial of 48 patients (45 male, 3 female) recruited from the Department of Rehabilitation Medicine, Hangang Sacred Heart Hospital, Korea, between November 2019 and April 2020. Our study was approved by the Ethics Committee of the Hangang Sacred Heart Hospital (HG2018-047) and registered in ClinicalTrials (NCT04138355). All patients provided written informed consent.

2.2. Study Group

Each of the 48 patients enrolled in the study were ≥18 years old and had sustained a deep partial-thickness (second-degree) burn or a full thickness (third-degree) burn involving only the right hand, which had been treated with a split-thickness skin graft (STSG) after the thermal injury, <6 months prior to enrollment. At the time of the study, all the patients were in the re-epithelialization phase of wound healing and had been transferred to the rehabilitation department, after acute burn treatment, to improve hand and wrist stiffness due to painful retracting scarring. The criteria for exclusion from the study were as follows: left-hand dominance; musculoskeletal diseases (fracture, amputation, rheumatoid arthritis, and degenerative joint diseases) of the right dominant hand; pregnancy; or potential for additional damage to the skin if exposed to ESWT and conventional occupational therapy.

The first 50 burn patients who met our inclusion/exclusion criteria were randomly allocated, using a computer program, to either the ESWT (n = 25) group or to the sham (n = 25) group. While all participants in the sham group completed the trial protocol, two patients in the ESWT group dropped out of the study because they did not want to undergo serial evaluations. Thus, 23 patients were ultimately included in the ESWT group, and 25 were included in the sham group (Figure 1).

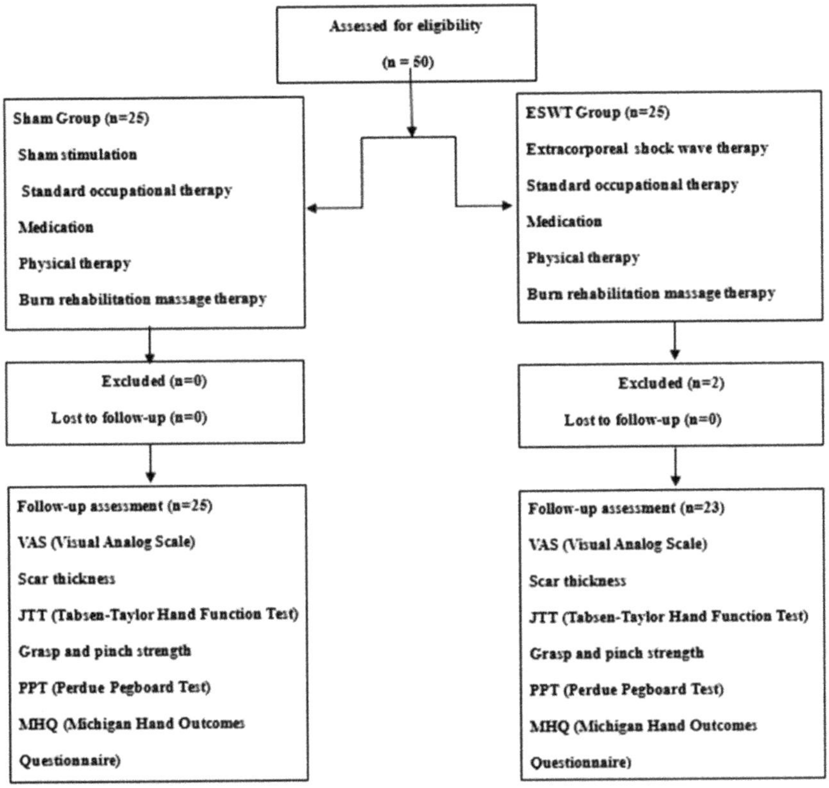

Figure 1. Diagram for subject enrollment, allocation, and follow-up.

2.3. Intervention

Patients in both groups received standard rehabilitation treatment for burn injuries to the hands, including medication, scar lubrication, massage therapy to the scars, and occupational therapy to improve hand function. Occupational therapy treatment consisted of 20 sessions (30 min per day, five days a week) for four weeks. Every effort was made to provide the same exercise rehabilitation for both groups and to adapt the level of difficulty of the exercises prescribed to each patient's performance. Patients received one ESWT or sham treatment session per week for four weeks.

Patients in the ESWT group were asked to select the most hypertrophic and retracting scar on their dominant right hand for treatment. ESWT was conducted using the Duolith SD-1 device (StorzMedical, Tägerwilen, Switzerland), with an electromagnetic cylindrical coil source used to focus the shock wave (Figure 2). ESWT was performed around the primary treatment site, at an intensity of 100 impulses/cm^2, an energy flux density (EFD) of 0.05 to 0.30 mJ/mm^2, and a frequency of 4 Hz. Between 1000 to 2000 impulses were administered per session, for four sessions held at one week intervals. In the sham group, the same shock wave equipment, with the same-shaped adapter, as in the experimental group was used, but with no energy emitted (Figure 3).

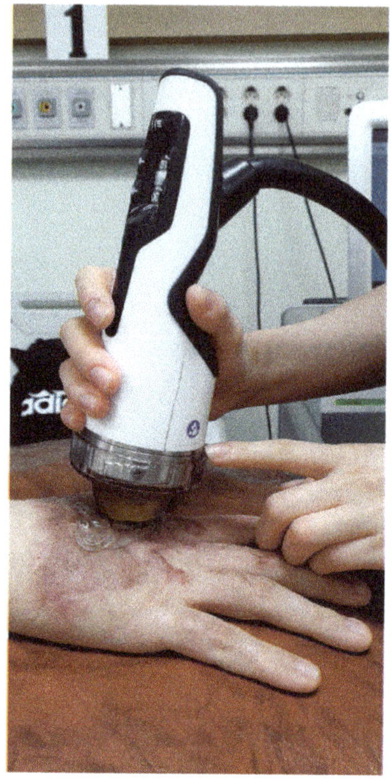

Figure 2. The extracorporeal shock wave therapy was administered to burn patients. The administered shock wave dose was 100 impulses/cm^2 at 0.05 to 0.30 mJ/mm^2 with a total of 1000 to 2000 impulses per treatment.

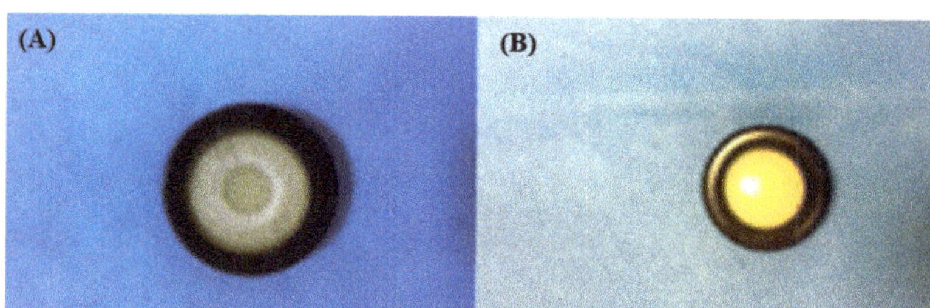

Figure 3. Sham adapter: (**A**) inside view; (**B**) outside view.

2.4. Outcome Measures

In order to evaluate the effect of ESWT, we compared the change in the severity of pain, scar thickness, and hand function between the ESWT and sham groups, from baseline measures taken immediately before the intervention and measures taken immediately after session 4. The 10-point visual analogue scale (VAS) was used to measure self-reported pain severity, with ratings from 0 (no pain) to 10 (unbearable pain). The Vancouver scar scale (VSS), an observer-dependent scale of the macroscopic appearance of scarring, was used to measure changes in the scar over the four week period of treatment [14]. The VSS consists of four parameters (vascularity, height, pliability, and pigmentation), scored in total on a 14-point scale, with a higher score indicative of a better outcome. The thickness of the scar was objectively quantified by ultrasound (128 BW1 US system, Medison, Korea). Grip and pinch strength were quantified using a hand-held dynamometer (Lafayette Instrument, USA). The Michigan hand outcomes questionnaire (MHQ) was used to assess a patient's perception of hand function on a scale of 0–100, with a higher score indicative of a better outcome [15]. The Jebsen–Taylor hand function test (JTT) was used to measure the performance speed of standardized tasks. The JTT consists of seven subtests, each scored on a scale of 0–15, with a higher score indicative of better hand function [16]. In the Perdue pegboard test (PPT), motor function is measured by the number of pins that can be placed in the board (along two parallel rows with 25 holes each) in 30 s, and dexterity is measured by the number of pins, washers, and collars that can be assembled in 60 s. Scores were evaluated for the affected right (dominant) hand and both hands [17]. Outcome measurements and data analyses were performed by a trained and blinded outcome assessor who was not involved in the intervention. Possible complications (pain, ecchymosis, skin abrasion, and swelling) were observed.

2.5. Statistical Analysis

Statistical analyses were performed using SPSS, version 23 (IBM Corp., Armonk, NY, USA). Fisher's exact test was used to evaluate the homogeneity of the distribution of sex and burn types between the two groups before treatment, and the independent t-test was used to evaluate the homogeneity of distribution of the total burn surface area (TBSA), scar thickness, total VSS, dominant-hand and bilateral PPT scores, and the score for picking up small objects subtest of the JTT. A between-group p-value < 0.05 was deemed significant. The pre- to post-treatment scores were evaluated between the two groups using the Mann–Whitney or independent t-test, as appropriate for the variable type and distribution, with a p-value < 0.05 deemed significant.

3. Results

There were no differences between the two groups in terms of demographic and clinical characteristic before treatment ($p > 0.05$ for all comparisons; Table 1). There were no differences in the measured outcomes before treatment between the two groups ($p > 0.05$ for all comparisons; Table 2).

Table 1. Baseline characteristics of the study group.

	ESWT Group (n = 23)	Sham Group (n = 25)	p-Value
Male:Female	22:1	23:2	0.53
Age (years)	47.09 ± 11.09	48.56 ± 11.18	0.94
Cause of burn			0.43
Flame burn	15	18	
Electrical burn	1	3	
Contact burn	0	1	
Scalding burn	3	1	
Spark burn	4	2	
Time to treatment (days)	64.04 ± 36.62	63.48 ± 14.43	0.12
TBSA (%)	28.39 ± 17.86	27.80 ± 19.46	0.91

ESWT, Extracorporeal shock wave therapy; TBSA, total burn surface area. Values are presented as mean ± standard deviation. The p-values were calculated using Fisher's exact test, the Mann–Whitney test, or Student's t-test as appropriate.

Table 2. Outcome measures at baseline.

	ESWT Group (n = 23)	Sham Group (n = 25)	*p*-Value
VAS	7.00 ± 1.24	6.96 ± 1.21	0.84
Thickness (cm)	0.21 ± 0.11	0.19 ± 0.06	0.36
	Vancouver Scar Scale		
Pigmentation	3.00 ± 0.00	2.92 ± 0.28	0.17
Pliability	1.87 ± 0.76	2.20 ± 0.76	0.14
Height	1.43 ± 0.51	1.56 ± 0.58	0.33
Vascularity	2.17 ± 0.72	2.32 ± 0.75	0.45
Total	8.48 ± 1.70	9.00 ± 1.85	0.32
	Grasp and Pinch Power Test		
Grasp (kg)	7.50 ± 7.40	5.81 ± 7.72	0.38
Lateral Pinch (kg)	3.21 ± 1.67	3.58 ± 5.21	0.43
Tip Pinch (kg)	1.40 ± 0.91	1.32 ± 1.33	0.56
	Jebsen–Taylor Hand Function Test		
Writing	11.04 ± 4.80	10.64 ± 3.49	0.10
Cards	3.57 ± 2.78	3.04 ± 2.42	0.53
Small	5.57 ± 3.86	5.04 ± 4.23	0.66
Checkers	9.26 ± 4.11	8.00 ± 5.38	0.72
Feeding	10.09 ± 4.07	8.88 ± 5.23	0.73
Light	8.78 ± 4.52	9.68 ± 3.69	0.60
Heavy	8.52 ± 4.33	8.08 ± 4.47	0.76
	Perdue Pegboard Test		
Affected hand	7.78 ± 5.51	8.52 ± 3.37	0.58
Both hands	5.78 ± 4.49	6.36 ± 2.61	0.59
Assembly	12.13 ± 12.33	14.00 ± 8.45	0.26
	Michigan Hand Outcomes Questionnaire		
Function	21.09 ± 12.96	23.80 ± 10.54	0.30
ADL	21.52 ± 12.38	23.20 ± 12.74	0.49
Work	15.57 ± 14.24	15.20 ± 18.06	0.63
Pain	34.35 ± 28.13	24.92 ± 21.27	0.22
Esthetics	12.36 ± 16.36	10.08 ± 13.78	0.74
Satisfaction	24.96 ± 12.35	25.08 ± 14.10	0.75

VAS, visual analogue scale; ESWT, extracorporeal shock wave therapy. Values are presented as the mean ± standard deviation. The *p*-values were calculated using Fisher's exact test, the Mann–Whitney test, or Student's t-test as appropriate.

More reductions were found in the ESWT group than in the sham group for the pre- to post-treatment change in the VAS score ($p = 0.001$) and vascularity VSS score ($p = 0.0015$) (Table 3). There was a slight decrease in the pre- to post-treatment change of scar thickness ($p = 0.018$) for the ESWT group over the sham group (Table 3). However, there were no significant differences in the change score between the two groups for scar pigmentation ($p = 0.19$), pliability ($p = 0.78$), height ($p = 0.66$), and the total VSS score ($p = 0.19$; Table 3). Similarly, grip strength improved in both groups, without a difference in the change scores between the two groups (grasp, $p = 0.99$; lateral pinch, $p = 0.46$; and tip pinch, $p = 0.26$; Table 3). For the JTT, the change scores were significantly greater for the ESWT than the sham group for the subtasks of simulated card-turning ($p = 0.02$) and picking up small objects ($p = 0.004$), with no between-group differences in the change score for the remaining subtasks (writing, $p = 0.12$; stacking checkers, $p = 0.15$; simulated feeding, $p = 0.99$; picking up large light objects, $p = 0.16$; and picking up large heavy objects, $p = 0.90$; Table 3). For the PPT, there were no significant differences in the change scores for the affected hand ($p = 0.12$), both hands ($p = 0.97$), and assembly ($p = 0.44$; Table 3). Furthermore, there were no between-group differences in any of the subscores of the MHQ (Table 3): function ($p = 0.17$); activities of daily living, ADL ($p = 0.51$); work ($p = 0.12$); pain ($p = 0.45$); esthetics ($p = 0.06$); and satisfaction ($p = 0.15$).

Table 3. Change score (pre- to post-treatment) on measured outcomes.

	ESWT Group (n = 23)	Sham Group (n = 25)	p-Value
VAS	−1.48 ± 1.04	−0.52 ± 0.77	0.001 **
Scar thickness (cm)	0.01 ± 0.07	0.07 ± 0.07	0.018 **
	Vancouver Scar Scale		
Pigmentation	−0.04 ± 0.21	−0.16 ± 0.37	0.19
Pliability	0.13 ± 0.81	0.08 ± 1.08	0.78
Height	0.09 ± 0.60	0.44 ± 0.58	0.06
Vascularity	−0.52 ± 0.73	−0.04 ± 0.61	0.015 **
Total	−0.35 ± 1.61	0.32 ± 1.75	0.19
	Grasp and Pinch Power Test		
Grasp (kg)	4.71 ± 4.90	4.71 ± 3.77	0.99
Lateral Pinch (kg)	1.10 ± 1.69	0.74 ± 1.61	0.46
Tip Pinch (kg)	0.80 ± 1.13	0.48 ± 0.78	0.26
	Jebsen−Taylor Hand Function Test		
Writing	1.57 ± 4.11	0.88 ± 3.43	0.12
Cards	2.48 ± 3.54	0.40 ± 2.22	0.02 *
Small	3.70 ± 4.30	0.16 ± 2.87	0.004 **
Checkers	1.30 ± 4.48	3.32 ± 4.40	0.15
Feeding	1.70 ± 3.97	1.48 ± 2.38	0.99
Light	1.78 ± 4.77	0.04 ± 2.17	0.16
Heavy	1.39 ± 5.06	0.60 ± 1.68	0.90
	Perdue Pegboard Test		
Affected hand	2.26 ± 3.51	0.00 ± 3.65	0.12
Both hands	1.61 ± 2.97	1.44 ± 4.23	0.97
Assembly	4.04 ± 10.55	1.72 ± 10.15	0.44
	Michigan Hand Outcomes Questionnaire		
Function	13.78 ± 18.12	8.60 ± 15.65	0.17
ADL	11.74 ± 20.43	12.20 ± 20.77	0.51
Work	19.22 ± 19.47	13.72 ± 22.91	0.12
Pain	−9.39 ± 24.78	−6.48 ± 18.45	0.45
Esthetics	10.55 ± 16.46	9.60 ± 21.33	0.15
Satisfaction	22.86 ± 21.59	10.30 ± 19.37	0.06

VAS, visual analogue scale; ESWT, extracorporeal shock wave therapy. Values are presented as the mean ± standard deviation. The p-values for between-group differences were calculated using the Mann–Whitney test (**, $p < 0.05$) and independent t-test (*, $p < 0.05$), as appropriate.

4. Discussion

We evaluated the effectiveness of ESWT on the hypertrophic scars of hand burns that required STSG. Therapeutic effects were evaluated by the change in scar pain, thickness, esthetic characteristics, and hand function after a four week period of treatment. The ESWT treatment of hypertrophic scarring after a burn injury to the hands provided significant benefits in improving hand function, decreasing pain, and suppressing hypertrophic scar growth.

Cho et al. [12] have reported on the effects of ESWT applied to the area of most severe pain after complete epithelialization on pain outcomes (ESWT dose: EFD, 0.05 to 0.15 mJ/mm^2; frequency, 4 Hz; and three sessions at one week intervals). The authors proposed that measured improvement in pain control with ESWT had resulted from a decrease in the number of unmyelinated nerve fibers; inhibition of nociceptors from repeated stimulation; regulation of neuroinflammatory molecules, such as substance P; and increased blood flow, facilitating tissue regeneration via an increase in endothelial nitric oxide synthase (eNOS). Joo et el. applied ESWT to burn scars with severe pruritus, using the same protocol as described by Cho et al., and found ESWT to be effective in reducing the severity of pruritus and improving ADLs [13]. Epithelial–mesenchymal transition (EMT), in which epithelial cells lose the inclination to reproduce, is known to have a role in fibrogenesis during hypertrophic scarring [18]. Seo et el. [1] identified that ESWT (EFD of 0.03, 0.1, and 0.3 mJ/mm^2; a frequency of 4 Hz; and a volume of 1000 pulses) suppressed EMT by inhibiting the EMT inducer [1].

In our study, we used an intensity and frequency of ESWT previously shown to have a therapeutic effect for burns. Previous research has shown the effectiveness of low dose ESWT (0.1 mJ/mm^2) in suppressing hypertrophic scar formation through inhibition of α-SMA expression [19,20]. Meirer et al. reported that ESWT, applied to partial-thickness burns, three and seven days after the burn injury (1500 impulses at 0.11 mJ/mm^2), reduced the need for surgery and decreased scar formation during the six month follow-up period [21].

In our study, we also identified a significant benefit of ESWT in improving vascularization of the scar tissue, measured using the VSS. Previous research has investigated the mechanisms underlying the mechanosensitive feedback between ESWT and stimulated cells [22]. Nitric oxide (NO) production contributes to an increase in perfusion, with the improved blood supply preventing ischemia [22,23]. The accelerated epithelialization after ESWT can be explained by multiple factors, including neovascularization, increased granulation, and increased epithelial cell proliferation in the burn wound [8,9,24]. High-energy ESWT (0.3 mJ/mm^2, frequency 4 Hz) increased the perfusion at remote sites via an increase of the NO and of vascular endothelial growth factor (VEGF) [25]. Davis et al. also demonstrated that the application of ESWT at 1 h postinjury significantly blunted the activity of inflammatory cells [26], although in clinical practice, hyperemia may occur at the site of ESWT due to an increase in local blood flow [6,13]. Overall, decreasing the healing time would be an important factor in reducing the risk of undesirable scarring and decreasing pain.

ESWT is known to be effective for reducing pain and improving function on orthopedic injuries [27]. Substance P may play a role in pain mediation in small unmyelinated C fibers. An intradermal injection of substance P causes a flare-up in pain, swelling, and pruritus. On the other hand, calcitonin gene-related peptide (CGRP) is a well-known marker of unmyelinated C fibers and thinly myelinated Aδ fibers, both of which are important in nociception. The loss of nerve fibers and the depletion of neuropeptides with ESWT might be effective in decreasing pain. A low dose of ESWT (0.08 mJ/mm^2, frequency 4 Hz) applied to a knee as a treatment for osteoarthritis reduced neuropeptide expression, which was associated with improved pain and gait function [28]. More substance P and CGRP are observed in painful hypertrophic scars compared to normal skin [29]. This evidence reinforces the idea that the pain-control effect of ESWT is likely to be mediated by its effect on pain mediators, and substance P and CGRP more specifically. The clinical benefits of ESWT have been reported for a range of orthopedic disorders and associated with self-reported improvements in function and quality of life [30–32].

ESWT has been widely used in treatment of various tendinopathies in upper limbs. Steroids limit tenocyte function by reducing proteoglycan and collagen synthesis, which reduce mechanical strength. Unlike steroid therapy, ESWT studies have shown that ESWT affects tenocyte regeneration, leading to an improvement in muscle strength. The effectiveness of ESWT compared with that of local steroid injections showed that ESWT had favorable effects on resolution of pain and improvement of grip strength [33,34]. In our study, we identified improvements in grip strength with ESWT, as well as improvement in simulated card-turning and the picking up of small objects. This improved function might be related to improvements in the pliability of the scar because of ESWT breaking down collagen fibers to induce scar remodeling. The increased pliability of the scars with ESWT, with a less evident effect on coloration, has already been reported [11]. A previous study [4] has also indicated that unfocused application of shock waves (EFD, 0.13 mJ/mm^2; frequency, 6 Hz; two sessions per week for five weeks) was effective in significantly improving VSS scores, scarring pain, and the range of movement of the hand. These clinical benefits of ESWT were thought to be mediated by stimulation of dermal fibroblasts, neoangiogenesis, and improvement in the parallel organization of collagen fibers within the skin. Similarly, a beneficial effect of ESWT has been reported for the treatment of trigger finger complaints, resulting from enhanced repair and healing of the degenerated tendon [34]. Overall, as pain, pruritus, and decreased function negatively impact the quality of life after a burn, ESWT may have a global effect in improving quality of life after burn injuries [35].

This study requires cautious interpretation of the data, for reasons of small sample size, a short follow-up period, and the absence of detailed measurement of range of motion in the affected hand. Future studies with a longer time frame and more detailed assessment are needed to confirm our findings. Continued basic research into the mechanisms underlying the clinical effects of ESWT are needed to determine optimal parameters for the clinical management of hypertrophic scars.

5. Conclusions

In making the comparison of ESWT with a sham stimulation therapy for the treatment of hypertrophic scarring of the hand after a burn injury, we identified a clinically beneficial effect of ESWT in promoting hand function, improving scarring, and alleviating scar-related pain. This indicates the clinical usefulness of the intensity and frequency parameters of ESWT that we used in our study. It is important to point out that the optimal frequency and intensity of ESWT for the treatment of hypertrophic scars of the hands after a burn remain to be determined. Our findings, however, do provide experimenters with the option to use ESWT for its potential to improve the management and treatment of hand burn scars after STSG.

Author Contributions: C.H.S. contributed as corresponding author of this work. S.Y.J. and S.Y.L. contributed equally to the conception, design, data analysis, and interpretation of results. Y.S.C. contributed to revising the article critically for important intellectual content. All authors contributed to the writing of the manuscript. All authors have read and agreed to the published version of the manuscript.

Funding: This research was supported by the National Research Foundation of Korea (NRF) grant funded by the Korean government (MSIT) (NRF-2018R1C1B6008584) and the Soonchunhyang University Research Fund.

Conflicts of Interest: The authors declare no potential conflict of interest.

References

1. Cui, H.S.; Hong, A.R.; Kim, J.B.; Yu, J.H.; Cho, Y.S.; Joo, S.Y.; Seo, C.H. Extracorporeal Shock Wave Therapy Alters the Expression of Fibrosis-Related Molecules in Fibroblast Derived from Human Hypertrophic Scar. *Int. J. Mol. Sci.* **2018**, *19*, 124. [CrossRef]
2. Arno, A.; Garcia, O.; Hernan, I.; Sancho, J.; Acosta, A.; Barret, J.P. Extracorporeal shock waves, a new non-surgical method to treat severe burns. *Burns J. Int. Soc.* **2010**, *36*, 844–849. [CrossRef]
3. Van der Veer, W.M.; Bloemen, M.C.; Ulrich, M.M.; Molema, G.; van Zuijlen, P.P.; Middelkoop, E.; Niessen, F.B. Potential cellular and molecular causes of hypertrophic scar formation. *Burns J. Int. Soc.* **2009**, *35*, 15–29. [CrossRef] [PubMed]
4. Saggini, R.; Saggini, A.; Spagnoli, A.M.; Dodaj, I.; Cigna, E.; Maruccia, M.; Soda, G.; Bellomo, R.G.; Scuderi, N. Extracorporeal Shock Wave Therapy: An Emerging Treatment Modality for Retracting Scars of the Hands. *Ultrasound Med. Biol.* **2016**, *42*, 185–195. [CrossRef] [PubMed]
5. Nuchtern, J.G.; Engrav, L.H.; Nakamura, D.Y.; Dutcher, K.A.; Heimbach, D.M.; Vedder, N.B. Treatment of fourth-degree hand burns. *J. Burn Care Rehabil.* **1995**, *16*, 36–42. [CrossRef] [PubMed]
6. De Lima Morais, T.M.; Meyer, P.F.; de Vasconcellos, L.S.; e Silva, J.C.; e Andrade, I.F.; de Farias, V.A.F.; da Silva, I.C.; Araújo, R.M.F.G.; da Silva, R.M.V.; Pacheco, E.F.; et al. Effects of the extracorporeal shock wave therapy on the skin: An experimental study. *Lasers Med. Sci.* **2019**, *34*, 389–396. [CrossRef]
7. Kuo, Y.R.; Wu, W.S.; Hsieh, Y.L.; Wang, F.S.; Wang, C.T.; Chiang, Y.C.; Wang, C.J. Extracorporeal shock wave enhanced extended skin flap tissue survival via increase of topical blood perfusion and associated with suppression of tissue pro-inflammation. *J. Surg. Res.* **2007**, *143*, 385–392. [CrossRef]
8. Djedovic, G.; Kamelger, F.S.; Jeschke, J.; Piza-Katzer, H. Effect of extracorporeal shock wave treatment on deep partial-thickness burn injury in rats: A pilot study. *Plast. Surg. Int.* **2014**, *2014*, 495967. [CrossRef]
9. Haupt, G.; Chvapil, M. Effect of shock waves on the healing of partial-thickness wounds in piglets. *J. Surg. Res.* **1990**, *49*, 45–48. [CrossRef]
10. Aguilera-Saez, J.; Munoz, P.; Serracanta, J.; Monte, A.; Barret, J.P. Extracorporeal shock wave therapy role in the treatment of burn patients. A systematic literature review. *Burns J. Int. Soc.* **2019**. [CrossRef]
11. Fioramonti, P.; Cigna, E.; Onesti, M.G.; Fino, P.; Fallico, N.; Scuderi, N. Extracorporeal shock wave therapy for the management of burn scars. *Dermatol. Surg.* **2012**, *38*, 778–782. [CrossRef] [PubMed]

12. Cho, Y.S.; Joo, S.Y.; Cui, H.; Cho, S.R.; Yim, H.; Seo, C.H. Effect of extracorporeal shock wave therapy on scar pain in burn patients: A prospective, randomized, single-blind, placebo-controlled study. *Medicine* **2016**, *95*, e4575. [CrossRef] [PubMed]
13. Joo, S.Y.; Cho, Y.S.; Seo, C.H. The clinical utility of extracorporeal shock wave therapy for burn pruritus: A prospective, randomized, single-blind study. *Burns J. Int. Soc.* **2018**, *44*, 612–619. [CrossRef] [PubMed]
14. Fang, Z.; Yang, X.; Wu, G.; Liu, M.; Han, J.; Tao, K.; Hu, D. The use of autologous platelet-rich plasma gel increases wound healing and reduces scar development in split-thickness skin graft donor sites. *J. Plast. Surg. Hand Surg.* **2019**, *53*, 356–360. [CrossRef]
15. Cowan, A.C.; Stegink-Jansen, C.W. Rehabilitation of hand burn injuries: Current updates. *Injury* **2013**, *44*, 391–396. [CrossRef]
16. Joo, S.Y.; Cho, Y.S.; Lee, S.Y.; Seok, H.; Seo, C.H. Effects of Virtual Reality-Based Rehabilitation on Burned Hands: A Prospective, Randomized, Single-Blind Study. *J. Clin. Med.* **2020**, *9*, 731. [CrossRef]
17. Schoneveld, K.; Wittink, H.; Takken, T. Clinimetric evaluation of measurement tools used in hand therapy to assess activity and participation. *J. Hand* **2009**, *22*, 221–235. [CrossRef]
18. Kalluri, R.; Neilson, E.G. Epithelial-mesenchymal transition and its implications for fibrosis. *J. Clin. Investig.* **2003**, *112*, 1776–1784. [CrossRef]
19. Zhao, J.C.; Zhang, B.R.; Hong, L.; Shi, K.; Wu, W.W.; Yu, J.A. Extracorporeal shock wave therapy with low-energy flux density inhibits hypertrophic scar formation in an animal model. *Int. J. Mol. Med.* **2018**, *41*, 1931–1938. [CrossRef]
20. Zhao, J.C.; Zhang, B.R.; Shi, K.; Wang, J.; Yu, Q.H.; Yu, J.A. Lower energy radial shock wave therapy improves characteristics of hypertrophic scar in a rabbit ear model. *Exp. Ther. Med.* **2018**, *15*, 933–939. [CrossRef]
21. Meirer, R.; Kamelger, F.S.; Piza-Katzer, H. Shock wave therapy: An innovative treatment method for partial thickness burns. *Burns J. Int. Soc.* **2005**, *31*, 921–922. [CrossRef] [PubMed]
22. Ottomann, C.; Hartmann, B.; Tyler, J.; Maier, H.; Thiele, R.; Schaden, W.; Stojadinovic, A. Prospective randomized trial of accelerated re-epithelization of skin graft donor sites using extracorporeal shock wave therapy. *J. Am. Coll. Surg.* **2010**, *211*, 361–367. [CrossRef] [PubMed]
23. Ottomann, C.; Stojadinovic, A.; Lavin, P.T.; Gannon, F.H.; Heggeness, M.H.; Thiele, R.; Schaden, W.; Hartmann, B. Prospective randomized phase II Trial of accelerated reepithelialization of superficial second-degree burn wounds using extracorporeal shock wave therapy. *Ann. Surg.* **2012**, *255*, 23–29. [CrossRef] [PubMed]
24. Meirer, R.; Kamelger, F.S.; Huemer, G.M.; Wanner, S.; Piza-Katzer, H. Extracorporal shock wave may enhance skin flap survival in an animal model. *Br. J. Plast. Surg.* **2005**, *58*, 53–57. [CrossRef] [PubMed]
25. Kisch, T.; Sorg, H.; Forstmeier, V.; Knobloch, K.; Liodaki, E.; Stang, F.; Mailänder, P.; Krämer, R. Remote effects of extracorporeal shock wave therapy on cutaneous microcirculation. *J. Tissue Viability* **2015**, *24*, 140–145. [CrossRef] [PubMed]
26. Davis, T.A.; Stojadinovic, A.; Anam, K.; Amare, M.; Naik, S.; Peoples, G.E.; Tadaki, D.; Elster, E.A. Extracorporeal shock wave therapy suppresses the early proinflammatory immune response to a severe cutaneous burn injury. *Int. Wound J.* **2009**, *6*, 11–21. [CrossRef]
27. Pinitkwamdee, S.; Laohajaroensombat, S.; Orapin, J.; Woratanarat, P. Effectiveness of Extracorporeal Shockwave Therapy in the Treatment of Chronic Insertional Achilles Tendinopathy. *Foot Ankle Int.* **2020**. [CrossRef]
28. Ochiai, N.; Ohtori, S.; Sasho, T.; Nakagawa, K.; Takahashi, K.; Takahashi, N.; Murata, R.; Moriya, H.; Wada, Y.; Saisu, T. Extracorporeal shock wave therapy improves motor dysfunction and pain originating from knee osteoarthritis in rats. *Osteoarthr. Cartil.* **2007**, *15*, 1093–1096. [CrossRef]
29. Henderson, J.; Terenghi, G.; McGrouther, D.A.; Ferguson, M.W. The reinnervation pattern of wounds and scars may explain their sensory symptoms. *J. Plast. Reconstr. Aesthetic Surg.* **2006**, *59*, 942–950. [CrossRef]
30. Dedes, V.; Stergioulas, A.; Kipreos, G.; Dede, A.M.; Mitseas, A.; Panoutsopoulos, G.I. Effectiveness and Safety of Shockwave Therapy in Tendinopathies. *Mater. Sociomed.* **2018**, *30*, 131–146. [CrossRef]
31. Dedes, V.; Tzirogiannis, K.; Polikandrioti, M.; Dede, A.M.; Mitseas, A.; Panoutsopoulos, G.I. Comparison of radial extracorporeal shockwave therapy with ultrasound therapy in patients with lateral epicondylitis. *J. Med. Ultrason.* **2020**, *47*, 319–325. [CrossRef] [PubMed]
32. Padua, R.; Bondi, R.; Ceccarelli, E.; Ripanti, S.; Bondi, L.; Campi, A. Extracorporeal shock wave therapy for chronic calcifying tendinitis of the shoulder. *J. Orthop. Traumatol.* **2002**, *2*, 147–150. [CrossRef]

33. Seok, H.; Kim, S.H. The effectiveness of extracorporeal shock wave therapy vs. local steroid injection for management of carpal tunnel syndrome: A randomized controlled trial. *Am. J. Phys. Med. Rehabil.* **2013**, *92*, 327–334. [CrossRef] [PubMed]
34. Zyluk, A.; Mosiejczuk, H. Outcomes of the treatment of trigger digits by extracorporal shock wave therapy (ESWT). *Handchir. Mikrochir. Plast. Chir.* **2020**, *52*, 25–28. [CrossRef] [PubMed]
35. Samhan, A.F.; Abdelhalim, N.M. Impacts of low-energy extracorporeal shockwave therapy on pain, pruritus, and health-related quality of life in patients with burn: A randomized placebo-controlled study. *Burns J. Int. Soc. Burn Inj.* **2019**, *45*, 1094–1101. [CrossRef] [PubMed]

Journal of
Clinical Medicine

MDPI

Article

Post-Traumatic Sepsis Is Associated with Increased C5a and Decreased TAFI Levels

Jan Tilmann Vollrath [1], Ingo Marzi [1], Anna Herminghaus [2], Thomas Lustenberger [1] and Borna Relja [1,3,*]

1 Department of Trauma, Hand and Reconstructive Surgery, Goethe University, 60590 Frankfurt, Germany; Tilmann.Vollrath@kgu.de (J.T.V.); Ingo.Marzi@kgu.de (I.M.); Thomas.Lustenberger@kgu.de (T.L.)
2 Department of Anesthesiology, Duesseldorf University Hospital, 40225 Duesseldorf, Germany; Anna.Herminghaus@med.uni-duesseldorf.de
3 Experimental Radiology, Department of Radiology and Nuclear Medicine, Otto von Guericke University, 39120 Magdeburg, Germany
* Correspondence: Borna.Relja@med.ovgu.de; Tel.: +49-391-67-282-42

Received: 8 March 2020; Accepted: 20 April 2020; Published: 24 April 2020

Abstract: Background: Sepsis frequently occurs after major trauma and is closely associated with dysregulations in the inflammatory/complement and coagulation system. Thrombin-activatable fibrinolysis inhibitor (TAFI) plays a dual role as an anti-fibrinolytic and anti-inflammatory factor by downregulating complement anaphylatoxin C5a. The purpose of this study was to investigate the association between TAFI and C5a levels and the development of post-traumatic sepsis. Furthermore, the predictive potential of both TAFI and C5a to indicate sepsis occurrence in polytraumatized patients was assessed. Methods: Upon admission to the emergency department (ED) and daily for the subsequent ten days, circulating levels of TAFI and C5a were determined in 48 severely injured trauma patients (injury severity score (ISS) ≥ 16). Frequency matching according to the ISS in septic vs. non-septic patients was performed. Trauma and physiologic characteristics, as well as outcomes, were assessed. Statistical correlation analyses and cut-off values for predicting sepsis were calculated. Results: Fourteen patients developed sepsis, while 34 patients did not show any signs of sepsis (no sepsis). Overall injury severity, as well as demographic parameters, were comparable between both groups (ISS: 25.78 ± 2.36 no sepsis vs. 23.46 ± 2.79 sepsis). Septic patients had significantly increased C5a levels (21.62 ± 3.14 vs. 13.40 ± 1.29 ng/mL; $p < 0.05$) and reduced TAFI levels upon admission to the ED (40,951 ± 5637 vs. 61,865 ± 4370 ng/mL; $p < 0.05$) compared to the no sepsis group. Negative correlations between TAFI and C5a ($p = 0.0104$) and TAFI and lactate ($p = 0.0423$) and positive correlations between C5a and lactate ($p = 0.0173$), as well as C5a and the respiratory rate ($p = 0.0266$), were found. In addition, correlation analyses of both TAFI and C5a with the sequential (sepsis-related) organ failure assessment (SOFA) score have confirmed their potential as early sepsis biomarkers. Cut-off values for predicting sepsis were 54,857 ng/mL for TAFI with an area under the curve (AUC) of 0.7550 ($p = 0.032$) and 17 ng/mL for C5a with an AUC of 0.7286 ($p = 0.034$). Conclusion: The development of sepsis is associated with early decreased TAFI and increased C5a levels after major trauma. Both elevated C5a and decreased TAFI may serve as promising predictive factors for the development of sepsis after polytrauma.

Keywords: polytrauma; sepsis; complement; patients

---

1. Introduction

Trauma is responsible for one out of 10 deaths worldwide and is among the most frequent causes of mortality, notably among young people [1]. Traumatized patients who survive the initial post-injury phase are at high risk to die from late-occurring complications such as multiple organ failure (MOF), respiratory complications, and/or sepsis [2–5]. During sepsis, the activation of both coagulation and complement systems, which can be triggered by a pathogen itself or damaged tissues, is essential as a reaction to tissue injury and for an adequate host defense against pathogens [6,7]. Nevertheless, abnormalities in the well-regulated interactions between these systems or their excessive activation can be harmful and lead to thrombosis or disseminated intravascular coagulation [6,7].

Thrombin-activatable fibrinolysis inhibitor (TAFI), a procarboxypeptidase 2 or carboxypeptidase U, is a carboxypeptidase B-like proenzyme with a molecular weight of 56 kDa [8]. Upon activation by the thrombin-thrombomodulin complex at the vascular endothelial surface, its activated TAFI form (TAFIa) inhibits fibrinolysis by removing C-terminal lysines from fibrin, which are imperative for the efficient formation of plasmin [8,9]. In a septic rat model with *Pseudomonas aeruginosa*, the inhibition of TAFIa reduced the systemic inflammatory response, thus suggesting that TAFI plays an important role in the deterioration of organ dysfunction in sepsis [10]. In a rat model of a sepsis-complicating burn injury, TAFI was elevated after 24 and 72 h, confirming the close link between inflammation and coagulation [11]. Septic patients, as well as healthy study subjects with low-grade lipopolysaccharide (LPS)-induced endotoxemia, showed decreased levels of TAFI [12,13], and in polytraumatized patients, TAFI levels inversely correlated with the inflammation-associated development of complications [14].

Anaphylatoxin C5a is a strong chemoattractant signal that is involved in the regulation of the innate immune system, playing a key role in host homeostasis, inflammation, and defense against pathogens [15–19]. Upon activation through the cleavage of C5 to C5a and C5b by the C5-convertase, C5a takes part in the recruitment and activation of inflammatory cells like neutrophils, eosinophils, T lymphocytes, and monocytes [19,20]. Recently, in a baboon model of *Escherichia coli* bacteremia, it was shown that complement-mediated bacteriolysis had a detrimental effect by inducing a release of LPS and fulminant inflammation [21]. The inhibition of C5 cleavage blocked sepsis-induced inflammation, decreased the associated consumptive coagulopathy, and protected organ functions, resulting in improved survival [21].

Besides its role in coagulation, TAFI has been shown to have anti-inflammatory properties, thus being able to inactivate activated complement factors C3a and C5a [22,23]. Therefore, in the present study, we included severely injured trauma patients with sepsis to determine whether TAFI might represent a possible link between inflammation/complement and coagulation in sepsis.

2. Materials and Methods

2.1. Ethics

This study was performed at the University Hospital of the Goethe University Frankfurt with the institutional ethical approval in accordance with the Declaration of Helsinki and following the Strengthening the Reporting of Observational Studies in Epidemiology (STROBE) guidelines (167/05). Written informed consent was obtained from all enrolled patients in accordance with ethical standards. All patients signed the informed consent forms themselves, or informed consent was obtained from the nominated legally authorized representative consenting on the behalf of participants, as approved by the ethical committee.

2.2. Patients

Patients were included according to the following criteria: history of penetrating or blunt trauma with an injury severity score (ISS) ≥ 16 and between 18 and 80 years of age. Patients with pre-existing immunological disorders, concomitant acute myocardial infarction, immunosuppressive or anticoagulant medication, burns, thromboembolic events, and/or lethal injury were excluded. All patients were treated according to the Advanced Trauma Life Support (ATLS®) standards and the polytrauma guidelines. While haemodynamically instable patients received immediate surgery, haemodynamically stable patient underwent whole-body computed tomography. Upon arrival to the emergency room, the following demographic and clinical data were collected: age; gender; blood pressure; respiratory rate; heart rate; temperature; mechanism of injury; abbreviated injury scale for each body region (head, chest, abdomen, and extremity); and the general injury severity (ISS), as described before [24]. Routine blood gas analysis (including pH and lactate) was performed upon admission to the hospital. The numbers of fresh frozen plasma (FFP) and packed red blood cell (PRBC) units transfused within the first 24 h and during further clinical course were recorded. The diagnose of sepsis was assessed by both the 2005 criteria outlined by the International Sepsis Forum [25], as well as by the revised definition criteria according to the Sepsis-3 criteria [26,27]. Systemic inflammatory response syndrome (SIRS) was defined by fulfilling at least two of the following criteria: heart rate > 90 beats per minute, respiratory rate > 20 per minute or arterial carbon dioxide tension ($PaCO_2$) < 32 mm Hg, body temperature >38 °C or <36 °C, and white blood cell count >12,000 cells/mm^3 or <4000 cells/mm^3 or with >10% immature forms. According to the old definition, sepsis was diagnosed when the patients fulfilled criteria for SIRS and had evidence for an infection. However, limitations of that definition, including an excessive focus on inflammation and the inadequate specificity and sensitivity of the SIRS criteria, led to the Sepsis-3 definition, in which sepsis was defined as life-threatening organ dysfunction caused by a dysregulated host response to infection. The authors have summarized that, for clinical operationalization, organ dysfunction can be represented by an increase in the sequential (sepsis-related) organ failure assessment (SOFA) score of 2 points or more, which is associated with an enhanced in-hospital mortality risk [26,27]. Medical records were analyzed regarding length of in-hospital stay, length of ICU stay, and in-hospital mortality.

2.3. Blood Processing and Analysis

Blood samples were obtained from 48 severely traumatized patients as early as possible after admission to the emergency department (ED) and until day ten daily in pre-chilled ethylene-diaminetetraacetic acid (EDTA) or heparin vacuum tubes (BD vacutainer; Becton Dickinson Diagnostics, Aalst, Belgium) for routine diagnostics or for laboratory investigations and were kept on ice until centrifugation at 2000× *g* for 15 min at 4 °C. Afterwards, supernatants were stored at −80 °C until analysis. The mean time between injury and acquisition of the blood sample was 81 ± 8 min.

TAFI levels were measured by using a commercially available ELISA (IMUCLONE™ TAFI ELISA; American Diagnostica Inc., Stamford, CT, USA) according to the manufacturer's instructions. The TAFI antigen level is expressed as a percentage of normal pooled plasma. C5a levels were determined using a commercially available Human C5a ELISA kit II (BD Biosciences, Heidelberg, Germany) according to the manufacturer's instructions. Blood counts were measured using the Sysmex XE-2100 automated blood cell counter (Sysmex Europe GmbH, Norderstedt, Germany). pH, lactate, and $PaCO_2$ were determined using a standard clinical blood gas analysis device (ABL800 Flex, Radiometer, Krefeld, Germany).

2.4. Statistics

All data were tested for normal distribution by a Kolmogorov-Smirnov-Lillieford's test. Continuous variables were compared using the Mann-Whitney U test, and categorical variables were analyzed with the two-sided Fisher's exact test. Data are presented as the mean ± standard error of the mean (SEM) unless otherwise stated. Receiver-operator curves (ROC) were calculated to analyze the optimal cut-off values. The sample size was performed based on the mean TAFI data obtained from the pilot study in Relja et al. [14]. Based on the mean values, a Cohen's d of 1.060 and an effect size of $r = 0.468$ were calculated. Applying a power of 0.8, a group size of 15 per group is necessary to reach significant results in an unpaired *t*-test ($\alpha = 0.05$). Results were considered as statistically significant when the *p*-value was <0.05. Statistical analysis was performed using GraphPad Prism 5.0 software (GraphPad Software Inc., San Diego, CA, USA).

3. Results

Main Findings

A cohort of 48 patients (33 male) met the inclusion criteria and were included in the study. Mean patient age was 52.23 ± 2.74 years, and all patients were substantially injured with a mean ISS of 24.95 ± 1.75. Of these, 14 patients with an ISS of 23.36 ± 2.79 developed sepsis during the clinical course, while 34 patients with an ISS of 25.78 ± 2.36 did not develop sepsis or septic complications. Table 1 summarizes the general patient and injury characteristics of the study population. There were no significant differences between the sepsis and no sepsis group with regard to the general patient and injury characteristics. The mean time between the onset of trauma and arrival to the ED was 66.17 ± 4.85 min. The mean time until admission to the ED between the cohort of septic patients vs. not septic patients did not statistically differ (65.40 ± 11.55 vs. 66.50 ± 5.17 min).

Table 1. Demographic and trauma characteristics of the study population. Data are given as mean ± standard error of the mean; $p < 0.05$. Abbreviations: a, no sepsis group; AIS, abbreviated injury scale; b, sepsis group; ISS, injury severity score; and ns, no significance.

Subjects and Trauma Characteristics	Total (n = 48)	No Sepsis [a] (n = 34)	Sepsis [b] (n = 14)	$p < 0.05$ a vs. b
age (years), mean ± sem	52.23 ± 2.74	48.45 ± 3.74	56,54 ± 3.68	ns
gender (male, %)	33 (68.75%)	22 (64.71%)	11 (78.57%)	ns
trauma mechanism (falls)	23 (47.92%)	16 (47.06%)	7 (50.00%)	ns
ISS	24.95 ± 1.75	25.78 ± 2.36	23.46 ± 2.79	ns
AIS ≥ 3 (n, %)				
Head	22 (45.83%)	16 (47.06%)	6 (42.86%)	ns
Chest	16 (33.33%)	11 (32.35%)	5 (35.71%)	ns
Abdomen	7 (14.58%)	4 (11.76%)	3 (21.43%)	ns
Extremity	10 (20.83%)	7 (20.59%)	3 (21.43%)	ns

To investigate the influence of blood transfusions concerning the development of sepsis after polytrauma, the number of fresh frozen plasma (FFP) and packed red blood cells (PRBC) during the first 24 h after admittance to the emergency department and during the whole clinical course were determined. Patients belonging to the sepsis group received significantly more units of packed red blood cells during the whole clinical treatment compared to the no sepsis group (10.50 ± 2.50 vs. 5.46 ± 21.74; $p < 0.05$). As depicted in Table 2, there were no significant differences between these two groups concerning the units of packed red blood cells during the first 24 h, the systolic blood pressure <90 mm Hg at admittance to the ED, the number of transfused units of fresh frozen plasma within 24 h or during the whole clinical course, or the body temperature at admittance to the ED. Furthermore, no significant differences among the groups in the international normalized ratio (INR), activated partial thromboplastin time (PTT), or platelet counts (PLT) were assessed.

Table 2. Physiologic characteristics of the study population. Data are given as mean ± standard error of the mean; $p < 0.05$. Abbreviations: a, no sepsis group; b, sepsis group; ED, emergency department; FFP, fresh frozen plasma; INR, international normalized ratio; ns, no significance; PLT, platelet; PRBC, packed red blood cells; PTT, activated partial thromboplastin time; and SBP, systolic blood pressure.

Physiologic Characteristics	Total ($n = 48$)	No Sepsis [a] ($n = 34$)	Sepsis [b] ($n = 14$)	$p < 0.05$ a vs. b
SBP < 90 mm Hg (ED, n, %)	5 (10.42%)	2 (5.71%)	3 (21.43%)	ns
PRBC transfusion within 24 h (Units)	4.84 ± 1.18	3.81 ± 1.53	7.14 ± 2.01	ns
PRBC transfusion total (Units)	6.98 ± 1.41	5.46 ± 21.74	10.50 ± 2.50	<0.05
FFP transfusion within 24 h (Units)	2.54 ± 0.69	1.65 ± 0.71	4.31 ± 1.45	ns
FFP transfusion total (Units)	2.68 ± 0.75	1.73 ± 0.75	4.43 ± 1.56	ns
INR (ED)	1.34 ± 0.08	1.36 ± 0.11	1.31 ± 0.06	ns
PTT (ED, s)	36.13 ± 2.79	37.12 ± 3.88	33.72 ± 1.62	ns
PLT count (ED, × $10^3/\mu L$)	201.40 ± 10.34	198.00 ± 12.44	210.30 ± 18.97	ns

A significantly prolonged stay in the intensive care unit was observed in septic patients (22.14 ± 4.12 days vs. 7.00 ± 1.16; $p < 0.0001$), and in-hospital stays lasted significantly longer for this group (41.07 ± 6.43 vs. 19 ± 2.90; $p < 0.001$) compared to the group without septic complications. A total of six patients (12.5%) died, with a significantly higher number of patients in the sepsis group compared with the no sepsis group (four vs. two; $p < 0.05$; Table 3).

Table 3. Outcome of the study population. Data are given as mean ± standard error of the mean; $p < 0.05$. Abbreviations: a, no sepsis group; b, sepsis group; ICU, intensive care unit.

Outcome	Total ($n = 48$)	No Sepsis [a] ($n = 34$)	Sepsis [b] ($n = 14$)	$p < 0.05$ a vs. b
ICU stay (days)	11.71 ± 1.82	7.00 ± 1.16	22.14 ± 4.12	<0.0001
in-hospital stay (days)	25.67 ± 3.13	19.00 ± 2.90	41.07 ± 6.43	<0.001
in-hospital mortality (n, %)	6 (12.5%)	2 (5.88%)	4 (28.57%)	<0.05

In order to further investigate the differences of clinical features at admission to the ED between patients developing sepsis during the clinical course and patients who did not develop sepsis, we compared lactate concentrations and pH values in the blood, heart rate, and respiratory rate in our study cohort. As shown in Figure 1, patients who developed sepsis had significantly higher amounts of lactate in their blood and a more acidic constellation of their acid bases balance, as depicted by significantly lower pH values ($p < 0.05$; Figure 1A,B). Furthermore, patients who developed sepsis during the clinical course had significant changes of their vital parameters, as they had higher respiratory and heart rates at their admission to the ED ($p < 0.05$; Figure 1C,D).

In order to investigate changes in coagulation and inflammation, we measured TAFI and C5a levels at admission to the ED. Patients belonging to the sepsis group had significantly lower TAFI levels and significantly higher C5a levels compared to the no sepsis group, as shown in Figure 2A,B, respectively ($p < 0.05$). Moreover, patients from the sepsis group showed significantly increased leukocytes counts compared with the no sepsis group ($p < 0.05$; Figure 2C).

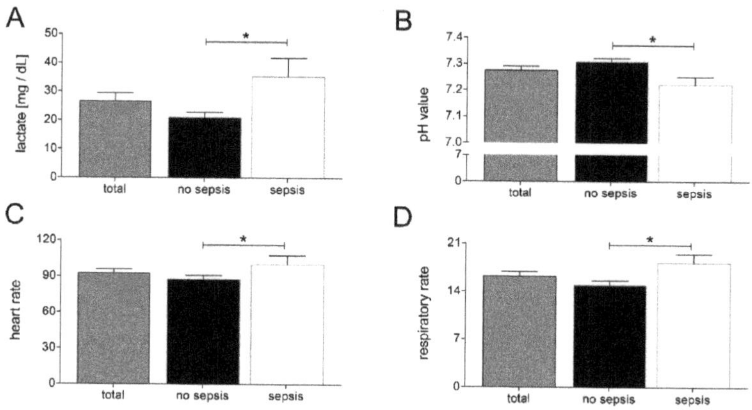

Figure 1. Upon admission of severely injured trauma patients ($n = 48$) to the emergency department, lactate levels (**A**), pH values (**B**), heart rate (**C**), and respiratory rate (**D**) were measured. Patients were stratified to those who developed sepsis in their clinical course (sepsis, $n = 14$) vs. those who did not develop infectious complications (no sepsis, $n = 34$). Data are shown as mean ± SEM. * $p < 0.05$ sepsis vs. no sepsis.

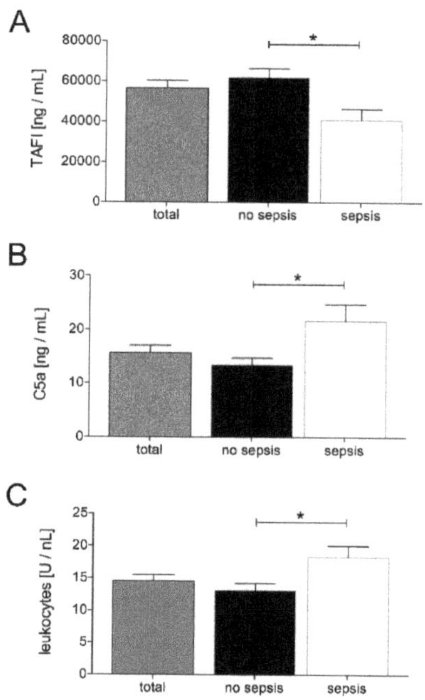

Figure 2. Upon admission of severely injured trauma patients ($n = 48$) to the emergency department, plasma thrombin-activatable fibrinolysis inhibitor (TAFI) levels (**A**), plasma C5a levels (**B**), and leukocyte counts (**C**) were determined. Patients were stratified to those who developed sepsis in their clinical course (sepsis, $n = 14$) vs. those who did not develop infectious complications (no sepsis, $n = 34$). Data are shown as mean ± SEM. * $p < 0.05$ sepsis vs. no sepsis.

In addition, we analyzed correlations between TAFI and/or C5a and clinical (heart and respiratory rate) or laboratory parameters (pH value, leukocyte count, lactate value, INR, thromboplastin time (TPT), PTT, and PLT) and the SOFA score. TAFI and C5a, as well as TAFI and lactate, have shown a significant negative correlation (TAFI and C5a: Pearson $r = -0.4933$, $p < 0.0104$ and TAFI and lactate: Pearson $r = -0.4268$, $p < 0.0423$; Table 4 and Figure 3A,B). Furthermore, C5a and lactate, as well as C5a and the respiratory rate, had a significant correlation (C5a and lactate: Pearson $r = 0.4542$, $p < 0.0173$ and C5a and respiratory rate: Pearson $r = 0.4185$, $p < 0.0266$; Table 4 and Figure 3C,D). In addition, correlation analysis of TAFI and C5a with the SOFA score have shown a significant negative correlation of TAFI with the SOFA score (Pearson $r = -0.3865$, $p = 0.0422$) and a significant positive correlation of C5a with the SOFA score (Pearson $r = 0.3795$, $p = 0.0386$) (Table 4).

Table 4. Correlation analyses between thrombin-activatable fibrinolysis inhibitor (TAFI), C5a, leukocyte counts, lactate levels, pH values, heart and respiratory rates, sequential (sepsis-related) organ failure assessment (SOFA) score, international normalized ratio (INR), thromboplastin time (TPT), partial thromboplastin time (PTT), and platelet (PLT). $p < 0.05$: statistically significant.

Correlation Analysis	Pearson *r*	*p*-Value	Number of Pairs
TAFI and C5a	−0.4933	0.0104	26
TAFI and leukocytes	−0.2442	0.1855	31
TAFI and lactate	−0.4268	0.0423	23
TAFI and pH	0.2079	0.3532	22
TAFI and heart rate	−0.2603	0.2304	23
TAFI and respiratory rate	−0.3685	0.0915	22
TAFI and SOFA score	−0.3865	0.0422	28
TAFI and INR	−0.0499	0.7860	32
TAFI and TPT	0.0299	0.8750	30
TAFI and PTT	0.0369	0.8409	32
TAFI and PLT	−0.3048	0.0085	33
C5a and leukocytes	−0.2260	0.1918	35
C5a and lactate	0.4542	0.0173	27
C5a and pH	−0.0805	0.6839	28
C5a and heart rate	0.2416	0.2068	29
C5a and respiratory rate	0.4185	0.0266	28
C5a and SOFA score	0.3795	0.0386	30
C5a and INR	−0.0199	0.9055	38
C5a and TPT	−0.2056	0.2291	36
C5a and PTT	0.0731	0.6629	38
C5a and PLT	0.0138	0.9353	37

To investigate which of the examined parameters in this study (TAFI, C5a, leukocytes count, lactate, heart rate, and respiratory rate) could provide a prognostic marker for the development of sepsis after polytrauma, the predictive power of each parameter has been calculated using ROC analyses. While the ROC analysis for lactate did not show a statistically significant area under the ROC curve ($p = 0.052$), TAFI showed an optimal cut-off for predicting sepsis on admission to the ED at 54,857 ng/mL, with a sensitivity of 64% and specificity of 87.50%. The AUC was 0.7550 (95% CI: 0.585 to 0.925; $p < 0.032$; Table 5 and Figure 4A). C5a showed an optimal cut-off at 17 ng/mL on admission to the ED for predicting sepsis in the clinical course, with a sensitivity of 75.00%, specificity of 70.00%, and an AUC of 0.7286 (95% CI: 0.547 to 0.910; $p < 0.034$; Table 5 and Figure 4B). Leukocytes showed an optimal cut-off at 14.50 U/nl, with a sensitivity of 65.63%, specificity of 69.23%, and an AUC of 0.7043 (95% CI: 0.527 to 0.882; $p < 0.033$; Table 5 and Figure 4C). The heart rate showed an optimal cut-off at 102.5/min on admission to the ED for predicting sepsis in the clinical course, with a sensitivity of 86.96%, specificity of 64.29%, and an AUC of 0.6957 (95% CI: 0.490 to 0.902; $p < 0.049$; Table 5 and Figure 4E). The respiratory rate showed an optimal cut-off at 15/min, with a sensitivity of 63.64% and a specificity of 64.29%. The AUC was 0.7029 (95% CI: 0.511 to 0.895; $p < 0.043$; Table 5 and Figure 4F).

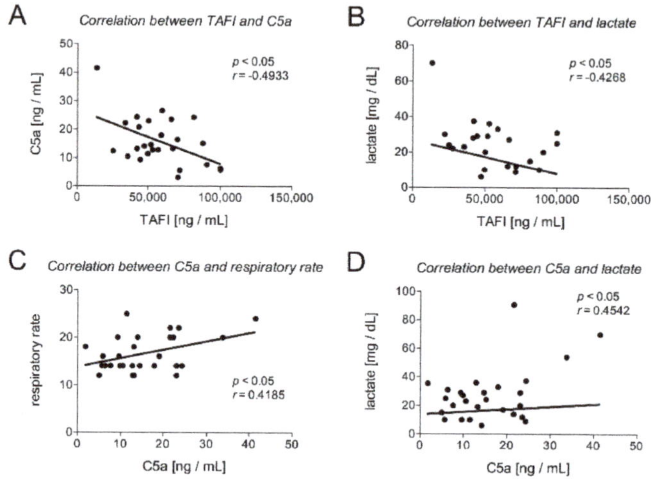

Figure 3. Correlation analysis between TAFI and C5a (**A**), TAFI and lactate (**B**), C5a and respiratory rate (**C**), and C5a and lactate (**D**) are shown. *r*: Pearson coefficient.

Table 5. Receiver-operator curve (ROC) analyses on TAFI, C5a, leukocyte count, lactate level, heart rate, and respiratory rate at admission to the emergency department to predict the development of sepsis after polytrauma. Sensitivity and specificity are given as percentage values. Abbreviations: AUC, area under the curve and CI, confidence interval.

Parameter	Cut-Off Value	Sensitivity % (95% CI)	Specificity % (95% CI)	AUC (95% CI)	*p*-Value
TAFI [ng/mL]	>54857	64.00 (42.52 to 82.03)	87.50 (47.35 to 99.68)	0.7550 (0.585 to 0.925)	0.032
C5a [ng/mL]	<17.00	75.00 (55.13 to 89.31)	70.00 (34.75 to 93.33)	0.7286 (0.547 to 0.910)	0.034
leukocytes [U/nL]	<14.50	65.63 (46.81 to 81.43)	69.23 (38.57 to 90.91)	0.7043 (0.527 to 0.882)	0.033
lactate [mg/dL]	<28.50	78.26 (56.30 to 92.54)	69.23 (38.57 to 90.91)	0.6973 (0.500 to 0.895)	0.052
heart rate	<102.5	86.96 (66.41 to 97.22)	64.29 (35.14 to 87.24)	0.6957 (0.490 to 0.902)	0.049
respiratory rate	<15.00	63.64 (40.66 to 82.80)	64.29 (35.14 to 87.24)	0.7029 (0.511 to 0.895)	0.043

The results in Figure 5 reflect the dynamic course of both parameters after trauma and sepsis. The distribution of the TAFI and C5a values in the samples obtained in the ED and subsequent daily measurements for ten consecutive days show that the TAFI was significantly decreased on admission, day 2, and on day 9 in the sepsis group compared to the control group without sepsis ($p < 0.05$; Figure 5A). On the contrary, the C5a values were significantly increased on admission, days 2–6, and on day 9 in the sepsis group compared to the control group without sepsis ($p < 0.05$; Figure 5B).

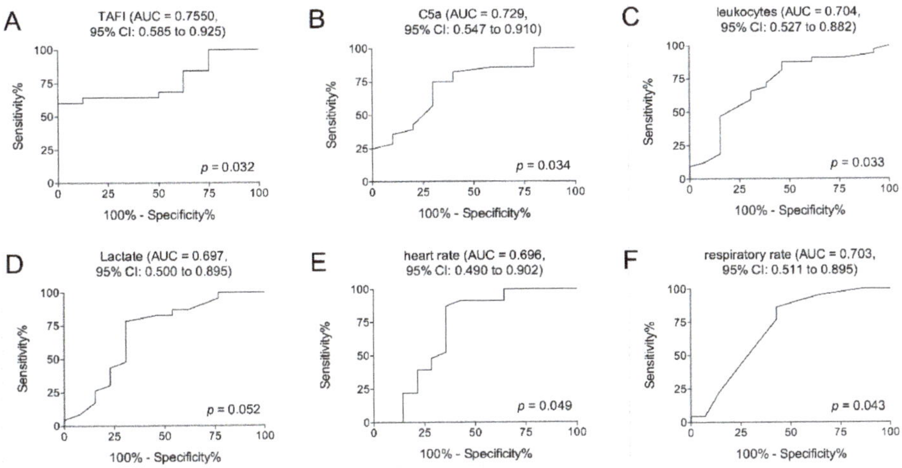

Figure 4. Receiver operating curve analyses on TAFI (**A**), C5a (**B**), leukocyte counts (**C**), lactate levels (**D**), heart rate (**E**), and respiratory rate (**F**) at admission to the emergency department to predict the development of sepsis after polytrauma are demonstrated. $p < 0.05$: statistically significant, AUC: area under the curve, and CI: confidence interval.

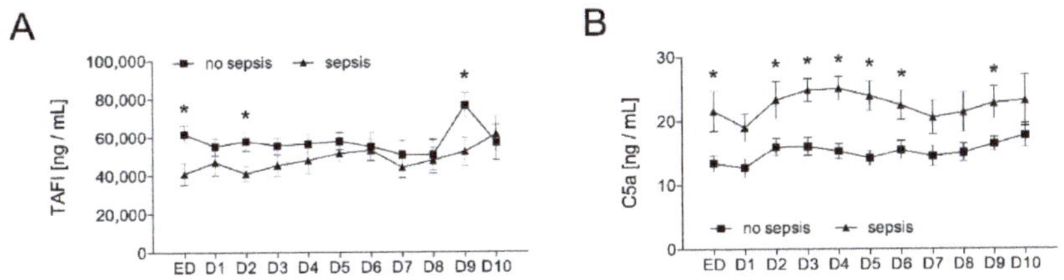

Figure 5. Upon admission of severely injured trauma patients (n = 48) to the emergency department (ED), plasma TAFI levels (**A**) and plasma C5a levels (**B**) were determined daily for ten days (D1–D10). Patients were stratified to those who developed sepsis in their clinical course (sepsis, n = 14) vs. those who did not develop infectious complications (no sepsis, n = 34). Data are shown as mean ± SEM. * $p < 0.05$ sepsis vs. no sepsis at the indicated time.

4. Discussion

Polytraumatized patients who survive the initial post-injury phase are at a serious risk to die from septic complications during their further clinical treatment [18]. Both the inflammatory/complement and the coagulation systems contribute to these harmful events. Regarding this, it is important to note that the cross-talk between the inflammation/complement and the coagulation occurs in both directions, as coagulation can affect the inflammatory activity as well as inflammation is able to activate coagulation [14,28,29]. TAFI is a carboxypeptidase B-like proenzyme, which, on the one hand, upon its activation to TAFIa by the thrombin-thrombomodulin complex inhibits fibrinolysis by removing C-terminal lysines from fibrin [8,9]. On the other hand, activated complement factors C3a and C5a can be inactivated by TAFIa [22,30]. The data suggests that TAFI may be a potential link between the inflammation/complement and the coagulation systems.

In the underlying study, we observed significantly reduced TAFI levels in patients developing sepsis during their clinical course after polytrauma compared to polytraumatized patients without septic complications. This difference occurred early upon admission of the patients to the ED. In contrast, C5a levels were significantly increased in septic patients after polytrauma. A significant negative correlation between TAFI and C5a levels was found. In addition, the correlation analyses of TAFI and C5a with the SOFA score have demonstrated a significant negative correlation of TAFI and a significant positive correlation of C5a with the SOFA score. These findings enhance markedly the impact of both TAFI and C5a as biomarkers, which may indicate later-occurring development of the post-traumatic sepsis. However, whether reduced TAFI levels in septic patients after polytrauma derive from, e.g., consumption in the course of coagulopathy or whether initially reduced TAFI levels potentially put patients at risk for septic complications still remains elusive. It can be speculated that maybe upon reduced TAFI levels, missing inactivation of C3a and C5a may lead to an immunological imbalance and an excessive immunological reaction. As nicely reviewed and originally published by the expert group around Huber-Lang, anaphylatoxin C5a appears in the circulation of humans within 20 min post-polytrauma, and its levels have been related to the mortality rate [31,32]. That data indicated an almost synchronical rapid activation and dysfunction of the complement, suggesting a trauma-induced complementopathy early after injury [32]. Furthermore, the authors suggest that these events may participate in the impairment of the post-traumatic innate immune response. Within the time latency between 20 min of the complement activation, as shown by Huber-Lang, and 66 min until admission of patients to the ED, as shown in our study, certainly, a trauma-induced complementopathy may have occurred. Thus, levels of both TAFI and C5a may have been different at the onset of trauma, and we cannot exclude any alterations which may have emerged until the blood sampling in the ED was performed. Thus, the latency between the timepoint of trauma and sampling in the ED must be taken into account when interpreting the results. Relja et al. reported elevated TAFI levels in polytraumatized patients with and without infectious complications but with a significantly higher increase in both TAFI and TAFIa in patients without infectious complications [14]. This supports the hypothesis that reduced TAFI levels may increase the risk for the development of septic complications. In line with these findings, Zeerleder et al. as well reported significantly decreased TAFI levels in septic patients compared to healthy controls [33]. Interestingly, in our pilot study, we found that TAFI levels at admission to the ED and at day 4 after the trauma were significantly lower in the smaller cohort of patients with complications compared to the control group [14]. In that study, we were able to demonstrate that TAFI levels inversely correlated with the inflammation-associated development of not-further-defined complications after major trauma. Furthermore, coagulopathic patients, however, experienced significantly lower levels of activated TAFI on admission and on days six to eight [34]. Based on those results, the finding that TAFI and C5a levels immediately at admission to the ED can stratify patients who are going to develop sepsis in their clinical course is certainly a promising result in terms of a search for early sepsis biomarkers. Yet, it remains to be noted that, in our study, we did not prospectively evaluate the levels of both potential biomarkers and that this remains to be elucidated in further studies.

Naito et al. investigated the link between C5a and TAFI with regard to acute lung injury and demonstrated that, in TAFI-deficient mice, LPS treatment induced a more severe acute lung injury (ALI) compared to wild-type mice [35]. Furthermore, the authors observed significantly higher concentrations of IL-1beta, TNF-beta, and IL-6, along with increased lung infiltration of neutrophils, in TAFI-deficient mice [35]. Naito et al. concluded that TAFI plays a critical role in the pathogenesis of ALI via its ability to regulate the activity of complement factor C5a [35]. Nishimura et al. reported worse alveolitis in TAFI knock-out mice than in wild-type (WT) mice with C5a instillation directly into the lungs [36]. In line with these results, we observed decreased TAFI levels and elevated C5a levels in patients who developed septic complications after polytrauma. More importantly, TAFI correlated negatively with C5a. Fujiwara et al. investigated the role of TAFI in allergic bronchial asthma and showed significantly worse airway responsiveness and increased pulmonary concentrations of IL-5 and osteopontin in a TAFI-deficient mouse model [37]. Pretreatment with a C5a antibody significantly attenuated these effects, and thus, the authors concluded that TAFI plays a protective role in the pathogenesis of allergic inflammation, probably by inhibiting the complement system [37]. In a model of inflammatory arthritis (anticollagen antibody–induced arthritis (CAIA)), Song et al. investigated the role of TAFI and showed that TAFI deficiency exacerbated inflammatory arthritis and, furthermore, that the cleavage of C5a by TAFI suppressed the ability of C5a to recruit immune cells to the affected joint [38]. Interestingly, the authors showed that the expression of both TAFI and C5a in synovial fluid was higher in patients with autoimmune arthritis than in those with osteoarthritis and concluded that TAFI plays an important role in attenuating local C5a-mediated inflammation and, thus, represents a molecular link between inflammation and coagulation in autoimmune arthritis [38].

While the above-mentioned studies all unanimously reported that decreased/lower levels of TAFI led to aggravated disease severity, Mook-Kanamori et al. showed that higher protein levels of TAFI in cerebrospinal fluid were significantly associated with systemic complications in patients with bacterial meningitis [39]. The authors observed survival benefits in TAFI-deficient mice in a pneumococcal meningitis mouse model as compared to wild-type mice and concluded that, during the initial phase of infection, a low level or an absence of TAFI results in initially increased complement levels, which may improve survival (in the animal model) and reduce systemic complications in humans suffering from bacterial meningitis [39]. Taken together, it still remains elusive whether TAFI acts as an acute reactant marker that links homeostasis and inflammation or whether a lack of TAFI plays an active role in the development of septic complications after polytrauma.

Most clinical studies examining anticoagulant effects on thrombo-inflammation have been performed in the context of sepsis, although some specific examples relevant to ischemia/reperfusion injuries are also reported. Unfortunately, the data in septic patients in which inhibitors of thrombin have been applied, as well as their efficiency, are limited [40]. As an example, the overall benefit of low molecular weight heparin in patients with sepsis remains, despite considerable investigations, uncertain [40]. Although initial trials with the IV infusion to restore plasma ATIII levels were promising, larger studies did not provide any benefit for overall mortality, and consequently, Rhodes et al. have made specific recommendations against the use of ATIII in the updated International Guidelines for the Management of Sepsis and Septic Shock [40,41]. The use of other anticoagulant agents, e.g., recombinant human activated protein C, have failed to consistently demonstrate a reduction in 28-day all-cause mortality in clinical trials [42]. Currently, soluble recombinant human thrombomodulin (rhTM) is undergoing clinical evaluation for the treatment of severe sepsis [40]. ART-123, an rhTM, appears to be a safe intervention in critically ill sepsis patients in phase 2b trials [40,43].

Although this study has several limitations—of those, the most important, the limited sample size—it must be considered that there is no significant difference between demographic and trauma characteristics between evaluated groups, which certainly ensures better compatibility of assessed data. Nevertheless, it has to be taken into account that patients in the sepsis group received significantly more PRBC during the whole clinical course, while there was no significant difference within the first 24 h (Table 2). Sadjadi et al. reported that, in trauma patients, infection was associated with the transfusion of PRBC and that transfused patients had eight times the increased risk of infection independently of their injury severity [44]. Likewise, Claridge et al. reported a dose-dependent correlation between transfusions of PRBC and the development of infection in traumatized patients [45]. Based on the data of our study, we cannot fully exclude an effect of transfused PRBC either on TAFI or on C5a, and this remains to be elaborated in future works. Although several studies have reported that a PRBC transfusion can negatively affect clinical outcomes [46,47], it still remains unclear if TAFI is an acute phase reactant that links hemostasis and inflammation or whether it plays an active role in the development of post-traumatic sepsis. With regard to the effects of PRBC transfusions on, e.g., the complement, certain clinical syndromes such as transfusion-related acute lung injury (TRALI) and transfusion-associated circulatory overload (TACO) that occur within 6 h of blood transfusions indicate an association [48,49]. The major drivers of those complications and their pathogenesis, however, are complex and incompletely understood. The potential connection between the complement system and neutrophils is given, as well as the parallels between these syndromes and other acute pulmonary disorders, which are known for their involvement of the complement. Yet, similar to TAFI, we cannot exclude a direct impact of the PRBS transfusion on C5a levels or its activity; however, since the transfusion rates within the first 24 h after the trauma did not differ between the septic and nonseptic group, we believe that the data as demonstrated are plausible. Moreover, C5a levels remain increased in septic patients nearly throughout the complete observational period, and thus, we believe that this effect is associated with inflammatory changes caused by sepsis rather than with PRBC transfusions, which, anyway, were initially not significantly enhanced. However, the increased amount of totally transfused PRBC in our study must therefore be considered as a disturbing variable by interpreting the data. Further limitations of the study include the study setting, since this study was conducted in a single center. In addition, the heterogeneity of the traumatized patients, as well as the variable timing of measurements, must be carefully considered in data interpretation. Although there were sufficient measurements made later after the trauma to determine the roles of TAFI and C5a as indicators of sepsis, a long-term study also including septic patients from other pathologies is necessary, but this was not the aim of the study.

Early recognition and effective management of patients at risk for infectious complications are essential for improved outcomes. However, early recognition specifically of post-traumatic sepsis is impeded by the lack of clinically proven and utilized biomarkers. The current work in clinical settings has not yielded the requisite gold standards for the diagnosis and monitoring of post-traumatic sepsis. Yet, identifying patients at risk for the development of sepsis during their clinical course is of great importance for further clinical treatment. TAFI and C5a may be helpful, specifically in, e.g., decision-making about the timing for post-traumatic surgeries or indicate patients that should early receive antibiotic therapy or undergo further specific clinical tests of sepsis markers. With regard to complement factors or TAFI as potential biomarkers in general, clinical studies with large subject numbers are needed to obtain the complete temporal profiles of, e.g., activation of the complement factors or factor dynamics in the course of sepsis development. Presumably, this should provide a multipanel set of biomarkers, which can be coupled with routine lab tests and blood cultures for the diagnosis and monitoring of sepsis.

Taken together, in the underlying study, we were able to show that the development of sepsis after major trauma is associated with decreased TAFI levels and increased C5a levels. The significant negative correlation between TAFI and C5a supports the concept that reduced TAFI levels may lead to an exacerbation of septic complications and that TAFI might play a protective role by downregulating inflammation. Furthermore, irrespective of their possible pathomechanistical roles in the onset of sepsis, both TAFI and C5a might serve as very early diagnostic markers to detect patients at risk for the development of sepsis or septic complications.

Author Contributions: Conceptualization, B.R. and T.L.; methodology, J.T.V. and B.R.; formal analysis, A.H. and B.R.; investigation, J.T.V.; data curation, B.R.; writing—original draft preparation, J.T.V.; writing—review and editing, I.M., A.H., T.L., and B.R.; visualization, A.H. and B.R.; supervision, B.R.; and project administration, B.R. All authors have read and agreed to the published version of the manuscript.

Funding: This research received no external funding.

Acknowledgments: We thank Kerstin Wilhelm, Minhong Wang, and Alexander Schaible for their outstanding technical assistance.

Conflicts of Interest: The authors declare no conflict of interest.

References

1. Norton, R.; Kobusingye, O. Injuries. *N. Engl. J. Med.* **2013**, *368*, 1723–1730. [CrossRef]
2. Osborn, T.M.; Tracy, J.K.; Dunne, J.R.; Pasquale, M.; Napolitano, L.M. Epidemiology of sepsis in patients with traumatic injury. *Crit. Care Med.* **2004**, *32*, 2234–2240. [CrossRef]
3. Relja, B.; Land, W.G. Damage-associated molecular patterns in trauma. *Eur. J. Trauma Emerg. Surg.* **2019**, 1–25. [CrossRef]
4. Relja, B.; Mors, K.; Marzi, I. Danger signals in trauma. *Eur. J. Trauma Emerg. Surg.* **2018**, *44*, 301–316. [CrossRef]

5. Nast-Kolb, D.; Aufmkolk, M.; Rucholtz, S.; Obertacke, U.; Waydhas, C. Multiple organ failure still a major cause of morbidity but not mortality in blunt multiple trauma. *J. Trauma* **2001**, *51*, 835–841, discussion 41-2. [CrossRef]
6. Markiewski, M.M.; DeAngelis, R.A.; Lambris, J.D. Complexity of complement activation in sepsis. *J. Cell Mol. Med.* **2008**, *12*, 2245–2254. [CrossRef]
7. Ward, P.A. The harmful role of c5a on innate immunity in sepsis. *J. Innate Immun.* **2010**, *2*, 439–445. [CrossRef]
8. Foley, J.H.; Kim, P.Y.; Mutch, N.J.; Gils, A. Insights into thrombin activatable fibrinolysis inhibitor function and regulation. *J. Thromb. Haemost.* **2013**, *11* (Suppl. 1), 306–315.
9. Bouma, B.N.; Mosnier, L.O. Thrombin activatable fibrinolysis inhibitor (TAFI) at the interface between coagulation and fibrinolysis. *Pathophysiol. Haemost. Thromb.* **2003**, *33*, 375–381. [CrossRef]
10. Muto, Y.; Suzuki, K.; Iida, H.; Sakakibara, S.; Kato, E.; Itoh, F.; Kakui, N.; Ishii, H. EF6265, a novel inhibitor of activated thrombin-activatable fibrinolysis inhibitor, protects against sepsis-induced organ dysfunction in rats. *Crit. Care Med.* **2009**, *37*, 1744–1749. [CrossRef]
11. Ravindranath, T.M.; Goto, M.; Demir, M.; Tobu, M.; Kujawski, M.F.; Hoppensteadt, D.; Samonte, V.; Iqbal, O.; Sayeed, M.M.; Fareed, J. Tissue factor pathway inhibitor and thrombin activatable fibrinolytic inhibitor plasma levels following burn and septic injuries in rats. *Clin. Appl Thromb. Hemost.* **2004**, *10*, 379–385. [CrossRef]
12. Verbon, A.; Meijers, J.C.; Spek, C.A.; Hack, C.E.; Pribble, J.P.; Turner, T.; Dekkers, P.E.; Axtelle, T.; Levi, M.; van Deventer, S.J.; et al. Effects of IC14, an anti-CD14 antibody, on coagulation and fibrinolysis during low-grade endotoxemia in humans. *J. Infect. Dis.* **2003**, *187*, 55–61. [CrossRef]
13. Watanabe, R.; Wada, H.; Watanabe, Y.; Sakakura, M.; Nakasaki, T.; Mori, Y.; Nishikawa, M.; Gabazza, E.C.; Nobori, T.; Shiku, H. Activity and antigen levels of thrombin-activatable fibrinolysis inhibitor in plasma of patients with disseminated intravascular coagulation. *Thromb. Res.* **2001**, *104*, 1–6. [CrossRef]
14. Relja, B.; Lustenberger, T.; Puttkammer, B.; Jakob, H.; Morser, J.; Gabazza, E.C.; Takei, Y.; Marzi, I. Thrombin-activatable fibrinolysis inhibitor (TAFI) is enhanced in major trauma patients without infectious complications. *Immunobiology* **2013**, *218*, 470–476. [CrossRef]
15. Ricklin, D.; Hajishengallis, G.; Yang, K.; Lambris, J.D. Complement: A key system for immune surveillance and homeostasis. *Nat. Immunol.* **2010**, *11*, 785–797. [CrossRef]
16. Ajona, D.; Ortiz-Espinosa, S.; Pio, R. Complement anaphylatoxins C3a and C5a: Emerging roles in cancer progression and treatment. *Semin. Cell Dev. Biol.* **2019**, *85*, 153–163. [CrossRef]
17. Blatt, A.Z.; Saggu, G.; Kulkarni, K.V.; Cortes, C.; Thurman, J.M.; Ricklin, D.; Lambris, J.D.; Valenzuela, J.G.; Ferreira, V.P. Properdin-Mediated C5a Production Enhances Stable Binding of Platelets to Granulocytes in Human Whole Blood. *J. Immunol.* **2016**, *196*, 4671–4680. [CrossRef]
18. Satyam, A.; Graef, E.R.; Lapchak, P.H.; Tsokos, M.G.; Dalle Lucca, J.J.; Tsokos, G.C. Complement and coagulation cascades in trauma. *Acute Med. Surg.* **2019**, *6*, 329–335. [CrossRef]
19. Guo, R.F.; Ward, P.A. Role of C5a in inflammatory responses. *Ann. Rev. Immunol.* **2005**, *23*, 821–852. [CrossRef]
20. Clarke, A.R.; Christophe, B.R.; Khahera, A.; Sim, J.L.; Connolly, E.S., Jr. Therapeutic Modulation of the Complement Cascade in Stroke. *Front. Immunol.* **2019**, *10*, 1723. [CrossRef]
21. Keshari, R.S.; Silasi, R.; Popescu, N.I.; Patel, M.M.; Chaaban, H.; Lupu, C.; Coggeshall, K.M.; Mollnes, T.E.; DeMarco, S.J.; Lupu, F. Inhibition of complement C5 protects against organ failure and reduces mortality in a baboon model of *Escherichia coli* sepsis. *Proc. Natl. Acad. Sci. USA* **2017**, *114*, E6390–E6399. [CrossRef]
22. Declerck, P.J. Thrombin activatable fibrinolysis inhibitor. *Hamostaseologie* **2011**, *31*, 165–166;168–173. [CrossRef]
23. Hugenholtz, G.C.; Meijers, J.C.; Adelmeijer, J.; Porte, R.J.; Lisman, T. TAFI deficiency promotes liver damage in murine models of liver failure through defective down-regulation of hepatic inflammation. *Thromb. Haemost.* **2013**, *109*, 948–955. [CrossRef]
24. Eguchi, A.; Franz, N.; Kobayashi, Y.; Iwasa, M.; Wagner, N.; Hildebrand, F.; Takei, Y.; Marzi, I.; Relja, B. Circulating Extracellular Vesicles and Their miR "Barcode" Differentiate Alcohol Drinkers with Liver Injury and Those Without Liver Injury in Severe Trauma Patients. *Front. Med.* **2019**, *6*, 30. [CrossRef]
25. Calandra, T.; Cohen, J. International Sepsis Forum Definition of Infection in the ICUCC. The international sepsis forum consensus conference on definitions of infection in the intensive care unit. *Crit. Care Med.* **2005**, *33*, 1538–1548. [CrossRef]

26. Shankar-Hari, M.; Phillips, G.S.; Levy, M.L.; Seymour, C.W.; Liu, V.X.; Deutschman, C.S.; Angus, D.C.; Rubenfeld, G.D.; Singer, M.; Sepsis Definitions Task, F. Developing a New Definition and Assessing New Clinical Criteria for Septic Shock: For the Third International Consensus Definitions for Sepsis and Septic Shock (Sepsis-3). *JAMA* **2016**, *315*, 775–787. [CrossRef]
27. Singer, M.; Deutschman, C.S.; Seymour, C.W.; Shankar-Hari, M.; Annane, D.; Bauer, M.; Bellomo, R.; Bernard, G.R.; Chiche, J.D.; Coopersmith, C.M.; et al. The Third International Consensus Definitions for Sepsis and Septic Shock (Sepsis-3). *JAMA* **2016**, *315*, 801–810. [CrossRef]
28. Levi, M.; Nieuwdorp, M.; van der Poll, T.; Stroes, E. Metabolic modulation of inflammation-induced activation of coagulation. *Semin. Thromb. Hemost.* **2008**, *34*, 26–32. [CrossRef]
29. Okamoto, T.; Tanigami, H.; Suzuki, K.; Shimaoka, M. Thrombomodulin: A bifunctional modulator of inflammation and coagulation in sepsis. *Crit. Care Res. Pract.* **2012**, *2012*, 614545. [CrossRef]
30. Myles, T.; Nishimura, T.; Yun, T.H.; Nagashima, M.; Morser, J.; Patterson, A.J.; Pearl, R.G.; Leung, L.L. Thrombin activatable fibrinolysis inhibitor, a potential regulator of vascular inflammation. *J. Biol. Chem.* **2003**, *278*, 51059–51067. [CrossRef]
31. Chakraborty, S.; Karasu, E.; Huber-Lang, M. Complement After Trauma: Suturing Innate and Adaptive Immunity. *Front. Immunol.* **2018**, *9*, 2050. [CrossRef] [PubMed]
32. Burk, A.M.; Martin, M.; Flierl, M.A.; Rittirsch, D.; Helm, M.; Lampl, L.; Bruckner, U.; Stahl, G.L.; Blom, A.M.; Perl, M.; et al. Early complementopathy after multiple injuries in humans. *Shock* **2012**, *37*, 348–354. [CrossRef] [PubMed]
33. Zeerleder, S.; Schroeder, V.; Hack, C.E.; Kohler, H.P.; Wuillemin, W.A. TAFI and PAI-1 levels in human sepsis. *Thromb. Res.* **2006**, *118*, 205–212. [CrossRef] [PubMed]
34. Lustenberger, T.; Relja, B.; Puttkammer, B.; Gabazza, E.C.; Geiger, E.; Takei, Y.; Morser, J.; Marzi, I. Activated thrombin-activatable fibrinolysis inhibitor (TAFIa) levels are decreased in patients with trauma-induced coagulopathy. *Thromb. Res.* **2013**, *131*, e26–e30. [CrossRef]
35. Naito, M.; Taguchi, O.; Kobayashi, T.; Takagi, T.; D'Alessandro-Gabazza, C.N.; Matsushima, Y.; Boveda-Ruiz, D.; Gil-Bernabe, P.; Matsumoto, T.; Chelakkot-Govindalayathil, A.L.; et al. Thrombin-activatable fibrinolysis inhibitor protects against acute lung injury by inhibiting the complement system. *Am. J. Respir. Cell Mol. Biol.* **2013**, *49*, 646–653. [CrossRef]
36. Nishimura, T.; Myles, T.; Piliponsky, A.M.; Kao, P.N.; Berry, G.J.; Leung, L.L. Thrombin-activatable procarboxypeptidase B regulates activated complement C5a in vivo. *Blood* **2007**, *109*, 1992–1997. [CrossRef]
37. Fujiwara, A.; Taguchi, O.; Takagi, T.; D'Alessandro-Gabazza, C.N.; Boveda-Ruiz, D.; Toda, M.; Yasukawa, A.; Matsushima, Y.; Miyake, Y.; Kobayashi, H.; et al. Role of thrombin-activatable fibrinolysis inhibitor in allergic bronchial asthma. *Lung* **2012**, *190*, 189–198. [CrossRef]
38. Song, J.J.; Hwang, I.; Cho, K.H.; Garcia, M.A.; Kim, A.J.; Wang, T.H.; Lindstrom, T.M.; Lee, A.T.; Nishimura, T.; Zhao, L.; et al. Plasma carboxypeptidase B downregulates inflammatory responses in autoimmune arthritis. *J. Clin. Investig.* **2011**, *121*, 3517–3527. [CrossRef]
39. Mook-Kanamori, B.B.; Valls Seron, M.; Geldhoff, M.; Havik, S.R.; van der Ende, A.; Baas, F.; van der Poll, T.; Meijers, J.C.; Morgan, B.P.; Brouwer, M.C.; et al. Thrombin-activatable fibrinolysis inhibitor influences disease severity in humans and mice with pneumococcal meningitis. *J. Thromb. Haemost.* **2015**, *13*, 2076–2086. [CrossRef]
40. Jackson, S.P.; Darbousset, R.; Schoenwaelder, S.M. Thromboinflammation: Challenges of therapeutically targeting coagulation and other host defense mechanisms. *Blood* **2019**, *133*, 906–918. [CrossRef]
41. Rhodes, A.; Evans, L.E.; Alhazzani, W.; Levy, M.M.; Antonelli, M.; Ferrer, R.; Kumar, A.; Sevransky, J.E.; Sprung, C.L.; Nunnally, M.E.; et al. Surviving Sepsis Campaign: International Guidelines for Management of Sepsis and Septic Shock: 2016. *Intensive Care Med.* **2017**, *43*, 304–377. [CrossRef] [PubMed]
42. Bernard, G.R.; Vincent, J.L.; Laterre, P.F.; LaRosa, S.P.; Dhainaut, J.F.; Lopez-Rodriguez, A.; Steingrub, J.S.; Garber, G.E.; Helterbrand, J.D.; Ely, E.W.; et al. Efficacy and safety of recombinant human activated protein C for severe sepsis. *N. Engl. J. Med.* **2001**, *344*, 699–709. [CrossRef] [PubMed]
43. Vincent, J.L.; Ramesh, M.K.; Ernest, D.; LaRosa, S.P.; Pachl, J.; Aikawa, N.; Hoste, E.; Levy, H.; Hirman, J.; Levi, M.; et al. A randomized, double-blind, placebo-controlled, Phase 2b study to evaluate the safety and efficacy of recombinant human soluble thrombomodulin, ART-123, in patients with sepsis and suspected disseminated intravascular coagulation. *Crit. Care Med.* **2013**, *41*, 2069–2079. [CrossRef] [PubMed]

44. Sadjadi, J.; Cureton, E.L.; Twomey, P.; Victorino, G.P. Transfusion, not just injury severity, leads to posttrauma infection: A matched cohort study. *Am. Surg.* **2009**, *75*, 307–312. [PubMed]
45. Claridge, J.A.; Sawyer, R.G.; Schulman, A.M.; McLemore, E.C.; Young, J.S. Blood transfusions correlate with infections in trauma patients in a dose-dependent manner. *Am. Surg.* **2002**, *68*, 566–572. [PubMed]
46. Taylor, R.W.; O'Brien, J.; Trottier, S.J.; Manganaro, L.; Cytron, M.; Lesko, M.F.; Arnzen, K.; Cappadoro, C.; Fu, M.; Plisco, M.S.; et al. Red blood cell transfusions and nosocomial infections in critically ill patients. *Crit. Care Med.* **2006**, *34*, 2302–2308, quiz 9. [CrossRef]
47. Patel, S.V.; Kidane, B.; Klingel, M.; Parry, N. Risks associated with red blood cell transfusion in the trauma population, a meta-analysis. *Injury* **2014**, *45*, 1522–1533. [CrossRef]
48. Jongerius, I.; Porcelijn, L.; van Beek, A.E.; Semple, J.W.; van der Schoot, C.E.; Vlaar, A.P.J.; Kapur, R. The Role of Complement in Transfusion-Related Acute Lung Injury. *Trans. Med. Rev.* **2019**, *33*, 236–242. [CrossRef]
49. Semple, J.W.; Rebetz, J.; Kapur, R. Transfusion-associated circulatory overload and transfusion-related acute lung injury. *Blood* **2019**, *133*, 1840–1853. [CrossRef]

Journal of
Clinical Medicine

MDPI

Article

Regulatory T Cells Modulate CD4 Proliferation after Severe Trauma via IL-10

Ramona Sturm [1], Lara Xanthopoulos [1,2], David Heftrig [2,3], Elsie Oppermann [4], Teodora Vrdoljak [5], Ildiko Rita Dunay [6], Ingo Marzi [1] and Borna Relja [2,*]

1 Department of Trauma Surgery, Goethe University, 60590 Frankfurt, Germany; Ramona.Sturm@kgu.de (R.S.); lara_x_@hotmail.de (L.X.); Ingo.Marzi@kgu.de (I.M.)
2 Experimental Radiology, Department of Radiology and Nuclear Medicine, Otto von Guericke University, 39120 Magdeburg, Germany; davidheftrig@googlemail.com
3 Clinic for Radiology, Neuroradiology and Nuclear Medicine, Klinikum Frankfurt Höchst, 60590 Frankfurt, Germany
4 Department of General and Visceral Surgery, University Hospital Frankfurt, Goethe-University, 60590 Frankfurt, Germany; Oppermann@em.uni-frankfurt.de
5 Department of Diagnostic and Interventional Radiology, University Hospital Dubrava, University of Zagreb School of Medicine, 10000 Zagreb, Croatia; Tea.Vrdoljak@gmail.com
6 Institute of Inflammation and Neurodegeneration, Otto von Guericke University Magdeburg, 39120 Magdeburg, Germany; ildiko.dunay@med.ovgu.de
* Correspondence: Borna.Relja@med.ovgu.de; Tel.: +49-391-67-28242

Received: 7 March 2020; Accepted: 3 April 2020; Published: 8 April 2020

Abstract: Objective: Severely injured patients frequently develop an immunological imbalance following the traumatic insult, which might result in infectious complications evoked by a persisting immunosuppression. Regulatory T cells (Tregs) maintain the immune homeostasis by suppressing proinflammatory responses, however, their functionality after trauma is unclear. Here, we characterized the role of Tregs in regulating the proliferation of $CD4^+$ lymphocytes in traumatized patients (TP). Methods: Peripheral blood was obtained daily from 29 severely injured TP (Injury Severity Score, ISS ≥16) for ten days following admission to the emergency department (ED). Ten healthy volunteers (HV) served as controls. The frequency and activity of Tregs were assessed by flow cytometry. Proliferation of $CD4^+$ cells was analyzed either in presence or absence of Tregs, or after blocking of either IL-10 or IL-10R1. Results: The frequencies of $CD4^+CD25^{high}$ and $CD4^+CD25^+CD127^-$ Tregs were significantly decreased immediately upon admission of TP to the ED and during the following 10 post-injury days. Compared with HV $CD4^+$ T cell proliferation in TP increased significantly upon their admission and on the following days. As expected, $CD4^+CD25^+CD127^-$ Tregs reduced the proliferation of $CD4^+$ cells in HV, nevertheless, $CD4^+$ proliferation in TP was increased by Tregs. Neutralization of IL-10 as well as blocking the IL-10R1 increased further $CD4^+$ T cell proliferation in Tregs-depleted cultures, thereby confirming an IL-10-mediated mechanism of IL-10-regulated $CD4^+$ T cell proliferation. Neutralization of IL-10 in TP decreased $CD4^+$ T cell proliferation in Tregs-depleted cultures, whereas blocking of the IL-10R1 receptor had no significant effects. Conclusions: The frequency of Tregs in the $CD4^+$ T lymphocyte population is reduced after trauma; however, their inductiveness is increased. The mechanisms of deregulated influence of Tregs on $CD4^+$ T cell proliferation are mediated via IL-10 but not via the IL-10R1.

Keywords: proliferation; lymphocytes; regulatory T cells; polytrauma; IL-10

1. Introduction

With an incidence of 10%, trauma represents one of the most common causes of death worldwide, and it remains the leading cause of death in young patients (<40 years of age) [1,2]. The most frequent causes of post-traumatic mortality which occurs within the first 72 h after the insult are caused by severe injuries to the central nervous system and/or hemorrhagic shock due to a significant blood loss. On the contrary, late post-injury mortality is often caused by secondary complications including sepsis, acute respiratory distress syndrome, and/or multiple organ dysfunction syndrome [3–5]. In the past, significant improvements in pre-clinical and clinical treatment strategies slightly reduced the post-traumatic mortality, particularly by addressing hemorrhagic shock, however, the rate of multiple organ failure induced by infectious complications has increased [5,6].

The multifactorial biological response to tissue injury after severe trauma triggers an uncontrolled inflammatory reaction. Endogenous damage-associated molecular patterns as well as pathogen-associated molecular patterns activate effector cells of the innate immunity [7–13]. In parallel, a counterbalancing anti-inflammatory response syndrome (CARS) can develop [12,14]. Thus, traumatized patients remain at risk for the development of a persistent inflammation, immunosuppression and catabolism syndrome (PICS) [15]. Neither cellular nor humoral mechanisms of the post-traumatic immunosuppression are fully understood. Depending on the prevailing cytokine milieu T cells develop either into the proinflammatory TH1 or the anti-inflammatory TH2 cell type. IL-10 and its inhibitory potency have been associated with a TH1/TH2 shift, which seems to be mediated by regulatory T cells (Tregs) [16–19]. In 1995, Sakaguchi et al. identified a subpopulation of $CD4^+$ T cells in mice that continuously expressed the α-chain of the IL-2 receptor (CD25) [20]. These Tregs can also be defined by the absence of the α-chain of the IL-7 receptor (CD127) [21,22] and by the expression of the transcription factor Forkhead box (Fox)P3 [23]. In the field of trauma research, different combinations mainly of the cellular surface markers have been applied to detect Tregs, however, a unified definition of Tregs according to their antigen expression has not been found yet [24,25]. With regard to their functions, it is known that Tregs can modulate and kill antigen presenting cells as well as effector T cells, and thus, that they may affect both innate and adaptive immunity [26]. It was demonstrated that the activity and percentage of Tregs were increased after trauma, but that their absolute numbers were reduced [25,27]. Interestingly, it was shown that anti-inflammatory cytokine IL-10 increased significantly in septic patients [28–30]. Stratifying major surgical patients to those who develop sepsis versus those without complications has uncovered that the last had significantly reduced IL-10 levels [31]. Aligned with these findings, IL-10 levels were elevated in traumatized patients with complications compared to those without complication [32]. Taken together, previous reports suggest that IL-10 is critically involved in immunosuppression following trauma, and further, that it is associated with the occurrence of post-traumatic complications. While the production of IL-10 by $CD4^+CD25^+$ cells was significantly reduced, the IL-10 production by Tregs was increased after trauma [24]. Thus, it appears reasonable that both IL-10 and Tregs play significant roles in the onset of post-traumatic immunosuppression. Yet, whether the inhibition of T cell-mediated inflammation is potentially regulated by Tregs or IL-10 itself deriving from other cells still remains unclear. However, to prevent infectious complications in traumatized patients, it is crucial to understand the mechanistical background of the post-traumatic immunosuppression.

2. Experimental Section

2.1. Ethics

This study was performed in the University Hospital of the Goethe-University Frankfurt with institutional ethics committee approval (312/10) in accordance with the Declaration of Helsinki and following the Strengthening the Reporting of Observational Studies in Epidemiology guidelines [33]. All enrolled patients or their legally authorized representative and all healthy volunteers signed the written informed consent form.

2.2. Study Setting and Population

Twenty-nine severely injured traumatized patients (TP) between 18 and 80 years of age with an Injury Severity Score (ISS) ≥16 were enrolled into this study immediately at admittance to the emergency department (ED). Inclusion criteria covered acute blunt or penetrating trauma. Exclusion criteria were pre-existing immunological disorders, HIV, infectious hepatitis, immune-suppressive medication, acute myocardial infarction, burns and/or thromboembolic events. Ten healthy volunteers served as controls.

2.3. Study Protocol

At admittance to the ED all TP were treated according to the polytrauma guidelines. Vital parameters were recorded. The ISS was determined based on the Abbreviated Injury Scale [34,35] of the six body regions. The sum of the squares of the three most severely injured body regions was applied to generate the overall injury severity (ISS).

2.4. Blood Sampling

Blood samples were taken as early as possible after admittance of the patient to the ED and daily for the following ten days between 7 and 11 a.m. Blood was withdrawn in ethylenediaminetetraacetic acid (EDTA) tubes (Sarstedt, Nürmbrecht, Germany) and kept either at room temperature for functional assays or on ice for flow cytometric analyses.

2.5. Analyses of Cell Surface Receptors

After the blood samples (100 µl) were transferred into polystyrene Falcon tubes (BD PharMingen, San Diego, CA, USA), they were diluted with 395 µl RPMI 1640 (Gibco) and finally 5 µl of the leukocyte activation cocktail (LAC, BD PharMingen, San Diego, CA, USA) were added. The samples were incubated for 5 h at 37 °C and 5% CO_2. Corresponding samples without stimulation served as controls. Centrifugation continued at 400× *g* for 5 min and the supernatants were removed. One hundred microliters of the Fix & Perm Solution A (Fix & Perm (R) ADG-GAS-002) for the intracellular staining were added. After 15 min at room temperature, cells were washed with phosphate-buffered saline (PBS), and centrifugation step followed at 400× *g* for 5 min. The supernatants were removed and 100 µL of the Fix & Perm Solution B were added. The samples were incubated for 30 min at room temperature in the dark with mouse anti-human CD4 Brilliant Violett (Clone RPA-T4, BD Bioscience, San Diego, CA, USA), mouse anti-human CD127 PerCP-Cy5.5 (Clone HIL-7R-M21, BD Bioscience, San Diego, CA, USA), mouse anti-human CD25 APC-Cy7 (Clone BC 96, BD Bioscience, San Diego, CA, USA), and mouse anti-human FoxP3 PE-Cy7 (Clone PCH101, BD Bioscience, San Diego, CA, USA) antibodies. Subsequently, 2 mL of the FACS lysing solution (BD PharMingen, San Diego, CA, USA) were added for additional 10 min. Then samples were washed twice with FACS buffer (PBS supplemented with 0.5% bovine serum albumin, BSA). Supernatants were removed, cells were diluted in 300 µl FACS buffer and immediately subjected to flow cytometric analyses with a BD FACS Canto II using a FACS DIVA software (BD, San Diego, CA, USA). The lymphocytes were defined by gating $CD4^+$ cells in the corresponding forward and side scatter scan. Positively gated cells were determined by their absolute cell numbers and the percentage of the selected parietal cell population were measured. Gating strategy is shown in Figure 1.

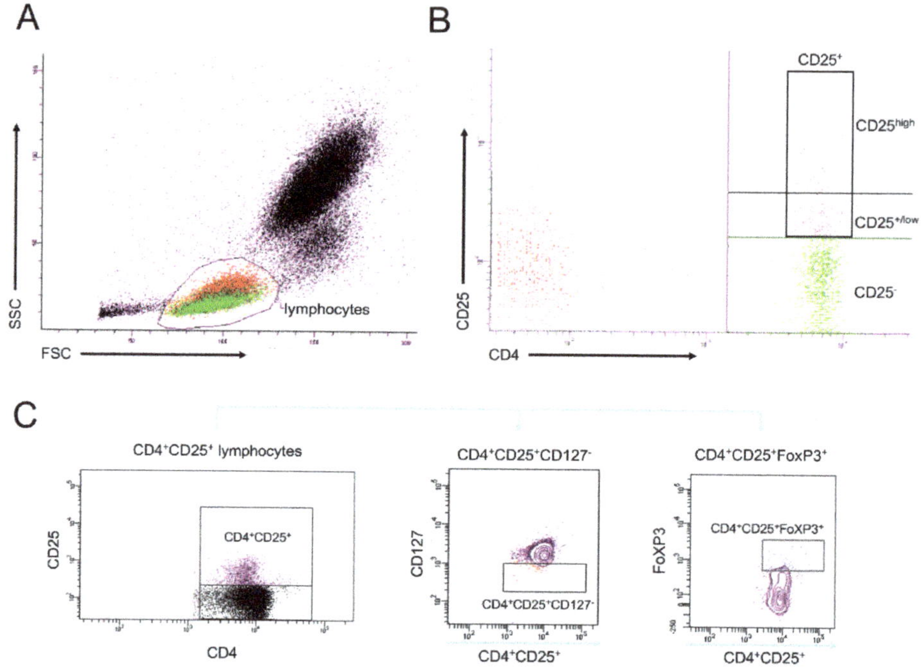

Figure 1. Gating strategy for the flow cytometric analysis. (**A**): Gating of the lymphocyte fraction in peripheral blood according to the forward and side scatter. (**B**): Gating for the detection of $CD4^+CD25^+$ cells. (**C**): Gating of the lymphocytes according to their CD4 and CD25 expression and subsequently of CD127 and FoxP3 expressing cells.

2.6. Isolation of $CD4^+$ Cells Including Tregs

$CD4^+$ leukocytes were isolated using Ficoll density gradient centrifugation (Ficoll solution, 1.077 g/mL; Biochrom GmbH, Berlin, Germany) at 800× g for 20 min at room temperature without break. Then, the mononuclear cell layer in the interface was removed and cells were washed twice with MACS buffer (PBS + BSA 0.5% + EDTA 2 mM). Leukocytes were isolated by negative selection using a Biotin-Antibody-Cocktail including CD8a, CD14, CD15, CD16, CD19, CD36, CD56, CD132, TcRγ/δ, and CD235a (CD4 T-cell Isolation Kit, Miltenyi Biotec, Bergisch Gladbach, Germany) according to the manufacturer's instructions. Also, CD71 and CD8 were removed by using CD71 and CD8 MicroBeads (Miltenyi Biotec Bergisch Gladbach, Germany). Subsequently, cells were applied for the proliferation assay of $CD4^+$ cells including Tregs.

2.7. Isolation of $CD4^+$ Cells without Tregs

After their isolation, $CD4^+$ cells were incubated with CD127 MicroBeads (Miltenyi Biotec, Bergisch Gladbach, Germany) for negative selection. $CD4^+CD127^+$ cells were removed from the column and placed on ice. Briefly, Tregs were isolated by incubating the $CD4^+CD127^-$ cells with CD25 MicroBeads (Miltenyi Biotec, Bergisch Gladbach, Germany) by positive selection. The flow through with $CD4^+CD127^-CD25^-$ cells constituted with pre-gained $CD4^+CD127^+$ cells the $CD4^+$ leukocyte population without Tregs.

2.8. Proliferation of Lymphocytes in a CD4$^+$ Culture with and without Tregs

Following their isolation, CD4$^+$ T cells with Tregs as well as CD4$^+$ T cells without Tregs were immediately used for experiments. 50,000 cells were diluted in 200 µl RPMI-1640 (with supplements of penicillin-streptomycin, gentamycinsulfate, and heat inactivated FBS) and seeded in 96-well plates (BD Biosciences, Franklin Lakes, NJ, USA). Previously, the wells were coated with anti-CD3 (2 µg/mL, BD PharMingen, Heidelberg, Germany) for 24 h at 4 °C. For co-stimulation of T cells, anti-CD28 (100 µg/mL, BD PharMingen, San Diego, CA, USA) was applied at the experimental day. IgG1κ Isotype Control Purified and NA/LE Mouse 107.3 were used as corresponding isotype controls (BD PharMingen, San Diego, CA, USA). For IL-10 neutralization or IL-10 receptor blocking, anti-IL-10 (JES3-19F1) or anti-IL10-receptor (3F9, 500 µg/mL, BD Bioscience, San Diego, CA, USA) antibodies were added. IgG2a Isotype Control Purified NA/LE Rat R35-95 antibody was used as control (BD PharMingen, San Diego, CA, USA). After 24 h at 37 °C and 5% CO_2 100 µl of the culture medium were replaced and either the anti-IL-10 or the anti-IL10-receptor antibody were added again. After 48 h supernatants were removed and cells were treated with the BrdU labeling solution (Cell Proliferation ELISA BrdU, La Roche, Basel, Switzerland) according to the manufacturer's instructions. The proliferation rates were detected by measuring the colorimetry using a Tecan microplate reader and Magellan software.

2.9. Statistical Analysis

GraphPad Prism 6.0 software (GraphPad Software Inc. San Diego, CA, USA) was used to perform the statistical analysis. Data are given as mean ± standard error of the mean (SEM) or as absolute cell numbers calculated in percent. A Student's *t*-test with Welch correction and one-way analysis of variance (ANOVA) with a Dunn post-hoc test was used for comparisons among the groups. A p value below 0.05 was considered statistically significant.

3. Results

3.1. Main Findings

3.1.1. Study Population

Twenty-nine patients with severe trauma (TP) and 10 healthy volunteers (HV) were enrolled in this study. The mean age of the patients was 44.6 ± 2.3 versus 37.6 ± 1.7 years of age. Seventy-five percent of patients were male. All patients were substantially injured with an ISS of 30.3 ± 2.3. The mean stay in the intensive care unit was 9.7 ± 2.6 days, and the total duration of the in-hospital stay was 19.3 ± 3.4 days. The data is comparable to mean values of the multiply injured trauma patients as demonstrated before [36,37].

3.1.2. Frequencies of Differentially Defined Tregs after Trauma

Of all CD4$^+$ lymphocytes from HV, 6.9% had low CD25 expression. TPs had significantly lower percentage of CD4$^+$CD25$^{+/low}$ lymphocytes in total leukocyte population at admission to the ED compared to ctrl ($p < 0.05$, Figure 2A), and this difference persisted during the complete observational time course (Figure 2A). LAC stimulation increased significantly the presence of CD4$^+$CD25$^{+/low}$ in HV to 12.9% compared to unstimulated samples from ctrl ($p < 0.05$). The low presence of CD4$^+$CD25$^{+/low}$ cells in TP was significantly enhanced after LAC stimulation compared to unstimulated samples from TP during the complete observational course ($p < 0.05$). Upon stimulation, the presence of CD4$^+$CD25$^{+/low}$ increased significantly compared to unstimulated samples over the ten days course and remained in the range of stimulated samples from HV (Figure 2A).

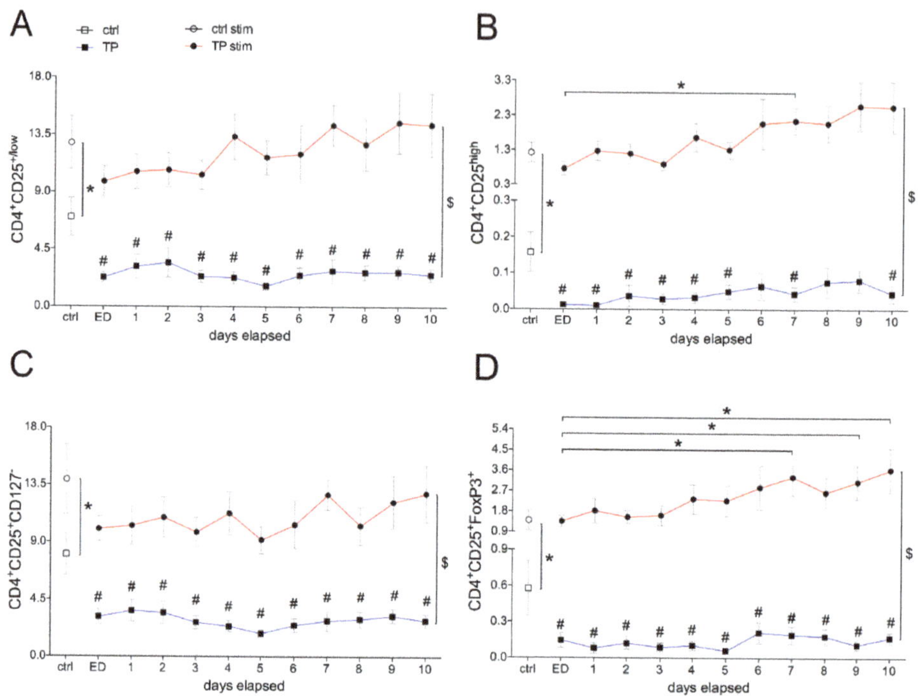

Figure 2. Whole blood from healthy volunteers (ctrl, $n = 10$, clear symbols) or major trauma patients (TP, $n = 29$, black symbols) was analyzed by flow cytometry over a 10-day time course after admission (emergency department, ED-10). Regulatory T cells (Tregs) were detected using anti-human CD4 and CD25 in the corresponding side and forward scatter. Unstimulated (square) and stimulated (circle, stim) cells were measured. Data are shown as mean ± SEM percentage of lymphocytes. (**A**): $CD4^+CD25^{+/low}$ Tregs to $CD4^+$ lymphocytes; (**B**): $CD4^+CD25^{+/high}$ Tregs to $CD4^+$ lymphocytes; (**C**): $CD4^+CD25^+CD127^-$ Tregs to $CD4^+$ lymphocytes; (**D**): $CD4^+CD25^+FoxP3^+$ Tregs to $CD4^+$ lymphocytes. $p < 0.05$ * vs. indicated #; unstimulated TP vs. unstimulated crtl $; stimulated TP vs. unstimulated TP.

The proportion of $CD4^+CD25^{+/high}$ cells was significantly reduced compared to ctrl immediately upon admission to the ED and remained diminished during the complete observational period (Figure 2B). In vitro stimulation increased significantly the proportion of $CD4^+CD25^{+/high}$ cells compared with unstimulated samples in both groups. Upon stimulation at post-injury day 7, the presence of $CD4^+CD25^{+/high}$ cells in TP was significantly enhanced compared to stimulated samples from ctrl (Figure 2B).

During the whole observational period, the ratio of $CD4^+CD25^+CD127^-$ cells to total CD4 lymphocytes remained significantly lower in TP compared to ctrl ($p < 0.05$, Figure 2C). After the in vitro stimulation with LAC, $CD4^+CD25^+CD127^-$ cells increased significantly in both TP and ctrl compared to the corresponding unstimulated samples ($p < 0.05$, Figure 2C).

During the whole observational period of ten days, the ratio of $CD4^+CD25^+FoxP3^+$ cells to total CD4 lymphocytes remained significantly lower in TP compared to ctrl ($p < 0.05$, Figure 2D). After the in vitro stimulation with LAC, $CD4^+CD25^+FoxP3^+$ cells increased significantly in both TP and ctrl compared to the corresponding unstimulated samples ($p < 0.05$, Figure 2D). Upon stimulation at post-injury days 7, 9, and 10, the presence of $CD4^+CD25^+FoxP3^+$ cells in TP was significantly enhanced compared to stimulated samples from ctrl ($p < 0.05$, Figure 2D).

3.1.3. Proliferation of CD4+ Cells Depending on Tregs

Depletion of Tregs out of the CD4+ lymphocyte population significantly increased the CD4+ T cell proliferation compared to CD4+ cells which still contained the Tregs fraction ($p < 0.05$, Figure 3A).

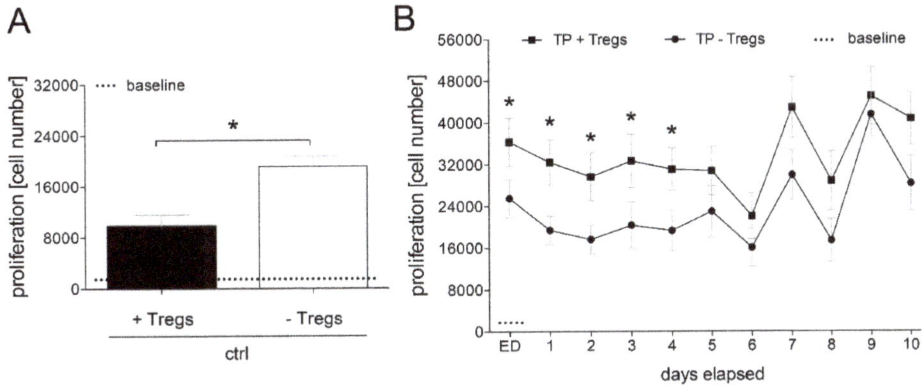

Figure 3. CD4+ T lymphocytes were isolated from healthy volunteers (ctrl) or major trauma patients (TP) and depleted from regulatory T cells (Tregs) over a 10-day time course after admission (emergency department, ED-10). (**A**): The proliferation rates in absolute cell numbers of CD4+ cells with (+) and without (−) Tregs in healthy volunteers and in (**B**): severely traumatized patients is shown. Data are shown as mean ± SEM. $p < 0.05$ *; +Tregs vs. −Tregs.

The proliferation rate of CD4+ cells containing the Tregs fraction was significantly enhanced in TP during the whole observational period compared to ctrl ($p < 0.05$). Immediately at admission of the TP to the ED as well as during the first four post-injury days, depletion of Tregs out of the CD4+ lymphocyte population significantly decreased the CD4+ T cell proliferation compared to CD4+ with Tregs ($p < 0.05$, Figure 3B).

3.1.4. Tregs-Mediated Proliferation of CD4+ Cells Depends on IL-10

The proliferation rate of CD4+ lymphocytes depleted from Tregs was significantly increased compared to the co-culture of CD4+ cells and Tregs in HV ctrl ($p < 0.05$, Figure 4). The proliferation rate of CD4+ lymphocytes depleted from Tregs was significantly decreased compared to the co-culture of CD4+ cells and Tregs in TP at admission to the ED ($p < 0.05$, Figure 4).

To determine the infuence of IL-10 on the Tregs regulated proliferative behavior of CD4+ cells, either IL-10 was neutralized or the IL-10R1 has been blocked. In the ctrl group, both neutralization of IL-10 as well as blocking the IL-10R1 in Tregs-depleted CD4+ cultures increased further and significantly the proliferation rates compared to the proliferation rate of the Tregs depleted CD4+ culture ($p < 0.05$). No significant differences in proliferation were observed between the IL-10-neutralized or IL-10R1-blocked Tregs-depleted CD4+ cells in ctrl (Figure 4). Furthermore, the control experiments with CD4+ cells containing Tregs population and undergoing both IL-10 as well as IL-10R1 neutralization show that Tregs apparently suppress the T cell proliferation by direct cell contacts, since the results were comparable to proliferation rates from the untreated controls without Tregs depletion. However, considering the above described results, both IL-10 or IL-10R1 do play a suppressive role in T cell proliferation under control conditions.

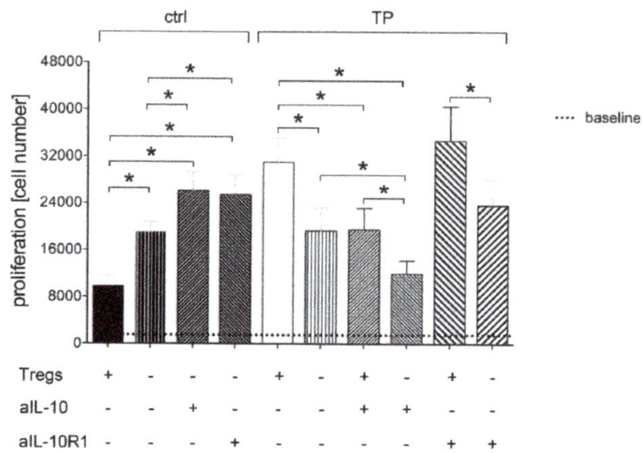

Figure 4. The proliferation rates in absolute cell numbers of $CD4^+$ cells with (+) and without (−) regulatory T cells (Tregs) in healthy volunteers (ctrl, $n = 10$) and severely traumatized patients (TP, $n = 25$) as well as depending on IL-10 neutralization (aIL-10) and IL-10 receptor blockade (aIL-10R1) is shown. Data are shown as mean ± SEM. $p < 0.05$ * vs. indicated.

Significantly increased proliferation rate of $CD4^+$ lymphocytes including Tregs versus Tregs-depleted $CD4^+$ cells in TP was significantly decreased upon the neutralization of IL-10 ($p < 0.05$, Figure 4). There was no difference in the proliferation rate between Tregs-containing $CD4^+$ cell culture with IL-10 neutralization and Tregs-depleted $CD4^+$ cell culture without IL-10 neutralization in TP. Nevertheless, the proliferation rate in Tregs-depleted $CD4^+$ cell culture with IL-10 neutralization was significantly reduced compared to Tregs-depleted $CD4^+$ cell culture in TP at ED ($p < 0.05$, Figure 4). The data indicate that IL-10 can reduce the $CD4^+$ lymphocyte proliferation irrespective of the presence of Tregs in the cell culture in TP at ED.

Significantly increased proliferation rate of $CD4^+$ lymphocytes including Tregs versus Tregs-depleted $CD4^+$ cells in TP was not changed upon blocking of the IL-10R1 in TP at ED (Figure 4). These data indicate that IL-10R1 does not mediate the effects on the $CD4^+$ lymphocyte proliferation in TP at ED which were induced by Tregs.

Briefly, the proliferation rate of Tregs-depleted $CD4^+$ lymphocytes was statistically comparable between ctrl and TP (Figure 4). However, while the neutralization of IL-10 in Tregs-depleted $CD4^+$ lymphocytes significantly increased the proliferation rate in ctrl, the same approach significantly reduced the proliferation of Tregs-depleted $CD4^+$ lymphocytes in TP at ED ($p < 0.05$, Figure 4).

While blocking of the IL-10R1 in Tregs-depleted $CD4^+$ lymphocytes significantly increased the proliferation rate in ctrl ($p < 0.05$), the same experimental approach resulted in comparable results in cells which were obtained from TP at ED, although the last was not significant (Figure 4).

4. Discussion

Aim of the present study was to phenotype Tregs after polytrauma and to determine their ratio in the cellular fraction of $CD4^+$ lymphocytes over an observational period of ten post-injury days. In addition, the underlying mechanism of Tregs-modulated proliferation of T cells via IL-10 or the IL-10 receptor, respectively, were elaborated after polytrauma.

Particularly the functions of $CD4^+$ T cells, which are essential for an effective defense against invading pathogens after trauma are reduced during CARS or PICS [15]. Thus, this immunological imbalance might result in serious complications, sepsis and (multiple) organ failure in the later post-injury phase. T cell suppression was associated with an increased rate of complications as well as enhanced mortality rates after severe injury [32]. Interestingly, an increased number of Tregs, which can inhibit T cell proliferation and their functions via IL-10 as well as increased IL-10 levels were associated with the development of post-traumatic complications and mortality [25,38–40]. A reduced number of Tregs with their increased activity after trauma were reported [27]. Previous studies report an increased proportion of Tregs in the CD4$^+$ T cell population after polytrauma [24]. Still, there is a lack of continuous follow-up studies regarding the frequency of Tregs in the CD4$^+$ T cell population and a comparison of the differentially and still inconsistently defined Tregs populations after polytrauma. Besides, it is also unclear whether Tregs exerts their inhibiting effects on the proliferative capacity of CD4$^+$ lymphocytes via IL-10 after severe injury. There are suggestions that Tregs inhibit T cell proliferation via TGF-β and IL-10 [39,41]. However, other studies propose that Tregs inhibit T cell proliferation via direct cell contacts independently of IL-10 [42]. Our control experiments also show that Tregs apparently suppress the T cell proliferation by direct cell contacts as already demonstrated by Levings et al. [42]. Although the authors suggest that Tregs inhibit T cell proliferation via direct cell contacts independently of IL-10, in our study both IL-10 or IL-10R1 do play a suppressive role in T cell proliferation under control conditions. Despite the depletion of Tregs, neutralization of both IL-10 as well as IL-10R1 further increased T cell proliferation. On the contrary, the suppressive activity of Tregs on T cell proliferation might not be triggered by direct cell contacts. Under traumatic conditions depletion of Tregs reduced T cell proliferation, which is a paradox in their natural and characteristic functions. In line with this, the presence of Tregs increased T cell proliferation. Blocking IL-10 in presence of Tregs reduced proliferation, though a depletion of Tregs with IL-10 blocking further decreased T cell proliferation. In summary, the direct proliferation-suppression which is observed under control conditions in healthy volunteers appears to be deregulated in trauma, and in this setting, IL-10 may be involved in the changed functionality of Tregs. Since IL-10R1 blockade under traumatic conditions has provided comparable results to healthy volunteers, the data suggest that the receptor exerts its functions. Thus, the results propose that the cell contact dependent suppression of T cell proliferation via Tregs may be closely linked to IL-10, and furthermore, that it may be associated with its unknown functions under traumatic conditions. Thus, the impact of Tregs on the T cell proliferation in polytraumatized patients and potential role of IL-10 still remain unknown.

MacConmara et al. examined the distribution and activation markers of Tregs in the lymphocyte population using peripheral blood from 19 polytraumatized patients (ISS: 36.6 ± 13.9) within 24 h after admission to the emergency department and after 7 days [24]. In contrast to the results of our study, the proportion of CD25-expressing cells immediately after trauma was comparable to healthy volunteers. At day 7, the proportion of CD25$^+$ cells and CD25$^{+/high}$ cells increased significantly, data that were not confirmed by our study since we did not observe an increase in the CD25$^+$ population. On the contrary, this specific population was reduced immediately at admission and during the ten post-injury days. However, the ex vivo in vitro stimulation induced Tregs. In the paper by MacConmara et al., the higher injury severity of their patients with enhanced complication rates may have induced these cells.

Hein et al. demonstrated that the absolute number of CD4$^+$CD25$^+$CD127$^-$ Tregs decreased immediately after a septic shock, but their proportion out of CD4$^+$ cells remained the same compared to healthy volunteers [25]. After 3 days, however, both the proportion and their absolute number increased. One week later, the absolute number of Tregs was comparable to healthy volunteers, but their percentage remained elevated due to the severe lymphopenia in septic patients [25]. In our study, there was a significant decrease of CD4$^+$CD25$^+$CD127$^-$ and CD4$^+$CD25$^{+/high}$ Tregs already at admission to the emergency department which persisted for the following 10 days. The data from Hein et al. demonstrated that lymphopenia was more pronounced in septic patients compared to non-septic patients, which actually have been mainly analyzed in our study. This might explain why the percentage of Tregs in our work was lower. Thus, based on the current literature, Tregs do have an important but not yet profoundly characterized role during the post-traumatic inflammation. They may be an important determinant of both extent and severity of the post-traumatic immunosuppression [18,43]. Since most patients dying from severe clinical problems including sepsis show signs of immunosuppression [44], there are reasonable suggestions that Tregs play an important role in the development of infectious complications after trauma. It has been demonstrated that both their number and functions increase following the onset of severe sepsis or septic shock [43]. In burn trauma models it has been shown that severe burn injury per se could change Tregs activities. As demonstrated by increased levels of cytokines produced by those cells and their activation markers, they might play an important role in the pathogenesis of sepsis as well as mortality in patients suffering from burn injuries [45]. Recently, Kramer et al. have demonstrated that the depletion of Tregs attenuated T cell brain infiltration, reactive astrogliosis, interferon-γ gene expression, and transiently motor deficits in murine acute traumatic brain injury [46]. Thus, the current literature does suggest that regulatory T cells contribute to post-traumatic complications, however, in our study only two patients during their stay in the intensive care unit have been diagnosed with sepsis. It is not possible to perform any statistical evaluations based on two patients, and therefore, further studies with a larger number of septic patients after trauma are required to clarify the importance of Tregs in post-traumatic sepsis.

Interestingly, our results are comparable to data obtained from a trauma model in rats consisting of a bilateral femoral fracture and hemorrhagic shock [47]. Four hours after trauma induction, the number of $CD4^+CD25^{+/high}FoxP3^+$ Tregs in peripheral blood was significantly lower compared to controls. In addition, the number of Tregs correlated negatively with the histological extent of injury severity [47].

When interpreting our data regarding the cell phenotype, we must indicate the application of LAC with Phorbol 12-Myristate 13-Acetate (PMA) and a calcium ionophore Ionomycin (PMA/Iono) for stimulation, which is commonly used for the detection of intracellular accumulations of cytokines by intracellular staining. Although the applied PMA/Iono stimulation is mainly utilized to elicit a primary cytokine response or intracellular proteins from T cells, its use does also activate Tregs. In line, Wang et al. have shown that regulatory T cells of the $CD4^+CD25^+FoxP3^+CD127^-$ phenotype were inducible by PMA/Iono stimulation [48]. This phenotype is comparable to those that have been detected in our study. Although CD3CD4 expression was suppressed by PMA/Iono, the proportion of CD4CD25FoxP3CD127 increased after PMA/Iono stimulation as shown by Wang et al. [48]. In addition, this data demonstrates that polyclonal stimulation using PMA/Iono can induce CD4CD25FoxP3IL-2 Treg in vitro. Another study described four phenotypically determined regulatory T cell phenotypes in peripheral blood lymphocytes, which were commonly characterized as $CD4^+CD25^{high}$, $CD4^+CD25^{high}FoxP3^+$, $CD4^+CD25^{high}CD127^-$, or $CD4^+CD25^{high}FoxP3^+CD127^-$ cells were increased upon PMA/Iono stimulation [49]. Importantly, PMA/Iono can also reduce antigen surface expression and specifically CD4 expression as demonstrated by Wang et al. and others [50–52]. Importantly, it has also been shown that the proportion of $FoxP3^+CD127^-$ peripheral blood lymphocytes increased with the quantity of CD25 on stimulated $CD4^+$ peripheral blood lymphocytes, and was highest in $CD25^{high}$ peripheral blood lymphocytes, emphasizing the relevance of $CD25^{high}$ as regulatory T cell marker [49]. Briefly, the data show that although CD3CD4 expression is suppressed by PMA/Iono, the proportion of CD4CD25FoxP3CD127 increases after PMA/Iono stimulation. These data as well as considering that the ratio of regulatory T cells to lymphocytes specifically expressing CD4 was evaluated in our study, the approach is reasonable. However, PMA/Iono as the standard polyclonal stimulus for T cell and inducible Treg [53] down-regulating CD4 expression quickly and severely must be considered as an important disadvantage for certain studies requiring separation of regulatory T cells. This was considered in our methodological settings, and therefore, Tregs have been separated from the T cell population before any stimuli were applied.

A post-traumatic anergy of $CD4^+$ T cells with their reduced numbers and activity has been described. Interestingly, despite CD3/CD28 stimulation, T cells isolated from severely injured patients with multiple organ dysfunction syndromes were not able to proliferate post-traumatically. In the present study, however, a significant post-traumatic increase in $CD4^+$ T cell proliferation was observed. Only by depleting Tregs from the $CD4^+$ T cell population reduced their proliferative capacity after trauma. With regard to the post-traumatic $CD4^+$ T cells anergy, it must be considered that no distinction was made between different T cell subgroups, and thus, only certain $CD4^+$ T cell subsets may have shown post-traumatically altered proliferation.

Beacher-Allan et al. have shown that the suppressive properties of $CD4^+CD25^{+/high}$ Tregs and the suppressed proliferation depended on the concentration of the applied stimulant [38]. In summary, Tregs have a contrary effect on T cell proliferation in trauma patients compared to healthy volunteers. This effect may be caused by an altered functionality of Tregs or by an altered effect of Tregs-associated cytokines on $CD4^+$ T cells. IL-10 mediated inhibition of T cells mainly leads to the inhibition of TH1 cells and their pro-inflammatory cytokines such as IFN-γ [54]. Waal Malefyt et al. demonstrated that although T cell proliferation was stimulated by monocytes, IL-10 significantly inhibited the proliferation depending on its concentration [55]. Our results show that the inhibitory effect of Tregs on T cell proliferation can be eliminated by IL-10 neutralization in healthy volunteers. Taken together, the data suggests that Tregs may exert their inhibitory effects on T cell proliferation via IL-10, contradicting the assumption that Tregs act independently of IL-10. In trauma patients, increased IL-10 levels were associated with enhanced complication rates of sepsis, CARS and increased mortality [28,29]. Remarkably, our data indicate that IL-10 exerted proliferation-increasing effects, since its neutralization reduced proliferation rates after trauma. This intriguing observation in Tregs depleted $CD4^+$ cultures may have been caused by other proliferation-inhibiting $CD4^+$ T cell types that potentially produced IL-10. Our results suggest that Tregs inhibit T cell proliferation via IL-10. However, IL-10 mainly affects TH1 cells rather than TH2 and in trauma there are reports suggesting a shift of TH1 towards TH2 cells. This may explain why Tregs cannot affect T cell proliferation after trauma to the same extent as in healthy individuals.

With regard to the functions of IL-10 receptor in polytraumatized patients, there are only sparse data in the literature. Wang et al. described that the continuous IL-10R blockade in spleen cells of infected mice significantly increased the IL-10 concentration compared to healthy mice [56]. In addition, IL-10R blockade increased the secretion of pro-inflammatory cytokines, reduced the survival time as well as the amount and efficacy of Tregs [56]. However, we did not observe any significant differences in proliferative capacity after receptor blockade. The proliferation-increasing effect induced by Tregs after trauma was detectable despite blocking the IL-10 receptor. Thus, blocking the IL-10 receptor does not result in the same effects as IL-10 neutralization in traumatized patients. To define the exact role of IL-10 and its receptor in Tregs after polytrauma further in vivo studies will be required.

Limitations of this study certainly include the confined number of traumatized patients that have been involved. In addition, only two patients developed septic complications during their stay in the intensive care unit and two patients died. This kind of study utilizes medical personnel as well as costs to a great extent, since the development of post-traumatic complications is not predictable, and thus all patients must be included prospectively in the analyses before they develop complications. Thus, clarifying the specific role of Tregs as well as their altered functions in sepsis development or mortality after polytrauma must be elaborated in larger studies in future. Also, further in vivo studies to evaluate the mechanistical and pathophysiological role of IL-10 as well as assessing of potential therapeutic targeting strategies in this setting are necessary. Besides, with regard to the definition of Tregs in general, so far, no consensus was reached on the use of a specific set of markers when identifying Tregs in human and mice. We have chosen CD25 to stratify the different phenotypes and their dynamics, yet, it remains to be noted that we did not evaluate the direct immunosuppressive activity and functionality of different phenotypes, and that this remains to be elucidated in further studies as well.

Taken together, both regulatory T cells as well as IL-10 have different effects on $CD4^+$ T cell proliferation after trauma compared to healthy controls. Here, Tregs-induced $CD4^+$ T cell proliferation after trauma may be mediated by IL-10. On the contrary, IL-10 receptor does not appear to be directly involved in those effects of Tregs after trauma. The potential involvement of another receptor for IL-10 remains to be elaborated in further studies.

Author Contributions: Conceptualization, B.R.; methodology, R.S., L.X., D.H. and E.O.; formal analysis, B.R.; investigation, R.S.; data curation, R.S.; writing—original draft preparation, R.S.; writing—review and editing, T.V., I.R.D. and I.M.; visualization, T.V. and I.R.D.; supervision, B.R.; project administration, B.R. All authors have read and agreed to the published version of the manuscript.

Funding: This research received no external funding.

Acknowledgments: We thank the student assistants of the Department of Trauma, Hand and Reconstructive Surgery, Goethe University Frankfurt for their help in obtaining samples from patients. We thank Kerstin Kontradowitz and Katrin Jurida for their outstanding technical assistance.

Conflicts of Interest: The authors declare no conflict of interest.

References

1. Peden, M.; Hyder, A. Road traffic injuries are a global public health problem. *BMJ* **2002**, *324*, 1153. [CrossRef]
2. World Health Organization. *Injuries and Violence: The Facts 2014*; World Health Organization: Geneva, Switzerland, 2014; Available online: https://apps.who.int/iris/handle/10665/149798. (accessed on 7 March 2020).
3. Acosta, J.A.; Yang, J.C.; Winchell, R.J.; Simons, R.K.; Fortlage, D.A.; Hollingsworth-Fridlund, P.; Hoyt, D.B. Lethal injuries and time to death in a level I trauma center. *J. Am. Coll. Surg.* **1998**, *186*, 528–533. [CrossRef]
4. Pfeifer, R.; Tarkin, I.S.; Rocos, B.; Pape, H.C. Patterns of mortality and causes of death in polytrauma patients–has anything changed? *Injury* **2009**, *40*, 907–911. [CrossRef]
5. Probst, C.; Pape, H.C.; Hildebrand, F.; Regel, G.; Mahlke, L.; Giannoudis, P.; Krettek, C.; Grotz, M.R. 30 years of polytrauma care: An analysis of the change in strategies and results of 4849 cases treated at a single institution. *Injury* **2009**, *40*, 77–83. [CrossRef]
6. Spahn, D.R.; Bouillon, B.; Cerny, V.; Coats, T.J.; Duranteau, J.; Fernandez-Mondejar, E.; Filipescu, D.; Hunt, B.J.; Komadina, R.; Nardi, G.; et al. Management of bleeding and coagulopathy following major trauma: An updated European guideline. *Crit. Care* **2013**, *17*, R76. [CrossRef]
7. Giannoudis, P.V.; Mallina, R.; Harwood, P.; Perry, S.; Sante, E.D.; Pape, H.C. Pattern of release and relationship between HMGB-1 and IL-6 following blunt trauma. *Injury* **2010**, *41*, 1323–1327. [CrossRef]
8. Seong, S.Y.; Matzinger, P. Hydrophobicity: An ancient damage-associated molecular pattern that initiates innate immune responses. *Nat. Rev. Immunol.* **2004**, *4*, 469–478. [CrossRef]
9. Wutzler, S.; Lustenberger, T.; Relja, B.; Lehnert, M.; Marzi, I. Pathophysiology of multiple trauma: Intensive care medicine and timing of treatment. *Chirurg* **2013**, *84*, 753–758. [CrossRef]
10. Zhang, Q.; Raoof, M.; Chen, Y.; Sumi, Y.; Sursal, T.; Junger, W.; Brohi, K.; Itagaki, K.; Hauser, C.J. Circulating mitochondrial DAMPs cause inflammatory responses to injury. *Nature* **2010**, *464*, 104–107. [CrossRef]
11. Lenz, A.; Franklin, G.A.; Cheadle, W.G. Systemic inflammation after trauma. *Injury* **2007**, *38*, 1336–1345. [CrossRef]
12. Relja, B.; Land, W.G. Damage-associated molecular patterns in trauma. *Eur. J. Trauma Emerg. Surg.* **2019**, 1–25. [CrossRef] [PubMed]
13. Relja, B.; Mors, K.; Marzi, I. Danger signals in trauma. *Eur. J. Trauma Emerg. Surg.* **2018**, *44*, 301–336. [CrossRef] [PubMed]
14. Kasten, K.R.; Goetzman, H.S.; Reid, M.R.; Rasper, A.M.; Adediran, S.G.; Robinson, C.T.; Cave, C.M.; Solomkin, J.S.; Lentsch, A.B.; Johannigman, J.A.; et al. Divergent adaptive and innate immunological responses are observed in humans following blunt trauma. *BMC Immunol.* **2010**, *11*, 4. [CrossRef] [PubMed]
15. Gentile, L.F.; Cuenca, A.G.; Efron, P.A.; Ang, D.; Bihorac, A.; McKinley, B.A.; Moldawer, L.L.; Moore, F.A. Persistent inflammation and immunosuppression: A common syndrome and new horizon for surgical intensive care. *J. Trauma Acute Care Surg.* **2012**, *72*, 1491–1501. [CrossRef]
16. Fiorentino, D.F.; Bond, M.W.; Mosmann, T.R. Two types of mouse T helper cell. IV. Th2 clones secrete a factor that inhibits cytokine production by Th1 clones. *J. Exp. Med.* **1989**, *170*, 2081–2095. [CrossRef]
17. Marik, P.E.; Flemmer, M. The immune response to surgery and trauma: Implications for treatment. *J. Trauma Acute Care Surg.* **2012**, *73*, 801–808. [CrossRef]
18. Venet, F.; Chung, C.S.; Monneret, G.; Huang, X.; Horner, B.; Garber, M.; Ayala, A. Regulatory T cell populations in sepsis and trauma. *J. Leukoc. Biol.* **2008**, *83*, 523–535. [CrossRef]

19. Monneret, G.; Venet, F.; Pachot, A.; Lepape, A. Monitoring immune dysfunctions in the septic patient: A new skin for the old ceremony. *Mol. Med.* **2008**, *14*, 64–78. [CrossRef]
20. Sakaguchi, S.; Sakaguchi, N.; Asano, M.; Itoh, M.; Toda, M. Immunologic self-tolerance maintained by activated T cells expressing IL-2 receptor alpha-chains (CD25). Breakdown of a single mechanism of self-tolerance causes various autoimmune diseases. *J. Immunol.* **1995**, *155*, 1151–1164.
21. Seddiki, N.; Santner-Nanan, B.; Martinson, J.; Zaunders, J.; Sasson, S.; Landay, A.; Solomon, M.; Selby, W.; Alexander, S.I.; Nanan, R.; et al. Expression of interleukin (IL)-2 and IL-7 receptors discriminates between human regulatory and activated T cells. *J. Exp. Med.* **2006**, *203*, 1693–1700. [CrossRef]
22. Liu, W.; Putnam, A.L.; Xu-Yu, Z.; Szot, G.L.; Lee, M.R.; Zhu, S.; Gottlieb, P.A.; Kapranov, P.; Gingeras, T.R.; Fazekas de St Groth, B.; et al. CD127 expression inversely correlates with FoxP3 and suppressive function of human CD4+ T reg cells. *J. Exp. Med.* **2006**, *203*, 1701–1711. [CrossRef]
23. Khattri, R.; Cox, T.; Yasayko, S.A.; Ramsdell, F. An essential role for Scurfin in CD4+CD25+ T regulatory cells. *Nat. Immunol.* **2003**, *4*, 337–342. [CrossRef] [PubMed]
24. MacConmara, M.P.; Maung, A.A.; Fujimi, S.; McKenna, A.M.; Delisle, A.; Lapchak, P.H.; Rogers, S.; Lederer, J.A.; Mannick, J.A. Increased CD4+ CD25+ T regulatory cell activity in trauma patients depresses protective Th1 immunity. *Ann. Surg.* **2006**, *244*, 514–523. [CrossRef]
25. Hein, F.; Massin, F.; Cravoisy-Popovic, A.; Barraud, D.; Levy, B.; Bollaert, P.E.; Gibot, S. The relationship between CD4+CD25+CD127- regulatory T cells and inflammatory response and outcome during shock states. *Crit. Care* **2010**, *14*, R19. [CrossRef] [PubMed]
26. Grant, C.R.; Liberal, R.; Mieli-Vergani, G.; Vergani, D.; Longhi, M.S. Regulatory T-cells in autoimmune diseases: Challenges, controversies and–yet–unanswered questions. *Autoimmun. Rev.* **2015**, *14*, 105–116. [CrossRef] [PubMed]
27. Venet, F.; Pachot, A.; Debard, A.L.; Bohe, J.; Bienvenu, J.; Lepape, A.; Monneret, G. Increased percentage of CD4+CD25+ regulatory T cells during septic shock is due to the decrease of CD4+CD25- lymphocytes. *Crit. Care Med.* **2004**, *32*, 2329–2331. [CrossRef] [PubMed]
28. Murphey, E.D.; Lin, C.Y.; McGuire, R.W.; Toliver-Kinsky, T.; Herndon, D.N.; Sherwood, E.R. Diminished bacterial clearance is associated with decreased IL-12 and interferon-gamma production but a sustained proinflammatory response in a murine model of postseptic immunosuppression. *Shock* **2004**, *21*, 415–425. [CrossRef] [PubMed]
29. Gogos, C.A.; Drosou, E.; Bassaris, H.P.; Skoutelis, A. Proversus anti-inflammatory cytokine profile in patients with severe sepsis: A marker for prognosis and future therapeutic options. *J. Infect. Dis.* **2000**, *181*, 176–180. [CrossRef]
30. Junger, W.G.; Hoyt, D.B.; Liu, F.C.; Loomis, W.H.; Coimbra, R. Immunosuppression after endotoxin shock: The result of multiple anti-inflammatory factors. *J. Trauma* **1996**, *40*, 702–709. [CrossRef]
31. Mokart, D.; Capo, C.; Blache, J.L.; Delpero, J.R.; Houvenaeghel, G.; Martin, C.; Mege, J.L. Early postoperative compensatory anti-inflammatory response syndrome is associated with septic complications after major surgical trauma in patients with cancer. *Br. J. Surg.* **2002**, *89*, 1450–1456. [CrossRef]
32. Menges, T.; Engel, J.; Welters, I.; Wagner, R.M.; Little, S.; Ruwoldt, R.; Wollbrueck, M.; Hempelmann, G. Changes in blood lymphocyte populations after multiple trauma: Association with posttraumatic complications. *Crit. Care Med.* **1999**, *27*, 733–740. [CrossRef] [PubMed]
33. Von Elm, E.; Altman, D.G.; Egger, M.; Pocock, S.J.; Gotzsche, P.C.; Vandenbroucke, J.P.; Initiative, S. The Strengthening the Reporting of Observational Studies in Epidemiology (STROBE) statement: Guidelines for reporting observational studies. *J. Clin. Epidemiol.* **2008**, *61*, 344–349. [CrossRef] [PubMed]
34. Rivkind, A.I.; Siegel, J.H.; Guadalupi, P.; Littleton, M. Sequential patterns of eicosanoid, platelet, and neutrophil interactions in the evolution of the fulminant post-traumatic adult respiratory distress syndrome. *Ann. Surg.* **1989**, *210*, 355–372. [CrossRef] [PubMed]
35. Baker, S.P.; O'Neill, B.; Haddon, W., Jr.; Long, W.B. The injury severity score: A method for describing patients with multiple injuries and evaluating emergency care. *J. Trauma* **1974**, *14*, 187–196. [CrossRef]
36. Relja, B.; Lustenberger, T.; Puttkammer, B.; Jakob, H.; Morser, J.; Gabazza, E.C.; Takei, Y.; Marzi, I. Thrombin-activatable fibrinolysis inhibitor (TAFI) is enhanced in major trauma patients without infectious complications. *Immunobiology* **2013**, *218*, 470–476. [CrossRef] [PubMed]

37. Relja, B.; Menke, J.; Wagner, N.; Auner, B.; Voth, M.; Nau, C.; Marzi, I. Effects of positive blood alcohol concentration on outcome and systemic interleukin-6 in major trauma patients. *Injury* **2016**, *47*, 640–645. [CrossRef]
38. Baecher-Allan, C.; Brown, J.A.; Freeman, G.J.; Hafler, D.A. CD4+CD25high regulatory cells in human peripheral blood. *J. Immunol.* **2001**, *167*, 1245–1253. [CrossRef]
39. Groux, H.; O'Garra, A.; Bigler, M.; Rouleau, M.; Antonenko, S.; de Vries, J.E.; Roncarolo, M.G. A CD4+ T-cell subset inhibits antigen-specific T-cell responses and prevents colitis. *Nature* **1997**, *389*, 737–742. [CrossRef]
40. Giannoudis, P.V.; Smith, R.M.; Perry, S.L.; Windsor, A.J.; Dickson, R.A.; Bellamy, M.C. Immediate IL-10 expression following major orthopaedic trauma: Relationship to anti-inflammatory response and subsequent development of sepsis. *Intensive Care Med.* **2000**, *26*, 1076–1081. [CrossRef] [PubMed]
41. Kitani, A.; Chua, K.; Nakamura, K.; Strober, W. Activated self-MHC-reactive T cells have the cytokine phenotype of Th3/T regulatory cell 1 T cells. *J. Immunol.* **2000**, *165*, 691–702. [CrossRef]
42. Levings, M.K.; Sangregorio, R.; Roncarolo, M.G. Human cd25(+)cd4(+) t regulatory cells suppress naive and memory T cell proliferation and can be expanded in vitro without loss of function. *J. Exp. Med.* **2001**, *193*, 1295–1302. [CrossRef] [PubMed]
43. Jiang, L.N.; Yao, Y.M.; Sheng, Z.Y. The role of regulatory T cells in the pathogenesis of sepsis and its clinical implication. *J. Interferon Cytokine Res.* **2012**, *32*, 341–349. [CrossRef] [PubMed]
44. Monneret, G.; Lepape, A.; Voirin, N.; Bohe, J.; Venet, F.; Debard, A.L.; Thizy, H.; Bienvenu, J.; Gueyffier, F.; Vanhems, P. Persisting low monocyte human leukocyte antigen-DR expression predicts mortality in septic shock. *Intensive Care Med.* **2006**, *32*, 1175–1183. [CrossRef] [PubMed]
45. Huang, L.F.; Yao, Y.M.; Dong, N.; Yu, Y.; He, L.X.; Sheng, Z.Y. Association between regulatory T cell activity and sepsis and outcome of severely burned patients: A prospective, observational study. *Crit. Care* **2010**, *14*, R3. [CrossRef]
46. Kramer, T.J.; Hack, N.; Bruhl, T.J.; Menzel, L.; Hummel, R.; Griemert, E.V.; Klein, M.; Thal, S.C.; Bopp, T.; Schafer, M.K.E. Depletion of regulatory T cells increases T cell brain infiltration, reactive astrogliosis, and interferon-gamma gene expression in acute experimental traumatic brain injury. *J. Neuroinflamm.* **2019**, *16*, 163. [CrossRef]
47. Dai, H.; Sun, T.; Liu, Z.; Zhang, J.; Zhou, M. The imbalance between regulatory and IL-17-secreting CD4(+)T cells in multiple-trauma rat. *Injury* **2013**, *44*, 1521–1527. [CrossRef]
48. Wang, H.; Daniel, V.; Sadeghi, M.; Opelz, G. Differences in the induction of induced human CD4(+) CD25(+) FoxP3(+) T-regulatory cells and CD3(+) CD8(+) CD28(-) T-suppressor cells subset phenotypes in vitro: Comparison of phorbol 12-myristate 13-acetate/ionomycin and phytohemagglutinin stimulation. *Transpl. Proc.* **2013**, *45*, 1822–1831. [CrossRef] [PubMed]
49. Wang, H.; Daniel, V.; Sadeghi, M.; Opelz, G. Plasticity and overlap of in vitro-induced regulatory T-cell markers in healthy humans. *Transpl. Proc.* **2013**, *45*, 1816–1821. [CrossRef]
50. Anderson, S.J.; Coleclough, C. Regulation of CD4 and CD8 expression on mouse T cells. Active removal from the cell surface by two mechanisms. *J. Immunol.* **1993**, *151*, 5123–5134. [PubMed]
51. Petersen, C.M.; Christensen, E.I.; Andresen, B.S.; Moller, B.K. Internalization, lysosomal degradation and new synthesis of surface membrane CD4 in phorbol ester-activated T-lymphocytes and U-937 cells. *Exp. Cell Res.* **1992**, *201*, 160–173. [CrossRef]
52. O'Neil-Andersen, N.J.; Lawrence, D.A. Differential modulation of surface and intracellular protein expression by T cells after stimulation in the presence of monensin or brefeldin A. *Clin. Diagn. Lab. Immunol.* **2002**, *9*, 243–250. [CrossRef]
53. Mukherjee, S.; Maiti, P.K.; Nandi, D. Role of CD80, CD86, and CTLA4 on mouse CD4(+) T lymphocytes in enhancing cell-cycle progression and survival after activation with PMA and ionomycin. *J. Leukoc. Biol.* **2002**, *72*, 921–931. [PubMed]
54. Fiorentino, D.F.; Zlotnik, A.; Vieira, P.; Mosmann, T.R.; Howard, M.; Moore, K.W.; O'Garra, A. IL-10 acts on the antigen-presenting cell to inhibit cytokine production by Th1 cells. *J. Immunol.* **1991**, *146*, 3444–3451. [PubMed]

55. De Waal Malefyt, R.; Haanen, J.; Spits, H.; Roncarolo, M.G.; te Velde, A.; Figdor, C.; Johnson, K.; Kastelein, R.; Yssel, H.; de Vries, J.E. Interleukin 10 (IL-10) and viral IL-10 strongly reduce antigen-specific human T cell proliferation by diminishing the antigen-presenting capacity of monocytes via downregulation of class II major histocompatibility complex expression. *J. Exp. Med.* **1991**, *174*, 915–924. [CrossRef] [PubMed]
56. Wang, G.G.; Chen, G.; Feng, H.; Liu, J.; Jiang, Y.J.; Shang, H.; Cao, Y.M. Plasmodium chabaudi AS: Distinct CD4(+)CD25(+)Foxp3(+) regulatory T cell responses during infection in DBA/2 and BALB/c mice. *Parasitol. Int.* **2013**, *62*, 24–31. [CrossRef] [PubMed]

Journal of
Clinical Medicine

MDPI

Article

Arthroscopy-Assisted Corrective Osteotomy, Reduction, Internal Fixation and Strut Allograft Augmentation for Tibial Plateau Malunion or Nonunion

Jr-Yi Wang [1,2], Chun-Ying Cheng [3,4], Alvin Chao-Yu Chen [3,4] and Yi-Sheng Chan [3,4,*]

1 Department of Orthopedics, Shuang Ho Hospital, Taipei Medical University, Taipei 11031, Taiwan; active9102078@gmail.com
2 Department of Orthopedics, School of Medicine, College of Medicine, Taipei Medical University, Taipei 11031, Taiwan
3 Department of Orthopedic Surgery, Chang Gung Memorial Hospital and Chang Gung University College of Medicine, Taoyuan 333, Taiwan; orthhand@cgmh.org.tw (C.-Y.C.); alvin_ortho@yahoo.com (A.C.-Y.C.)
4 Bone and Joint Research Center, Chang Gung Memorial Hospital, Taoyuan 333, Taiwan
* Correspondence: chan512@cgmh.org.tw

Received: 18 February 2020; Accepted: 30 March 2020; Published: 1 April 2020

Abstract: Purpose: The purpose of this study was to present the results of arthroscopy-assisted corrective osteotomy (AACO), reduction, internal fixation, and strut allograft augmentation for tibial plateau malunion or nonunion. Methods: Fifty-eight patients, mean age 49 ± 11.9 years old, with tibial plateau malunion ($n = 44$) or nonunion ($n = 14$), were included in this study. There were 19 Schatzker type II fractures (32.7%), 2 type III fractures (3.4%), 7 type IV fractures (12%), 20 type V fractures (34.5%), and 10 type VI fractures (17.2%). The mean follow-up period was 46.2 ± 17.6 months. Clinical and radiologic outcomes were scored by the Rasmussen system. Articular depression was measured from computed tomography. Secondary osteoarthritis was diagnosed when radiographs showed a narrowed joint space in the injured knee at follow-up. Results: Mean clinical score improved from 15.4 ± 3.9 (pre-revision) to 23.2 ± 4.5 (post-revision). Mean radiologic score improved from 7.7 ± 2.5 (pre-revision) to 12.0 ± 3.9 (post-revision). Fifty-six fractures achieved successful union. The average union time was 19.6 ± 7.5 weeks. Post-revision, 81% had good or excellent clinical results and 62% had good or excellent radiological results. Secondary osteoarthritis (OA) was noted in 91% of all injured knees, where 25.8% were mild OA, 25.8 % were moderate OA, and 38% were severe OA. There were 6 cases of deep infection (10.3%) and 1 case of wound edge necrosis (1.7%). Five cases were converted to total knee replacement after the index surgery with an average period of 13.5 months (range 8–24 months). Conclusions: Arthroscopy-assisted corrective osteotomy, reduction, internal fixation, and strut allograft augmentation can restore tibial plateau malunion/nonunion with well-documented radiographic healing and good clinical outcomes.

Keywords: Arthroscopy-assisted corrective osteotomy; tibial plateau malunion; tibial plateau nonunion

---

1. Introduction

Management of tibial plateau fractures is challenging. Malreduction, improper fixation, neglected intra-articular lesions, and inadequate management of bone defects lead to the failure of surgical treatment [1–5]. Traditionally, open corrective osteotomy with bone grafting is the standard of care following malunion [2,4–9]. However, arthrotomy with wide soft tissue dissection may have the higher incidence of complications and longer recovery time for the patient [2,4,5,9].

The advantage of arthroscopically-assisted osteosynthesis of fractures of the tibial plateau are direct visualization of intra-articular fractures, accurate fracture reduction, reduced morbidity in comparison with arthrotomy, simplified diagnosis and treatment of meniscal and ligamentous injuries, thorough-joint lavage, and removal of loose fragments [10–16]. Good early to medium-term results of arthroscopically-assisted osteosynthesis of tibial plateau fractures have been reported previously [10,11,17–20]. The purpose of this study was to present the radiological and clinical results of tibial plateau malunion or nonunion treated with arthroscopically-assisted corrective osteotomy (AACO) surgery. To our knowledge, this unique and novel method is not reported in the literature. We hypothesized that AACO surgery for tibial plateau malunion or nonunion wound allow accurate, stable alignment and articular surface reduction with minimal dissection and a satisfactory outcome.

2. Materials and Methods

From January 2002 to July 2013, 63 consecutive patients with tibial plateau fracture malunion or nonunion underwent arthroscopically-assisted corrective osteotomy (AACO). Fifty-eight patients (92%) who were followed up for over 24 months were enrolled in this retrospective case series. All patients were given a consent form before surgery and underwent the same treatment protocol for arthroscopy-assisted corrective osteotomy, reduction, internal fixation, and strut allograft augmentation for tibial plateau malunion or nonunion. The study was conducted in accordance with the Declaration of Helsinki, and the protocol was approved by the Ethics Committee of Chang Gung Memorial Hospital (Project identification code 104-8592B). The mean age at operation was 49 ± 11.9 years old (range: 22 to 75 years). The follow-up period was 46.2 ± 17.6 months. No patients were lost to follow-up in this consecutive case series. Tibial plateau fractures were categorized by the Schatzker classification according to initial fracture patterns [21]. Table 1 lists patient demographics. Indications for operative fixation included any varus instability exceeding 10° of medial tibial plateau fracture at full extension or lateral plateau fracture with valgus instability exceeding 10° and articular step-off exceeding 3 mm or tibial condylar widening exceeding 5 mm. Patients were excluded if they had any of the following features: active or previous infection in the affected knee joint, poor soft-tissue status, knee ankylosis, bad compliance, morbid obesity, severe systemic illness (diabetic mellitus under poor control, liver cirrhosis Child B/C, active cancer, chemotherapy, hemophilia, or a medical contraindication for surgery). Those who followed up for more than 24 months were enrolled in this study.

Table 1. Demographics of surgical patients: Schatzker classification of fracture types and associated soft-tissue injuries.

	Type II	Type III	Type IV	Type V	Type VI	Total
No. of patients (%)	19 (32.7%)	2 (3.4%)	7 (12%)	20 (34.5%)	10 (17.2%)	58 (100%)
Mean age (yr)	49.8 ± 12.9	34 ± 16.9	49.3 ± 7.2	49.5 ± 13.4	49.2 ± 8.3	49 ± 11.9
Gender (M/F)	5/14	0/2	1/6	6/14	4/6	16/42
Side (R/L)	7/12	0/2	0/7	9/11	7/3	23/35
Preoperative condition						
Range of motion	1.3 ± 3.3~102.3 ± 30.6	0.0 ± 0.0~110.0 ± 28.3	3.6 ± 6.3~115.0 ± 15.0	4.0 ± 7.7~93.7 ± 27.9	12.5 ± 16.2~84.0 ± 28.6	4.4 ± 9.18~98.0 ± 28.5
Mean depression plateau (mm)	15.9 ± 6.2	7.5 ± 3.53	16.4 ± 3.77	19.5 ± 7.7	20.7 ± 5.6	17.7 ± 6.8
Mean tibiofemoral angle	7.3 ± 3.3	8.0 ± 2.8	−2.4 ± 5.44	−1.5 ± 9.6	0.4 ± 7.6	-

Table 1. *Cont.*

	Type II	Type III	Type IV	Type V	Type VI	Total
Postoperative condition						
Range of motion (latest follow up)	1.1 ± 3.1~111.6 ± 22.4	0.0 ± 0.0~130.0 ± 0.0	0.0 ± 0.0~122.8 ± 7.6	1.3 ± 3.9~112.3 ± 17.0	4.5 ± 6.0~105.0 ± 19.0	1.5 ± 4.0~112.7 ± 18.8
Mean depression plateau (mm)	2.8 ± 3.6	0.0 ± 0.0	2.7 ± 4.0	5.1 ± 4.9	5.5 ± 3.4	3.9 ± 4.2
Mean tibiofemoral angle	6.7 ± 5.7	6.0 ± 0.0	4.6 ± 4.3	3.4 ± 9.3	1.0 ± 7.5	-
Associated injuries						
High grade chondral injury (Outerbridge Gr 3, Gr 4) (%)	11(57.9%)	0	2 (28.6%)	9 (45%)	6 (60%)	28 (48.3%)
Meniscus (%)	10	1	3	8	4	26 (44.8%)
ACL (%)	1	0	1	4	2	8 (13.8%)
PCL (%)	1	0	1	3	0	5 (8.6%)
MCL (%)	0	0	0	1	0	1 (1.7%)
Frequency of patients involved (%)	52.6% (10/19)	50%	57.1% (4/7)	55.5% (11/20)	50% (5/10)	53.4% (31/58)

ACL: anterior cruciate ligament, PCL: posterior cruciate ligament; MCL: medial collateral ligament.

Preoperative evaluations included detailed physical examination of the condition of the soft-tissue envelope, sensory-motor function of the limb, and vascular status in terms of pulsation over the dorsalis pedis and posterior tibialis arteries. All patients underwent plain film study in anteroposterior and lateral views as well as computed tomography of each knee. The mean duration between the first time surgery to revision surgery was 9.2 ± 5.7 months. All preoperative evaluations and surgical procedures were performed by a single surgeon (Y-S.C.).

2.1. Surgical Technique

The patients were positioned supine on the operating table and given general endotracheal anesthesia. Before surgery, a complete knee evaluation was performed with the patient under anesthesia. A pneumatic tourniquet was applied to the thigh, but a leg holder was not required because most arthroscopic manipulation was conducted in the "figure 4" position. The anterolateral and anteromedial portals were used to insert the arthroscope as well as working instruments. The arthroscopic joint inspection permitted evaluation of the cartilage condition, debridement of fibrous tissue, and localization of fracture malunion site (Figure 1A). The cartilage injury grading was recorded as Outerbridge classification [22]. The capsuloligamentous structures were then probed and the associated intra-articular lesions were evaluated. Incisions were made on the side of the fracture directly medial-lateral (types I through IV) and bilaterally for types V and VI, starting from approximately 1 cm proximal to the articular surface and extending approximately 8 cm distally. The previous plate and screw were removed and wound culture was done routinely. The tibial metaphysis was carefully exposed and care was taken to avoid arthrotomy and minimize periosteal stripping. The depressed fragment or malunited area was located with a standard tibial guide for anterior cruciate ligament (ACL) reconstruction and a Kirschner wire was inserted through the metaphysis into the edge of malunited fracture line (Figure 1B). Another Kirschner wire repeated the aforementioned procedure. Then, a 0.5 cm osteotome was started at the metaphyseal area to the articular area on the plane that the two Kirschner wires created to completely separate the bone malunion area (Figure 1C). The method was repeated several times until the depressed articular fragment was freely elevated by bone tamp (Figure 1E) and using Kirschner wire to temporarily fix the elevated fragment. The articular height was checked under fluoroscope exam and arthroscopically.

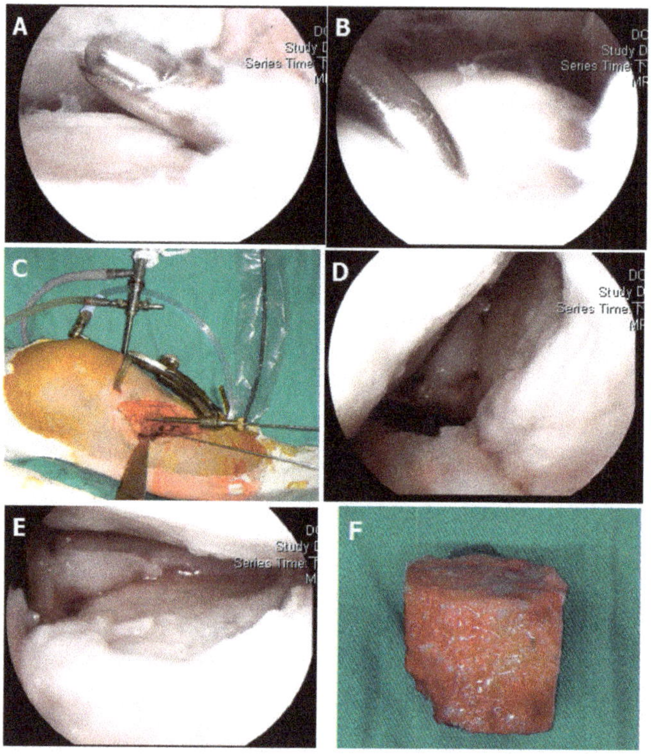

Figure 1. Operative procedure: (**A**) Arthroscopic documentation and debridement. (**B**) Use of a microfracture awl to identify the intra-articular depression zone. (**C**) Anterior cruciate ligament (ACL) tibial guiding for osteotomy axis and location, where two parallel Kirschner wire determined one plane, the 5 mm osteotome started from the metaphysic area to the articular surface. (**D**) The malunited fracture area was completely released. (**E**) The depressed articular fragments were elevated with bone tamp under direct arthroscopically inspection. (**F**) Bone grafting of the metaphyseal defect with structural allograft femoral head.

The metaphyseal area may have revealed a huge bone defect. We measured the length, width, and depth of the defect area. Then, the fresh frozen femoral head allograft were defrosted and cut by oscillator saw to fit the previous measured bone defect. The overlying cartilage were removed as cleanly as possible. Then, this cancellous strut allograft was impacted into the metaphyseal bone defect area (Figure 1F). The residual small defect was filled with artificial bone graft and GeneX (Biocomposites Ltd., Staffordshire, UK) putty (β-tricalcium phosphate/calcium sulfate hemihydrate compound) mixed with vancomycin powder. Internal fixation was applied with either a nonlocking L buttress plate (Depuy Synthes 4.5 mm L buttress plate) or a locking plate (Depuy Synthes LCP Proximal Tibial Plate 3.5) and interfragmentary screw (Depuy Synthes Standard screws 3.5 mm, cortical or cancellous) fixation. Intraoperative radiographs were routinely taken for all types of fractures to reconfirm adequate reduction before wound closure.

The associated intra-articular pathology was treated in the appropriate sequence after fracture fixation. Meniscal tears were repaired when they were within 5 mm of the meniscosynovial junction.

Degenerative meniscus tears were debrided and trimmed to stable end. ACL injuries were treated by arthroscopy-assisted fixation of the ACL avulsion fracture in a 1-stage surgical procedure and second-stage reconstruction after fracture healing for complete ACL tears.

2.2. Clinical and Radiologic Assessment

The pre-revision and post-revision clinical and radiologic scales were recorded according to the Rasmussen system (Tables 2 and 3) [23]. The post-revision scales was recorded at the latest followed up outpatient department visit. The Rasmussen system was intended to improve upon the Hohl and Luck system [24] by making it more quantitative. The advantage of the Rasmussen system is its analysis of both functional and anatomic end results for tibial plateau fractures after treatment. This scoring system is widely used in related studies of tibial plateau fractures [11,25–28]. The follow-up protocol included analysis of subjective complaints and objective clinical findings. All 58 patients completed a questionnaire regarding their overall function. Subjective data were collected to assess swelling, difficulty climbing stairs, joint stability, ability to work and participate in sports, and overall patient satisfaction with recovery. Range of motion (ROM) of the knee joint was measured with the patient in a prone position with test-side ankle off plinth. A goniometer axis was placed at the skin prominence of lateral epicondyle of the femur. A stationary arm was placed along the femur to greater trochanter. A movement arm was placed along the fibula to lateral malleolus. Measurement of ROM was documented at each OPD visit. We only presented the preoperative ROM and most recent postoperative follow-up ROM. All patients were evaluated by the senior author (Y-S.C.).

Table 2. Criteria for clinical assessment.

Clinical Parameter	Points	Excellent	Good	Fair	Poor
Subjective					
Pain		5	4	2	0
None	6				
Occasional pain, needs no medication	5				
Stabbing pain	4				
Intense, activity-related	2				
Night pain, at rest	0				
Walking capacity		6	4	2	1
Normal	6				
Outdoors >1 h	4				
Outdoors >15 min	2				
Indoors only	1				
Wheelchair/bedridden	0				
Objective					
Extension		6	4	2	2
Normal	6				
<10° loss	4				
>10° loss	2				
Total range of motion		5	4	2	1
>140°	6				
>120°	5				
>90°	4				
>60°	2				
>30°	1				
0°	0				
Stability		5	4	2	2
Normal	6				
Abnormal in 20° flexion	5				
Instability in extension <10°	4				
Instability in extension >10°	2				
Total (minimum)		30–27	26–20	19–10	9–6

Table 3. Criteria for radiologic assessment.

Radiological Parameter	Points	Excellent	Good	Fair	Poor
Depression		6	4	2	0
None	6				
<6 mm	4				
6–10 mm	2				
>10 mm	0				
Condylar widening		6	4	2	0
None	6				
<6 mm	4				
6–10 mm	2				
>10 mm	0				
Angulation (valgus/varus)		6	4	2	0
Normal	6				
<10°	4				
10°–20°	2				
>20°	0				
Total (minimum)		18	17–12	11–6	5–0

A radiographic evaluation, including bipedal examination and examination of both knees, was done preoperatively, at 3 months, 6 months, and 1 year postoperatively, and then annually thereafter. Long-leg standing films (with standing scanography used to measure the tibio-femoral angle) were obtained annually postoperatively.

In each case, preoperative and postoperative articular depression were measured from the Computed tomography (CT) coronal series. The amount of articular depression was measured from the opposite remaining articular surface. A line was drawn at the level of the normal articular surface and extended across the depressed area. A measurement was made from this line to the point of maximum depression. When both plateaus were involved, a line was drawn at the level of the femoral condyles and another line parallel to it was drawn through the base of the tibial spine, then lines were drawn to the point of maximum depression of both plateaus. Magnetic resonance imaging scans were used to identify meniscal disorders and ligamentous injuries.

Union was defined as the presence of a bridging callus on 2 radiographic views [29]. Nonunion was defined as a failure of progressive radiographic healing over a 1 year period [2]. Osteoarthritic changes were judged according to Ahlbäck's scale [30] and the mechanical axis was measured by radiography. On the basis of Ahlbäck's scale, osteoarthritis was estimated by narrowing of the joint space. Secondary osteoarthritis was defined as follows: if the radiograph showed a narrowed joint space in the injured knee at follow-up, the comparison was with the film taken at the time of injury. If the findings were comparable, no secondary degenerative change was recorded. If relative narrowing was noted, comparison was then made with the film of the uninjured knee. Relative narrowing of the joint space by less than 50% was considered mild, relative narrowing by greater than 50% was considered moderate, and 100% (i.e., obliterated) narrowing was considered severe [31].

2.3. Statistical Methods

Each radiograph was evaluated by 5 observers (visiting orthopedic staff) in a blinded fashion to assess interobserver variance. The 5 observers also classified fracture type and measured articular depression in the 58 patients. Statistical analysis determined the interobserver variance in the diagnosis for secondary osteoarthritis, fracture type, and articular depression. The interobserver variability by use of the kappa method in the diagnosis of secondary osteoarthritis, fracture type, and articular depression was in all cases insignificant ($p < 0.05$). The Mann–Whitney U test was used for comparing preoperative and postoperative clinical and radiological outcomes. $P < 0.05$ was recognized as significance.

3. Results

Data of the surgical patients are shown in Table 1. There was no significant relation between fracture type and patient age, gender, or injured limb ($p > 0.05$). The average range of motion was 4.4 ± 9.18 to 98.0 ± 28.5 preoperatively and 1.5 ± 4.0 to 112.7 ± 18.8 postoperatively. The tibial-femoral angles were 7.3 ± 3.3 (type II), 8.0 ± 2.8 (type III), −2.4 ± 5.44 (type IV), −1.5 ± 9.6 (type V), and 0.4 ± 7.6 (type VI) preoperatively and were corrected to 6.7 ± 5.7 (type II), 6.0 ± 0.0 (type III), 4.6 ± 4.3 (type IV), 3.4 ± 9.3 (type V), and 1.0 ± 7.5 (type VI) postoperatively. The preoperative depression of the plateaus were 15.9 ± 6.2 (type II), 7.5 ± 3.5 (type III), 16.4 ± 3.8 (type IV), 19.5 ± 7.7 (type V), and 20.7 ± 5.6 (type VI) and were reduced to 2.8 ± 3.6 (type II), 0.0 ± 0.0 (type III), 2.7 ± 4.0 (type IV), 5.1 ± 4.9 (type V), and 5.5 ± 3.4 (type VI) postoperatively. In total, the amount of depression of the plateaus were 17.7 ± 6.8 preoperatively and 3.9 ± 4.2 postoperatively. Significant difference was noted in type II, IV, V, VI, and overall (Figures 2 and 3).

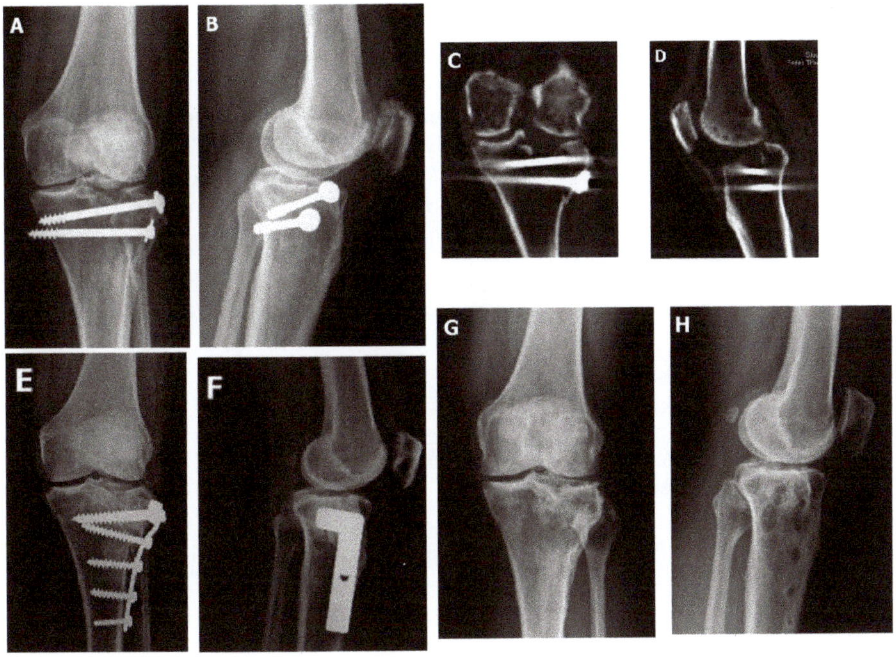

Figure 2. (**A**,**B**) This 43-year-old patient had a Type II fracture, where open reduction with internal fixation was done by two cannulated screws on the day of injury. This radiograph was checked four months after the initial surgery, where a lateral split with depression was noted. (**C**,**D**) CT revealed lateral plateau huge intraarticular split and depression. (**E**,**F**) Immediate postoperative radiograph after arthroscopically-assisted corrective osteotomy (AACO), bone grafting with structural allograft femoral head, and internal fixation by lateral plate. (**G**,**H**) 4 years after AACO, the plate was removed and the radiological score were excellent.

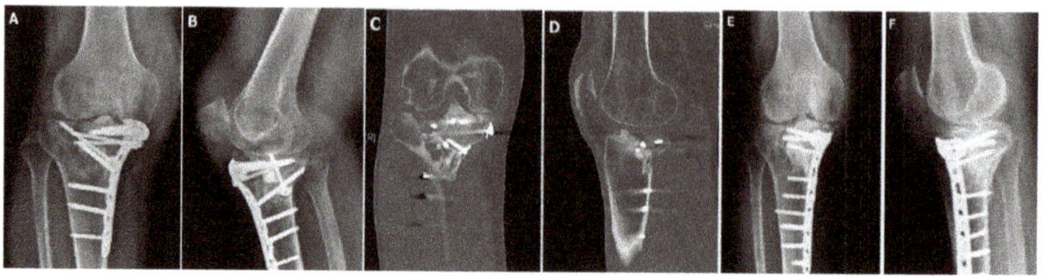

Figure 3. (**A**,**B**) This 57-year-old patient had a Type II fracture, where open reduction with internal fixation was done by medial locking plate 3 days after injury. When this radiograph was checked 14 months after the initial surgery, lateral plateau depression and widening were noted. (**C**,**D**) CT revealed lateral plateau huge intraarticular depression. (**E**,**F**) 2.5 years after AACO, the radiological score was excellent.

3.1. Clinical Assessment

Table 4 shows preoperative and postoperative clinical assessment results. Preoperatively, the clinical Rasmussen scores were 17.1 ± 1.9 (type II), 20.0 ± 4.2 (type III), 15.6 ± 4.4 (type IV), 14.9 ± 4.2 (type V), and 12.1 ± 4.1 (type VI). Postoperatively, the clinical scores increased to 22.6 ± 5.3 (type II), 26.0 ± 0.0 (type III), 25.3 ± 1.4 (type IV), 23.6 ± 4.0 (type V), and 21.6 ± 5.2 (type VI). In total, the clinical scores were 15.4 ± 3.9 preoperatively and 23.2 ± 4.5 postoperatively. Significant difference was noted in type II, IV, V, VI, and overall. The clinical satisfactory rate improved from 10.3% preoperatively to 81% postoperatively.

Table 4. Results of clinical assessment in 58 patients.

Fracture Type	No. of Patients	Average Clinical Score	Excellent	Good	Fair	Poor	Satisfactory Results
Type II	19	22.6 ± 5.3	4 (21%)	10 (52.6%)	5 (26.3%)	None	73.7%
Type III	2	26.0 ± 0.0	None	2 (100%)	None	None	100%
Type IV	7	25.3 ± 1.4	1 (14.3%)	6 (85.7%)	None	None	100%
Type V	20	23.6 ± 4.0	1 (5%)	17 (85%)	1 (5%)	1(5%)	90%
Type VI	10	21.6 ± 5.2	1 (10%)	5 (50%)	4 (40%)	None	60%
Total Injuries	58	23.2 ± 4.5	7(12%)	40(68.9%)	10(17.2%)	1(1.7%)	47(81%)

3.2. Radiologic Assessment

All 58 fractures, except 2, achieved successful union (these 2 nonunion cases shifted to total knee arthroplasty). The average union time was 19.6 weeks. Table 5 shows preoperative and postoperative radiologic assessment results. Preoperatively, the radiological Rasmussen scores were 8.9 ± 1.4 (type II), 13.0 ± 1.4 (type III), 8.0 ± 2.3 (type IV), 6.6 ± 2.6 (type V), and 6.2 ± 2.0 (type VI). Postoperatively, the radiological scores increased to 13.3 ± 3.2 (type II), 17.0 ± 1.4 (type III), 14.3 ± 3.3 (type IV), 10.7 ± 4.2 (type V), and 9.6 ± 2.6 (type VI). In total, the radiological scores were 7.7 ± 2.5 preoperatively and 12.0 ± 3.9 postoperatively. Significant difference was noted in type II, IV, V, VI, and overall. The radiological satisfactory rate improved from 8.6% preoperatively to 62% postoperatively.

Table 5. Results of radiological assessment in 25 patients.

Fracture Type	No. of Patients	Average Radiological Score	Excellent	Good	Fair	Poor	Satisfactory Results
Type IV	5	16 (range: 14–18)	3 (60%)	2 (40%)	None	None	100%
Type V	2	16.5 (range: 14–18)	1 (50%)	1 (50%)	None	None	100%
Type VI	18	15 (range: 10–18)	9 (34%)	8 (44%)	1 (22%)	None	94%
Total Injuries	25	15.8	13 (52%)	11 (44%)	1 (4%)	None	96% (24/25)

3.3. Associated Injuries and Procedures

Of the 58 patients in this series, 31 (53.4%) had associated intra-articular lesions (meniscus, cruciate ligament, collateral ligament) (Table 1). Among these 31 patients, the meniscal injury was noted in 25 knees. There were 7 medial and 21 lateral meniscal injuries. Three knees had both medial and lateral meniscal pathology. Five menisci were sutured, 23 were partially resected, and none were totally removed. Ligament injuries were noted in 11 knees with 17 lesions, including 4 ACL complete ruptures, 4 ACL partial ruptures, 1 PCL complete rupture, 3 PCL partial ruptures, and 1 medial collateral ligament partial rupture. There were 4 combined ligament injuries (ACL partial tear and PCL partial tear in three knees and ACL complete tear and PCL complete tear) in one knee. High-grade chondral injuries (Outerbridge Gr 3, Gr 4) were noted in 11 type II, 2 type IV, 9 type V, and 6 type VI fractures. In total, 28 (48.3%) knees had high-grade chondral injuries.

3.4. Complications

Secondary osteoarthritis was noted in 53 injured knees (91%). The relative narrowing of the joint space was mild in 15 knees (25.8%; 7 type II, 1 type IV, 4 type V, and 3 type VI), moderate in 3 knees (25.8 %; 4 type II, 4 type IV, 4 type V, and 3 type VI), and severe in 23 knees (38%; 6 type II, 1 type III, 2 type IV, 10 type V, and 4 type VI). In the 58 patients, deep infection was noted in 6 cases (10.3%). Wound debridement, sequestrum removal, and copious irrigation were done and parenteral antibiotics were used. The implants were removed if the screws were loosening and left in place if the screw and plate were stable. In the six cases of deep infection, five cases were cured without recurrent infection after one to two debridement surgeries. Two cases develop knee arthrofibrosis, with the range of motion only 0 to 30 degree. Arthroscopic release was done for these two patients at the same time when removing the locking plate and screws.

There was one case of wound edge necrosis that was noted 1 month after the index surgery. Rotation musculocutaneous flap was done for wound coverage. The flap and wound healed well. The osteotomy site healed well too.

Five cases (3 type II, 1 type V and 1 type VI) needed to shift to knee arthroplasty due to persistent pain, nonunion, and radiograph-confirmed severe post-traumatic osteoarthritis. The average interval between the index surgery to total knee arthroplasty was 13.5 months (range 8–24 months). No complications directly associated with arthroscopy were noted in any of the 58 patients.

4. Discussion

In this report, we presented the surgical technique and radiographic and clinical outcomes of arthroscopic-assisted corrective osteotomy in the treatment of tibial plateau fracture malunion or nonunion. Postoperatively, 81% patients achieved satisfactory clinical results and 61% patients achieved satisfactory radiographic results. Significant improvement was confirmed by comparing preoperative and postoperative conditions.

Complication after tibial plateau fracture surgery has been reported by several authors [1,3,32]. Papagelopoulos et al. divided the complications into early (i.e., loss of reduction, deep vein thrombosis, infection) or late (i.e., malunion and nonunion, implant breakage, post-traumatic arthritis) categories [1]. Huang et al. analyzed the causes of failure for their 25 patients who had failed tibia plateau surgery and revealed that 19 (76%) had inadequate fixation, 21 (84%) had malreduction, and 25 (100%) had bone defects [3].

Knee arthroplasty for post traumatic knee arthritis following tibial plateau fracture malunion or nonunion has been reported by many authors. However, according to different series, higher complication rates: 13.7%–34%, poor outcomes: 19%–23%, soft-tissue compromise: 5%–13%, stiff knee: 4%–11.5%, high revision rate 4%–11%, and deep infection: 3%–5% were noted, where all of the above were higher than primary knee arthroplasty for degenerative knee osteoarthritis [33–40]. Besides, 12%–13% of patients need semi-constrained or hinge knee implants for compensation of the post-traumatic articular depression and ligament imbalance.

Corrective osteotomy could maintain the native knee joint, restore lower extremity alignment, preserve the bone stock, delay joint replacement, and create better conditions for an eventual replacement. These reconstructive surgical strategies were mentioned in only a few studies [2,4,9]. Wu et al. presented their technique for correction of the tibia plateau fracture malunion with varus deformity by tibia shaft osteotomy distal to the tibial tubercle, realigning the lower extremity axis, and medial fixation by 95° angled blade plate [2]. Postoperatively, the proximal medial tibial angle (PMTA) was corrected to the acceptable range (80°–99°) in all patients and knee function improved in 88% patients. However, with this technique, intraarticular pathology, such as intraarticular step-off and associate intraarticular soft tissue pathology, cannot be managed properly. Kerkhoffs et al. reported their technique with combined intra-articular and varus opening wedge osteotomy for lateral depression and valgus malunion of the tibia plateau [4,5]. According to their technique, with a standard lateral arthrotomy, the anterior 50% to 60% of the lateral plateau can easily be visualized to expose more posteriorly situated depressions, an osteotomy of the Gerdy tubercle and reflection of the attached iliotibial tract allow visualization of approximately 80% of the lateral plateau, and an additional osteotomy of the fibular head allows full anterior dislocation of the lateral tibial plateau. An osteotomy of the tibial tuberosity is necessary when there is a combination of medial and lateral malunions. Although the authors reported that excellent results were achieved in 74% patients, possible disadvantages of extended arthrotomy and delayed healing of tibial tubercle osteotomy site may be encountered.

Recently, computer-assisted planning and patient-specific surgical guidelines have been proposed to correct tibial plateau post-traumatic malunion [41–43]. Initial results are encouraging. However, this technique must mobilize the soft tissue attachment to fully position the guide on the bone. This includes the pes anserinus and the ilio-tibial band. In addition, additional CTs will be required if the opposite side is used as a reconstruction template, resulting in increased radiation exposure.

We presented the surgical technique and radiographic and clinical outcomes of arthroscopic-assisted corrective osteotomy in the treatment of tibial plateau fracture malunion or nonunion. In our series, postoperatively, 81% patients achieved satisfactory clinical result and 61% patients achieved satisfactory radiographic result. Significant improvement was confirmed by comparing preoperative and postoperative conditions. This technique can be used in all type of tibial plateau malunion and nonunion fractures. Of the 58 patients, 51.7% suffered Schatzker type V or type VI fractures and could be managed by the technique very well with significant improvement both clinically and radiologically. However, according to the Rasmussen score of radiological results, fractures with type V or type VI would get relatively lower scores. This may explain why our series had only a 61% for satisfactory radiologic results.

By the assistance of arthroscopy, the fracture malunion site could be identified, the corrective osteotomy were created, and the depressed intraarticular fragment could be elevated under direct visualization. Besides, the diagnosis, documentation, and management of associate intraarticular soft tissue pathology could be performed smoothly under arthroscopy at one-stage surgery. Our technique avoided arthrotomy and fibulotomy. To the best of our knowledge, this is the first case series presenting the new technique.

In our series, we had five cases that needed to convert to total knee arthroplasty due to persistent pain, nonunion, and radiograph-confirmed severe post-traumatic osteoarthritis with a mean conversion time of 13.5 months (range: 8–24 months). Three cases used primary total knee replacement and two cases used constrained condylar knee prosthesis (LCCK; Zimmer) and there was no need for rotating hinge type revision total knee replacement. There was no further complication related to the arthroplasty procedure.

However, some limitations and weaknesses of this study must be acknowledged: there was no control group, this was not a randomized study, only a single surgeon was involved, all patients were rated by the same author, the sample size was limited, and follow-up to determine further osteoarthritic change needs to be longer.

5. Conclusions

Arthroscopy-assisted corrective osteotomy, reduction, internal fixation, and strut allograft augmentation is a unique and new method to restore tibial plateau malunion/nonunion with well-documented radiographic healing, good clinical outcomes, and low complication rates.

Author Contributions: J.-Y.W. and Y.-S.C. conceived and planned the study. J.-Y.W., C.-Y.C. and A.C.-Y.C. contributed to data acquisition and processing. J.-Y.W., and Y.-S.C. wrote the manuscript. All authors provided critical feedback and directed the research, analysis, and writing of the manuscript. All authors have read and agreed to the published version of the manuscript.

Funding: The authors did not receive any specific grant for this research from any funding agency in the public, commercial, or not-for-profit sectors.

Conflicts of Interest: The authors declare no conflict of interest.

References

1. Papagelopoulos, P.J.; Partsinevelos, A.A.; Themistocleous, G.S.; Mavrogenis, A.F.; Korres, D.S.; Soucacos, P.N. Complications after tibia plateau fracture surgery. *Injury* **2006**, *37*, 475–484. [CrossRef] [PubMed]
2. Wu, C.C. Salvage of proximal tibial malunion or nonunion with the use of angled blade plate. *Arch. Orthop. Trauma Surg.* **2006**, *126*, 82–87. [CrossRef] [PubMed]
3. Huang, P.-H.; Cheng, C.-Y.; Chen, Y.-J.; Chao-Yu Chen, A.; Hsu, K.-Y.; Chan, Y.-S.; Chen, W.-J. Reasons for failure of surgical treatment in 25 tibial plateau fractures. *Formos. J. Musculoskelet. Disord.* **2012**, *3*, 14–18. [CrossRef]
4. Kerkhoffs, G.M.; Rademakers, M.V.; Altena, M.; Marti, R.K. Combined intra-articular and varus opening wedge osteotomy for lateral depression and valgus malunion of the proximal part of the tibia. *JBJS* **2008**, *90*, 1252–1257. [CrossRef] [PubMed]
5. Kerkhoffs, G.M.; Rademakers, M.V.; Altena, M.; Marti, R.K. Combined intra-articular and varus opening wedge osteotomy for lateral depression and valgus malunion of the proximal part of the tibia. Surgical technique. *JBJS* **2009**, *91 Pt 1* (Suppl. 2), 101–115. [CrossRef]
6. Saengnipanthkul, S. Uni-condyle high tibial osteotomy for malunion of medial plateau fracture: Surgical technique and case report. *J. Med Assoc. Thail. Chotmaihet Thangphaet* **2012**, *95*, 1619–1624.
7. Prasad, G.; Zahn, H. Medial tibial hemi-condylar elevation osteotomy as an operative technique to treat varus mal-united tibial plateau fracture. *Musculoskelet. Surg.* **2012**, *96*, 63–66. [CrossRef]
8. Singh, H.; Singh, V.R.; Yuvarajan, P.; Maini, L.; Gautam, V.K. Open wedge osteotomy of the proximal medial tibia for malunited tibial plateau fractures. *J. Orthop. Surg.* **2011**, *19*, 57–59. [CrossRef]
9. Marti, R.K.; Kerkhoffs, G.M.; Rademakers, M.V. Correction of lateral tibial plateau depression and valgus malunion of the proximal tibia. *Oper. Orthop. Und Traumatol.* **2007**, *19*, 101–113. [CrossRef]
10. Hung, S.S.; Chao, E.K.; Chan, Y.S.; Yuan, L.J.; Chung, P.C.; Chen, C.Y.; Lee, M.S.; Wang, C.J. Arthroscopically assisted osteosynthesis for tibial plateau fractures. *J. Trauma* **2003**, *54*, 356–363. [CrossRef]

11. Chan, Y.S.; Yuan, L.J.; Hung, S.S.; Wang, C.J.; Yu, S.W.; Chen, C.Y.; Chao, E.K.; Lee, M.S. Arthroscopic-assisted reduction with bilateral buttress plate fixation of complex tibial plateau fractures. *Arthrosc. J. Arthrosc. Relat. Surg.* **2003**, *19*, 974–984. [CrossRef] [PubMed]
12. Chan, Y.S.; Chiu, C.H.; Lo, Y.P.; Chen, A.C.; Hsu, K.Y.; Wang, C.J.; Chen, W.J. Arthroscopy-assisted surgery for tibial plateau fractures: 2- to 10-year follow-up results. *Arthrosc. J. Arthrosc. Relat. Surg.* **2008**, *24*, 760–768. [CrossRef]
13. Suganuma, J.; Akutsu, S. Arthroscopically assisted treatment of tibial plateau fractures. *Arthrosc. J. Arthrosc. Relat. Surg.* **2004**, *20*, 1084–1089. [CrossRef] [PubMed]
14. Lubowitz, J.H.; Vance, K.J.; Ayala, M.; Guttmann, D.; Reid, J.B., 3rd. Interference screw technique for arthroscopic reduction and internal fixation of compression fractures of the tibial plateau. *Arthrosc. J. Arthrosc. Relat. Surg.* **2006**, *22*, 1359-e1. [CrossRef] [PubMed]
15. Cetik, O.; Cift, H.; Asik, M. Second-look arthroscopy after arthroscopy-assisted treatment of tibial plateau fractures. *Knee Surg. Sports Traumatol. Arthrosc. Off. J. Esska* **2007**, *15*, 747–752. [CrossRef] [PubMed]
16. Chan, Y.S. Arthroscopy- assisted surgery for tibial plateau fractures. *Chang. Gung. Med. J.* **2011**, *34*, 239–247. [CrossRef]
17. Van Glabbeek, F.; van Riet, R.; Jansen, N.; D'Anvers, J.; Nuyts, R. Arthroscopically assisted reduction and internal fixation of tibial plateau fractures: Report of twenty cases. *Acta Orthop. Belg.* **2002**, *68*, 258–264.
18. Fowble, C.D.; Zimmer, J.W.; Schepsis, A.A. The role of arthroscopy in the assessment and treatment of tibial plateau fractures. *Arthrosc. J. Arthrosc. Relat. Surg.* **1993**, *9*, 584–590. [CrossRef]
19. Guanche, C.A.; Markman, A.W. Arthroscopic management of tibial plateau fractures. *Arthrosc. J. Arthrosc. Relat. Surg.* **1993**, *9*, 467–471. [CrossRef]
20. Vangsness, C.T., Jr.; Ghaderi, B.; Hohl, M.; Moore, T.M. Arthroscopy of meniscal injuries with tibial plateau fractures. *J. Bone Jt. Surg. Br. Vol.* **1994**, *76*, 488–490. [CrossRef]
21. Schatzker, J.; McBroom, R.; Bruce, D. The tibial plateau fracture. The Toronto experience 1968–1975. *Clin. Orthop. Relat. Res.* **1979**, *138*, 94–104.
22. Outerbridge, R.E.; Dunlop, J.A. The problem of chondromalacia patellae. *Clin. Orthop. Relat. Res.* **1975**, 177–196. [CrossRef] [PubMed]
23. Rasmussen, P.S. Tibial condylar fractures. Impairment of knee joint stability as an indication for surgical treatment. *JBJS* **1973**, *55*, 1331–1350. [CrossRef]
24. Hohl, M. Tibial condylar fractures. *JBJS* **1967**, *49*, 1455–1467. [CrossRef]
25. Jensen, D.B.; Rude, C.; Duus, B.; Bjerg-Nielsen, A. Tibial plateau fractures. A comparison of conservative and surgical treatment. *J. Bone Jt. Surg. Br. Vol.* **1990**, *72*, 49–52. [CrossRef]
26. Lobenhoffer, P.; Schulze, M.; Gerich, T.; Lattermann, C.; Tscherne, H. Closed reduction/percutaneous fixation of tibial plateau fractures: Arthroscopic versus fluoroscopic control of reduction. *J. Orthop. Trauma* **1999**, *13*, 426–431. [CrossRef]
27. Hsu, C.J.; Chang, W.N.; Wong, C.Y. Surgical treatment of tibial plateau fracture in elderly patients. *Arch. Orthop. Trauma Surg.* **2001**, *121*, 67–70. [CrossRef]
28. Gill, T.J.; Moezzi, D.M.; Oates, K.M.; Sterett, W.I. Arthroscopic reduction and internal fixation of tibial plateau fractures in skiing. *Clin. Orthop. Relat. Res.* **2001**, 243–249. [CrossRef]
29. Whittle, A.P.; Russell, T.A.; Taylor, J.C.; Lavelle, D.G. Treatment of open fractures of the tibial shaft with the use of interlocking nailing without reaming. *JBJS* **1992**, *74*, 1162–1171. [CrossRef]
30. Ahlback, S. Osteoarthrosis of the knee. A radiographic investigation. *Acta Radiol. Diagn.* **1968**, *227* (Suppl. 277), 7–72.
31. Honkonen, S.E. Degenerative arthritis after tibial plateau fractures. *J. Orthop. Trauma* **1995**, *9*, 273–277. [CrossRef] [PubMed]
32. Rademakers, M.V.; Kerkhoffs, G.M.; Sierevelt, I.N.; Raaymakers, E.L.; Marti, R.K. Operative treatment of 109 tibial plateau fractures: Five- to 27-year follow-up results. *J. Orthop. Trauma* **2007**, *21*, 5–10. [CrossRef] [PubMed]
33. Scott, C.E.; Davidson, E.; MacDonald, D.J.; White, T.O.; Keating, J.F. Total knee arthroplasty following tibial plateau fracture: A matched cohort study. *Bone Jt. J.* **2015**, *97*, 532–538. [CrossRef] [PubMed]
34. Lizaur-Utrilla, A.; Collados-Maestre, I.; Miralles-Munoz, F.A.; Lopez-Prats, F.A. Total Knee Arthroplasty for Osteoarthritis Secondary to Fracture of the Tibial Plateau. A Prospective Matched Cohort Study. *J. Arthroplast.* **2015**, *30*, 1328–1332. [CrossRef]

35. Houdek, M.T.; Watts, C.D.; Shannon, S.F.; Wagner, E.R.; Sems, S.A.; Sierra, R.J. Posttraumatic Total Knee Arthroplasty Continues to Have Worse Outcome Than Total Knee Arthroplasty for Osteoarthritis. *J. Arthroplast.* **2015**. [CrossRef]
36. Abdel, M.P.; von Roth, P.; Cross, W.W.; Berry, D.J.; Trousdale, R.T.; Lewallen, D.G. Total Knee Arthroplasty in Patients With a Prior Tibial Plateau Fracture: A Long-Term Report at 15 Years. *J. Arthroplast.* **2015**, *30*, 2170–2172. [CrossRef]
37. Wasserstein, D.; Henry, P.; Paterson, J.M.; Kreder, H.J.; Jenkinson, R. Risk of total knee arthroplasty after operatively treated tibial plateau fracture: A matched-population-based cohort study. *JBJS* **2014**, *96*, 144–150. [CrossRef]
38. Parratte, S.; Bonnevialle, P.; Pietu, G.; Saragaglia, D.; Cherrier, B.; Lafosse, J.M. Primary total knee arthroplasty in the management of epiphyseal fracture around the knee. *Orthop. Traumatol. Surg. Res. Otsr* **2011**, *97*, S87–S94. [CrossRef]
39. Civinini, R.; Carulli, C.; Matassi, F.; Villano, M.; Innocenti, M. Total knee arthroplasty after complex tibial plateau fractures. *La Chir. Degli Organi Di Mov.* **2009**, *93*, 143–147. [CrossRef]
40. Saleh, K.J.; Sherman, P.; Katkin, P.; Windsor, R.; Haas, S.; Laskin, R.; Sculco, T. Total knee arthroplasty after open reduction and internal fixation of fractures of the tibial plateau: A minimum five-year follow-up study. *JBJS* **2001**, *83-a*, 1144–1148. [CrossRef]
41. Pagkalos, J.; Molloy, R.; Snow, M. Bi-planar intra-articular deformity following malunion of a Schatzker V tibial plateau fracture: Correction with intra-articular osteotomy using patient-specific guides and arthroscopic resection of the tibial spine bone block. *Knee* **2018**, *25*, 959–965. [CrossRef] [PubMed]
42. Wang, H.; Newman, S.; Wang, J.; Wang, Q.; Wang, Q. Corrective Osteotomies for Complex Intra-Articular Tibial Plateau Malunions using Three-Dimensional Virtual Planning and Novel Patient-Specific Guides. *J. Knee Surg.* **2018**, *31*, 642–648. [CrossRef] [PubMed]
43. Furnstahl, P.; Vlachopoulos, L.; Schweizer, A.; Fucentese, S.F.; Koch, P.P. Complex Osteotomies of Tibial Plateau Malunions Using Computer-Assisted Planning and Patient-Specific Surgical Guides. *J. Orthop. Trauma* **2015**, *29*, e270–e276. [CrossRef] [PubMed]

Journal of
Clinical Medicine

MDPI

Article

Validation of the mTICCS Score as a Useful Tool for the Early Prediction of a Massive Transfusion in Patients with a Traumatic Hemorrhage

Klemens Horst [1,*], Rachel Lentzen [1], Martin Tonglet [2], Ümit Mert [1], Philipp Lichte [1], Christian D. Weber [1], Philipp Kobbe [1], Nicole Heussen [3,4] and Frank Hildebrand [1]

1 Department of Trauma and Reconstructive Surgery, University Hospital, RWTH 52074 Aachen, Germany; rlentzen@ukaachen.de (R.L.); umert@ukaachen.de (Ü.M.); plichte@ukaachen.de (P.L.); chrweber@ukaachen.de (C.D.W.); pkobbe@ukaachen.de (P.K.); fhildebrand@ukaachen.de (F.H.)
2 Department of Emergency, Liege University Hospital, Domaine du Sart Tilman, 4000 Liege, Belgium; tongletm@yahoo.com
3 Department of Medical Statistics, RWTH Aachen University, 52074 Aachen, Germany; nheussen@ukaachen.de
4 Medical School, Sigmund Freud Private University, 1020 Vienna, Austria
* Correspondence: khorst@ukaachen.de

Received: 26 February 2020; Accepted: 27 March 2020; Published: 30 March 2020

Abstract: The modified Trauma-Induced Coagulopathy Clinical Score (mTICCS) presents a new scoring system for the early detection of the need for a massive transfusion (MT). While validated in a large trauma cohort, the comparison of mTICCS to established scoring systems is missing. This study therefore validated the ability of six scoring systems to stratify patients at risk for an MT at an early stage after trauma. A dataset of severely injured patients (ISS ≥ 16) derived from the database of a level I trauma center (2010–2015) was used. Scoring systems assessed were Trauma-Associated Severe Hemorrhage (TASH) score, Prince of Wales Hospital (PWH) score, Larson score, Assessment of Blood Consumption (ABC) score, Emergency Transfusion Score (ETS), and mTICCS. Demographics, diagnostic data, mechanism of injury, injury pattern (graded by AIS), and outcome (length of stay, mortality) were analyzed. Scores were calculated, and the area under the receiver operating characteristic curves (AUCs) were evaluated. From the AUCs, the cut-off point with the best relationship of sensitivity-to-specificity was used to recalculate sensitivity, specificity, positive predictive values (PPV), and negative predictive values (NPV). A total of 479 patients were included; of those, blunt trauma occurred in 92.3% of patients. The mean age of patients was 49 ± 22 years with a mean ISS of 25 ± 29. The overall MT rate was 8.4% ($n = 40$). The TASH score had the highest overall accuracy as reflected by an AUC of 0.782 followed by the mTICCS (0.776). The ETS was the most sensitive (80%), whereas the TASH score had the highest specificity (82%) and the PWH score had the lowest (51.83%). At a cut-off > 5 points, the mTICCS score showed a sensitivity of 77.5% and a specificity of 74.03%. Compared to sophisticated systems, using a higher number of weighted variables, the newly developed mTICCS presents a useful tool to predict the need for an MT in a prehospital situation. This might accelerate the diagnosis of an MT in emergency situations. However, prospective validations are needed to improve the development process and use of scoring systems in the future.

Keywords: mTICCS; TICCS; massive transfusion; shock; multiple trauma; polytrauma; bleeding; transfusion

1. Introduction

Traumatic hemorrhage still represents a challenging problem in injured patients [1,2]. In this context, uncontrolled bleeding is found in about 50% of patients, deceasing in the first 48 hours after trauma, thereby presenting one of the leading causes of early posttraumatic death. The main sources of severe bleeding are thoracic, abdominal, and pelvic injuries [3,4]. Although early laboratory diagnostics, including standard coagulation parameters, ROTEM®, and implementation of massive transfusion (MT) protocols, have been found to improve the outcome, prediction, and early identification of patients which need MT is still difficult [5–7]. For this purpose, several scores using clinical parameters, laboratory results, and imaging have been introduced and validated [8,9]. However, some of the relevant scoring parameters are not available before diagnostics in the emergency room have been finalized, which negatively affects their clinical utility for prediction of a necessary MT. In 2014, Tonglet et al. introduced the "Trauma-Induced Coagulopathy Clinical Score" (TICCS), which is based on the general injury severity assessment, blood pressure, and extent of bodily injury (Table 1) [10]. Due to its simplicity, this calculation is feasible on scene and allows for the timely identification of patients in need of the preclinical start of damage control resuscitation (DCR) and later, possibly, an MT. Modified Trauma-Induced Coagulopathy Clinical Score (mTICCS) was validated in 2017 in a population of 33,385 trauma patients [11]. The present work aims to compare the newly developed mTICCS with established and frequently used scoring systems to identify patients at risk for needing an MT.

2. Experimental Section

Severely injured patients (ISS ≥ 16) that were consecutively admitted to our trauma center (Level 1) between 2010 and 2015 were included in this study. Demographic data, as well as laboratory parameters (hemoglobin (Hb), lactate (Lac), partial thromboplastin time (PTT), International Normalized Ratio (INR)), and imaging data (focused assessment with sonography for trauma (FAST), X-ray, and CT), were collected. Furthermore, the mechanism of injury, injury pattern (graded by AIS), and outcome (length of stay, mortality) were recorded. Due to the retrospective nature of this study, ethical approval was not required.

2.1. Scores

Only scores including parameters that could be reproduced by the data captured in the hospital information system were considered. An MT was defined as the administration of 10 or more units of packed red blood cells (pRBC) in the first 24 h after arrival at the emergency room (ER). Scores were raised by two investigators (KH; RL). In case of discrepancies, results were discussed until consensus was achieved.

2.1.1. Trauma-Associated Severe Hemorrhage (TASH) Score

To identify the risk for needing an MT, the TASH score uses seven independent, weighted variables: systolic blood pressure, sex, hemoglobin, focused assessment for the sonography of trauma (FAST), heart rate, base excess (BE), and extremity or pelvic fractures. Using a logistic function, the TASH score is transformed into the probability of an MT. Consequently, a score ≥ 16 points indicates a > 50% probability of an MT. Furthermore, a score ≥ 27 points is associated with a 100% predicted and obtained risk for an MT [12,13].

2.1.2. Assessment of Blood Consumption (ABC) Score

The ABC score uses parameters: penetrating trauma mechanism, systolic blood pressure ≤ 90 mmHg on ER arrival, heart rate ≥ 120 bpm on ER arrival, and positive FAST examination, which are available during the first few minutes after hospital admission of a trauma patient, to assess the risk for an MT [14].

2.1.3. Larson Score

The Larson score is based on the "Joint Theater Trauma Registry" transfusion database, which includes data of US service personnel injured in combat scenarios during overseas deployment. The Larson score includes heart rate, systolic blood pressure, hemoglobin, and base deficit to identify the probability of an MT [15].

2.1.4. Prince of Wales Hospital (PWH) Score

The PWH score is based on data from 1891 civilian trauma patients admitted to The Prince of Wales Hospital in Hong Kong. Statistical analyses identified seven parameters: heart rate ≥ 120 bpm, systolic blood pressure ≤ 90 mmHg, Glasgow coma scale ≤ 8, displaced pelvic fracture, computer tomography (CT) scan or FAST-positive for fluid, base deficit > 5 mmol/L, hemoglobin ≤ 7 g/dL, and hemoglobin 7.1–10.0 g/dL, to predict the need for an MT [16].

2.1.5. Emergency Transfusion (ET) Score

Based on data from 1103 patients, nine parameters, with different predictive values indicating the need for a blood transfusion, were chosen for the ET score, including systolic blood pressure (SBP) < 90 mmHg or SBP 90–120 mmHg, free fluid on the abdominal ultrasound, clinically unstable pelvic ring fracture, aged 20–60 years or > 60 years, admission from scene of accident, traffic accident, and fall from > 3 m. Score values range from 1 (0.7% probability of an MT) to 9.5 (97% probability of an MT) points [17].

2.1.6. Modified Trauma-Induced Coagulopathy Clinical Score (mTICCS)

The mTICCS is a modified version of the TICCS [10]. There are three assessment criteria that form the score: the assessment of general severity, blood pressure, and the extent of body injury (Table 1). The original TICCS separated critical patients being admitted to the emergency room and noncritical patients without activation of the emergency room. If the emergency room was activated, 2 points were assigned, otherwise the patient was graded with 0 points. As severely injured patients are generally treated in emergency rooms, all patients were automatically assigned 2 points. Additionally, mTICCS does not discriminate between left and right extremity injuries but rather whether the injury affected the upper (left and/or right) or lower (left and/or right) extremities. In the modified scoring system, 1 point was attributed to a severe injury of the upper extremities and 1 point for a severe injury of the lower extremities.

Table 1. modified Trauma Induced Coagulopathy Clinical Score (Mticcs) criteria.

Criteria	Points
General Severity	
Admitted into resuscitation room with trauma team activation	2
Blood Pressure	
SBP * fell below 90 mmHg at least once	5
SBP * always above 90 mmHg	0
Extent of Significant Injuries	
Head and neck	1
Upper extremity (left or right)	1
Lower extremity (left or right)	1
Torso	2
Abdomen	2
Pelvis	2
Total Possible Score	2–16

* SBP: systolic blood pressure.

2.2. Statistical Analyses

Demographic data as well as injury mechanisms and pattern were described in tables by median and range or frequency and percentage. Comparisons between MT and no MT groups were performed by Wilcoxon rank-sum-test for continuous data or Chi-square-test. Results are presented as p-values.

mTICCS was compared to TASH, ABC, Larson, PWH, and ETS scores to evaluate its diagnostic accuracy. The different scores were evaluated with the need for an MT within the first 24 h after admission. The area under the receiver operating characteristic curve (AUC) was calculated for each score. The Youden Index was used to determine the cut-off point at which sensitivity and specificity were of equal diagnostic importance. The Youden Index specifies the optimal cut-off point by maximizing the difference between true positive and false positive ratings over all possible cut-off points. Prevalence, sensitivity, specificity, positive predicted values (PPV), and negative predicted values (NPV) with corresponding 95% confidence limits (95% CI) were used for the comparison of scores.

The AUC of the mTICCS was compared to the AUCs of TASH, ABC, Larson, PWH, and ETS scores to assess and compare the overall diagnostic accuracy. Results were reported as the AUC value with the corresponding 95% confidence limits and p-values. For all comparisons, the significance level was set to 5%, and due to the explorative nature of this study no adjustment was made to the significance level for multiple testing. All analyses were performed by SPSS 25.0 (IBM®, New York, NY, USA) and MedCalc®version 18.9.1 (MedCalc software, Ostend, Belgium).

3. Results

3.1. General Data

In total, 479 patients were included in this study. Demographic data, injury mechanisms, as well as mortality rates are displayed in Table 2. Overall, patients were discharged after 21 (29) days, of which they spent 14 (31) days in the intensive care unit. On average, patients were ventilated for 194 (398) hours. The overall MT rate was 8.4% (n = 40).

Table 2. Demographic data, injury mechanisms, and trauma severity.

Demographic Data	**No MT** n **= 439**	**MT** n **= 40**	p**-Value**
Age in years median (range)	50 (2–93)	42 (11–82)	0.536 †
Male sex in % (n)	70.6 (310)	80.0 (32)	0.209 §
‡ ISS median (range)	24 (16–75)	29 (17–59)	0.000 †
# NISS median (range)	27 (16–75)	31 (17–59)	0.011 †
RR * ≤ 90mmHg initial in % (n)	4.1 (18)	17.5 (7)	0.001 §
¥ BP in total ≤ 24 h median (range)	0 (0–9)	21.5 (10–106)	0.001 †
Overall mortality in % (n)	23.5 (103)	52.5 (21)	0.000§
Injury Mechanism (% n)			
Blunt	92.5 (406)	87.5 (35)	0.072 §
Car	17.3 (76)	15 (6)	0.710 §
Motorbike	11.2 (49)	17.5 (7)	0.232 §
Bicycle	7.5 (33)	0 (0)	0.072 §
Fall < 3 m	22.3 (98)	7.5 (3)	0.028 §
Fall > 3 m	16.2 (71)	20 (8)	0.532 §
Pedestrian	8.2 (36)	20 (8)	0.013 §
Burn	3 (13)	0 (0)	0.270 §
Other	14.1 (62)	20 (8)	0.314 §

Table 2. *Cont.*

Demographic Data	No MT $n = 439$	MT $n = 40$	p-Value
$ **AIS median (range)**			
Head	3 (0–5)	2 (0–5)	0.193 †
Face	0 (0–3)	0 (0–3)	0.444 †
Thorax	2 (0–5)	3 (0–5)	0.132 †
Abdomen	0 (0–5)	2 (0–5)	0.000 †
Extremities	2 (0–5)	3 (0–4)	0.000 †
External	0 (0–6)	0 (0–2)	0.624 †

* RR = blood pressure by Riva-Rocci in mmHg; ¥ BP = blood products; ‡ ISS = Injury Severity Scale; # NISS = New Injury Severity Scale; $ AIS = Abbreviated Injury Score. † Wilcoxon rank-sum-test for continuous data, § Chi-square-test.

3.2. AUC Analysis

For the tested scores, AUC analysis revealed values between 0.648 (PWH) and 0.782 (TASH) (Table 3; Figure 1). mTICCS had a significantly larger AUC than PWH (0.776, 95% CI: (0.736; 0.812) vs. 0.648, 95% CI: (0.603; 0.691); $p = 0.0103$). However, no significant difference was identified between the AUC of mTICCS and the AUCs of the other scores (Table 3).

Table 3. Comparative area under the curve (AUC) analysis.

Score	mTICCS	TASH	ABC	Larson	PWH	ETS
AUC	0.776	0.782	0.684	0.740	0.648	0.713
95% CI *	0.736; 0.812	0.743; 0.819	0.641; 0.726	0.698; 0.779	0.603; 0.691	0.670; 0.753
Cut-off	> 5	> 8	> 0	> 1	>2	> 2.5
p-value for the comparison of AUC to AUC of mTICCS		0.8852	0.0756	0.3839	0.0103	0.0804

* CI (confidence interval).

3.3. Prevalence, Sensitivity, Specificity, Positive, and Negative Predictive Values

Sensitivity was highest for ETS, followed by mTICCS, PWH, TASH, ABC, and Larson, respectively. However, specificity was highest for TASH, followed by Larson, ABC, mTICCS, ETC, and PWH (Table 4). TASH also presented with the highest PPV, while NPV was highest for mTICCS (Table 4).

Table 4. Prevalence, sensitivity, specificity, positive predictive value (PPV), and negative predictive value (NPV).

Score	mTICCS	TASH	ABC	Larson	PWH	ETS
Prevalence (%)	8.35	8.35	8.35	8.35	8.35	8.35
Sensitivity (%)	77.50	67.50	60.00	55.00	77.50	80.00
95% CI *	61.5; 89.2	50.9; 81.4	43.3; 75.1	38.5; 70.7	61.5; 89.2	64.4; 90.9
Specificity (%)	74.03	82.00	74.56	79.50	51.83	52.97
95% CI *	69.7; 78.1	78.1; 85.5	70.3; 78.6	75.4; 83.2	47.0; 56.5	48.2; 57.7
PPV (%)	21.4	25.5	17.8	19.6	12.8	13.4
95% CI *	17.8; 25.5	20.3; 31.4	13.8; 22.6	14.9; 25.5	10.8; 15.1	11.4; 15.7
NPV (%)	97.3	96.5	95.3	95.1	96.2	96.7
95% CI *	95.3; 98.5	94.5; 97.7	93.3; 96.8	93.2; 96.5	93.4; 97.8	93.9; 98.2

* CI (confidence interval).

Considering mTICCS as screening tool, 145 were identified at risk of MT (145 test positives among 479 screend patients), and among these 145 patients, 31 went on to need MT (PPV of 21%). In addition, of the 40 patients needing MT in our sample, 31 were correctly identified by mTICCS (sensitivity of

77.50%) while 9 patients were missed (false negative). On the other hand, of the 439 patients who do not need MT, 325 were correctly identified (specificity of 74.03%) while 114 were missed (false positive).

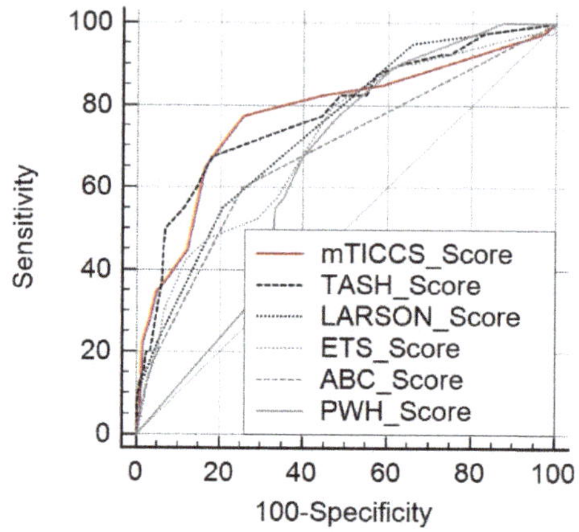

Figure 1. Area under the receiver operating characteristic curves (AUCs) for the mTICCS, Trauma-Associated Severe Hemorrhage (TASH), Assessment of Blood Consumption (ABC), Larson, Prince of Wales Hospital (PWH), and Emergency Transfusion Score (ETS) scores.

4. Discussion

Although early management of acute coagulopathy in trauma victims improves the outcome, timely identification and prediction of a trauma-induced hemorrhage and the associated need for an MT remains challenging [18,19]. Therefore, the present study compared the newly developed and easily applicable mTICCS to five established scoring algorithms in order to classify the relevance of mTICCS as a prediction method for an MT. Our results show that the AUC of the mTICCS was comparable to the TASH, Larson, ABC, and ETS scores and superior to the PHW score. mTICCS is calculated with the lowest number of assessment criteria, which are also easily accessible and gained early on in evaluation. These findings make mTICCS highly interesting for a clinical routine, as the assessment criteria of general trauma severity, blood pressure, and extent of body injury do not need sophisticated diagnostic tools and can easily be scored by paramedics as well as hospital staff.

In general, one could assume that more complex scores are superior for prediction of an MT when compared to more compact systems. Accordingly, the TASH score [12], which includes demographic data, physical variables, laboratory results, injury patterns, and sonography, was shown to represent the gold standard in the prediction of an MT with the highest AUC (0.889) when compared to the PWH (0.860) and the score of Vandromme et al (0.840) in a trauma cohort of 5147 patients [9]. The authors of this study concluded that weighted and more sophisticated systems like TASH and PWH scores, which include more and often similar variables, performed better than those that use simple, nonweighted models [9]. However, the PWH score did not perform well in our study and presented with a significantly lower AUC than mTICCS. This is interesting because the PWH score uses comparable components to the TASH score and applies weights to selected individual parameters to stratify patient' risk for an MT. Similar to the results found in our study, Mitra et al. showed, in a trauma cohort of 1234 Australian patients, that the PWH score was significantly less predictive for an MT than other scores [20]. The PWH score was initially developed and validated in the New Territories of Hong Kong, where 95% of the population are Chinese; therefore, ethical aspects might explain the observed differences between the scoring systems. Similarly, Singhal et al. showed that thromboelastography analysis of Asian and Caucasian patients revealed different hemostatic mechanisms [21]. In this context, Asians presented with significantly lower postoperative factor levels than Caucasians, and baseline comparisons of factor and serum levels revealed that Asians presented with the lowest thrombogenic profiles when compared to other ethnic groups. Further aspects in regard to different hemostatic mechanisms between the two races were confirmed [21,22]. In contrast to the PHW score, the well-performing TASH score was developed and validated in a Caucasian population; therefore, it may be assumed that ethnicity has a significant influence on the relevance of a score to evaluate the probability of an MT.

In addition to ethnicity, other aspects of the study population's composition need to be considered when comparing the predictive value of different scores. In this context, Brockamp et al. included patients with an ISS > 9 who survived until ICU admission [9]. Thus, it might be assumed that those scores were tested against a relatively "stable" cohort, with a lower risk for bleeding complications, compared to the scores included in the present study (ISS > 16, admission to shock room). This is supported by a higher percentage of MTs in the present study (8.4%) compared to 5.6%, which was reported by Brockamp et al. [9]. When considering the highly complex TASH and PWH scores, combat zones, as well as civilian scenarios with severely injured patients, recommend more simple tools to stratify patient' risk for an MT [14,15,17]. Other scores (Larson, ABC, and ET scores) have aimed to address this issue; however, these scores still use either laboratory (e.g., base deficit, hemoglobin) or other diagnostic (e.g., x-ray, FAST) variables, which are probably not available on scene or hamper timely identification of patients in need of the preclinical start of DCR and a future MT. Furthermore, although the data needed to calculate these scores may be available in a relatively short time after hospital admission, it still requires time to collect the data and calculate the score. This calls into question the utility of these scores as "early" identification tools and explains why these scores are not routinely used in clinical practice.

The original version of TICCS focused on easy and early application and could be determined before hospital admission [10,23]. Due to the known benefits of additional variables, like laboratory parameters or diagnostic imaging procedures, adding to the validity of prediction scores, Swerts et al. hypothesized that using BE and FAST would improve the predictive value of TICCS. Both parameters were chosen because they could theoretically be used in a prehospital setting. However, adding these variables to the original TICCS did not significantly improve the scoring system's ability to predict the need for an MT [24]. Unfortunately, the authors do not discuss possible reasons for their findings. BE has recently been discussed critically as a possible scoring variable [25], as it reflects the acid-base status and may increase during metabolic and respiratory acidosis and thus influence therapeutic resuscitation, such as fluid loading (chloride-induced acidosis) [26]. Moreover, in regard to additional imaging procedures, Becker et al. observed that the false-negative rate of FAST performed in blunt abdominal trauma patients with a high injury severity score (ISS > 25) is higher than that performed in patients with an ISS < 25 [27]. The authors demonstrated that the sensitivity of FAST is lower among patients with an ISS > 25 (65.1%) than patients with an ISS < 25 (86.4%). Becker at al. concluded that patients with a high ISS are at an increased risk of having ultrasound-occult injuries and have a lower accuracy during their ultrasound examination than patients with a low to moderate ISS [27]. Thus, including FAST into a scoring system for an MT prediction should be discussed carefully.

The original TICCS was adjusted to the modified version (mTICCS) in regard to the special characteristics of severely injured patients and the need to simplify predictions scores [11]. With this study we were able to show that despite its simplicity, the prognostic value (as indicated by the AUC) of mTICCS was not significantly different than that of the other scores. Thus, mTICCS might provide a useful tool to predict the need for an MT at a very early stage after trauma.

For the present analysis, a single dataset from a Level 1 trauma center was used, including a significant number of severely injured patients. All containing variables for the scoring systems and algorithms could be assessed. Furthermore, detailed data on transfusion practices and the use of blood products were available. However, data presented in the current study were collected from a retrospective database with information collected after hospital admission. Thus, information about prehospital applications of hemostatic agents with a potential influence on the amount of administered pRBCs was not available and might have caused some bias to the results. Furthermore, the score should be used by paramedics, nursing staff in the emergency room, as well as emergency physicians. Due to the retrospective nature of the study, an interrater liability might occur. Taking these shortcomings into account, prospective validation of the presented scores is urgently needed.

5. Conclusions

Based on its three assessment criteria, including the assessment of general severity, blood pressure, and extent of bodily injury, the mTICCS showed no significant difference in AUC when compared to the AUCs of other established and more sophisticated scores. Yet, due to mTICCS simple applicability, diagnosis can be made very early after hospital admission or even in the prehospital setting. Thus, mTICCS might provide a new useful diagnostic tool to detect patients with ongoing bleeding in need of an MT. Consequently, the time until therapy is initiated can be reduced. Prospective, follow-up studies are needed to determine the effect of this efficiency on outcome parameters.

Author Contributions: Conceptualization, K.H. and F.H.; Data curation, K.H., R.L., Ü.M., P.L., and C.D.W.; Formal analysis, K.H., M.T., P.L., and F.H.; Investigation, K.H., R.L., and Ü.M.; Methodology, K.H., C.D.W., and N.H.; Project administration, K.H. and F.H.; Resources, P.K. and F.H.; Supervision, K.H., N.H., P.K., and F.H.; Validation, K.H., M.T., P.L., C.D.W., P.K., and N.H.; Visualization, C.D.W. and N.H.; Writing—original draft, K.H. and M.T.; Writing—review and editing, N.H., P.K., and F.H. All authors have read and agreed to the published version of the manuscript.

Acknowledgments: The article was proofread by Proof-Reading-Service.com, Devonshire Business Centre, Works Road, Letchworth Garden City, SG6 1GJ, United Kingdom.

Conflicts of Interest: The authors declare no conflict of interest.

References

1. Pfeifer, R.; Tarkin, I.; Rocos, B.; Pape, H.C. Patterns of mortality and causes of death in polytrauma patients—Has anything changed? *Injury* **2009**, *40*, 907–911. [CrossRef] [PubMed]
2. Pfeifer, R.; Teuben, M.; Andruszkow, H.; Barkatali, B.M.; Pape, H.-C. Mortality Patterns in Patients with Multiple Trauma: A Systematic Review of Autopsy Studies. *PLoS ONE* **2016**, *11*, e0148844. [CrossRef] [PubMed]
3. Acosta, J.A.; Yang, J.C.; Winchell, R.J.; Simons, R.K.; A Fortlage, D.; Hollingsworth-Fridlund, P.; Hoyt, D.B. Lethal injuries and time to death in a level I trauma center. *J. Am. Coll. Surg.* **1998**, *186*, 528–533. [CrossRef]
4. Kauvar, D.S.; Lefering, R.; Wade, C.E. Impact of Hemorrhage on Trauma Outcome: An Overview of Epidemiology, Clinical Presentations, and Therapeutic Considerations. *J. Trauma Inj. Infect. Crit. Care* **2006**, *60*, S3–S11. [CrossRef]
5. Cohen, J.; Scorer, T.G.; Wright, Z.; Stewart, I.J.; Sosnov, J.; Pidcoke, H.; Fedyk, C.; Kwan, H.; Chung, K.K.; Heegard, K.; et al. A prospective evaluation of thromboelastometry (ROTEM) to identify acute traumatic coagulopathy and predict massive transfusion in military trauma patients in Afghanistan. *Transfusion* **2019**, *59*, 1601–1607. [CrossRef]
6. Prat, N.J.; Meyer, A.D.; Ingalls, N.K.; Trichereau, J.; DuBose, J.J.; Cap, A.P. Rotational thromboelastometry significantly optimizes transfusion practices for damage control resuscitation in combat casualties. *J. Trauma Acute Care Surg.* **2017**, *83*, 373–380. [CrossRef]
7. Murphy, C.H.; Hess, J.R. Massive transfusion: Red blood cell to plasma and platelet unit ratios for resuscitation of massive hemorrhage. *Curr. Opin. Hematol.* **2015**, *22*, 533–539. [CrossRef]
8. Tonglet, M. Early Prediction of Ongoing Hemorrhage in Severe Trauma: Presentation of the Existing Scoring Systems. *Arch. Trauma Res.* **2016**, *5*, 33377. [CrossRef]
9. Brockamp, T.; Nienaber, U.; Mutschler, M.; Wafaisade, A.; Peiniger, S.; Lefering, R.; Bouillon, B.; Maegele, M. Predicting on-going hemorrhage and transfusion requirement after severe trauma: A validation of six scoring systems and algorithms on the TraumaRegister DGU®. *Crit. Care* **2012**, *16*, R129. [CrossRef]
10. Tonglet, M.; Minon, J.-M.; Seidel, L.; Poplavsky, J.L.; Vergnion, M. Prehospital identification of trauma patients with early acute coagulopathy and massive bleeding: Results of a prospective non-interventional clinical trial evaluating the Trauma Induced Coagulopathy Clinical Score (TICCS). *Crit. Care* **2014**, *18*, 648. [CrossRef]

11. Tonglet, M.; Lefering, R.; Minon, J.-M.; Ghuysen, A.; D'Orio, V.; Hildebrand, F.; Pape, H.C.; Horst, K. Prehospital identification of trauma patients requiring transfusion: Results of a retrospective study evaluating the use of the trauma induced coagulopathy clinical score (TICCS) in 33,385 patients from the TraumaRegister DGU®. *Acta Chir. Belg.* **2017**, *117*, 385–390. [CrossRef] [PubMed]
12. Yucel, N.; Lefering, R.; Maegele, M.; Vorweg, M.; Tjardes, T.; Ruchholtz, S.; Neugebauer, E.A.M.; Wappler, F.; Bouillon, B.; Rixen, D. Trauma Associated Severe Hemorrhage (TASH)-Score: Probability of Mass Transfusion as Surrogate for Life Threatening Hemorrhage after Multiple Trauma. *J. Trauma: Inj. Infect. Crit. Care* **2006**, *60*, 1228–1237. [CrossRef] [PubMed]
13. Maegele, M.; Lefering, R.; Wafaisade, A.; Theodorou, P.; Wutzler, S.; Fischer, P.; Bouillon, B.; Paffrath, T.; Trauma Registry of Deutsche Gesellschaft für Unfallchirurgie (TR-DGU). Revalidation and update of the TASH-Score: A scoring system to predict the probability for massive transfusion as a surrogate for life-threatening haemorrhage after severe injury. *Vox Sang.* **2010**, *100*, 231–238. [CrossRef] [PubMed]
14. Nunez, T.C.; Voskresensky, I.V.; Dossett, L.A.; Shinall, R.; Dutton, W.D.; Cotton, B.A. Early Prediction of Massive Transfusion in Trauma: Simple as ABC (Assessment of Blood Consumption)? *J. Trauma Inj. Infect. Crit. Care* **2009**, *66*, 346–352. [CrossRef]
15. Larson, C.R.; White, C.E.; Spinella, P.C.; Jones, J.A.; Holcomb, J.B.; Blackbourne, L.H.; Wade, C.E. Association of Shock, Coagulopathy, and Initial Vital Signs with Massive Transfusion in Combat Casualties. *J. Trauma Inj. Infect. Crit. Care* **2010**, *69*, S26–S32. [CrossRef]
16. Rainer, T.; Ho, A.M.-H.; Yeung, J.H.; Cheung, N.K.; Wong, R.; Tang, N.; Ng, S.K.; Manoel, A.L.D.O.; Lai, P.B.; Graham, C.A. Early risk stratification of patients with major trauma requiring massive blood transfusion. *Resuscitation* **2011**, *82*, 724–729. [CrossRef]
17. Kuhne, C.A.; Zettl, R.; Fischbacher, M.; Lefering, R.; Ruchholtz, S. Emergency Transfusion Score (ETS): A Useful Instrument for Prediction of Blood Transfusion Requirement in Severely Injured Patients. *World J. Surg.* **2008**, *32*, 1183–1188. [CrossRef]
18. Chang, R.; Holcomb, J.B. Optimal Fluid Therapy for Traumatic Hemorrhagic Shock. *Crit. Care Clin.* **2017**, *33*, 15–36. [CrossRef]
19. Tran, A.; Matar, M.; Steyerberg, E.; Lampron, J.; Taljaard, M.; Vaillancourt, C. Early identification of patients requiring massive transfusion, embolization, or hemostatic surgery for traumatic hemorrhage: A systematic review protocol. *Syst. Rev.* **2017**, *6*, 80. [CrossRef]
20. Mitra, B.; Cameron, P.; Mori, A.; Maini, A.; Fitzgerald, M.; Paul, E.; Street, A. Early prediction of acute traumatic coagulopathy. *Resuscitation* **2011**, *82*, 1208–1213. [CrossRef]
21. Singhal, D.; Smorodinsky, E.; Guo, L. Differences in Coagulation Among Asians and Caucasians and the Implication for Reconstructive Microsurgery. *J. Reconstr. Microsurg.* **2010**, *27*, 57–62. [CrossRef] [PubMed]
22. Cheung, Y.F.; Chay, G.; Ma, E. Ethnic Differences in Coagulation Factor Abnormalities After the Fontan Procedure. *Pediatr. Cardiol.* **2006**, *27*, 96–101. [CrossRef] [PubMed]
23. Thorn, S.; Güting, H.; Maegele, M.; Gruen, R.L.; Mitra, B. Early Identification of Acute Traumatic Coagulopathy Using Clinical Prediction Tools: A Systematic Review. *Medicina* **2019**, *55*, 653. [CrossRef] [PubMed]
24. Swerts, F.; Mathonet, P.Y.; Ghuysen, A.; D´orio, V.; Minon, J.M.; Tonglet, M. Early identification of trauma patients in need for emergent transfusion: Results of a single-center retrospective study evaluating three scoring systems. *Eur. J. Trauma Emerg. Surg.* **2018**, *45*, 681–686. [CrossRef] [PubMed]
25. Raux, M.; Le Manach, Y.; Gauss, T.; Baumgarten, R.; Hamada, S.; Harrois, A.; Riou, B.; Duranteau, J.; Langeron, O.; Mantz, J.; et al. Comparison of the Prognostic Significance of Initial Blood Lactate and Base Deficit in Trauma Patients. *Anesthesiology* **2017**, *126*, 522–533. [CrossRef]
26. Berend, K.; De Vries, A.; Gans, R.O. Physiological Approach to Assessment of Acid–Base Disturbances. *N. Engl. J. Med.* **2014**, *371*, 1434–1445. [CrossRef]
27. Becker, A.; Lin, G.; McKenney, M.G.; Marttos, A.; Schulman, C. Is the FAST exam reliable in severely injured patients? *Injury* **2010**, *41*, 479–483. [CrossRef]

Journal of
Clinical Medicine

MDPI

Article

Effects of Virtual Reality-Based Rehabilitation on Burned Hands: A Prospective, Randomized, Single-Blind Study

So Young Joo [1], Yoon Soo Cho [1], Seung Yeol Lee [2], Hyun Seok [2,†] and Cheong Hoon Seo [1,*,†]

1 Department of Rehabilitation Medicine, Hangang Sacred Heart Hospital, College of Medicine Hallym University, Seoul 07247, Korea; anyany98@naver.com (S.Y.J.); yscho@hallym.or.kr (Y.S.C.)
2 Department of Physical Medicine and Rehabilitation, College of Medicine, Soonchunhyang University Hospital, Bucheon 14584, Korea; shouletz@gmail.com (S.Y.L.); 50503@schmc.ac.kr (H.S.)
* Correspondence: chseomd@gmail.com; Tel.: +82-2-2639-5738; Fax: +82-2-2635-7820
† H.S. and C.H.S. contributed equally as corresponding authors of this work.

Received: 31 January 2020; Accepted: 4 March 2020; Published: 9 March 2020

Abstract: Hands are the most frequent burn injury sites. Appropriate rehabilitation is essential to ensure good functional recovery. Virtual reality (VR)-based rehabilitation has proven to be beneficial for the functional recovery of the upper extremities. We investigated and compared VR-based rehabilitation with conventional rehabilitation (CON) in patients with burned hands. Fifty-seven patients were randomized into a VR or CON group. Each intervention was applied to the affected hand for four weeks, and clinical and functional variables were evaluated. Hand function was evaluated before intervention and four weeks after intervention using the Jebsen-Taylor hand function test (JTT), Grasp and Pinch Power Test, Purdue Pegboard test (PPT), and Michigan Hand Outcomes Questionnaire (MHQ). The JTT scores for picking up small objects and the MHQ scores for hand function, functional ADL, work, pain, aesthetics, and patient satisfaction were significantly higher in the VR group than in the CON group ($p < 0.05$). The results suggested that VR-based rehabilitation is likely to be as effective as conventional rehabilitation for recovering function in a burned hand. VR-based rehabilitation may be considered as a treatment option for patients with burned hands.

Keywords: virtual reality; burn; hand

1. Introduction

The distal parts of the upper extremities are the most common sites of thermal injury. The hand is one of the three most common joints of scar contracture deformity following a burn injury [1,2]. Some studies have reported that the total body surface area grafted and injury to the right dominant hand are some of the predictors of hand contracture [1]. The loss of hand function after a burn can have a crucial effect on the activities of daily living (ADL). Some reports have noted that two-thirds of the patients with deep hand burns change their profession because of their hand functional disorder [3]. Functionally, hand contractures may affect one's ability to perform ADL, such as dressing, eating, and grooming as well as fine motor tasks such as typing, writing, and occupational activities. Common complications after a burn to the hand include joint deformities, sensory impairment, scar contracture, and postburn edema [3].

Appropriate rehabilitation is important to ensure that good functional recovery is achieved [4,5]. Burned hands are usually treated and managed by a multidisciplinary team at a burn center to conservatively manage hypertrophic scars and soft tissue contractures. Rehabilitation of the burned hand should be initiated in the acute stages by means of individualized positioning, splinting, and exercise for improving functional activity [6,7]. Frequent exercise throughout the day is more beneficial than one session of intensive exercise [8,9]. Repeated range of motion (ROM) exercises are helpful in decreasing edema and conditioning the tissue. Despite rehabilitation of the burned hand, impaired hand function may remain [10]. Many interventions have been developed and tested for patients with burns; however, the strategies of hand rehabilitation remain controversial [11,12].

Recent studies have recommended repetitive exercises using virtual reality (VR) for functional recovery from upper extremity disorders [13,14] because the effectiveness of task-specific training improved when tasks were ordered in a random practice sequence using repetition and positive feedback. Many types of VR-based rehabilitation apparatus, from commercial video game equipment to robotics, are currently being developed and used. The RAPAEL Smart Glove™ (Neofect, Yong-in, Korea) is a VR rehabilitation tool designed for the distal upper extremities [15]. VR is an interactive and enjoyable intervention that creates a virtual rehabilitation scene in which the intensity of practice can be systemically manipulated [16]. Recently, VR has been used in burn studies mainly for pain reduction during acute burn dressing [17,18]. However, few studies have used VR systems for therapeutic purposes and functional assessments in burn patients. This study aimed to evaluate the effects of VR-based rehabilitation on burned hands and compare the results to those of matched conventional intervention (CON) rehabilitation in patients with burns.

2. Materials and Methods

The present study was a single-blind, randomized controlled trial. We recruited 57 (54 men and 3 women) patients from the Department of Rehabilitation Medicine at Hangang Sacred Heart Hospital in Korea between June and October 2019. Our study was registered on ClinicalTrials (NCT03865641). The study was registered at the Ethics Committee of the Hangang Sacred Heart Hospital (2014-081). Patients provided written informed consent. All participants' burn scars had re-epithelialized after split-thickness skin graft (STSG). To evaluate the effectiveness of VR rehabilitation accurately, the comparison was limited to the right hand and wrist. We included patients aged ≥18 years with a deep, partial-thickness (second-degree) burn or a full thickness (third-degree) burn with the involvement of >50% of the body surface area of the dominant right hand, with joint contracture (hand and wrist). In addition, these patients were transferred to the rehabilitation department after acute burn treatment and less than 6 months since the onset of the burn injury (Figure 1).

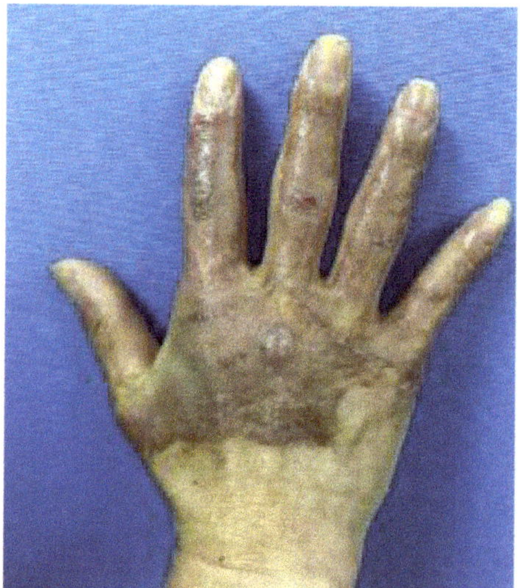

Figure 1. Patient with a deep partial-thickness burn or a full thickness burn with the involvement of >50% of the body surface area of the dominant right hand.

The study excluded patients who had fourth-degree burns (involving muscles, tendons, and bone injuries), musculoskeletal diseases (fracture, amputation, rheumatoid arthritis, and degenerative joint diseases) involving the burned hand, neurological diseases (such as peripheral nerve disorders), preexisting physical and psychologic disability (severe aphasia and cognitive impairment that could influence the intervention), or severe pain impeding hand rehabilitation. Numbers were assigned to 66 burn patients according to the order of admission who satisfied all the aforementioned criteria. A computer program was used to randomly divide them into the VR group (n = 32) or the CON group (n = 34). One patient in the VR group completed 17 sessions before dropping out due to scheduling conflict. Two patients in the CON group were forced to drop out before completing the study, including one who completed 11 sessions before dropping out due to unrelated medical issues and one who completed 18 sessions before dropping out due to a personal scheduling conflict. Three patients in the VR group and three patients in the CON group dropped out of the study because they recovered function in the injured hand after 20 sessions and could return to their daily life; therefore, they did not want to undergo serial evaluations and did not visit the outpatient clinic. Data from these subjects were not included in the analyses. Thus, patients were divided into two groups (28 patients in the VR group and 29 patients in the CON group) (Figure 2). All patients received a four-week intervention (20 sessions for 60 min per day). The VR group received 30-min standard therapy and 30-min VR-based rehabilitation. The CON group received 60-min standard therapy. The VR and CON interventions focused on the burned hand. Every effort was made to match the exercise rehabilitation in both groups and to adapt the level of difficulty to each patient's performance. The intervention frequency and duration did not differ between the VR and CON groups. The rehabilitation was supervised by three occupational therapists who had experience with VR rehabilitation tools and conventional therapy. Therefore, all factors, except for the use of the VR system, were consistent between the 2 groups.

We applied the RAPAEL Smart Glove^{TM} (Neofect, Yong-in, Korea) system, which combined the use of an exoskeleton type glove and the VR system (Figure 3). This tool can be operated only through active movement and not through passive movement. The software can be used to visualize the virtual hands in the VR tool according to the data gathered by a glove-shaped sensor device. The training programs demanded the following volitional movements: forearm pronation/supination, wrist flexion/extension, wrist radial/ulnar deviation, and finger flexion/extension (Figure 4). Visual and audio feedback informed the patients of success or failure. The patients were required to accurately complete a task in time and with proper power to obtain high scores. The standard therapy comprised range of motion (ROM) exercises for the burned hand, strengthening exercises of the upper extremities using tabletop activities, manual lymphatic drainage, and desensitizing sensory stimulation of hypertrophic scars.

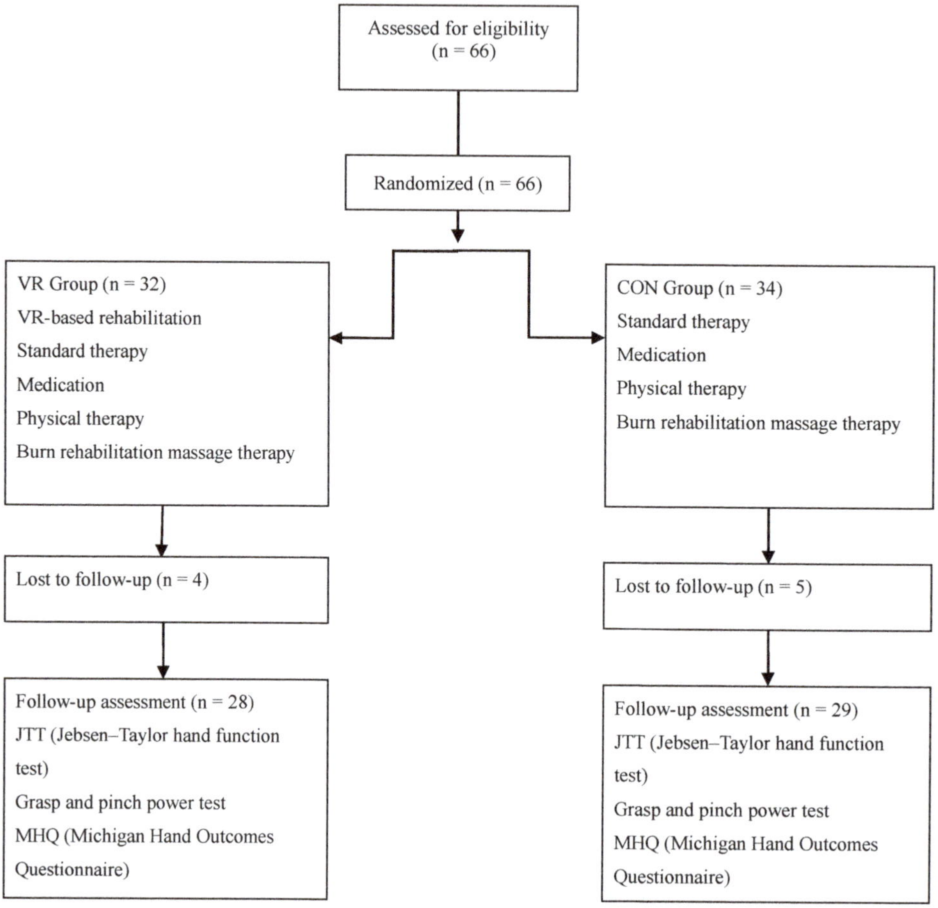

Figure 2. Diagram for subject enrollment, allocation, and follow-up. VR: virtual reality; CON: conventional rehabilitation

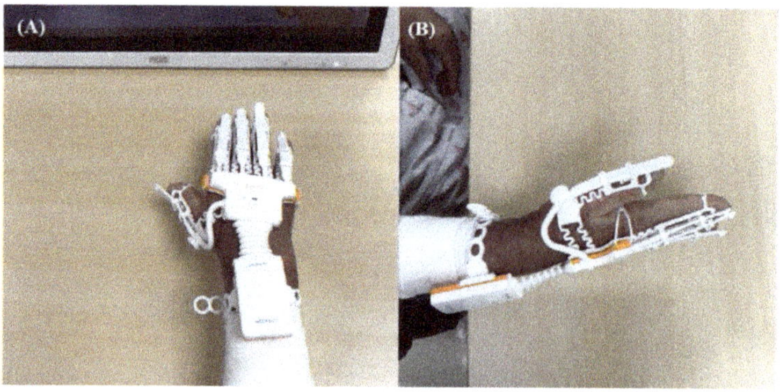

Figure 3. Virtual reality-based rehabilitation system on the burned hand of a study patient: (**A**) antero-posterior view (**B**) lateral view.

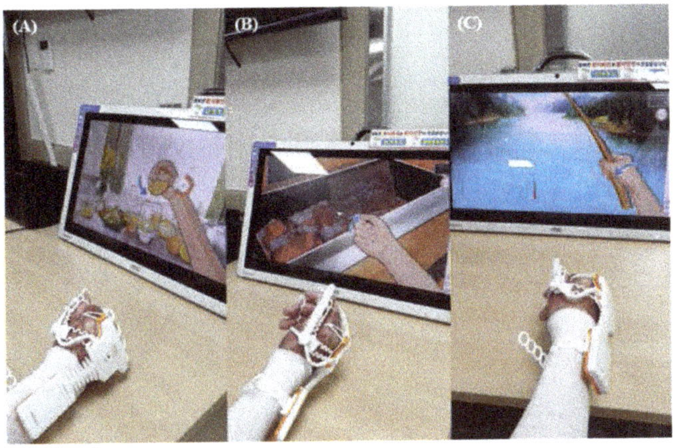

Figure 4. Volitional movements in the virtual reality-based rehabilitation system: (**A**) finger flexion/extension, (**B**) forearm pronation/supination, (**C**) wrist flexion/extension.

A squeeze dynamometer (Lafayette Instrument, Lafayette, IN, USA) was used to measure grip strength, and the Michigan Hand Outcomes Questionnaire (MHQ) [19] was used to assess a patient's perception of hand function. All MHQ scale scores are based on a scale from 0 to 100. For all scores, except for pain scores, higher scores indicate better hand performance. For the pain scale, lower scores indicate less pain. The Jebsen–Taylor hand function test (JTT) measured the performance speed of standardized tasks [20]. The JTT involves a series of 7 subtests. We used a scoring system in which each subtest score ranged from 0 to 15, and the total score ranged from 0 to 105. The Purdue Pegboard test (PPT) was used to measure fine hand motor functions and dexterity. The scores in the PPT indicate the numbers of pins placed in a board with 2 parallel rows of 25 holes within 30 s. The assembly score in the PPT is assessed for the number of assembled pins, washers, and collars in 60 s. We recorded scores for the right affected hand, both hands, and assembly. The grip strength, JTT, PPT, and MHQ scores were measured immediately before the intervention and after the 4-week intervention. Outcome measurements and data analyses were performed by a trained and blinded outcome assessor who was not involved in the intervention.

Statistical analysis was performed using SPSS, version 23 (International Business Machines (IBM) Corp., Armonk, NY, USA). Parametric data was analyzed using a paired t-test after testing for normality. Non-parametric data was analyzed using the Mann–Whitney test and the Wilcoxon signed-rank sum test. To examine the pretreatment homogeneity between the VR and CON groups, the Mann–Whitney test was used for age, time to treatment, Grasp and Pinch Power Test, PPT, all areas of the JTT, and all areas of the MHQ, with a significance level of $p < 0.05$. The changes before and after intervention were compared using the independent t-test for tip pinch strength between groups. The changes before and after intervention were compared using the Mann–Whitney test for all parameters except pinch strength, with a significance level of $p < 0.05$. The scores after intervention were compared between the two groups using the Mann–Whitney test for grasp strength, lateral pinch strength test, all areas of the PPT, all areas of the MHQ, and all areas of the JTT. As this was the first study to assess the efficacy of the VR-based rehabilitation in patients with burns, power calculation was based on a previous study, which applied VR-based rehabilitation for the distal upper extremity function in patients with stroke [15]. Accordingly, eighteen patients were required in each group to provide 80% power for efficacy evaluation, setting the α level at 0.05. We calculated that a minimum 52 patients were needed, considering a 30% dropout rate.

3. Results

Within six months after a burn injury, 57 patients had received rehabilitative therapy. Before the intervention, there were no differences in demographic and clinical characteristics between the patients in the VR and CON groups (Table 1).

Table 1. Baseline characteristics of the study patients.

	VR Group (n = 28)	CON Group (n = 29)	p-Value
Male: Female	28:0	26:3	0.24
Age (years)	48.07 ± 8.14	41.69 ± 14.05	0.21
Cause of burn			0.06
Flame burn	18	16	
Electrical burn	2		
Contact burn		6	
Scalding burn	2	4	
Spark burn	6	3	
Time to treatment (days)	74.79 ± 24.15	83.79 ± 46.22	0.98
TBSA (%)	27.71 ± 20.15	27.38 ± 20.65	
Grasp and Pinch Power Test			
Grasp (kg)	4.35 ± 4.73	4.59 ± 3.98	0.53
Lateral Pinch (kg)	3.23 ± 1.38	3.97 ± 2.04	0.05
Tip Pinch (kg)	1.66 ± 1.48	1.60 ± 0.95	0.74
Jebsen Hand Function Test			
Writing	11.71 ± 2.81	10.72 ± 4.73	0.78
Cards	4.21 ± 2.28	3.97 ± 3.18	0.43
Small	7.86 ± 2.21	8.41 ± 4.82	0.05
Checkers	10.43 ± 3.58	9.69 ± 4.45	0.60
Feeding	11.36 ± 3.00	11.45 ± 3.71	0.32
Light	10.21 ± 3.34	9.66 ± 5.61	0.38
Heavy	9.79 ± 3.27	9.41 ± 4.81	0.45
Perdue Pegboard Test			
Affected hand	8.64 ± 3.07	8.41 ± 6.12	0.40
Both hands	6.86 ± 2.14	5.55 ± 5.21	0.58
Assembly	16.43 ± 8.70	14.34 ± 12.94	0.63
Michigan Hand Outcomes Questionnaire			
Function	19.64 ± 17.16	18.10 ± 13.19	0.83
ADL	21.07 ± 20.38	20.69 ± 16.46	0.91
Work	23.21 ± 22.49	15.52 ± 18.19	0.20
Pain	50.71 ± 19.42	58.45 ± 17.38	0.16
Aesthetics	15.63 ± 19.95	16.16 ± 17.72	0.58
Satisfaction	19.64 ± 19.67	20.69 ± 16.46	0.73

VR, Virtual Reality; CON, conventional; TBSA, total burn surface area; ADL, activities of daily living; Values are presented as mean ± standard deviation, p-values were calculated using Fisher's exact test or a Mann–Whitney test and a Student's t-test.

There were significant improvements in the grasp, lateral pinch, and tip pinch strength changes taken before and after intervention in the VR group compared with the changes in the CON group ($p = 0.03$, $p = 0.002$, $p = 0.03$, respectively) (Table 2). There were no significant differences in the grasp, lateral pinch, and tip pinch strength between the two groups after intervention ($p = 0.13$, $p = 0.06$, and $p = 0.07$, respectively) (Table 3). In the JTT, the subtest scores for picking up small objects and simulated feeding in the VR group showed significant changes, compared with the changes in the CON group ($p < 0.001$ and $p = 0.04$) (Table 2). The subtest score for picking up small objects was significantly higher in the VR group than in the CON group after the intervention ($p = 0.01$) (Table 3). There were no significant changes between the groups in the affected hand, both hands, and assembly ($p = 0.58$, $p = 0.69$, and $p = 0.96$, respectively) (Table 2). There were no significant differences in the affected hand, both hands, and assembly between the two groups after intervention ($p = 0.74$, $p = 0.33$, and $p = 0.41$, respectively) (Table 3).

Table 2. The changes of pre-intervention and post-intervention in both groups.

	VR Group (n = 28)	CON Group (n = 29)	p-Value
Grasp and Pinch Power Test			
Grasp (kg)	3.71 ± 4.02	1.78 ± 3.17	** 0.03
Lateral Pinch (kg)	1.31 ± 1.42	−0.46 ± 2.41	** 0.002
Tip Pinch (kg)	0.95 ± 0.88	0.19 ± 0.95	* 0.03
Jebsen Hand Function Test			
Writing	0.64 ± 1.95	0.93 ± 1.87	0.23
Cards	0.07 ± 3.23	0.07 ± 3.13	0.96
Small	2.36 ± 2.45	−0.31 ± 3.24	** <0.001
Checkers	0.57 ± 3.71	0.62 ± 4.32	0.81
Feeding	0.64 ± 2.42	−0.24 ± 2.85	** 0.04
Light	1.00 ± 3.10	1.48 ± 5.47	0.69
Heavy	0.07 ± 3.16	1.14 ± 3.99	0.90
Perdue Pegboard Test			
Affected hand	1.86 ± 2.46	2.21 ± 4.39	0.58
Both hands	2.93 ± 4.40	2.17 ± 3.42	0.69
Assembly	5.86 ± 8.31	5.62 ± 10.54	0.96
Michigan Hand Outcomes Questionnaire			
Function	32.14 ± 11.50	26.72 ± 18.82	0.28
ADL	37.14 ± 15.95	22.59 ± 17.25	** 0.003
Work	26.64 ± 28.25	22.07 ± 17.55	0.37
Pain	−23.21 ± 24.62	−13.62 ± 21.25	0.12
Aesthetics	21.88 ± 24.62	15.22 ± 22.93	0.24
Satisfaction	30.95 ± 10.72	15.95 ± 17.22	** 0.001

VR: Virtual Reality; CON: conventional; * $p < 0.05$ independent t-test; measurements between groups were compared; ** $p < 0.05$ Mann–Whitney test; measurements between groups were compared.

Table 3. Scores of hand function tests and the Michigan Hand Outcomes Questionnaire after intervention.

	VR Group (n = 28)	CON Group (n = 29)	p-Value
Grasp and Pinch Power Test			
Grasp (kg)	8.06 ± 6.61	6.37 ± 5.91	0.13
Lateral Pinch (kg)	4.54 ± 1.75	3.50 ± 2.69	0.06
Tip Pinch (kg)	2.61 ± 1.83	1.80 ± 1.29	0.07
Jebsen Hand Function Test			
Writing	12.36 ± 1.31	11.66 ± 4.32	0.33
Cards	4.29 ± 3.14	4.03 ± 3.21	0.69
Small	10.21 ± 1.64	8.10 ± 3.49	* 0.01
Checkers	11.00 ± 3.08	10.31 ± 3.01	0.33
Feeding	12.00 ± 2.80	11.21 ± 3.81	0.55
Light	11.21 ± 2.56	11.14 ± 3.60	0.40
Heavy	9.86 ± 3.50	10.55 ± 3.55	0.39
Perdue Pegboard Test			
Affected hand	10.50 ± 3.24	10.62 ± 5.18	0.74
Both hands	9.79 ± 5.88	7.72 ± 4.53	0.33
Assembly	22.29 ± 8.20	19.97 ± 11.72	0.41
Michigan Hand Outcomes Questionnaire			
Function	51.79 ± 17.91	44.83 ± 19.34	0.16
ADL	58.21 ± 18.92	43.28 ± 18.48	* 0.005
Work	47.86 ± 19.88	37.59 ± 13.73	* 0.04
Pain	27.50 ± 16.64	44.83 ± 26.57	* 0.002
Aesthetics	37.50 ± 19.39	31.38 ± 20.17	0.25
Satisfaction	50.60 ± 18.35	36.64 ± 17.55	* 0.02

VR: Virtual Reality; CON: conventional; * $p < 0.05$ Mann–Whitney test; measurements before the intervention and immediately following the 4-week intervention were compared.

In the MHQ scores, the subtest scores for functional ADL and patient satisfaction in the VR group showed significant changes, compared with the changes in the CON group ($p = 0.003$ and $p = 0.001$) (Table 2). There were significant improvements in the MHQ scores for functional ADL, work, pain, and patient satisfaction differences between the two groups ($p = 0.005$, $p = 0.04$, $p = 0.002$, and $p = 0.02$) (Table 3) No patient experienced adverse events such as skin abrasions or worsening of joint pain during training. In addition, no surgery-related adverse events were reported.

4. Discussion

After the intervention, the subtest scores in the JTT (picking up small objects) and subscale scores for ADL, work, pain, and satisfaction in the MHQ were significantly higher in the VR group than in the CON group. Minimum clinically important changes for scoring system in the JTT and MHQ have not been established in patients with burns. However, results of the JJT and MHQ showed significantly the improvements in VR group [16,21]. Participants were able to engage with the VR system and complete the interventions without premature withdrawal or non-adherence. A previous study has emphasized the importance of robot-assisted rehabilitation in the acute phase after musculoskeletal injuries and reported that it allowed the patient to mobilize the affected arm early by reducing muscle mass loss and improving motor capacity [22]. Immobilization after burn injuries induces loss of muscle strength and flexibility in adjacent joints. Recent studies have emphasized acute rehabilitation in patients with burns [23]. Schwickert et al. reported that VR treatment immediately after orthopedic surgery suppressed pain perception as the patient's attention was highly focused on task completion [24]. The role of immersive VR in pain reduction has been proven during physical therapy and burn wound care in patients with burns [17,18,25]. These studies found that VR rehabilitation in the acute rehabilitation phase after STSG was well-tolerated by patients with burns.

Importantly, significant changes in multiple outcome measures were observed in the VR group after intervention. Jeffery et al. reported that the VR system can be modified to maximize therapeutic benefits such as improving the ROM of the shoulder and elbow joints after burn injury [26]. The tasks in the VR system include ADLs, such as cooking, cleaning windows, squeezing oranges, and turning over pages. The patients were required to accurately complete each task in time and with proper power, to gain high scores. This provides a feeling of satisfaction in the MHQ that leads to positive reinforcement. A recent randomized controlled study showed that the subtest scores in the JTT were greater in the VR rehabilitation group than in the CON rehabilitation group in patients with hand impairments after stroke [16]. In addition, our study found that VR-based rehabilitation may be more effective in improving hand function as CON rehabilitation, according to the JTT and MHQ scores (pain and satisfaction).

We found that VR rehabilitation was effective according to the MHQ scores for ADL and work. Park et al. reported that upper extremity rehabilitation improved hand function in patients, in addition to elbow and forearm improvement [27]. Functions that include grasp power are associated with proximal upper extremity functions. Previous studies have found that task-specific rehabilitation improved upper extremity functions [28]. Some reports have shown that the effects of VR-based upper extremity rehabilitation had been transferred to untrained tasks [13,16,29]. This study found generalized improvement in unpracticed motor tasks after intervention for ADL tasks.

Moreover, many reports regarding neurorehabilitation have suggested that for functional recovery in the upper and lower extremities, repetitive intervention using VR is helpful and induces neuroplasticity [14,30–32]. Saleh et al. observed the different mechanisms between robot-assisted VR training and conventional functional rehabilitation in patients with chronic stroke using functional magnetic resonance imaging (MRI). Their study concluded that the different neural reorganization was due to the greater visuomotor feedback of the robot-assisted VR system than that of the conventional functional rehabilitation [33]. Further studies are required to evaluate the changes in brain activity or peripheral neuromuscular functions to improve our understanding of the mechanisms of VR rehabilitation after musculoskeletal injury, including burns. This study has limitations that require cautious interpretation of the data, including a relatively small sample size and narrowly focused inclusion criteria. For evaluating the efficacy of VR rehabilitation in patients with burned hand, the hand ROM parameter could be analyzed. However, the hand ROM parameter was not included in the routine hand function evaluations in this study. Further studies are required to compare efficacy in terms of edema reduction and improvement in hand ROM between VR-based and CON rehabilitation and to determine appropriate intervention levels for burned hands.

5. Conclusions

VR-based rehabilitation may be as effective as conventional hand rehabilitation for improving hand power, hand function, and MHQ scores. Burn survivors with acute hand impairment after STSG were able to successfully use the VR system and had significantly better scores on pain, ADL, work and satisfaction scales on the MHQ than the control group. As a result of this study, VR-based intervention is likely to be a clinically useful rehabilitation tool for patients with burned hands. Furthermore, studies that include hand rehabilitation for fourth-degree burns with severe neuromuscular injuries along with treatment intensity, frequency, and VR-based intervention interval studies are needed.

Author Contributions: C.H.S. and H.S. contributed equally as corresponding authors of this work. S.Y.J. contributed to the conception, design, data analysis, and interpretation of results. Y.S.C. and S.Y.L. contributed to revising the article critically for important intellectual content. All authors contributed to the writing of the manuscript. All authors have read and agreed to the published version of the manuscript.

Funding: This research was supported by the National Research Foundation of Korea (NRF), funded by the Korea government (MSIT) (NRF-2018R1C1B6008584).

Conflicts of Interest: The authors declare no potential conflict of interest.

References

1. Schneider, J.C.; Holavanahalli, R.; Helm, P.; O'Neil, C.; Goldstein, R.; Kowalske, K. Contractures in burn injury part II: Investigating joints of the hand. *J. Burn Care Res.* **2008**, *29*, 606–613. [CrossRef]
2. Richard, R.L.; Lester, M.E.; Miller, S.F.; Bailey, J.K.; Hedman, T.L.; Dewey, W.S.; Greer, M.; Renz, E.M.; Wolf, S.E.; Blackbourne, L.H. Identification of cutaneous functional units related to burn scar contracture development. *J. Burn Care Res.* **2009**, *30*, 625–631. [CrossRef] [PubMed]
3. Nuchtern, J.G.; Engrav, L.H.; Nakamura, D.Y.; Dutcher, K.A.; Heimbach, D.M.; Vedder, N.B. Treatment of fourth-degree hand burns. *J. Burn Care Rehabil.* **1995**, *16*, 36–42. [CrossRef] [PubMed]
4. Moore, M.L.; Dewey, W.S.; Richard, R.L. Rehabilitation of the burned hand. *Hand Clin.* **2009**, *25*, 529–541. [CrossRef] [PubMed]
5. Richard, R.; Baryza, M.J.; Carr, J.A.; Dewey, W.S.; Dougherty, M.E.; Forbes-Duchart, L.; Franzen, B.J.; Healey, T.; Lester, M.E.; Li, S.K.; et al. Burn rehabilitation and research: Proceedings of a consensus summit. *J. Burn Care Res.* **2009**, *30*, 543–573. [CrossRef] [PubMed]
6. Sorkin, M.; Cholok, D.; Levi, B. Scar Management of the Burned Hand. *Hand Clin.* **2017**, *33*, 305–315. [CrossRef]
7. Serghiou, M.A.; Niszczak, J.; Parry, I.; Richard, R. Clinical practice recommendations for positioning of the burn patient. *Burns* **2016**, *42*, 267–275. [CrossRef]
8. Richard, R.L.; Miller, S.F.; Finley, R.K., Jr.; Jones, L.M. Comparison of the effect of passive exercise v static wrapping on finger range of motion in the burned hand. *J. Burn Care Rehabil.* **1987**, *8*, 576–578. [CrossRef]
9. Tanigawa, M.C.; O'Donnell, O.K.; Graham, P.L. The burned hand: A physical therapy protocol. *Phys. Ther.* **1974**, *54*, 953–958. [CrossRef]
10. Fufa, D.T.; Chuang, S.S.; Yang, J.Y. Postburn contractures of the hand. *J. Hand Surg. Am.* **2014**, *39*, 1869–1876. [CrossRef]
11. Schouten, H.J.; Nieuwenhuis, M.K.; van Zuijlen, P.P. A review on static splinting therapy to prevent burn scar contracture: Do clinical and experimental data warrant its clinical application? *Burns* **2012**, *38*, 19–25. [CrossRef] [PubMed]

12. Choi, J.S.; Mun, J.H.; Lee, J.Y.; Jeon, J.H.; Jung, Y.J.; Seo, C.H.; Jang, K.U. Effects of modified dynamic metacarpophalangeal joint flexion orthoses after hand burn. *Ann. Rehabil. Med.* **2011**, *35*, 880–886. [CrossRef] [PubMed]
13. Burgar, C.G.; Lum, P.S.; Shor, P.C.; Machiel Van der Loos, H.F. Development of robots for rehabilitation therapy: The Palo Alto VA/Stanford experience. *J. Rehabil. Res Dev.* **2000**, *37*, 663–673. [PubMed]
14. Placidi, G. A smart virtual glove for the hand telerehabilitation. *Comput. Biol. Med.* **2007**, *37*, 1100–1107. [CrossRef]
15. Shin, J.H.; Kim, M.Y.; Lee, J.Y.; Jeon, Y.J.; Kim, S.; Lee, S.; Seo, B.; Choi, Y. Effects of virtual reality-based rehabilitation on distal upper extremity function and health-related quality of life: A single-blinded, randomized controlled trial. *J. Neuroeng. Rehabil.* **2016**, *13*, 17. [CrossRef]
16. Thielbar, K.O.; Lord, T.J.; Fischer, H.C.; Lazzaro, E.C.; Barth, K.C.; Stoykov, M.E.; Triandafilou, K.M.; Kamper, D.G. Training finger individuation with a mechatronic-virtual reality system leads to improved fine motor control post-stroke. *J. Neuroeng. Rehabil.* **2014**, *11*, 171. [CrossRef]
17. Schmitt, Y.S.; Hoffman, H.G.; Blough, D.K.; Patterson, D.R.; Jensen, M.P.; Soltani, M.; Carrougher, G.J.; Nakamura, D.; Sharar, S.R. A randomized, controlled trial of immersive virtual reality analgesia, during physical therapy for pediatric burns. *Burns* **2011**, *37*, 61–68. [CrossRef]
18. Kipping, B.; Rodger, S.; Miller, K.; Kimble, R.M. Virtual reality for acute pain reduction in adolescents undergoing burn wound care: A prospective randomized controlled trial. *Burns* **2012**, *38*, 650–657. [CrossRef]
19. Cowan, A.C.; Stegink-Jansen, C.W. Rehabilitation of hand burn injuries: Current updates. *Injury* **2013**, *44*, 391–396. [CrossRef]
20. Schoneveld, K.; Wittink, H.; Takken, T. Clinimetric evaluation of measurement tools used in hand therapy to assess activity and participation. *J. Hand Ther.* **2009**, *22*, 221–235. [CrossRef]
21. Ayaz, M.; Karami, M.Y.; Deilami, I.; Moradzadeh, Z. Effects of Early Versus Delayed Excision and Grafting on Restoring the Functionality of Deep Burn-Injured Hands: A Double-Blind, Randomized Parallel Clinical Trial. *J. Burn Care Res.* **2019**, *40*, 451–456. [CrossRef] [PubMed]
22. Nerz, C.; Schwickert, L.; Becker, C.; Studier-Fischer, S.; Mussig, J.A.; Augat, P. Effectiveness of robot-assisted training added to conventional rehabilitation in patients with humeral fracture early after surgical treatment: Protocol of a randomised, controlled, multicentre trial. *Trials* **2017**, *18*, 589. [CrossRef] [PubMed]
23. Kornhaber, R.; Rickard, G.; McLean, L.; Wiechula, R.; Lopez, V.; Cleary, M. Burn care and rehabilitation in Australia: Health professionals' perspectives. *Disabil. Rehabil.* **2019**, *41*, 714–719. [CrossRef] [PubMed]
24. Schwickert, L.; Klenk, J.; Stahler, A.; Becker, C.; Lindemann, U. Robotic-assisted rehabilitation of proximal humerus fractures in virtual environments: A pilot study. *Z. Für Gerontol. Und Geriatr.* **2011**, *44*, 387–392. [CrossRef] [PubMed]
25. Carrougher, G.J.; Hoffman, H.G.; Nakamura, D.; Lezotte, D.; Soltani, M.; Leahy, L.; Engrav, L.H.; Patterson, D.R. The effect of virtual reality on pain and range of motion in adults with burn injuries. *J. Burn Care Res.* **2009**, *30*, 785–791. [CrossRef] [PubMed]
26. Schneider, J.C.; Ozsecen, M.Y.; Muraoka, N.K.; Mancinelli, C.; Della Croce, U.; Ryan, C.M.; Bonato, P. Feasibility of an Exoskeleton-Based Interactive Video Game System for Upper Extremity Burn Contractures. *PM & R* **2016**, *8*, 445–452.
27. Park, W.Y.; Jung, S.J.; Joo, S.Y.; Jang, K.U.; Seo, C.H.; Jun, A.Y. Effects of a Modified Hand Compression Bandage for Treatment of Post-Burn Hand Edemas. *Ann. Rehabil. Med.* **2016**, *40*, 341–350. [CrossRef]
28. French, B.; Leathley, M.J.; Sutton, C.J.; McAdam, J.; Thomas, L.H.; Forster, A.; Langhorne, P.; Price, C.; Walker, A.; Watkins, C.L. A systematic review of repetitive functional task practice with modelling of resource use, costs and effectiveness. *Health Technol. Assess.* **2008**, *12*, 1–17. [CrossRef]
29. Schaefer, S.Y.; Patterson, C.B.; Lang, C.E. Transfer of training between distinct motor tasks after stroke: Implications for task-specific approaches to upper-extremity neurorehabilitation. *Neurorehabil. Neural. Repair.* **2013**, *27*, 602–612. [CrossRef]
30. Saita, K.; Morishita, T.; Arima, H.; Hyakutake, K.; Ogata, T.; Yagi, K.; Shiota, E.; Inoue, T. Biofeedback effect of hybrid assistive limb in stroke rehabilitation: A proof of concept study using functional near infrared spectroscopy. *PLoS ONE* **2018**, *13*, e0191361. [CrossRef]
31. You, S.H.; Jang, S.H.; Kim, Y.H.; Hallett, M.; Ahn, S.H.; Kwon, Y.H.; Kim, J.H.; Lee, M.Y. Virtual reality-induced cortical reorganization and associated locomotor recovery in chronic stroke: An experimenter-blind randomized study. *Stroke* **2005**, *36*, 1166–1171. [CrossRef] [PubMed]

32. Xiao, X.; Lin, Q.; Lo, W.L.; Mao, Y.R.; Shi, X.C.; Cates, R.S.; Zhou, S.F.; Huang, D.F.; Li, L. Cerebral Reorganization in Subacute Stroke Survivors after Virtual Reality-Based Training: A Preliminary Study. *Behav. Neurol.* **2017**, *2017*, 6261479. [CrossRef] [PubMed]
33. Saleh, S.; Fluet, G.; Qiu, Q.; Merians, A.; Adamovich, S.V.; Tunik, E. Neural Patterns of Reorganization after Intensive Robot-Assisted Virtual Reality Therapy and Repetitive Task Practice in Patients with Chronic Stroke. *Front. Neurol.* **2017**, *8*, 452. [CrossRef] [PubMed]

Journal of
Clinical Medicine

MDPI

Article

Persistent Inflammation, Immunosuppression and Catabolism Syndrome (PICS) after Polytrauma: A Rare Syndrome with Major Consequences

Lillian Hesselink [1,2,†,*], Ruben J. Hoepelman [1,†], Roy Spijkerman [1,2], Mark C. H. de Groot [3], Karlijn J. P. van Wessem [1], Leo Koenderman [2,4], Luke P. H. Leenen [1] and Falco Hietbrink [1]

1 Department of Trauma Surgery, University Medical Center Utrecht, 3584 CX Utrecht, The Netherlands; rjhoepelman@gmail.com (R.J.H.); r.spijkerman-5@umcutrecht.nl (R.S.); kwessem@umcutrecht.nl (K.J.P.v.W.); l.p.h.leenen@umcutrecht.nl (L.P.H.L.); f.hietbrink@umcutrecht.nl (F.H.)

2 Center for Translational Immunology, Wilhelmina Children's Hospital, University Medical Center Utrecht, 3584 CX Utrecht, The Netherlands; l.koenderman@umcutrecht.nl

3 Department of Clinical Chemistry and Hematology, University Medical Center Utrecht, 3584 CX Utrecht, The Netherlands; M.C.H.deGroot-3@umcutrecht.nl

4 Department of Respiratory Medicine, University Medical Center Utrecht, 3584 CX Utrecht, The Netherlands

* Correspondence: lilianhesselink@gmail.com; Tel.: +31-88-755-9882

† Authors contributed equally to this study.

Received: 2 December 2019; Accepted: 7 January 2020; Published: 10 January 2020

Abstract: Nowadays, more trauma patients develop chronic critical illness (CCI), a state characterized by prolonged intensive care. Some of these CCI patients have disproportional difficulties to recover and suffer from recurrent infections, a syndrome described as the persistent inflammation, immunosuppression and catabolism syndrome (PICS). A total of 78 trauma patients with an ICU stay of ≥14 days (CCI patients) between 2007 and 2017 were retrospectively included. Within this group, PICS patients were identified through two ways: (1) their clinical course (≥3 infectious complications) and (2) by laboratory markers suggested in the literature (C-reactive protein (CRP) and lymphocytes), both in combination with evidence of increased catabolism. The incidence of PICS was 4.7 per 1000 multitrauma patients. The sensitivity and specificity of the laboratory markers was 44% and 73%, respectively. PICS patients had a longer hospital stay (median 83 vs. 40, $p < 0.001$) and required significantly more surgical interventions (median 13 vs. 3, $p = 0.003$) than other CCI patients. Thirteen PICS patients developed sepsis (72%) and 12 (67%) were readmitted at least once due to an infection. In conclusion, patients who develop PICS experience recurrent infectious complications that lead to prolonged hospitalization, many surgical procedures and frequent readmissions. Therefore, PICS forms a substantial burden on the patient and the hospital, despite its low incidence.

Keywords: PICS; trauma; immunology; infectious complications

1. Introduction

In recent decades, there has been much improvement in the clinical care for trauma patients, which has led to a decrease in mortality by exsanguination and life-threatening inflammatory complications, such as Acute Respiratory Distress Syndrome (ARDS), sepsis and multiple organ dysfunction syndrome (MODS) [1,2]. In particular, the initial approach and resuscitation, the introduction of standardized operating procedures, early hemorrhage control and improved clinical critical care have contributed to this decrease [3–6].

The increased survival directly upon trauma and the fact that fewer patients die of inflammatory complications nowadays has led to an increase in average intensive care unit (ICU) stay [7]. A prolonged

ICU stay is also referred to as a state of chronic critical illness (CCI) [8,9]. Although no consensus exists on the definition of CCI [10,11], >14 days ICU stay is often used in recent literature [8,9,12].

Some of these CCI patients suffer from poor wound healing, recurrent infections and a disproportionately slow recovery [7,8,13]. This syndrome has been described as the 'persistent inflammation, immunosuppression and catabolism syndrome' (PICS) [5,7,14], not to be confused with the post-intensive care syndrome [15]. PICS is characterized by chronic low-grade inflammation, suppressed host immunity and a loss of lean body mass, despite nutritional intervention [7,13]. It is not quite clear which patients develop PICS and what the clinical course of these patients is. As the course is suggested to be complicated with multiple infections and high mortality rates, it is essential to identify patients at risk for PICS as early as possible. Clinical risk factors described so far include a poor premorbid health status and an age of 65 years and above [8,13,16]. Also, previous studies investigated readily available laboratory markers to enable identification of PICS patients shortly after trauma. Markers suggested in the literature include decreased lymphocyte counts, increased elevated C-reactive protein (CRP) levels and substantial weight loss or persistent decreased albumin levels [5,7].

To date, perioperative care continues to improve, and the elderly population is growing. Although literature is scarce on the subject, it suggests that PICS will be an increasing problem for ICU patients [13]. Therefore, the objectives of this study were to investigate the incidence of PICS after trauma in a Level I trauma center to determine the clinical course of these patients and to test the postulated markers to identify PICS patients in this study population.

2. Materials and Methods

2.1. Study Design

We conducted a 11 year retrospective cohort study of severely injured trauma patients admitted to the University Medical Center Utrecht (UMCU) from 1 January 2007 to 31 December 2017. PICS patients were identified in two ways: (1) by their clinical course and (2) by markers described in the literature [5,7,16]. The incidence of PICS was calculated, and the sensitivity and specificity of the markers were analyzed.

2.2. Patients

As an intensive care stay of >2 weeks is the common denominator in most definitions of CCI and PICS, all patients ≥16 years of age with an ICU stay of 14 or more consecutive days during hospitalization were selected from the trauma registry database of the UMC Utrecht. Patients were excluded if they were admitted to the ICU for other reasons than critical illness (e.g., logistical reasons or requiring ventilation support due to spinal cord lesions). Also, patients with isolated neurotrauma (e.g., traumatic brain injury or spinal cord injury) were excluded because these patients often have a prolonged ICU stay in the absence of systemic pathologies. Isolated neurotrauma was defined as having brain injury without injuries in other regions with an abbreviated injury scale (AIS) ≤2 [17]. Patient characteristics and data concerning trauma mechanism, treatment and complications were obtained. These data were collected from the prospective trauma registry and supplemented with hematological data from the Utrecht Patient Oriented Database (UPOD) and clinical data from the medical record system. The technical details of the UPOD have been described elsewhere [18]. In short, this database is an infrastructure of relational databases that allows (semi) automated transfer, processing and storage of data, including administrative information, medical and surgical procedures, medication orders, and laboratory test results for all clinically admitted patients and patients attending the outpatient clinic of the UMC Utrecht since 2004.

2.3. Definitions, Variables and Outcomes

CCI is used for patients with a prolonged ICU stay and PICS is used for a subset of CCI patients who exhibit a clinical phenotype consisting of inflammation, immunosuppression and catabolism.

However, no uniform definitions exist for either CCI or PICS. An overview of the definitions used in this study is given in Figure 1. We defined CCI as an ICU stay of ≥14 days. Furthermore, we defined PICS clinically as: ICU stay of ≥14 days, ≥3 infectious complications and evidence of a catabolic state. A catabolic state was defined as either weight loss >10%, Body Mass Index (BMI) <18 or albumin <30 g/L during hospitalization [7]. If none of these markers for catabolic state were available (which was the case in 4/78 patients), the medical record system was searched for the nutritional state of the patient in dietitians' notes, explicitly stating if the patient was in a catabolic state or not. An infectious complication was defined as an infection during hospitalization which required some kind of intervention (either pharmacological, surgical or radiological) or a readmission due to an infection after discharge. Patients meeting these criteria were considered to be the "clinical PICS group". This group was compared to other CCI patients not meeting these criteria.

Secondly, an attempt was made to identify PICS using the markers suggested in the literature (the PICS markers-positive group) [5,7]. Patients were considered to be PICS markers-positive if they had ≥2 days of immunosuppression (lymphocyte count <0.8 × 10^9/L), ≥2 days of inflammation (CRP >50 mg/L) and a catabolic state as described above, during the first 30 days of hospitalization. PICS markers-positive patients were compared to other CCI patients not meeting these criteria (PICS markers-negative).

Infectious complications, hospital length of stay (LOS), ICU LOS, readmissions due to infectious complications, surgical procedures during hospitalization and surgical procedures after discharge, but related to the initial trauma or to acquired complications, were collected. Sepsis was defined as an increase in the sequential organ failure assessment (SOFA) score of 2 points or more in response to infection, according to the third international consensus definition for sepsis (Sepsis-3) [19]. Multitrauma was defined as Injury Severity Score (ISS) ≥ 16 [20]. Massive transfusion was defined as >10 units packed red blood cells within 24 h.

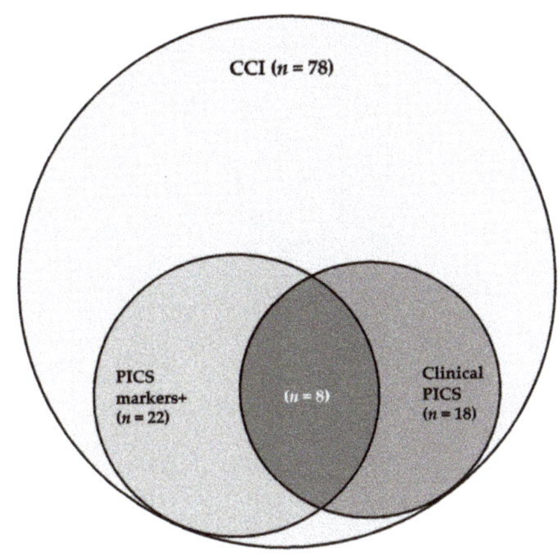

	CCI	PICS markers+	Clinical PICS
Persistent	≥ 14 days ICU	≥ 14 days ICU	≥ 14 days ICU
Inflammation		CRP > 50mg/L for ≥ 2 days	≥ 3 infectious complications
Immunosuppression		lymphocytes < 0.8 x 10^9/L for ≥ 2 days	
Catabolism		weight loss > 10% BMI < 18 albumin < 30 g/L	weight loss > 10% BMI < 18 albumin < 30 g/L

Figure 1. Overview of definitions used in this study and number of patients who fulfilled criteria according to these definitions. CCI = chronic critical illness, PICS = persistent inflammation, immunosuppression and catabolism syndrome, ICU = intensive care unit, BMI = Body Mass Index.

2.4. Statistical Analysis

All data were analyzed with IBM SPSS version 25(IBM Corporation, New York City, NY, USA). Distribution of normality was tested using the Shapiro–Wilk test. Continuous patient characteristics were presented as median with interquartile range (IQR) and compared using the Mann–Whitney U test, because the data were not normally distributed. The Fisher exact test was used to compare categorical patient data. Laboratory values are depicted as median with IQR because values were not normally distributed. Statistical significance was defined as a p-value < 0.05. Incidence was determined using the clinically identified PICS patients and calculated per 1000 trauma and multitrauma patients admitted to this hospital annually. The sensitivity and specificity of the markers were tested for our population using the clinical PICS group as gold standard. To compare lymphocytes and CRP between groups over time and to correlate for within-subject correlation, a linear generalized estimated equation (GEE) was used with an AR-1 correlation structure.

2.5. Ethics

A waiver was provided by the institutional medical ethics committee for this retrospective analysis of this prospectively collected database. In addition, in line with the academic hospital policy, an opt-out procedure was in place for use of patient data for research purposes. The process and storage of data were in accordance with privacy and ethics regulations. Data were analyzed anonymously.

3. Results

3.1. PICS Incidence

Between 2007 and 2017, 13,576 trauma patients were admitted to the UMC Utrecht. Of these patients, 3859 were multitrauma patients and a total of 183 patients were admitted to the ICU for 14 days or longer (Figure 2). Two patients were excluded because they had no ICU indication (but needed ventilation support due to preexisting pathologies, which could not be provided elsewhere due to logistical reasons), and a total of 103 patients were excluded because of isolated neurotrauma.

The remaining 78 patients fulfilled the criteria for CCI. The incidence of CCI in our trauma population was therefore 5.7 per 1000 trauma patients and 20 per 1000 multitrauma patients. Of the 78 CCI patients, 18 patients met the criteria for the "clinical PICS group" (Table 1) and 22 patients met the criteria for the "PICS markers-positive group" (Table 2). A total of eight patients fulfilled the criteria for both groups. Based on clinically identified PICS patients, the incidence of PICS was 1.3 per 1000 trauma patients and 4.7 per 1000 multitrauma patients were admitted to our center.

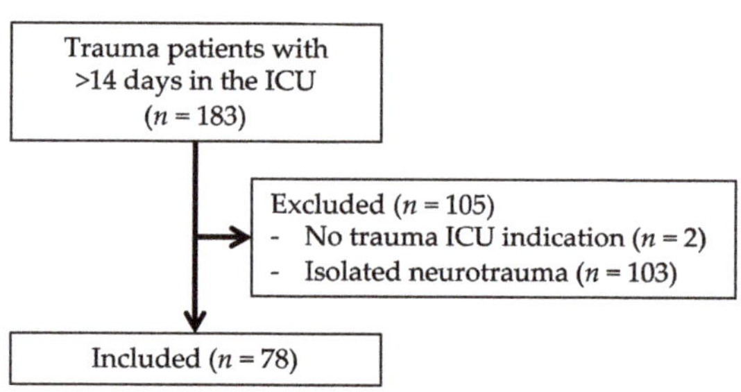

Figure 2. Flowchart of patient inclusion.

3.2. Clinical PICS Patients vs. Other CCI Patients

Clinical PICS patients received massive transfusion twice as often as the other CCI patients (67% vs. 33%, $p = 0.015$). Despite the long ICU stay in both groups, the clinical PICS patients were hospitalized twice as long as the other CCI patients (83 vs. 40 days, $p < 0.001$) (Table 1). ICU stay and duration of mechanical ventilation were also significantly longer for the clinical PICS group (30 vs. 19 days, $p = 0.006$ and 17 vs. 20 days, $p = 0.001$, respectively). Thirteen clinical PICS patients (72%) developed sepsis, while only 10 other CCI patients (17%) developed sepsis ($p < 0.001$). Also, PICS patients developed significantly more infections with multi-drug resistant organisms ($p = 0.000$). The number of readmissions due to infectious causes was significantly higher in the clinical PICS group (67% vs. 13%, $p < 0.001$). Surgical procedures during hospitalization were required for all (100%) clinical PICS patients and 61% needed additional surgical procedures after discharge related to the initial trauma or due to infectious complications. These percentages were significantly lower for the other CCI patients (73%, $p = 0.016$ and 22% $p = 0.001$). The number of surgical procedures per patient was higher in the PICS group too, both during hospitalization (eight vs. two, $p < 0.001$) as well as after discharge (three vs. 0, $p = 0.006$). During hospitalization, one clinical PICS patient died due to sepsis. Of the other CCI patients, three died due to irreversible neurological injuries and one due to sepsis during hospitalization. Within 3 years after trauma, an additional two clinical PICS patients died, one due to sepsis and one due to an unknown cause. Also, six other CCI patients died, one due to sepsis and five due to unknown causes.

3.3. PICS Markers-Positive Group vs. Other CCI Patients

Patients in the PICS markers-positive group had a significantly longer ICU stay than those not fulfilling the criteria (27 vs. 19 days, $p < 0.001$) (Table 2). Also, these patients more often required dialysis (five vs. 0, $p = 0.001$) and were significantly longer mechanically ventilated (27 versus 17 days, $p = 0.000$). Significantly more patients had infectious complications in the PICS markers-positive group (90% vs. 66%, $p = 0.045$) and there were more infectious complications per patient in the PICS markers-positive group (median of 2 vs. 0, $p = 0.008$). Sepsis also occurred more in the PICS markers-positive group (50% vs. 21%, $p = 0.025$). During hospitalization, three patients died in the PICS markers-positive group (two sepsis, one neurological injury) and two patients died in the PICS markers-negative group due to neurological injuries. Within 3 years after trauma, an additional two patients died in the PICS markers-positive group (one sepsis, one unknown) and six patients died in the PICS markers-negative group (one sepsis, five unknown).

Table 1. Patient characteristics of clinically identified PICS patients vs. other CCI patients.

Characteristics	Entire Cohort ($n = 78$)	No PICS ($n = 60$)	Clinical PICS ($n = 18$)	p-Value
Gender, male (%)	63 (80.8%)	48 (80.0%)	15 (83.3%)	0.999
Age	49 (32–65)	46 (28–62)	57 (45–68)	0.086
Injury severity score	34 (26–42)	34 (27–41)	29 (22–48)	0.548
Injury mechanism				
Traffic accident	51 (65.4%)	39 (65.0%)	12 (66.7%)	0.261
Fall from height	18 (23.1%)	15 (25.0%)	3 (16.7%)	
Crush injury	4 (5.1%)	2 (3.3%)	2 (11.1%)	
Other	5 (6.4%)	4 (6.9%)	1 (5.6%)	
Massive transfusion protocol	32 (41.0%)	20 (33.3%)	12 (66.7%)	**0.015**
Hospital days	43 (35–63)	40 (31–52)	83 (41–106)	**<0.001**
ICU days	20 (16–29)	19 (16–26)	30 (19–37)	**0.006**
Tracheostomy	45 (57.7%)	33 (55.0%)	12 (66.7%)	0.427
Mechanical ventilation days	20 (15–27)	17 (14–26)	20 (27–38)	**0.001**
Continuous veno-venous hemofiltration	5 (6.4%)	2 (3.3%)	3 (16.7%)	0.078
Infectious complications	57 (73.1%)	39 (65.0%)	18 (100%)	**0.002**
Per patient	1 (0–2)	1 (0–1)	3 (3–3)	**<0.001**
Sepsis *	23 (29.5%)	10 (16.7%)	13 (72.2%)	**<0.001**
Type of infections				
Pneumonia	40 (51.3%)	28 (46.7%)	12 (66.7%)	0.185
Surgical site infection	14 (17.9%)	6 (10.0%)	8 (44.4%)	**0.002**
Blood stream infection	15 (19.8%)	6 (10.0%)	9 (50.0%)	**0.001**
Infected OSM	7 (9.0%)	1 (1.7%)	6 (33.3%)	**<0.001**
UTI	5 (6.4%)	4 (6.7%)	1 (5.6%)	0.999
Abscess	4 (5.1%)	2 (3.3%)	2 (11.1%)	0.226
Other	12 (15.4%)	5 (8.3%)	7 (38.9%)	**0.005**

Table 1. *Cont.*

Characteristics	Entire Cohort (*n* = 78)	No PICS (*n* = 60)	Clinical PICS (*n* = 18)	*p*-Value
Multi-drug resistant organisms				
MRSA	1 (1.3%)	0 (0%)	1 (5.6%)	0.000
ESBL	5 (6.4%)	3 (5.0%)	2 (11.1%)	
MDR-GNB	5 (6.4%)	1 (1.7%)	4 (22.2%)	
Multi-drug resistant *Pseudomonas*	2 (2.6%)	0 (0%)	2 (11.1%)	
Multi-drug resistant *Acinobacter*	2 (2.6%)	1 (1.7%)	1 (5.6%)	
Infectious readmissions	20 (25.6%)	8 (13.3%)	12 (66.7%)	**<0.001**
Per patient	0 (0–0)	0 (0–0)	1 (0–3)	**<0.001**
Total infectious complications during or after hospitalization per patient	1 (0–3)	1 (0–2)	6 (3–7)	**<0.001**
Surgical procedures during hospitalization	62 (79.5%)	44 (73.3%)	18 (100%)	**0.016**
Per patient	3 (1–6)	2 (0–5)	8 (3–13)	**<0.001**
Surgical procedures after discharge	27 (34.6%)	16 (22.4%)	11 (61.1%)	**0.011**
Per patient	2 (0–2)	0 (0–1)	3 (0–5)	**0.006**
Total surgical procedures during or after hospitalization per patient	3 (1–7)	3 (1–5)	13 (2–22)	**0.003**
Discharge				
Other hospital	8 (10.3%)	7 (11.7%)	1 (5.6%)	0.931
Nursing home	11 (14.1%)	9 (15.0%)	2 (11.1%)	
Rehabilitation facility	27 (34.6%)	19 (31.7%)	8 (44.4%)	
Home (+/− additional care)	27 (34.6%)	21 (25.0%)	6 (33.3%)	
Total mortality	13 (16.6%)	10 (16.6%)	3 (16.7%)	1.000
In hospital	5 (6.4%)	4 (6.7%)	1 (5.6%)	1.000
<3 years	8 (10.3%)	6 (10.0%)	2 (11.1%)	1.000

All data are shown as n (%) or median (IQR). CCI = chronic critical illness. ICU = Intensive care unit. OSM = Osteosynthesis material. UTI = Urinary tract infection. MRSA = Methicillin-resistant *Staphylococcus aureus*. ESBL = Extended Spectrum Beta-Lactamase. MDR-GNB = Multidrug-resistant Gram-negative bacilli. Mortality <3 years does not include mortality during hospitalization. Variables are compared between patient meeting the clinical PICS criteria and those not meeting the clinical PICS criteria with a Fisher's exact test, a Mann–Whitney U test or a Student *T*-test * Sepsis = defined as an increase in SOFA score >2 within a day in response to infection.

Table 2. Characteristics of CCI patients with positive PICS markers vs. other CCI patients.

Characteristics	Entire Cohort (*n* = 78)	No PICS Markers (*n* = 56)	PICS Markers (*n* = 22)	*p*-Value
Gender, male (%)	63 (80.8%)	45 (80.4%)	18 (81.8%)	0.999
Age	49 (32–65)	49 (33–66)	40 (27–63)	0.512
Injury severity score	34 (26–42)	34 (29–43)	29 (20–42)	0.147
Injury mechanism				
Traffic accident	51 (65.4%)	36 (64.2%)	15 (68.2%)	0.702
Fall from height	18 (23.1%)	14 (25%)	4 (18.2%)	
Crush injury	4 (5.1%)	3 (5.4%)	1 (4.6%)	
Other	5 (6.4%)	3 (5.4%)	2 (9.1%)	
Massive transfusion protocol	32 (41.0%)	21 (37.5%)	11 (50.0%)	0.322
Hospital days	43 (35–63)	42 (34–60)	50 (35–93)	0.281
ICU days	20 (16–29)	19 (16–25)	27 (23–36)	**<0.001**
Tracheostomy	45 (57.7%)	31 (55.4%)	14 (63.6%)	0.613
Mechanical ventilation days	20 (15–27)	17 (14–26)	27 (22–37)	**0.000**
Continuous veno-venous hemofiltration	5 (6.4%)	0 (0%)	5 (22.7%)	**0.001**

Table 2. *Cont.*

Characteristics	Entire Cohort (n = 78)	No PICS Markers (n = 56)	PICS Markers (n = 22)	p-Value
Infectious complications	57 (73.1%)	37 (66%)	20 (90%)	**0.045**
Per patient	1 (0–2)	1 (0–2)	2 (1–3)	**0.008**
Sepsis *	23 (29.5%)	12 (21.4%)	11 (50%)	**0.025**
Type of infections				
Pneumonia	40 (51.3%)	24 (42.9%)	16 (72.7%)	**0.024**
Surgical site infection	14 (17.9%)	11 (9.6%)	3 (13.6%)	0.746
Blood stream infection	15 (19.8%)	8 (14.3%)	7 (31.8%)	0.110
Infected OSM	7 (9.0%)	3 (5.4%)	4 (18.2%)	0.094
UTI	5 (6.4%)	4 (7.1%)	1 (4.5%)	0.999
Abscess	4 (5.1%)	1 (1.8%)	3 (13.6%)	0.066
Other	12 (15.4%)	7 (12.5%)	5 (22.7%)	0.303
Multi-drug resistant organisms				0.233
MRSA	1 (1.3%)	1 (1.8%)	0 (0%)	
ESBL	5 (6.4%)	3 (5.4%)	1 (4.5%)	
MDR-GNB	5 (6.4%)	2 (3.6%)	1 (4.5%)	
Multi-drug resistant *Pseudomonas*	2 (2.6%)	1 (1.8%)	1 (4.5%)	
Multi-drug resistant *Acinobacter*	2 (2.6%)	1 (1.8%)	1 (4.5%)	
Infectious readmissions	20 (25.6%)	13 (23.2%)	7 (31.8%)	0.565
Per patient	0 (0–0.25)	0 (0–0)	0 (0–1)	0.246
Total infectious complications during or after hospitalization per patient	1 (0–3)	1 (0–2)	2 (1–5)	**0.018**
Surgical procedures during hospitalization	62 (79.5%)	46 (82.1%)	16 (72.7%)	0.365
Per patient	3 (1–6)	3 (1–5)	3 (0–9)	0.720
Surgical procedures after discharge	27 (34.6%)	20 (35.7%)	7 (31.8%)	0.797
Per patient	2 (0–2)	0 (0–1)	0 (0–2)	0.937
Total surgical procedures during or after hospitalization per patient	3 (1–7)	3 (1–7)	3 (0–14)	0.980
Discharge				0.488
Other hospital	8 (10.3%)	5 (8.9%)	3 (13.6%)	
Nursing home	11 (14.1%)	9 (16.1%)	2 (9.1%)	
Rehabilitation facility	27 (34.6%)	20 (35.7%)	7 (31.8%)	
Home (+/− additional care)	27 (34.6%)	20 (35.7%)	7 (31.8%)	
Totally mortality	13 (16.6%)	8 (14.3%)	5 (22.7%)	0.500
In hospital	5 (6.4%)	2 (3.6%)	3 (13.6%)	0.133
<3 years	8 (10.3%)	6 (10.7%)	2 (9.1%)	1.000

All data are shown as n (%) or median (IQR). CCI = chronic critical illness. ICU = Intensive care unit. OSM = Osteosynthesis material. UTI = Urinary tract infection. MRSA = Methicillin-resistant *Staphylococcus aureus*. ESBL = Extended Spectrum Beta-Lactamase. MDR-GNB = Multidrug-resistant Gram-negative bacilli. Mortality <3 years does not include mortality during hospitalization. Variables are compared between patient meeting the clinical PICS criteria and those not meeting the clinical PICS criteria with a Fisher's exact test, a Mann–Whitney U test or a Student *T*-test * Sepsis = defined as an increase in SOFA score >2 within a day in response to infection.

3.4. *Testing the Accuracy of PICS Markers*

3.4.1. Sensitivity and Specificity

The total population consisted of 78 patients. Eighteen PICS patients were clinically identified (clinical PICS). Of these patients, eight patients were also identified as PICS patients using the PICS markers. Therefore, of the 22 patients who were in the PICS markers-positive group, 14 did not have clinical evidence of PICS. This resulted in a sensitivity of 44% and a specificity of 77% in our study population (Table 3).

Table 3. PICS markers tested for sensitivity and specificity in the study population.

Total Cohort (n = 78)	Clinical PICS (n = 18)	Other CCI Patients (n = 60)	
PICS markers (n = 22)	n = 8	n = 14	Positive predictive value = 36%
No PICS markers (n = 56)	n = 10	n = 46	Negative predictive value = 82%
	Sensitivity = 44%	Specificity = 77%	

PICS markers+ = patients with positive PICS markers, PICS markers− = patients not fulfilling the PICS markers criteria. Sensitivity = 8/18 × 100. Specificity = 46/60 × 100. Positive predictive value = 8/22 × 100. Negative predictive value = 46/56 × 100.

3.4.2. Lymphocytes and CRP

No significant differences were found in lymphocyte count (β = 0.02, p = 0.999) and CRP levels (β = −0.12, p = 0.999) between patients who developed clinical PICS and patients who did not develop PICS. Median lymphocyte count was within criterion values (>0.8 × 10^9/L) and median CRP levels were outside criterion values (>50 mg/L) for both groups during the first month after trauma (Figure 3). Although not significant, there was a trend towards lower lymphocyte counts in clinical PICS patients during the first week after trauma. When comparing clinical PICS patients with lymphocytopenia (≥2 days of lymphocyte count <0.8 × 10^9/L) to clinical PICS patients without lymphocytopenia (Table 4), these patients did have a longer ICU stay (27 vs. 19, p = 0.001), longer duration of mechanical ventilation (35 vs. 21 days, p = 0.001), more infectious complications per patient (six vs. three, p = 0.020) and more surgical procedures per patient after initial discharge (0 vs. five, p = 0.037).

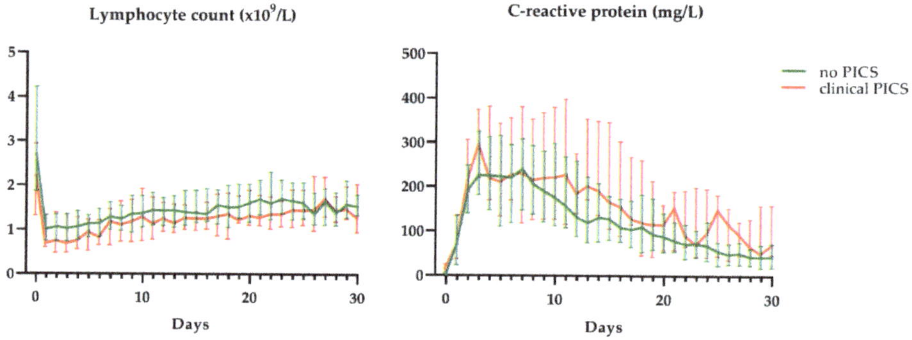

Figure 3. C-reactive protein levels and lymphocyte counts in clinically identified PICS patients (clinical PICS) in red and other CCI patients (no PICS) in green. Grey areas depict reference values. Data are presented as median with interquartile range.

Table 4. Outcome comparison of clinical PICS patients with lymphocytopenia ** versus clinical PICS patients without lymphocytopenia.

Characteristics	Normal Lymphocyte Count (n = 9)	Lymphocytopenia (n = 9)	p-Value
Hospital days	58 (40–128)	92 (71–110)	0.401
ICU days	19 (16–25)	27 (23–36)	**0.001**
Tracheostomy	4 (44.4%)	8 (88.9%)	0.131
Mechanical ventilation days	21 (16–27)	35 (31–60)	**0.001**
Continuous veno-venous hemofiltration	0 (0%)	3 (33.3%)	0.206
Infectious complications during hospitalization	9 (100%)	9 (100%)	0.999
Per patient	3 (3–3)	3 (3–4)	0.090

Table 4. *Cont.*

Characteristics	Normal Lymphocyte Count (n = 9)	Lymphocytopenia (n = 9)	p-Value
Multi-drug resistant organisms			
MRSA	1 (11.1%)	0 (0%)	0.217
ESBL	2 (22.2%)	0 (0%)	
MDR-GNB	1 (11.1%)	3 (33.3%)	
Multi-drug resistant *Pseudomonas*	0 (0%)	2 (22.2%)	
Multi-drug resistant *Acinobacter*	0 (0%)	1 (11.1%)	
Sepsis *	7 (77.8%)	6 (66.7%)	0.999
Infectious readmissions	5 (55.6%)	7 (77.8%)	0.620
Per patient	1 (0–1)	2 (1–5)	0.050
Total infectious complications during or after hospitalization per patient	3 (3–4)	6 (4–8)	**0.020**
Surgical procedures during hospitalization	9 (100%)	9 (100%)	0.999
Per patient	4 (2–10)	9 (6–15)	0.156
Surgical procedures after discharge	4 (44.4%)	7 (77.8%)	0.335
Per patient	0 (0–3)	5 (1–15)	**0.037**
Total surgical procedures during or after hospitalization per patient	7 (2–12)	17 (8–24)	0.051
Discharge			
Other hospital	1 (11.1%)	1 (11.1%)	0.091
Nursing home	1 (11.1%)	1 (11.1%)	
Rehabilitation facility	2 (22.2%)	6 (66.7%)	
Home (+/− additional care)	5 (55.6%)	1 (11.1%)	
Totally mortality	0 (0%)	2 (22.2%)	0.471
In hospital	0 (0%)	1 (11.1%)	0.999
<3 years	0 (0%)	1 (11.1%)	0.999

All data are shown as n (%) or median (IQR). ICU = Intensive care unit. OSM = Osteosynthesis material. UTI = Urinary tract infection. MRSA = Methicillin-resistant *Staphylococcus aureus*. ESBL = Extended Spectrum Beta-Lactamase. MDR-GNB = Multidrug-resistant Gram-negative bacilli. Mortality <3 years does not included mortality during hospitalization. Variables are compared between patient meeting the PICS markers criteria and those not meeting the PICS markers criteria with a Fisher's exact test, a Mann–Whitney U test or a Student *T*-test * Sepsis = defined as an increase in SOFA score >2 in response to infection. ** Lymphocytopenia = defined as lymphocyte count below 0.8×10^9/L for 2 or more consecutive days.

4. Discussion

In this study, we identified 18 PICS patients in eleven years, which translates to an incidence of 4.7 per 1000 multitrauma patients admitted to our level 1 trauma center annually. Both in-hospital mortality and 3 year mortality was low in the clinical PICS group. It may seem that PICS is a negligible problem with rather low incidence rates and high survival rates. However, PICS forms a substantial burden on the daily life of patients who develop the syndrome. These patients often require frequent and complex medical care up to 3 years after trauma. Also, they experience recurrent, sometimes life-threatening, recognition infections and require recurrent surgical procedures for this.

Costs of long-term medical care, and especially critical and surgical care, are high. The costs of an ICU and ward bed were recently calculated at approximately €2200 and €450 per day in the Netherlands, respectively [21]. Since PICS patients had an average of 30 days in the ICU and 83 days in the hospital, the average cost of total hospital stay is estimated at €89.850 per PICS patient. Compared to the average hospitalized trauma patient, these expanses are estimated to be a thirteen fold difference at least, based on average Dutch length of hospital and ICU stay reported in the literature [22,23]. This is a gross underestimation, since it does not include costs of imaging, medication, surgical procedures [24], readmissions and long-term care facilities. Therefore, PICS accounts for a substantial part of trauma-related expenses and forms an exuberant financial burden on the hospital, despite its low incidence.

The adverse outcomes associated with PICS were most evident in the clinically identified PICS patients. Outcomes of patients identified by the previously suggested markers were not as bad as those of the clinical PICS patients, but slightly worse than outcomes of other CCI trauma patients. This suggests that the PICS markers are not accurate enough to detect the clinically relevant PICS patients with the worst outcomes. This was supported by the low marker sensitivity and specificity found in this study.

Besides these laboratory markers, which are described to facilitate the detection of PICS, an ICU length of stay of 14 days or longer is a frequently described criterion for PICS [8]. Therefore, we used this as an inclusion criterion in our study to make a selection in the many trauma patients who were admitted over eleven years. However, ICU care differs greatly among countries, making a cut-off in ICU days an arguable criterion. In some countries, patients are not admitted to the ICU because of critical illness, but because a higher nurse to patient ratio is needed for other reasons or simple monitoring is required. In other countries however, patients are only admitted to the ICU when they are severely ill or require mechanical ventilation, such as in our hospital [25,26]. When there is no need for mechanical ventilation, but patients do need more care than a ward can deliver, patients are typically admitted to the intermediate care unit (IMCU) in our hospital. Therefore, it is possible that higher PICS incidence rates are found in countries with no IMCU or with different admission criteria for the ICU.

Furthermore, retrospective identification of a catabolic state in trauma patients can be challenging. Although BMI < 18 is a fairly undisputed criterion for poor nutritional state, body weight can, especially in the ICU, fluctuate daily (e.g., under influence of fluid in and output) [27]. Albumin (half-life of 14–20 days) is widely used to assess the nutritional status of patients, but is also a negative acute-phase protein and thus decreases when a patient experiences physiological stress (e.g., infection, surgery or trauma) [28]. Other markers for catabolism also included pre-albumin, retinol-binding protein (RBP) and creatinine-height index (CHI) [7], but these were not retrospectively available. Pre-albumin is also a negative acute phase protein, but with a shorter (2–3 days) half-life and smaller body pool, which theoretically makes it a more reliable indicator for nutrition. However pre-albumin, RBP and CHI, are all greatly influenced by renal function, infection and trauma as well [28,29].

It is not surprising that the specificity of these markers was low. CRP is an acute-phase protein, that is elevated due to many causes, including trauma, surgical procedures and infections [30–33]. Many PICS and other CCI patients underwent surgical procedures and developed infections in their first week after admission. Furthermore, lymphocytes are affected by trauma and infection and failure to normalize lymphopenia was described to increase mortality after trauma [34,35]. However, no significant difference in lymphocyte counts was found between PICS patients and other CCI patients, suggesting that this marker is not adequate to identify PICS. On the other hand, PICS patients who did have low lymphocyte counts had worse outcomes than PICS patients who did not have this. Therefore, although lymphocyte counts alone cannot be used to identify PICS, lymphocyte counts might be a useful addition to identify the PICS patients with the worst outcomes.

Hence, the PICS markers described so far are nonspecific, insensitive and arguable, and there is a need for better biomarkers to identify PICS. Recently, automated flow cytometry became available which enables fast and point-of-care analysis of receptor expression of immune cells [36,37]. Further research should investigate if such analyses can be used to identify patients at risk for PICS in an early stage. Early identification of patients at risk would enable earlier interventions. Although no specific treatment options exist so far, these patients might benefit from an immunoprotective protocol. Nowadays, trauma patients at risk for adverse inflammatory outcomes, often undergo damage control surgery, damage control orthopedics and damage control resuscitation [38,39]. Patients at risk for PICS are likely to benefit from these damage control strategies as well. In addition, limited evidence suggests that enhanced nutritional support (e.g., the addition of addition of arginine and glutamine [40]) and adjusted prophylactic antibiotic strategies [41,42] can have an immunoprotective effect in critically ill trauma patients. It is tempting to speculate that combining these interventions into an immunoprotective protocol, could improve clinical outcomes of patients at risk for PICS. Furthermore, it is remarkable that the mortality rate amongst PICS patients is low, in contrast to what was previously suggested in the literature [43]. This suggests that it is justified to keep continuing supportive treatment in PICS patients despite recurrent severe adverse outcomes.

The main limitation of this study was that there is no consensus on the definition for PICS in the literature. PICS is considered a clinical diagnosis, often recognized by a disproportionally long ICU/hospital stay, recurrent and nosocomial infections, failure to rehabilitate and disproportional weight loss. Physicians identify PICS patients through a combination of these characteristics, which to date, have not been well translated into criteria. The PICS definition for this study (≥3 infections, ICU stay of ≥14 days, evidence of catabolic state) was therefore based on the clinical course of the patients and was chosen during a consensus meeting with trauma surgeons treating these patients. Although this was needed to objectify the incidence of PICS, it is possible that this led to a slight overestimation or underestimation of the PICS incidence. Another limitation was the retrospective design of the study. Due to this, we were only able to obtain regular laboratory data. Genomic data or phenotypic cellular data were not available. Furthermore, other measures (e.g., urine 3-methylhistidine) or modalities (e.g., dedicated ultrasound) to detect disproportional muscle loss, were not available. Also, a limitation of a retrospective design is the change of missing values. However, because the data were extracted from the UPOD, and the UPOD contains all hematological parameters irrespective of the requested parameter, the number of missing values (e.g., lymphocyte counts and CRP levels) was limited. Moreover, laboratory values are generally requested daily for trauma patients in the ICU. Therefore, there were barely any missing values during the patients' ICU stay.

In conclusion, there is a need for a clear PICS definition and better markers to detect PICS. Patients who develop PICS experience recurrent inflammatory complications that lead to frequent readmissions and surgical procedures. Furthermore, infectious complications are frequently the result of multi-drug-resistant organisms. Therefore, PICS forms a substantial burden on the patient and a significant burden on hospitals, despite its low incidence.

Author Contributions: F.H., L.P.H.L., L.K., K.J.P.v.W., R.S., R.J.H. and L.H. developed the original study design. M.C.H.d.G. and R.J.H. performed the data extraction. R.J.H., L.H. and R.S. performed the analyses. All authors contributed to the interpretation of the data. R.J.H. and L.H. made the figures, tables and drafted the initial paper. All other authors made significant revisions to the manuscript. All authors have read and agreed to the published version of the manuscript.

Funding: This research received no external funding.

Conflicts of Interest: The authors declare no conflict of interest.

References

1. Jochems, D.; Leenen, L.P.H.; Hietbrink, F.; Houwert, R.M.; van Wessem, K.J.P. Increased reduction in exsanguination rates leaves brain injury as the only major cause of death in blunt trauma. *Injury* **2018**, *49*, 1661–1667. [CrossRef] [PubMed]
2. van Wessem, K.J.P.; Leenen, L.P.H. Reduction in Mortality Rates of Postinjury Multiple Organ Dysfunction Syndrome. *Shock* **2017**, *49*, 33–38. [CrossRef] [PubMed]
3. Lyons, T.; Balogh, Z.J.; Evans, J.A.; McDougall, D.; van Wessem, K.J.P.; Lee, K.A. Epidemiology of Traumatic Deaths: Comprehensive Population-Based Assessment. *World J. Surg.* **2009**, *34*, 158–163.
4. Radomski, M.; Zettervall, S.; Schroeder, M.E.; Messing, J.; Dunne, J.; Sarani, B. Critical Care for the Patient With Multiple Trauma. *J. Intensive Care Med.* **2016**, *31*, 307–318. [CrossRef]
5. Gentile, L.F.; Cuenca, A.G.; Vanzant, E.L.; Efron, P.A.; Mckinley, B.; Moore, F.; Moldawer, L.L. Persistent inflammation and immunosuppression: A common sydrome and new horizon for surgical intensive care. *J. Trauma Acute Care Surg.* **2012**, *72*, 1491–1501. [CrossRef]

6. Lansink, K.W.W.; Gunning, A.C.; Leenen, L.P.H. Cause of death and time of death distribution of trauma patients in a Level I trauma centre in the Netherlands. *Eur. J. Trauma Emerg. Surg.* **2013**, *39*, 375–383. [CrossRef]
7. Mira, J.C.; Brakenridge, S.C.; Moldawer, L.L.; Moore, F.A. Persistent Inflammation, Immunosuppression and Catabolism Syndrome (PICS). *Crit. Care Clin.* **2017**, *33*, 245–258. [CrossRef]
8. Mira, J.C.; Cuschieri, J.; Ozrazgat-Baslanti, T.; Wang, Z.; Ghita, G.L.; Loftus, T.J.; Stortz, J.A.; Raymond, S.L.; Lanz, J.D.; Hennessy, L.V.; et al. The epidemiology of chronic critical illness after severe traumatic injury at two level-one trauma centers. *Crit. Care Med.* **2017**, *45*, 1989–1996. [CrossRef]
9. Stortz, J.A.; Murphy, T.J.; Raymond, S.L.; Mira, J.C.; Ungaro, R.; Dirain, M.L.; Nacionales, D.C.; Loftus, T.J.; Wang, Z.; Ozrazgat-Baslanti, T.; et al. Evidence for persistent immune suppression in patients who develop chronic critical illness after sepsis. *Shock* **2018**, *49*, 249–258. [CrossRef]
10. Nelson, J.E.; Cox, C.E.; Hope, A.A.; Carson, S.S. Concise Clinical Review: Chronic Critical Illness. *Am. J. Respir. Crit. Care Med.* **2010**, *182*, 1–9. [CrossRef]
11. Carson, S.S. Definitions and epidemiology of the chronically critically ill. *Respir. Care* **2012**, *57*, 848–858. [CrossRef] [PubMed]
12. Gardner, A.K.; Ghita, G.L.; Wang, Z.; Ozrazgat-Baslanti, T.; Raymond, S.L.; Mankowski, R.T.; Brumback, B.A.; Efron, P.A.; Bihorac, A.; Moore, F.A.; et al. The Development of Chronic Critical Illness Determines Physical Function, Quality of Life, and Long-Term Survival Among Early Survivors of Sepsis in Surgical ICUs. *Crit. Care Med.* **2019**, *47*, 566–573. [CrossRef] [PubMed]
13. Rosenthal, M.D.; Moore, F.A. Persistent inflammatory, immunosuppressed, catabolic syndrome (PICS): A new phenotype of multiple organ failure. *J. Adv. Nutr. Hum. Metab.* **2015**, *1*, 1–16.
14. Loftus, T.J.; Moore, F.A.; Moldawer, L.L. ICU-Acquired Weakness, Chronic Critical Illness, and the Persistent Inflammation-Immunosuppression and Catabolism Syndrome. *Crit. Care Med.* **2017**, *45*, e1184. [CrossRef] [PubMed]
15. Rawal, G.; Yadav, S.; Kumar, R. Post-intensive care syndrome: An overview. *J. Transl. Intern. Med.* **2017**, *5*, 90–92. [CrossRef] [PubMed]
16. Vanzant, E.L.; Lopez, C.M.; Ozrazgat-baslanti, T.; Davis, R.; Cuenca, A.G.; Gentile, L.F.; Dina, C.; Cuenca, A.L.; Bihorac, A.; Leeuwenburgh, C.; et al. Persistent Inflammation, Immunosuppression and Catabolism Syndrome after Severe Blunt Trauma. *J. Trauma Acute Care Surg.* **2014**, *76*, 21–30. [CrossRef]
17. Gennarelli, T.A.; Wodzin, E. AIS 2005: A contemporary injury scale. *Injury* **2006**, *37*, 1083–1091. [CrossRef]
18. ten Berg, M.J.; Huisman, A.; Van den Bemt, P.M.L.A.; Schobben, A.F.A.M.; Egberts, A.C.G.; van Solinge, W.W. Linking laboratory and medication data: New opportunities for pharmacoepidemiological research. *Clin. Chem. Lab. Med.* **2007**, *45*, 13–19. [CrossRef]
19. Singer, M.; Deutschmann, C.S.; Seymour, C.W.; Shanka-hari, M.; Annane, D.; Bauer, M. The Third International Consensus Definitions for Sepsis and Septic Shock (Sepsis-3). *JAMA* **2016**, *315*, 801–810. [CrossRef]
20. Baker, S.P.; O'Neill, B.; Haddon, W.; Long, W.B. The injury severity score: A method for describing patients with multiple injuries and evaluating emergency care. *J. Trauma* **1974**, *14*, 187–196. [CrossRef]
21. Plate, J.D.J.; Peelen, L.M.; Leenen, L.P.H.; Hietbrink, F. The intermediate care unit as a cost-reducing critical care facility in tertiary referral hospitals: A single-centre observational study. *BMJ Open* **2019**, *9*, 1–5. [CrossRef]
22. Eurostat Hospital Discharges and Length of Stay Statistics. Available online: https://ec.europa.eu/eurostat/statistics-explained/index.php/Hospital_discharges_and_length_of_stay_statistics (accessed on 10 August 2019).
23. Lansink, K.W.W.; Gunning, A.C.; Spijkers, A.T.E.; Leenen, L.P.H. Evaluation of Trauma Care in a Mature Level I Trauma Center in The Netherlands: Outcomes in a Dutch Mature Level I Trauma. *World J. Surg.* **2013**, *37*, 2353–2359. [CrossRef]
24. Childers, C.P.; Maggard-Gibbons, M. Understanding costs of care in the operating room. *JAMA Surg.* **2018**, *153*, e176233. [CrossRef] [PubMed]
25. Murthy, S.; Wunsch, H. Clinical review: International comparisons in critical care-lessons learned. *Crit. Care* **2012**, *16*, 218. [CrossRef] [PubMed]
26. Wunsch, H.; Angus, D.C.; Harrison, D.A.; Collange, O.; Fowler, R.; Hoste, E.A.J.; De Keizer, N.F.; Kersten, A.; Linde-Zwirble, W.T.; Sandiumenge, A.; et al. Variation in critical care services across North America and Western Europe. *Crit. Care Med.* **2008**, *36*, 2787–2793. [CrossRef] [PubMed]

27. You, J.W.; Lee, S.J.; Kim, Y.E.; Cho, Y.J.; Jeong, Y.Y.; Kim, H.C.; Lee, J.D.; Kim, J.R.; Hwang, Y.S. Association between weight change and clinical outcomes in critically ill patients. *J. Crit. Care* **2013**, *28*, 923–927. [CrossRef]
28. Bharadwaj, S.; Ginoya, S.; Tandon, P.; Gohel, T.D.; Guirguis, J.; Vallabh, H.; Jevenn, A.; Hanouneh, I. Malnutrition: Laboratory markers vs nutritional assessment. *Gastroenterol. Rep.* **2016**, *4*, 272–280. [CrossRef]
29. Alpers, D.H.; Stenson, W.F.; Taylore, B.E.; Bier, D.M. Manual of nutritional therapeutics. In *Manual of Nutrional Therapeutics*; LWW: Philadelphia, UK, 2008; pp. 104–105.
30. Gosling, P.; Dickson, G.R. Serum c-reactive protein in patients with serious trauma. *Injury* **1992**, *23*, 483–486. [CrossRef]
31. Simon, L.; Gauvin, F.; Amre, D.; Saint-Louis, P. Serum Procalcitonin and C-Reactive Protein Levels as Markers of Bacterial Infection: A Systematic Review and Meta-analysis. *Clin. Infect. Dis.* **2014**, *39*, 206–217. [CrossRef]
32. Santonocito, C.; De Loecker, I.; Donadello, K.; Moussa, M.D.; Markowicz, S.; Gullo, A.; Vincent, J.L. C-reactive protein kinetics after major surgery. *Anesth. Analg.* **2014**, *119*, 624–629. [CrossRef]
33. Sabino, H.; Moreira, P.; Mealha, R.; Fernandes, A.; Coelho, L.; Almeida, E.; Póvoa, P. C-reactive protein as a marker of infection in critically ill patients. *Clin. Microbiol. Infect.* **2005**, *11*, 101–108.
34. Huber-Lang, M.; Lambris, J.D.; Ward, P.A. Innate immune responses to trauma. *Nat. Immunol.* **2018**, *19*, 327–341. [CrossRef] [PubMed]
35. Heffernan, D.S.; Monaghan, S.F.; Cioffi, W.G.; Machan, J.T.; Thakkar, R.K.; Ayala, A. Failure to normalize lymphopenia following trauma is associated with increased mortality, independent of the leukocytosis pattern. *Crit. Care* **2012**, *16*, R12. [CrossRef] [PubMed]
36. Hesselink, L.; Spijkerman, R.; Van Wessem, K.J.P.; Koenderman, L.; Leenen, L.P.H.; Huber-lang, M.; Hietbrink, F. Neutrophil heterogeneity and its role in infectious complications after severe trauma. *World J. Emerg. Surg.* **2019**, *14*, 24. [CrossRef] [PubMed]
37. Spijkerman, R.; Hesselink, L.; Hellebrekers, P.; Vrisekoop, N.; Hietbrink, F.; Leenen, L.P.H.; Koenderman, L. Automated flow cytometry enables high performance point-of-care analysis of leukocyte phenotypes. *J. Immunol. Methods* **2019**, *474*, 112646. [CrossRef]
38. Pape, H.C. Effects of changing strategies of fracture fixation on immunologic changes and systemic complications after multiple trauma: Damage control orthopedic surgery. *J. Orthop. Res.* **2008**, *26*, 1478–1484. [CrossRef]
39. Lamb, C.M.; Macgoey, P.; Navarro, A.P.; Brooks, A.J. Damage control surgery in the era of damage control resuscitation. *Br. J. Anaesth.* **2014**, *113*, 242–249. [CrossRef]
40. Jacobs, D.; Jacobs, D.; Kudsk, K.; Moore, F.; Oswanski, M.; Poole, G.; Sacks, G.; Scherer, L., 3rd; Sinclair, K.; EAST Practice Management Guidelines Work Group. Practice management guidelines for nutritional support of the trauma patient. *J. Trauma Acute Care Surg.* **2004**, *57*, 660–679. [CrossRef]
41. de Smet, A.; Kluytmans, J.; Cooper, B.S.; Mascini, E.M.; Van Der Werf, T.S.; Van Der Hoeven, J.G.; Pickkers, P.; Bernards, A.T.; Kuijper, E.J.; Hall, M.A.L.; et al. Decontamination of the Digestive Tract and Oropharynx in ICU Patients. *N. Engl. J. Med.* **2009**, *360*, 20–31. [CrossRef]
42. Oostdijk, E.A.N.; Kesecioglu, J.; Schultz, M.J.; Visser, C.E.; De Jonge, E.; Van Essen, E.H.R.; Bernards, A.T.; Purmer, I.; Brimicombe, R.; Bergmans, D.; et al. Effects of decontamination of the oropharynx and intestinal tract on antibiotic resistance in icus a randomized clinical trial. *JAMA J. Am. Med. Assoc.* **2014**, *312*, 1429–1437. [CrossRef]
43. Rosenthal, M.D.; Moore, F.A. Persistent Inflammation, Immunosuppression, and Catabolism: Evolution of Multiple Organ Dysfunction. *Surg. Infect.* **2016**, *17*, 167–172. [CrossRef] [PubMed]

Journal of
Clinical Medicine

MDPI

Review

Neuroendocrine Modulation of the Immune Response after Trauma and Sepsis: Does It Influence Outcome?

Philipp Kobbe [1], Felix M. Bläsius [1], Philipp Lichte [1], Reiner Oberbeck [2] and Frank Hildebrand [1,*]

[1] Deparment of Trauma and Reconstructive Surgery, University Hospital RWTH Aachen, D-52074 Aachen, Germany; p.kobbe@ukaachen.de (P.K.); fblaesius@ukaachen.de (F.M.B.); plichte@ukaachen.de (P.L.)

[2] Deparment of Trauma and Hand Surgery, Wald-Klinikum, 07548 Gera, Germany; reiner.oberbeck@wkg.srh.de

* Correspondence: fhildebrand@ukaachen.de; Tel.: +49-241-89350

Received: 19 June 2020; Accepted: 16 July 2020; Published: 18 July 2020

Abstract: Although the treatment of multiple-injured patients has been improved during the last decades, sepsis and multiple organ failure (MOF) still remain the major cause of death. Following trauma, profound alterations of a large number of physiological systems can be observed that may potentially contribute to the development of sepsis and MOF. This includes alterations of the neuroendocrine and the immune system. A large number of studies focused on posttraumatic changes of the immune system, but the cause of posttraumatic immune disturbance remains to be established. However, an increasing number of data indicate that the bidirectional interaction between the neuroendocrine and the immune system may be an important mechanism involved in the development of sepsis and MOF. The aim of this article is to highlight the current knowledge of the neuroendocrine modulation of the immune system during trauma and sepsis.

Keywords: trauma; sepsis; DHEA; steroids; catecholamine

---

1. Introduction

Despite profound improvements in the initial care and in the treatment of multiple injured patients that follows, MOF and sepsis represent an ongoing threat [1,2]. It is assumed that the posttraumatic changes of the immune system crucially contribute to the development of these complications in multiple-injured patients. This includes pro- and anti-inflammatory changes of the immune system while an excessive reaction of both of the components leads to a massive disturbance of the immunological homeostasis [2–4].

Parallel to the changes of the immune system in multiple-injured as well as in septic patients, neuroendocrine systems are activated. Activation of the sympatho-adrenergic system (SAS) leads to a massively increased release of the catecholamines adrenaline and noradrenaline into the circulation [5,6]. The released adrenaline mainly originates from the adrenal medulla, and the noradrenaline mainly originates from the postganglionic sympathetic nerve fibers [6]. An increased release of catecholamines occurs in the initial stage as well as in the acute and late stage of sepsis and is enhanced by the released pro-inflammatory cytokines (Interleukin (IL)-6, Tumor Necrosis Factor (TNF)-α) [6]. Furthermore, the spleen, the lung and the gut-associated lymphoid tissue (GALT) are tightly sympathetically innervated and play a crucial role with respect to the adrenergic modulation of the immune system. In addition, it could be demonstrated that most of the cells of the immune system are equipped with α- as well as β-adrenergic receptors on their cell surface and that many of these cells are able to synthesize catecholamines themselves [7].

Apart from the activation of the SAS, a massive release of hormones of the hypothalamic–pituitary–adrenal axis (HPA-axis) or the hypothalamic–gonadal axis (HPG-axis) is found [5,6]. Activation of the HPA-axis is detectable after severe traumata as well as in septic patients and is responsible for a massive increase of cortisol and its release hormone ACTH. Here, the stimulation of the HPA-axis by pro-inflammatory cytokines like TNF-α, IL-1 and IL-6 plays a crucial role [8]. Between the amount of the cortisol level and the severity of the illness, a positive correlation exists. In cases of a prolonged course of disease, a peripheral glucocorticoid resistance develops characterized by normal or decreased ACTH and elevated cortisol levels [6].

With regard to the HPG-axis, which is likewise controlled by the release of hormones of the hypothalamus, decreased testosterone levels could be found in men after severe trauma and during sepsis whereas women react with an increase of their estrogen levels, presumably based on an increased aromatizing of androgens. In this case, it also comes to an influence of pro-inflammatory cytokines on hormone release [9].

Blood levels of the steroid hormone Dehydroepiandrosterone (DHEA) and its sulphated pattern (DHEA-S) are significantly decreased in critically ill and septic patients [10,11]. DHEA is the quantitatively most important human steroid hormone, which is produced mostly in the adrenal gland but also in the gonads. DHEA has not only a potent immunomodulatory activity by itself, but it is also considered to be a precursor of the androgen and estrogen biosynthesis [12]. During sepsis and trauma, a dissociation of cortisol and DHEA is found, which leads to an imbalance between immune-suppressive and immune-stimulating steroid hormones [8,13]. In accordance with this, it was shown that depressed levels of circulating DHEA in patients with sepsis are positively correlated to the risk of death [14,15].

Until now, it was assumed that the activation of neuroendocrine systems (SAS, HPA-axis, HPG-axis, DHEA) during trauma and sepsis serves the adaption of physiological systems like metabolism, heart/circulation, tissue regeneration and the central nervous system onto the elevated requirements.

The aim of this review is, on the one hand, to highlight current insights on how neuroendocrine released messengers are responsible for immunomodulation following severe trauma and during sepsis and, on the other hand, to find out whether this knowledge has been transferred into clinical practice.

2. Hypothalamic–Pituitary–Adrenal (HPA) Axis

Trauma and sepsis cause complex alterations of the hypothalamic–pituitary–adrenal axis and glucocorticoid signaling [16]. The immunomodulatory effects of glucocorticoids are well described. On the one hand, glucocorticoids inhibit the release of pro-inflammatory cytokines from T helper-1 (Th1) and antigen-presenting cells (APCs), and on the other hand, glucocorticoids induce the release of anti-inflammatory cytokines from T helper-2 (Th2) cells [17]. Through thismechanism glucocorticoids cause a Th1/Th2-shift of the immunological response. Additionally, glucocorticoids inhibit the function of neutrophil and eosinophil granulocytes as well as macrophages [18,19]. Glucocorticoid-induced immune suppression is used in autoimmune disorders and after organ transplant, and theoretically, these immunomodulatory effects may attenuate the overwhelming inflammatory response following severe trauma or during sepsis. Especially under consideration that critical ill patients show signs of relative adrenal insufficiency by suppression of the HPG axis due to the critical illness as well as sedative/analgesic drugs [16,20], the systemic substitution of glucocorticoids and the modulation of the metabolism of glucocorticoids appears reasonable. Recently, the role of 11β-Hydroxysteroid dehydrogenase type 1 (11β-HSD1) in acute and chronic inflammation has been pointed out [21–23]. 11β-HSD1 causes an intracellular conversion of inactive cortisone to the active cortisol. Therefore, 11β-HSD1 is an intracellular gate-keeper for glucocorticoid action [22]. Interestingly, the expression of 11β-HSD1 is greatly up-regulated during differentiation of monocytes into macrophages thus theoretically curbing the inflammatory potency of these cells [21]. However, it appears that this intracellular immunomodulation by 11β-HSD1 is disturbed during trauma and hemorrhage resulting in an inefficacy of released glucocorticoids to modulate the inflammatory response [24].

There are numerous animal studies in which corticosteroid administration consistently protected against lethal sepsis; however, clinical trials in sepsis found much less consistency in survival benefits from corticosteroids, although most trials demonstrated faster resolution in shock and organ dysfunction [25]. The Corticosteroid Therapy of Septic Shock (CORTICUS) study showed no benefit of hydrocortisone on survival or reversal of shock in patients with septic shock [26]. Although hydrocortisone treatment of patients in septic shock resulted in faster improvement of organ function, mainly of the cardiovascular system, this had no effect on mortality [27]. The HYPOLYTE (Hydrocortisone Polytraumatise) study showed that in intubated trauma patients hydrocortisone significantly reduced the risk of hospital-acquired pneumonia, however, again without altering the mortality rate [28]. Critics of glucocorticoid application argue that acute-phase sepsis is associated with increased glucocorticoid receptor expression and cortisol concentrations, possibly implying no need for exogenous substitution, which may even increase glucocorticoid resistance through a negative feedback mechanism [29]. Furthermore, glucocorticoid application is known to have potential hazardous side-effects, especially a slight increase of the incidence of clinically important gastrointestinal bleeding in critical ill patients [30].

Despite above mentioned findings of single studies, recent data from meta-analyses suggests with a low- to moderate-quality evidence that a long course of low-dose corticosteroids reduces 28-day mortality without inducing major complications [25,31–33]. Nonetheless, corticosteroid therapy for septic and trauma patients remains controversial despite general agreement that corticosteroids improve sepsis-associated comorbidities, such as shock, organ dysfunction, and length of hospital stay.

An immunomodulatory effect is also found for other hormones of the anterior pituitary gland as ACTH, β-endorphin, and prolactin. The administration of prolactin during experimental polymicrobial sepsis in mice increased the mortality rate from 47% to 81%. This effect was paralleled by a significant increase of splenocyte apoptosis rate and a marked depression of splenocyte proliferation. Furthermore, prolactin administration profoundly affected cellular cytokine release (IL-2, IL-6, IFN-γ) 48 h after induction of sepsis by cecal ligation and puncture [34]. However, the available literature about the immunomodulatory effects of pituitary hormones is controversial despite the suppressive effects on the immune cell proliferation and activity or rather the release of pro-inflammatory cytokines predominantly shown (Table 1) [35].

Table 1. Clinical studies.

Insult	Author	Type of Study	Number of Included Patients	Medication/Substance	Result
HPA Axis					
Sepsis	Sprung et al.	multicenter, randomized, double-blind, placebo-controlled	499	Hydrocortisone	no improvement of survival
					no improvement of reversal of shock
Sepsis	Lian et al.	meta-analysis	10,044	Corticosteroids	reduction of 28-day mortality
Sepsis	Fang et al.	meta-analysis	9564	Corticosteroids	reduction of 28-day mortality
Trauma	Roquilly et al.	multicenter, randomized, double-blind, placebo-controlled	149	Hydrocortisone	reduction of hospital-acquired pneumonia
HPG Axis					
Insult	**Author**	**Type of Study**	**Number of Included Patients**	**Medication/Substance**	**Result**
Surgical patients	Bulger et al.	randomized, double-blind, placebo-controlled	41	Oxandrolone	prolonged CMV, no improved outcome
Trauma/Sepsis	Frink et al.	monocenter, comparative study	143	none	lower MODS and sepsis rates in females
Trauma/Sepsis	Offner et al.	monocenter, comparative study	545	none	male gender is associated with infections
Trauma/Sepsis	Trentzsch et al.	retrospective, multicenter, comparative study	29,353	none	male gender is associated with higher MOF, sepsis and mortality rates
Trauma/Sepsis	Trentzsch et al.	retrospective, multicenter, comparative study	10,334	none	female gender is associated with improved organ function and lower sepsis rates
Trauma/Sepsis	Schoeneberg et al.	retrospective, multicenter, comparative study	962	none	female gender is associated with lower sepsis rates
Surcical patients	Wichmann et al.	monocenter, comparative study	40	none	lower IL-6 concentrations in women compared to men after surgery
Surgical patients/Sepsis	Wichmann et al.	monocenter, comparative study	4218	none	lower sepsis incidence in women
Trauma/Sepsis	Deitch et al.	monocenter, comparative study	5192	none	hormonally active women had a better physiological response

Table 1. *Cont.*

HPG Axis					
Insult	**Author**	**Type of Study**	**Number of Included Patients**	**Medication/Substance**	**Result**
Trauma	Haider et al.	retrospective, multicenter, comparative study	48,394	none	hormonally active women showed an improved survival
Trauma	Wohltmann	retrospective, multicenter, comparative study	20,261	none	hormonally active womed showed an improved survival
Trauma	Oberholzer et al.	monocenter, comparative study	1276	none	females showed an decreased posttraumatic morbidity
Trauma	George et al.	retrospective, multicenter, comparative study	155,691	none	females showed an improved survival
Trauma/Sepsis	Rappold et al.	monocenter, comparative study	1229	none	female gender offered no protection from ARDS, pneumonia, sepsis or death
Trauma	Gannon et al.	retrospective, multicenter, comparative study	22,332	none	no influence of female gender on outcome
Sepsis	Eachempati et al.	prospective, monocenter, comparative study	1348	none	female gender is an independent predictor of increased mortality
Trauma	Napolitano et al.	monocenter, comparative study	18,892	none	no influence of female gender on outcome
Trauma	Dossett et al.	prospective, multicenter, comparative study	991	none	serum estradiol levels were a marker for injury severity and a predictor of death
Sepsis	Sakr et al.	prospective, multicenter, comparative study	3902	none	women had a lower sepsis prevalence
DHEA					
Insult	**Author**	**Type of Study**	**Number of Included Patients**	**Medication/Substance**	**Result**
Influence of trauma on systemic DHEA/DHEAS levels	Foster et al.	prospective, monocenter, comparative study	95 patients	DHEA/DHEAS	1. Rapid decrease of DHEA after trauma with recovery to the normal range by 3 months 2. DHEAS rapidly reduced after trauma with no recovery until 6 months after trauma

Table 1. *Cont.*

DHEA					
Insult	**Author**	**Type of Study**	**Number of Included Patients**	**Medication/Substance**	**Result**
Influence of trauma on systemic DHEA/DHEAS levels	Brorsson et al.	prospective, monocenter, comparative study	50 patients	DHEA/DHEAS	1. Significant decrease of DHEA and DHEAS over the observation period of 5 days
Effects of sepsis and trauma on DHEA/DHEAS after ACTH stimulation	Arlt et al.	prospective, monocenter, comparative study	212 patients	DHEA/DHEAS	1. Decreased DHEAS levels after trauma and sepsis 2. Increased DHEA levels after sepsis, decreased levels after trauma 3. No increase of DHEA after ATCH-application in septic patients
SAS/PCS					
Insult	**Author**	**Type of Study**	**Number of Included Patients**	**Medication/Substance**	**Result**
Sepsis	Macchia et al.	retrospective, multicenter, comparative study	9465	beta-blocker	reduction of 28-day mortality
Sepsis	Morelli et al.	prospective, randomized, monocenter, comparative study	154	beta-blocker (esmolol)	reduction of mortality
Trauma	Bukur et al.	monocenter, retrospective, comparative study	663	beta-blocker	reduction of mortality

3. Hypothalamic–Pituitary–Gonadal (HPG) Axis

A relevant interaction between the HPG-axis and severe trauma and infections has been well described. On the one hand, traumatic and infectious insults induce a central suppression of the HPG axis with reduced gonadal androgen production and an associated state of catabolism (reduction of muscle mass, increased nitrogen loss) [36]. Therefore, the therapeutic use of a synthetic androgen (oxandrolone) has been investigated to support the switch to an anabolic situation. However, in contrast to burn injuries, it was not found to exert beneficial effects after major trauma [37]. On the other hand, sex hormones have the potential to significantly influence the posttraumatic course [11]. The so-called gender-dependent dimorphism of morbidity and mortality after trauma and sepsis is mainly based on experimental data indicating that sex hormones have relevant effects on various organs and the immune system after trauma and sepsis [38]. In general, 17-β-estradiol (E2) and estrogen-receptor agonists were shown to have beneficial effects on organ function, tissue damage (e.g., neutrophil infiltration, edema formation) and the immune response, whereas androgens (e.g., testosterone) were associated with enhanced organ damage and a dysfunctional immune system [39–42]. For example, E2 was shown to be beneficial for cardiac function after trauma-hemorrhage (TH) (e.g., increased cardiac output) due to protective effects on myocardial mitochondria, induction of heme oxygenase-1 (HO-1) [43], downregulation of nuclear factor kappa-light-chain-enhancer of activated B-cells (NF-κB) and the modulation of inflammatory mediators, such as heat shock proteins (HSP) and cytokines. In this context, E2 decreased the likelihood of cardiomyocyte necrosis by increasing HSP70 levels [44]. Furthermore, an E2-associated reduction of pulmonary damage after TH with a decrease of edema and neutrophil infiltration was observed [45,46]. As potential mechanisms for the beneficial hepatic effects of E2, a restoration of liver metabolism (normalization of adenosine triphosphate) and a reduction of apoptosis by up-regulation of Bcl-2 and induction of HO-1, heat shock proteins (HSP) and p38 mitogen activated protein kinase (p38 MAPK) was discussed. E2 attenuated acute renal injury by reducing apoptosis, endothelial cell damage and inflammation. Moreover, the intestine benefits from posttraumatic E2-application due to an increased blood flow and a decrease of neutrophil infiltration [45,47,48]. Furthermore, sex hormones significantly modulated cellular and humoral immune functions after TH. Interestingly, enzymes relevant for the synthesis of sex steroids were also found in immune cells (e.g., T-cells). The expression and activity of these enzymes were modulated by TH and differed between males and proestrus females. In males, TH resulted in increased levels of 5α-reductase which catalyzes the synthesis of 5α-dihydrotestosterone (5α-DHT). 5α-DHT itself is well known to exert even more pronounced immunosuppressive effects than testosterone. In contrast, in proestrus females, an enhanced aromatase activity was observed which resulted in an increased E2 synthesis [49]. Thus, these changes might contribute to the gender-related differences found after TH and sepsis [40]. Focusing on specific immune cells, macrophages from different tissue compartments were shown to respond differently following TH with an increased productive capacity for TNF-α and IL-6 of hepatic (Kupffer cells) and alveolar macrophages and a decreased synthesis of splenic and peritoneal macrophages [40]. Administration of E2 resulted in a normalization of the productive capacity but also in a beneficial modulation of toll-like receptor (TLR) and iNOS synthesis [48]. Furthermore, both dendritic (reduced antigen presentation) and T-cell function (shift from T-helper (Th) 1 to Th2-cell) were impaired after TH, which was assumed to contribute to the increased susceptibility for infectious complications after trauma. Again, these changes were especially pronounced in males and were reversed by E2-treatment [50,51]. In addition, an E2-induced interference with the apoptosis rate of immune cells and the synthesis of HSP was verified [2,39,51].

It has been proven that these effects of sex hormones are mediated by specific androgen- (AR) and estrogen (ER) receptors, which are expressed by almost all cells. For AR no further major subdivision is reported, whereas ER are subdivided in two major subtypes, ERα- and ER-β. The distribution of these ER is organ specific. In both, lung and heart, the effects of E2 seem to be mediated via ER-β [52]. In the liver, ER-α dependent effects were primarily described; however, ER-α-independent effects were also found [53]. Moreover, in the intestine, ERα- and ER-β mediated effects of E2 were found [54]. Hepatic and splenic macrophages and T-cells seem to preferably express ER-α and show improved function after administration of E2 or the selective ER-α-agonist propyl pyrazole triol (PPT) [42], whereas alveolar macrophages normalized posttraumatic function after application of a ER-β-agonist [40]. Based on the aforementioned results, it seems likely that ER subtypes may have tissue-specific roles in mediating the effects of E2 after TH.

All these aforementioned, beneficial effects on the various organs and the immune system might contribute to the improved survival observed after E2-application in animal models of TH even without large volume fluid resuscitation. In these studies, an E2-associated shift of the remaining blood into heart, liver and kidney has been discussed as a further favorable aspect [55–57].

Although sex hormones have been described to also influence human immune cell function, knowledge about these effects after TH and sepsis is relatively sparse. After infections, human mononuclear cells from males were shown to produce lower levels of type I interferons (IFN) in response to TLR-7 ligands and higher IL-10 in response to TLR-9 ligands as compared to females [58]. Furthermore, women were shown to have an enhanced capability of producing antibodies [59,60]. Clinical studies also described effects on the humoral immune response after multiple trauma and sepsis [61,62]. In this context, females younger than 50 years with an ISS > 25 had significantly lower plasma cytokines after multiple trauma [62].

Furthermore, diverse clinical studies found evidence for a more favorable clinical course after trauma and sepsis for females. In this context, female gender was associated with a lower incidence of posttraumatic infections (e.g., pneumonia, sepsis) and multiple organ failure (MOF) [63–68]. As a result, less requirements for intensive care were associated in female patients [69].

In some studies, however, only premenopausal females (in most studies defined as <50 years) showed lower incidences of posttraumatic complications (e.g., sepsis, MOF, mortality), a reduction of lactate levels and decreased blood transfusion requirements compared to males of the same age [62,65,66,70–73]. This might support the findings of the aforementioned experimental studies indicating a beneficial effect of E2 on the further clinical course. However, both, reduced sepsis rates and survival benefits have also been described for postmenopausal women [61,74,75]. Here, persistently increased androgen levels and the associated immunosuppression in males might play a role.

In the search for the mechanisms of the immunomodulating effect of estrogen, myeloid-derived suppressor cells (MDSC), a heterogeneous population of the myeloid lineage, which modulate the adaptive immune response, have attracted the focus of research efforts [76]. These cell subtypes have been shown to constitute a crucial component of the innate immune system in various inflammatory states. During systemic inflammation, MDSCs are recruited from the bone marrow [77]. In this respect, it could be shown in different mouse models that after CLP procedure and recruitment, an accumulation of MDSCs takes place in secondary lymphatic organs. The recruitment of MDSCs is mediated by MAMPs (e.g., LPS) and DAMPs (e.g., HMGB1) [77–79]. Furthermore, MDSC are induced and activated in the presence of estrogen and cytokines, such as IL-6, IFN-γ and IL-1β, and strongly contribute to T-cell dysfunction in various diseases such as sepsis, tumorigenesis and trauma [80–82]. Especially in the case of estrogen, a direct activation of the STAT3 signaling pathway and upregulation of JAK2 and SRC in MDSCs and a consecutive anti-inflammatory function of MDSCs could be demonstrated [83].

However, results on sex-related differences after trauma and sepsis are not unequivocal. Some studies found no differences for complications (e.g., sepsis) and mortality after blunt trauma [62,67,70,84,85], whereas even increased mortality rates for females with an age around 80 years were observed by Eachempati et al. [86]. Without specifically considering patient's age, also others described an increased mortality rate in females after development of infections (e.g., pneumonia, sepsis) or after major surgery [86,87]. In a study of Dossett et al. increasing levels of E2 were even associated to a higher mortality rate of critically ill patients [88].

There might be different reasons for these partly divergent results. Despite significant effects of the estrous cycle on E2 levels, none of the aforementioned studies has determined the cycle phase, some did not consider age. In addition, the effects of co-morbidities, pre-medication (e.g., oral contraceptives, hormone replacement therapy), injury severity and distribution (e.g., traumatic brain injury, TBI) have not been considered so far. In this context, it is well known that TBI has the potential to depress systemic E2 levels; however, this association has not been taken into account in most of the studies [89]. Consideration of patients with mild or moderate trauma and a low risk of adverse outcome might keep gender-related effects from becoming visible [65]. In this regard, diverse studies found gender-associated divergences only in patients with a high overall injury severity [62,73,90].

In conclusion, particularly based on experimental but also indirectly from clinical studies [62,65], it is likely that not the gender itself, but sex hormones influence the immune response, the incidence of complications and the outcome after trauma and sepsis [9,89]. Therefore, consideration of the sex hormone status could be an important step for an individual therapeutic approach after trauma. Therapeutic utilization of the interaction of E2/testosterone with the immune system after trauma and sepsis may offer new strategies. These include the application of E2, ER-agonists, androgen receptor antagonists and α-reductase-inhibitors, which prevent the conversion of testosterone into highly active dihydrotestosterone. However, up until now, no clinical trials have been published investigating the clinical value of these approaches (Table 1).

4. Dehydroepiandrosterone (DHEA)

DHEA, the most abundant circulating steroid in humans is mainly synthesized in the adrenal cortex. It has been well described to be involved in the response to trauma and sepsis [91]. Beside trauma- and sepsis-related effects on DHEA-synthesis and -metabolism, an immunomodulatory potency of DHEA under the aforementioned conditions has been proven in experimental studies. In this context, a beneficial effect of DHEA on the incidence of complications, the clinical status, survival and immune function after hemorrhagic shock, infections and a combination of these insults has been described [13,92,93]. Furthermore, an improved function of the cellular immune system, which includes a marked improvement of the proliferation rate of lymphocytes with a simultaneous decrease of the apoptosis rate of lymphocytes, was observed. At the same time, a varied pattern of cytokine release with a DHEA-induced inhibition of TNF-α, IL-6 and IL-10 release was found [13,92]. Accordingly, administration of DHEA immediately before induction of TH normalized immune cell migration (NK-cells, CD4+ and CD8+ lymphocytes) and splenocyte apoptosis rate in a murine model of hemorrhagic shock [94]. In a murine model of bilateral femoral fractures DHEA suppressed the serum levels of proinflammatory cytokines (IL-6, TNF-α, MCP-1) and also of IL-10 but did not improve markers of pulmonary inflammation [95]. Same effects of DHEA were found in case of neuroinflammation after TBI. In addition, DHEA resulted in improved long-term cognitive and behavioral outcome [96]. DHEA-treatment after infections displayed an increased survival rate, reduced bacterial contamination in the peritoneal fluid, decreased pro-inflammatory (e.g., TNF-α, IL-6) and enhanced anti-inflammatory cytokine release (e.g., IL-4, IL-10). These DHEA-associated changes of the inflammatory response were supposed to be caused by suppressed NO-secretion and a shift towards the Th2 response. Furthermore, an improved delayed-type of hypersensitivity reaction after DHEA-application was observed, demonstrating that apart from the innate immune system, also a modulation of the acquired part of the immune system is initiated [97,98]. In contrast, administration of DHEA in a murine sepsis model of cecal ligation and puncture revealed that there was no difference in the survival rate, the cellular proliferation and apoptosis rate whether mice received DHEA immediately before induction of a polymicrobial sepsis or after the development of the first septic symptoms [97]. The way of DHEA administration might represent a potential reason for these different findings. In this context, it was shown that subcutaneous administration of DHEA was accompanied by an improved survival and normalized immune functions whereas intravenous or intraperitoneal treatment with DHEA failed to exert the expected effects on the survival rate and immune functions of septic mice. Moreover, a varyingly strong activation of the HSP-70 release in the different shock organs (lunge, liver, kidney) could be detected in septic mice dependent on the way of DHEA administration [99].

However, it is of major relevance to note that transfer of animal data to the human situation has to be interpreted with caution. In this context, rodent adrenal DHEA production is modest compared to that of humans. Furthermore, these animals have the ability to convert exogenous DHEA to sex steroids. Therefore, studies specifically focusing on the human situation are of upmost importance. However, in vitro and clinical studies on the effects of DHEA on immune cells after trauma and sepsis are rare. In an in vitro study, DHEA-S was able to stimulate the synthesis of reactive oxygen species (ROS) via NADPH oxidase activation directly and thereby improve neutrophil function [100]. Neutrophils hold a unique position among the leukocytes, since they are the only subpopulation with an active transporter, the organic anion-transporting polypeptide D (OATP-D). Furthermore, neutrophils do not have steroid sulfatase, which activates DHEAS to DHEA. The effect of DHEA consequently must be a direct one. In addition, in case of primary adrenal insufficiency with a frequently associated deficit of DHEA/DHEAS, an impaired natural killer cell cytotoxic function was found. However, this impaired function was not influenced by longstanding DHEA-therapy [101]. Apart from this direct influence of DHEA on immune cells, an intracellular metabolization into sex steroids was postulated. In this respect, DHEA related activation of monocytes and their interaction with endothelial cells was shown to depend on the conversion to androgens and subsequent binding on androgen receptors [102]. DHEA may also antagonize the effects of glucocorticoids but also act as an inhibitor of the glucose-6-phosphatase in the hyperglycemic environments that are common after trauma [103]. Additionally, it was shown that cells of the immune system are able to synthesize DHEA, which could influence the cell function in an autocrine control loop [13].

In this context, it could be shown that the GR receptor is also expressed on circulating MDSCs. Lu et al. could show in an experimental study on a liver injury mouse model that the modulating effect of glucocorticoids is caused by suppression/activation of HIF1α and HIF1α-dependent glycolysis [104]. Based on these observations, the modulation of MDSC function by systemic steroids may represent a new therapeutic target, although detailed data on the timing of use and type of steroid are still lacking. Furthermore, the function of MDSC in sepsis and trauma has not been sufficiently studied [105,106]. The vast majority of data are based on studies in tumors, although an increasing number of studies highlight the role of MDSC subtypes in the resolution of inflammation after severe sepsis and trauma [106,107].

In the clinical setting, DHEA and DHEAS serum levels have been shown to immediately decrease in multiple trauma patients, indicating an early trauma-related reduction of adrenal androgen synthesis [11,20]. In the further clinical course, a stepwise recovery towards pre-traumatic levels over a period of several months was described. Interestingly, this recovery was significantly influenced by the medication over the clinical course, e.g., with a relevant delay in case of opioid treatment [11]. The decline of DHEAS was both, more pronounced and permanent compared to DHEA, suggesting an additional downregulation of DHEA sulfation after trauma [11,108]. As particularly low levels of DHEAS have been associated with an impaired immune function and higher complications rates (e.g., infections, mortality) [11,109], substitution of DHEAS or DHEA with stimulation of its sulfation might represent promising approaches for a beneficial modulation of the posttraumatic course. This is also true for septic patients who also demonstrated a significant reduction of DHEAS levels [108].

Cortisol and DHEAS appear to be the antagonists. DHEAS has the potential to counteract the immunosuppressive effect of cortisol. In post-traumatic and septic conditions, a decrease in DHEAS has been shown to enhance the immunosuppressive effect of cortisol [110].

Under additional consideration of the positive modulatory influence of DHEA on the immune system without proven significant adverse effects in experimental studies, a clinical utilization of DHEA or DHEA-S within the framework of controlled test conditions, for example, in septic or trauma patients, would be a possible step to prove the efficiency of this new therapeutic approach. However, interventional clinical studies so far only exist for healthy volunteers and patients with autoimmune disorders or osteoporosis who showed beneficial effects on immune response or the underlying disease (e.g., reduced inflammatory response, increased bone mass) [12,13]. For practicality of DHEA supplementation in case of trauma or sepsis, specific considerations in terms of dosing, delivery and safety under specific posttraumatic or -infectious conditions (e.g., polypharmacy, impaired hepatic function) are obligatory needed (Table 1).

5. Sympathetic-Adrenergic (SAS) and Parasympathetic-Cholinergic (PCS) System

The immunomodulatory effect of the activation of the sympatho-adrenergic system (SAS) by catecholamines has been known for a long time and has been proven by several animal and human studies. Likewise, the expression of α- as well as β-adrenergic receptors, those in a higher density, on the surface of nearly all cells of the immune system could be validated [111]. The subcutaneous or intravenous administration of the catecholamines adrenalin and noradrenalin leads to marked changes of the migration behavior and activity of circulating T- and NK-cells in healthy volunteers. This effect was inhibited by the administration of a non-selective but not of a β1-selective antagonist, which indicates that the effect might be mediated by β2-receptors [112]. Even after release of endogenous catecholamines, similar effects could be found [111]. Furthermore, it could be shown that catecholamines influence the release of pro- (IL-1β, IL-2, IL-6, IL-12, TNF-α) as well as anti-inflammatory cytokines (IL-10), and these effects could also be inhibited by the administration of β-adrenergic antagonists. Considering a synopsis of current literature, concerning TH1-cytokines, a rather inhibiting impact could be observed whereas with the release of TH2-cytokines, an activating impact seems to predominate [111,113]. Overall, catecholamines in vitro inhibit the adaptive immunity by reducing the proliferation of T helper, T cytotoxic and B-cells and shifting the TH1/TH2 balance towards Th2 cells [114]. In this context, it should be mentioned that the catecholamine dopamine is a potent inhibitor of the MDSC-mediated immunosuppression via the DA and D1-like receptors [115]. MDSCs have been shown to play a central role in the regulation of the pro-inflammation response in the early stage of sepsis. Their function seems to be the limitation of hyperinflammation by L-arginine degradation, production of ROS and NO, the secretion of anti-inflammatory cytokines like IL-10, inducing apoptosis mediated by FAS-FASL, and the activation of T regulatory cells (Tregs) [116–119]. On the other hand, this anti-inflammatory role seems to be disadvantageous in the later course of sepsis [120]. A function of MDSCs that has been insufficiently investigated so far involves the cell–cell crosstalk with macrophages, the induction of an M2 phenotype and the associated influence of MDSCs on the resolution of inflammation [121]. In the context of a consecutive chronic critical illness and a persistent inflammation immunosuppression and catabolism syndrome, MDSCs appear to be essential for the preservation of existing immunosuppression by suppression of the lymphocyte proliferation [120].

It was shown that adrenaline and noradrenaline are able to influence the release of pro- and anti-inflammatory cytokines, and it was postulated that both catecholamines are involved in the dysregulation of the immune system [111]. Accordingly, an animal model of hemorrhagic shock showed that the shock-induced mobilization of immune cells is blocked independently of the blood pressure by pharmacological blocking of adrenergic β-receptors. Additionally, an increased apoptosis rate of splenocytes was documented [122]. In another study using a murine sepsis model, the pharmacological blocking of adrenergic β-receptors led to an inhibition of the proliferation as well as an increased apoptosis rate of splenocytes and a varied release of cytokines (IFN-γ, IL-6). These immunological effects were accompanied by an increased mortality rate and a deteriorated clinical situation of the mice [123]. Similar results have been shown after selective inhibition of β2-receptors in a mouse sepsis model [122,124]. The exogenous infusion of adrenaline led to significant changes of the distribution of immune cells in the blood of septic mice. The apoptosis and proliferation rate of splenocytes and the release of cytokines were also significantly different without effects on the mortality rate or clinical situation. Additional administration of propranolol intensified the adrenergic effects on the apoptosis of immune cells, antagonized the adrenalin-induced cell mobilization and led to an increased release of IL-6. These effects were accompanied by a markedly increased mortality. Further studies about the pharmacological blocking of adrenergic β-receptors in animal models of sepsis prove a modulation of the release of pro- and anti-inflammatory cytokines even though the results are partially controversial [124].

The impact of circulating catecholamines or the blocking of adrenergic receptors on the immune system could also be shown under conditions of hemorrhagic shock and sepsis. Most of these data are based on animal studies, but in a small prospective study in trauma patients, it could be shown that administration of β-receptor blockers decreased serum IL-6 levels and that patients pretreated with β-receptor blockers had lower initial base deficits after trauma [125]. Clinical studies concerning the immunomodulatory effects of catecholamines in multiple-injured or septic patients are rare, because the use of hypotensive drugs, such as β-blockers in severe sepsis and septic shock, raises justified safety issues. Beyond that, the administration of catecholamines or of β-adrenergic antagonists is often clinically without alternative. A retrospective study reported that critically ill trauma patients receiving β-blockers had a significantly lower in-hospital mortality compared to patients with similar ISS scores not receiving β-blockers (11% vs. 19%) [126]. In general, β-blockers are used in sepsis under the intention to modulate the cardiovascular system but not to influence the inflammatory response; nonetheless β-blockade resulted in a decreased 28 day mortality in septic patients treated with esmolol [127]. Critically ill septic patients with chronic β-blocker prescriptions had lower 28 day mortality than sensitivity and pair-matched controls [128]. These improved outcomes with β-blockers could be due to decreased myocardial oxygen demand [129], improved myocardial oxygen utilization [130] and/or immunomodulation of hypercatecholaminemia [131].

Although several beneficial effects of β-blockers in trauma and sepsis have been described, including restoration of normal cellular metabolism, improved glucose regulation and improved cardiac function [132], the consequences of this interaction for the clinical treatment of patients after multiple trauma or during sepsis in terms of immunomodulation are not clear. The effects of β- blockade on infectious outcomes following the systemic inflammatory response syndrome (SIRS) [133] and the compensatory anti-inflammatory response syndrome (CARS) [134] are unknown. Therefore, more basic research is needed to elucidate the intra- and extracellular mechanisms of immunomodulation of β-blockers. Further, it has to be determined which patients may benefit and especially at which timepoint in the treatment course since an initial sympathetic activation after injury is beneficial but a persistent severe overactivation detrimental. Therefore, the immune suppressive side effects of the β-adrenergic antagonists should be critically included in the therapy decision.

Besides the sympathetic-adrenergic system, also the parasympathetic-cholinergic system (PCS) is able to modulate the inflammatory response [135,136]. The activation of the parasympathetic-cholinergic system via the release of the neurotransmitter acetylcholine (ACh) results in an immune-suppression by inhibition of cytokine production [137]. ACh binds to both nicotinic and muscarinic cholinergic receptors. The main nicotinic cholinergic receptor found on macrophages is the α7 nicotinic ACh receptor subunit (α7nAChR) [137]. It is believed that cholinergic agonists through the activation of α7nACh receptors inhibit NF-κB activation and hence downregulate the production of pro- inflammatory cytokines, such as TNFα [137]. Cholinergic stimulation has been shown to reduce pro- inflammatory cytokine production and prevent lethal tissue injury in multiple models of local and systemic inflammation and sepsis, including acute lung injury, hemorrhagic shock or polymicrobial sepsis [136]. These findings encouraged researchers to assess the therapeutic potential of vagus nerve stimulation (VNS) in attenuating the systemic inflammatory responses evoked by endotoxemia [137]. Direct electrical stimulation of the peripheral vagus nerve in vivo during lethal endotoxemia in rats inhibited TNFα synthesis in the liver, attenuated peak serum TNFα amounts and prevented the development of shock [137]. A beneficial effect of VNS immunomodulation has been reported in other studies for different immunological pathologies [137]. Interestingly, the immunomodulatory effect of vagus nerve stimulation in terms of systemic TNFα reduction is dependent on the spleen, since it fails to work in splenectomized animals [136]. Interruption of the common celiac branch of the abdominal vagus nerve abolishes vagal anti-inflammatory effects, suggesting that cholinergic signaling targets the spleen via this specific branch of the vagus nerve [136].

To date, there are no human studies reporting on the specific pharmacological stimulation of the parasympathetic-cholinergic system in order to modulate the inflammatory response in trauma or septic patients. Nonetheless, transcutaneous mechanical vagus nerve stimulation can exhibit anti-inflammatory effects that may be considered in the clinical setting under special circumstances (Table 1).

6. Conclusions

With the exception of corticosteroids, up-to-date proactive modulation of the inflammatory response following trauma and sepsis has not been introduced into clinical practice. Although animal studies show great potential of neuroendocrine immune modulation following trauma and sepsis, knowledge concerning dosage and timing in clinical practice remains unclear. Especially the potential of severe side-effects caused by modulation of this highly complex and dynamic inflammatory response cannot be predicted so far. Future studies are required to achieve the transfer of promising data from bench to bedside.

Author Contributions: Conceptualization, P.K. and F.H.; resources, F.H.; writing—original draft preparation, P.K. and F.H.; writing—review and editing, F.M.B., P.L., R.O. and F.H.; supervision, F.H. All authors have read and agreed to the published version of the manuscript.

Funding: This research received no external funding.

Conflicts of Interest: The authors declare no conflict of interest.

References

1. Nast-Kolb, D.; Aufmkolk, M.; Rucholtz, S.; Obertacke, U.; Waydhas, C. Multiple organ failure still a major cause of morbidity but not mortality in blunt multiple trauma. *J. Trauma* **2001**, *51*, 835–841. [CrossRef] [PubMed]
2. Neunaber, C.; Zeckey, C.; Andruszkow, H.; Frink, M.; Mommsen, P.; Krettek, C.; Hildebrand, F. Immunomodulation in polytrauma and polymicrobial sepsis—Where do we stand? *Recent Pat. Inflamm. Allergy Drug Discov.* **2011**, *5*, 17–25. [CrossRef] [PubMed]
3. Hildebrand, F.P.H.K.C. Die Bedeutung der Zytokine in der posttraumatischen Entzündungsreaktion. *Unfallchirurg* **2005**, *108*, 793–803. [CrossRef] [PubMed]
4. Kirchhoff, C.; Biberthaler, P.; Mutschler, W.E.; Faist, E.; Jochum, M.; Zedler, S. Early down-regulation of the pro-inflammatory potential of monocytes is correlated to organ dysfunction in patients after severe multiple injury: A cohort study. *Crit. Care* **2009**, *13*, R88. [CrossRef]
5. Gann, D.S.; Lilly, M.P. The neuroendocrine response to multiple trauma. *World J. Surg.* **1983**, *7*, 101–118. [CrossRef]
6. Kumar, V.; Sharma, A. Is neuroimmunomodulation a future therapeutic approach for sepsis? *Int. Immunopharmacol.* **2010**, *10*, 9–17. [CrossRef]
7. Madden, K.S.; Sanders, V.M.; Felten, D.L. Catecholamine influences and sympathetic neural modulation of immune responsiveness. *Annu. Rev. Pharmacol. Toxicol.* **1995**, *35*, 417–448. [CrossRef]
8. Vermes, I.; Beishuizen, A. The hypothalamic-pituitary-adrenal response to critical illness. *Best Pract. Res. Clin. Endocrinol. Metab.* **2001**, *15*, 495–511. [CrossRef]
9. Bösch, F.; Angele, M.K.; Chaudry, I.H. Gender differences in trauma, shock and sepsis. *Mil. Med. Res.* **2018**, *5*, 35. [CrossRef]
10. Beishuizen, A.; Thijs, L.G.; Vermes, I. Decreased levels of dehydroepiandrosterone sulphate in severe critical illness: A sign of exhausted adrenal reserve? *Crit. Care* **2002**, *6*, 434–438. [CrossRef]
11. Foster, M.A.; Taylor, A.E.; Hill, N.E.; Bentley, C.; Bishop, J.; Gilligan, L.C.; Shaheen, F.; Bion, J.F.; Fallowfield, J.L.; Woods, D.R.; et al. Mapping the steroid response to major trauma from injury to recovery: A prospective cohort study. *J. Clin. Endocrinol. Metab.* **2020**, *105*, 925–937. [CrossRef] [PubMed]

12. Williams, J.R. The effects of dehydroepiandrosterone on carcinogenesis, obesity, the immune system, and aging. *Lipids* **2000**, *35*, 325–331. [CrossRef]
13. Oberbeck, R.; Kobbe, P. Dehydroepiandrosterone (DHEA): A steroid with multiple effects. Is there any possible option in the treatment of critical illness? *Curr. Med. Chem.* **2010**, *17*, 1039–1047. [CrossRef] [PubMed]
14. Dhatariya, K.K. Is there a role for dehydroepiandrosterone replacement in the intensive care population? *Intensive Care Med.* **2003**, *29*, 1877–1880. [CrossRef] [PubMed]
15. Marx, C.; Petros, S.; Bornstein, S.R.; Weise, M.; Wendt, M.; Menschikowski, M.; Engelmann, L.; Höffken, G. Adrenocortical hormones in survivors and nonsurvivors of severe sepsis: Diverse time course of dehydroepiandrosterone, dehydroepiandrosterone-sulfate, and cortisol. *Crit. Care Med.* **2003**, *31*, 1382–1388. [CrossRef]
16. Marik, P.E. Glucocorticoids in sepsis: Dissecting facts from fiction. *Crit. Care* **2011**, *15*, 158. [CrossRef]
17. Elenkov, I.J. Glucocorticoids and the Th1/Th2 balance. *Ann. N. Y. Acad. Sci.* **2004**, *1024*, 138–146. [CrossRef]
18. Ronchetti, S.; Ricci, E.; Migliorati, G.; Gentili, M.; Riccardi, C. How glucocorticoids affect the neutrophil life. *Int. J. Mol. Sci.* **2018**, *19*, 4090. [CrossRef]
19. Joyce, D.A.; Steer, J.H.; Abraham, L.J. Glucocorticoid modulation of human monocyte/macrophage function: Control of TNF-α secretion. *Inflamm. Res.* **1997**, *46*, 447–451. [CrossRef]
20. Brorsson, C.; Dahlqvist, P.; Nilsson, L.; Thunberg, J.; Sylvan, A.; Naredi, S. Adrenal response after trauma is affected by time after trauma and sedative/analgesic drugs. *Injury* **2014**, *45*, 1149–1155. [CrossRef]
21. Thieringer, R.; Le Grand, C.B.; Carbin, L.; Cai, T.Q.; Wong, B.; Wright, S.D.; Hermanowski-Vosatka, A. 11 Beta-hydroxysteroid dehydrogenase type 1 is induced in human monocytes upon differentiation to macrophages. *J. Immunol.* **2001**, *167*, 30–35. [CrossRef] [PubMed]
22. Chapman, K.; Holmes, M.; Seckl, J. 11β-hydroxysteroid dehydrogenases: Intracellular gate-keepers of tissue glucocorticoid action. *Physiol. Rev.* **2013**, *93*, 1139–1206. [CrossRef] [PubMed]
23. Chapman, K.E.; Coutinho, A.E.; Zhang, Z.; Kipari, T.; Savill, J.S.; Seckl, J.R. Changing glucocorticoid action: 11β-hydroxysteroid dehydrogenase type 1 in acute and chronic inflammation. *J. Steroid. Biochem. Mol. Biol.* **2013**, *137*, 82–92. [CrossRef] [PubMed]
24. Wang, P.; Ba, Z.F.; Jarrar, D.; Cioffi, W.G.; Bland, K.I.; Chaudry, I.H. Mechanism of adrenal insufficiency following trauma and severe hemorrhage: Role of hepatic 11beta-hydroxysteroid dehydrogenase. *Arch. Surg.* **1999**, *134*, 394–401. [CrossRef]
25. Annane, D. The role of acth and corticosteroids for sepsis and septic shock: An update. *Front. Endocrinol.* **2016**, *7*, 70. [CrossRef]
26. Sprung, C.L.; Annane, D.; Keh, D.; Moreno, R.; Singer, M.; Freivogel, K.; Weiss, Y.G.; Benbenishty, J.; Kalenka, A.; Forst, H.; et al. Hydrocortisone therapy for patients with septic shock. *N. Engl. J. Med.* **2008**, *358*, 111–124. [CrossRef]
27. Rhodes, A.; Chiche, J.D.; Moreno, R. Improving the quality of training programs in intensive care: A view from the ESICM. *Intensive Care Med.* **2011**, *37*, 377–379. [CrossRef]
28. Roquilly, A.; Mahe, P.J.; Seguin, P.; Guitton, C.; Floch, H.; Tellier, A.C.; Merson, L.; Renard, B.; Malledant, Y.; Flet, L.; et al. Hydrocortisone therapy for patients with multiple trauma: The randomized controlled HYPOLYTE study. *JAMA* **2011**, *305*, 1201–1209. [CrossRef]
29. Vardas, K.; Ilia, S.; Sertedaki, A.; Charmandari, E.; Briassouli, E.; Goukos, D.; Apostolou, K.; Psarra, K.; Botoula, E.; Tsagarakis, S.; et al. Increased glucocorticoid receptor expression in sepsis is related to heat shock proteins, cytokines, and cortisol and is associated with increased mortality. *Intensive Care Med. Exp.* **2017**, *5*, 10. [CrossRef]
30. Butler, E.; Møller, M.H.; Cook, O.; Granholm, A.; Penketh, J.; Rygård, S.L.; Aneman, A.; Perner, A. The effect of systemic corticosteroids on the incidence of gastrointestinal bleeding in critically ill adults: A systematic review with meta-analysis. *Intensive Care Med.* **2019**, *45*, 1540–1549. [CrossRef]
31. Lian, X.J.; Huang, D.Z.; Cao, Y.S.; Wei, Y.X.; Lian, Z.Z.; Qin, T.H.; He, P.C.; Liu, Y.H.; Wang, S.H. Reevaluating the role of corticosteroids in septic shock: An updated meta-analysis of randomized controlled trials. *Biomed. Res. Int.* **2019**, *2019*, 3175047. [CrossRef] [PubMed]
32. Fang, F.; Zhang, Y.; Tang, J.; Lunsford, L.D.; Li, T.; Tang, R.; He, J.; Xu, P.; Faramand, A.; Xu, J.; et al. Association of corticosteroid treatment with outcomes in adult patients with sepsis: A systematic review and meta-analysis. *JAMA Intern. Med.* **2019**, *179*, 213–223. [CrossRef]

33. Annane, D.; Bellissant, E.; Bollaert, P.E.; Briegel, J.; Confalonieri, M.; De Gaudio, R.; Keh, D.; Kupfer, Y.; Oppert, M.; Meduri, G.U. Corticosteroids in the treatment of severe sepsis and septic shock in adults: A systematic review. *JAMA* **2009**, *301*, 2362–2375. [CrossRef]
34. Oberbeck, R.; Schmitz, D.; Wilsenack, K.; Schüler, M.; Biskup, C.; Schedlowski, M.; Nast-Kolb, D.; Exton, M.S. Prolactin modulates survival and cellular immune functions in septic mice. *J. Surg. Res.* **2003**, *113*, 248–256. [CrossRef]
35. Schleimer, R.P. An overview of glucocorticoid anti-inflammatory actions. *Eur. J. Clin. Pharmacol.* **1993**, *45* (Suppl. 1), S3–S7. [CrossRef] [PubMed]
36. McCann, S.M.; Kimura, M.; Karanth, S.; Yu, W.H.; Mastronardi, C.A.; Rettori, V. The mechanism of action of cytokines to control the release of hypothalamic and pituitary hormones in infection. *Ann. N. Y. Acad. Sci.* **2000**, *917*, 4–18. [CrossRef]
37. Bulger, E.M.; Jurkovich, G.J.; Farver, C.L.; Klotz, P.; Maier, R.V. Oxandrolone does not improve outcome of ventilator dependent surgical patients. *Ann. Surg.* **2004**, *240*, 472–478. [CrossRef]
38. Angele, M.K.; Schwacha, M.G.; Ayala, A.; Chaudry, I.H. Effect of gender and sex hormones on immune responses following shock. *Shock* **2000**, *14*, 81–90. [CrossRef]
39. Bird, M.D.; Karavitis, J.; Kovacs, E.J. Sex differences and estrogen modulation of the cellular immune response after injury. *Cell. Immunol.* **2008**, *252*, 57–67. [CrossRef]
40. Choudhry, M.A.; Bland, K.I.; Chaudry, I.H. Trauma and immune response—Effect of gender differences. *Injury* **2007**, *38*, 1382–1391. [CrossRef]
41. Sperry, J.L.; Minei, J.P. Gender dimorphism following injury: Making the connection from bench to bedside. *J. Leukoc. Biol.* **2008**, *83*, 499–506. [CrossRef] [PubMed]
42. Weniger, M.; Angele, M.K.; Chaudry, I.H. The role and use of estrogens following trauma. *Shock* **2016**, *46* (Suppl. 1), 4–11. [CrossRef] [PubMed]
43. Szalay, L.; Shimizu, T.; Schwacha, M.G.; Choudhry, M.A.; Loring WRue, I.; Bland, K.I.; Chaudry, I.H. Mechanism of salutary effects of estradiol on organ function after trauma-hemorrhage: Upregulation of heme oxygenase. *Am. J. Physiol. Heart Circ. Physiol.* **2005**, *289*, H92–H98. [CrossRef]
44. Voss, M.R.; Stallone, J.N.; Li, M.; Cornelussen, R.N.; Knuefermann, P.; Knowlton, A.A. Gender differences in the expression of heat shock proteins: The effect of estrogen. *Am. J. Physiol. Heart. Circ. Physiol.* **2003**, *285*, H687–H692. [CrossRef] [PubMed]
45. Kawasaki, T.; Chaudry, I.H. The effects of estrogen on various organs: Therapeutic approach for sepsis, trauma, and reperfusion injury. Part 2: Liver, intestine, spleen, and kidney. *J. Anesth.* **2012**, *26*, 892–899. [CrossRef] [PubMed]
46. Frink, M.; Thobe, B.M.; Hsieh, Y.C.; Choudhry, M.A.; Schwacha, M.G.; Bland, K.I.; Chaudry, I.H. 17β-Estradiol inhibits keratinocyte-derived chemokine production following trauma-hemorrhage. *Am. J. Physiol. Lung Cell. Mol. Physiol.* **2007**, *292*, L585–L591. [CrossRef] [PubMed]
47. Yu, H.P.; Pang, S.T.; Chaudry, I.H. Hepatic gene expression patterns following trauma-hemorrhage: Effect of posttreatment with estrogen. *Shock* **2013**, *39*, 77–82. [CrossRef] [PubMed]
48. Yu, H.P.; Hsieh, Y.C.; Suzuki, T.; Choudhry, M.A.; Schwacha, M.G.; Bland, K.I.; Chaudry, I.H. Mechanism of the nongenomic effects of estrogen on intestinal myeloperoxidase activity following trauma-hemorrhage: Up-regulation of the PI-3K/Akt pathway. *J. Leukoc. Biol.* **2007**, *82*, 774–780. [CrossRef]
49. Samy, T.S.A.; Zheng, R.; Matsutani, T.; Loring, W.; Rue, I.; Bland, K.I.; Chaudry, I.H. Mechanism for normal splenic T lymphocyte functions in proestrus females after trauma: Enhanced local synthesis of 17β-estradiol. *Am. J. Physiol.Cell Physiol.* **2003**, *285*, C139–C149. [CrossRef]
50. Angele, M.K.; Knöferl, M.W.; Ayala, A.; Bland, K.I.; Chaudry, I.H. Testosterone and estrogen differently effect Th1 and Th2 cytokine release following trauma-haemorrhage. *Cytokine* **2001**, *16*, 22–30. [CrossRef]
51. Choudhry, M.A.; Schwacha, M.G.; Hubbard, W.J.; Kerby, J.D.; Rue, L.W.; Bland, K.I.; Chaudry, I.H. Gender differences in acute response to trauma-hemorrhage. *Shock* **2005**, *24* (Suppl. 1), 101–106. [CrossRef]
52. Yu, H.P.; Hsieh, Y.C.; Suzuki, T.; Shimizu, T.; Choudhry, M.A.; Schwacha, M.G.; Chaudry, I.H. Salutary effects of estrogen receptor-beta agonist on lung injury after trauma-hemorrhage. *Am. J. Physiol. Lung Cell. Mol. Physiol.* **2006**, *290*, L1004–L1009. [CrossRef] [PubMed]
53. Hsieh, Y.C.; Yu, H.P.; Frink, M.; Suzuki, T.; Choudhry, M.A.; Schwacha, M.G.; Chaudry, I.H. G protein-coupled receptor 30-dependent protein kinase A pathway is critical in nongenomic effects of estrogen in attenuating liver injury after trauma-hemorrhage. *Am. J. Pathol.* **2007**, *170*, 1210–1218. [CrossRef]

54. Yu, H.P.; Shimizu, T.; Hsieh, Y.C.; Suzuki, T.; Choudhry, M.A.; Schwacha, M.G.; Chaudry, I.H. Tissue-specific expression of estrogen receptors and their role in the regulation of neutrophil infiltration in various organs following trauma-hemorrhage. *J. Leukoc. Biol.* **2006**, *79*, 963–970. [CrossRef] [PubMed]
55. Hubbard, W.; Keith, J.; Berman, J.; Miller, M.; Scott, C.; Peck, C.; Chaudry, I.H. 17α-Ethynylestradiol-3-sulfate treatment of severe blood loss in rats. *J. Surg. Res.* **2015**, *193*, 355–360. [CrossRef] [PubMed]
56. Kim, H.; Chen, J.; Zinn, K.R.; Hubbard, W.J.; Fineberg, N.S.; Chaudry, I.H. Single photon emission computed tomography demonstrated efficacy of 17β-estradiol therapy in male rats after trauma-hemorrhage and extended hypotension. *J. Trauma* **2010**, *69*, 1266–1273. [CrossRef]
57. Miller, M.; Keith, J.; Berman, J.; Burlington, D.B.; Grudzinskas, C.; Hubbard, W.; Peck, C.; Scott, C.; Chaudry, I.H. Efficacy of 17α-ethynylestradiol-3-sulfate for severe hemorrhage in minipigs in the absence of fluid resuscitation. *J. Trauma Acute Care Surg.* **2014**, *76*, 1409–1416. [CrossRef]
58. Tayel, S.S.; Helmy, A.A.; Ahmed, R.; Esmat, G.; Hamdi, N.; Abdelaziz, A.I. Progesterone suppresses interferon signaling by repressing TLR-7 and MxA expression in peripheral blood mononuclear cells of patients infected with hepatitis C virus. *Arch. Virol.* **2013**, *158*, 1755–1764. [CrossRef]
59. Bouman, A.; Heineman, M.J.; Faas, M.M. Sex hormones and the immune response in humans. *Hum. Reprod. Update* **2005**, *11*, 411–423. [CrossRef]
60. Taneja, V. Sex hormones determine immune response. *Front. Immunol.* **2018**, *9*, 1931. [CrossRef]
61. Schröder, J.; Kahlke, V.; Staubach, K.H.; Zabel, P.; Stüber, F. Gender differences in human sepsis. *Arch. Surg.* **1998**, *133*, 1200–1205. [CrossRef]
62. Frink, M.; Pape, H.C.; van Griensven, M.; Krettek, C.; Chaudry, I.H.; Hildebrand, F. Influence of sex and age on mods and cytokines after multiple injuries. *Shock* **2007**, *27*, 151–156. [CrossRef] [PubMed]
63. Offner, P.J.; Moore, E.E.; Biffl, W.L. Male gender is a risk factor for major infections after surgery. *Arch. Surg.* **1999**, *134*, 935–938. [CrossRef] [PubMed]
64. Gannon, C.J.; Pasquale, M.; Tracy, J.K.; McCarter, R.J.; Napolitano, L.M. Male gender is associated with increased risk for postinjury pneumonia. *Shock* **2004**, *21*, 410–414. [CrossRef] [PubMed]
65. Trentzsch, H.; Lefering, R.; Nienaber, U.; Kraft, R.; Faist, E.; Piltz, S. The role of biological sex in severely traumatized patients on outcomes: A matched-pair analysis. *Ann. Surg.* **2015**, *261*, 774–780. [CrossRef] [PubMed]
66. Trentzsch, H.; Nienaber, U.; Behnke, M.; Lefering, R.; Piltz, S. Female sex protects from organ failure and sepsis after major trauma haemorrhage. *Injury* **2014**, *45* (Suppl. 3), S20–S28. [CrossRef] [PubMed]
67. Schoeneberg, C.; Kauther, M.D.; Hussmann, B.; Keitel, J.; Schmitz, D.; Lendemans, S. Gender-specific differences in severely injured patients between 2002 and 2011: Data analysis with matched-pair analysis. *Crit. Care* **2013**, *17*, R277. [CrossRef]
68. Wichmann, M.W.; Müller, C.; Meyer, G.; Adam, M.; Angele, M.K.; Eisenmenger, S.J.; Schildberg, F.W. Different immune responses to abdominal surgery in men and women. *Langenbecks Arch. Surg.* **2003**, *387*, 397–401. [CrossRef]
69. Wichmann, M.W.; Inthorn, D.; Andress, H.J.; Schildberg, F.W. Incidence and mortality of severe sepsis in surgical intensive care patients: The influence of patient gender on disease process and outcome. *Intensive Care Med.* **2000**, *26*, 167–172. [CrossRef] [PubMed]
70. Mostafa, G.; Huynh, T.; Sing, R.F.; Miles, W.S.; Norton, H.J.; Thomason, M.H. Gender-related outcomes in trauma. *J. Trauma* **2002**, *53*, 430–434. [CrossRef]
71. Deitch, E.A.; Livingston, D.H.; Lavery, R.F.; Monaghan, S.F.; Bongu, A.; Machiedo, G.W. Hormonally active women tolerate shock-trauma better than do men: A prospective study of over 4000 trauma patients. *Ann. Surg.* **2007**, *246*, 447–453. [CrossRef] [PubMed]
72. Haider, A.H.; Crompton, J.G.; Chang, D.C.; Efron, D.T.; Haut, E.R.; Handly, N.; Cornwell, E.E., 3rd. Evidence of hormonal basis for improved survival among females with trauma-associated shock: An analysis of the National Trauma Data Bank. *J. Trauma* **2010**, *69*, 537–540. [CrossRef] [PubMed]
73. Wohltmann, C.D.; Franklin, G.A.; Boaz, P.W.; Luchette, F.A.; Kearney, P.A.; Richardson, J.D.; Spain, D.A. A multicenter evaluation of whether gender dimorphism affects survival after trauma. *Am. J. Surg.* **2001**, *181*, 297–300. [CrossRef]
74. Oberholzer, A.; Keel, M.; Zellweger, R.; Steckholzer, U.; Trentz, O.; Ertel, W. Incidence of septic complications and multiple organ failure in severely injured patients is sex specific. *J. Trauma* **2000**, *48*, 932–937. [CrossRef]

75. George, R.L.; McGwin, G.; Jr Metzger, J.; Chaudry, I.H.; Rue, L.W., 3rd. The association between gender and mortality among trauma patients as modified by age. *J. Trauma* **2003**, *54*, 464–471. [CrossRef]
76. Hüsecken, Y.; Muche, S.; Kustermann, M.; Klingspor, M.; Palmer, A.; Braumüller, S.; Huber-Lang, M.; Debatin, K.-M.; Strauss, G. MDSCs are induced after experimental blunt chest trauma and subsequently alter antigen-specific T cell responses. *Sci. Rep.* **2017**, *7*, 12808. [CrossRef]
77. Ray, A.; Chakraborty, K.; Ray, P. Immunosuppressive MDSCs induced by TLR signaling during infection and role in resolution of inflammation. *Front. Cell. Infect. Microbiol.* **2013**, *3*, 52. [CrossRef]
78. Bayik, D.; Tross, D.; Klinman, D.M. Factors influencing the differentiation of human monocytic myeloid-derived suppressor cells into inflammatory macrophages. *Front. Immunol.* **2018**, *9*, 608. [CrossRef]
79. Greifenberg, V.; Ribechini, E.; Rössner, S.; Lutz, M.B. Myeloid-derived suppressor cell activation by combined LPS and IFN-gamma treatment impairs DC development. *Eur. J. Immunol.* **2009**, *39*, 2865–2876. [CrossRef]
80. Condamine, T.; Gabrilovich, D.I. Molecular mechanisms regulating myeloid-derived suppressor cell differentiation and function. *Trends Immunol.* **2011**, *32*, 19–25. [CrossRef]
81. Uhel, F.; Azzaoui, I.; Grégoire, M.; Pangault, C.; Dulong, J.; Tadié, J.M.; Gacouin, A.; Camus, C.; Cynober, L.; Fest, T.; et al. Early expansion of circulating granulocytic myeloid-derived suppressor cells predicts development of nosocomial infections in patients with sepsis. *Am. J. Respir. Crit. Care Med.* **2017**, *196*, 315–327. [CrossRef] [PubMed]
82. Cuenca, A.G.; Delano, M.J.; Kelly-Scumpia, K.M.; Moreno, C.; Scumpia, P.O.; Laface, D.M.; Heyworth, P.G.; Efron, P.A.; Moldawer, L.L. A paradoxical role for myeloid-derived suppressor cells in sepsis and trauma. *Mol. Med.* **2011**, *17*, 281–292. [CrossRef]
83. Svoronos, N.; Perales-Puchalt, A.; Allegrezza, M.J.; Rutkowski, M.R.; Payne, K.K.; Tesone, A.J.; Nguyen, J.M.; Curiel, T.J.; Cadungog, M.G.; Singhal, S.; et al. Tumor cell-independent estrogen signaling drives disease progression through mobilization of myeloid-derived suppressor cells. *Cancer Discov.* **2017**, *7*, 72–85. [CrossRef] [PubMed]
84. Rappold, J.F.; Coimbra, R.; Hoyt, D.B.; Potenza, B.M.; Fortlage, D.; Holbrook, T.; Minard, G. Female gender does not protect blunt trauma patients from complications and mortality. *J. Trauma* **2002**, *53*, 436–441. [CrossRef]
85. Gannon, C.J.; Napolitano, L.M.; Pasquale, M.; Tracy, J.K.; McCarter, R.J. A statewide population-based study of gender differences in trauma: Validation of a prior single-institution study. *J. Am. Coll. Surg.* **2002**, *195*, 11–18. [CrossRef]
86. Eachempati, S.R.; Hydo, L.; Barie, P.S. Gender-based differences in outcome in patients with sepsis. *Arch. Surg.* **1999**, *134*, 1342–1347. [CrossRef] [PubMed]
87. Napolitano, L.M.; Greco, M.E.; Rodriguez, A.; Kufera, J.A.; West, R.S.; Scalea, T.M. Gender differences in adverse outcomes after blunt trauma. *J. Trauma* **2001**, *50*, 274–280. [CrossRef] [PubMed]
88. Dossett, L.A.; Swenson, B.R.; Heffernan, D.; Bonatti, H.; Metzger, R.; Sawyer, R.G.; May, A.K. High levels of endogenous estrogens are associated with death in the critically injured adult. *J. Trauma* **2008**, *64*, 580–585. [CrossRef]
89. Weniger, M.; D'Haese, J.G.; Angele, M.K.; Chaudry, I.H. Potential therapeutic targets for sepsis in women. *Exp. Opin. Ther. Targets* **2015**, *19*, 1531–1543. [CrossRef]
90. Magnotti, L.J.; Fischer, P.E.; Zarzaur, B.L.; Fabian, T.C.; Croce, M.A. Impact of gender on outcomes after blunt injury: A definitive analysis of more than 36,000 trauma patients. *J. Am. Coll. Surg.* **2008**, *206*, 984–991. [CrossRef]
91. Bentley, C.; Hazeldine, J.; Greig, C.; Lord, J.; Foster, M. Dehydroepiandrosterone: A potential therapeutic agent in the treatment and rehabilitation of the traumatically injured patient. *Burns Trauma* **2019**, *7*, 26. [CrossRef] [PubMed]
92. Hildebrand, F.; Pape, H.-C.; Hoevel, P.; Krettek, C.; van Griensven, M. The importance of systemic cytokines in the pathogenesis of polymicrobial sepsis and dehydroepiandrosterone treatment in a rodent model. *Shock* **2003**, *20*, 338–346. [CrossRef] [PubMed]
93. Barkhausen, T.; Hildebrand, F.; Krettek, C.; van Griensven, M. DHEA-dependent and organ-specific regulation of TNF-alpha mRNA expression in a murine polymicrobial sepsis and trauma model. *Crit. Care* **2009**, *13*, R114. [CrossRef] [PubMed]

94. Oberbeck, R.; Nickel, E.; von Griensven, M.; Tschernig, T.; Wittwer, T.; Schmitz, D.; Pape, H.C. The effect of dehydroepiandrosterone on hemorrhage-induced suppression of cellular immune function. *Intensive Care Med.* **2002**, *28*, 963–968. [CrossRef]
95. Lichte, P.; Pfeifer, R.; Werner, B.E.; Ewers, P.; Tohidnezhad, M.; Pufe, T.; Hildebrand, F.; Pape, H.C.; Kobbe, P. Dehydroepiandrosterone modulates the inflammatory response in a bilateral femoral shaft fracture model. *Eur. J. Med. Res.* **2014**, *19*, 27. [CrossRef] [PubMed]
96. Yilmaz, C.; Karali, K.; Fodelianaki, G.; Gravanis, A.; Chavakis, T.; Charalampopoulos, I.; Alexaki, V.I. Neurosteroids as regulators of neuroinflammation. *Front. Neuroendocrinol.* **2019**, *55*, 100788. [CrossRef] [PubMed]
97. Schmitz, D.; Kobbe, P.; Wegner, A.; Hammes, F.; Oberbeck, R. Dehydroepiandrosterone during sepsis: Does the timing of administration influence the effectiveness. *J. Surg. Res.* **2010**, *163*, e73–e77. [CrossRef]
98. Zhao, J.; Cao, J.; Yu, L.; Ma, H. Dehydroepiandrosterone resisted *E. Coli* O157:H7-induced inflammation via blocking the activation of p38 MAPK and NF-κB pathways in mice. *Cytokine* **2020**, *127*, 154955. [CrossRef]
99. Oberbeck, R.; Deckert, H.; Bangen, J.; Kobbe, P.; Schmitz, D. Dehydroepiandrosterone: A modulator of cellular immunity and heat shock protein 70 production during polymicrobial sepsis. *Intensive Care Med.* **2007**, *33*, 2207–2213. [CrossRef]
100. Radford, D.J.; Wang, K.; McNelis, J.C.; Taylor, A.E.; Hechenberger, G.; Hofmann, J.; Chahal, H.; Arlt, W.; Lord, J.M. Dehydroepiandrosterone sulfate directly activates protein kinase C-β to increase human neutrophil superoxide generation. *Mol. Endocrinol.* **2010**, *24*, 813–821. [CrossRef]
101. Bancos, I.; Hazeldine, J.; Chortis, V.; Hampson, P.; Taylor, A.E.; Lord, J.M.; Arlt, W. Primary adrenal insufficiency is associated with impaired natural killer cell function: A potential link to increased mortality. *Eur. J. Endocrinol.* **2017**, *176*, 471–480. [CrossRef] [PubMed]
102. Corsini, E.; Galbiati, V.; Papale, A.; Kummer, E.; Pinto, A.; Serafini, M.M.; Guaita, A.; Spezzano, R.; Caruso, D.; Marinovich, M.; et al. Role of androgens in dhea-induced rack1 expression and cytokine modulation in monocytes. *Immunity Ageing I A* **2016**, *13*, 20. [CrossRef] [PubMed]
103. Perner, A.; Nielsen, S.E.; Rask-Madsen, J. High glucose impairs superoxide production from isolated blood neutrophils. *Intensive Care Med.* **2003**, *29*, 642–645. [CrossRef]
104. Lu, Y.; Liu, H.; Bi, Y.; Yang, H.; Li, Y.; Wang, J.; Zhang, Z.; Wang, Y.; Li, C.; Jia, A.; et al. Glucocorticoid receptor promotes the function of myeloid-derived suppressor cells by suppressing HIF1α-dependent glycolysis. *Cell. Mol. Immunol.* **2018**, *15*, 618–629. [CrossRef]
105. Jiang, J.K.; Fang, W.; Hong, L.J.; Lu, Y.Q. Distribution and differentiation of myeloid-derived suppressor cells after fluid resuscitation in mice with hemorrhagic shock. *J. Zhejiang Univ. Sci. B* **2017**, *18*, 48–58. [CrossRef] [PubMed]
106. Cheng, L.; Xu, J.; Chai, Y.; Wang, C.; Han, P. Dynamic changes in trauma-induced myeloid-derived suppressor cells after polytrauma are associated with an increased susceptibility to infection. *Int. J. Clin. Exp. Pathol.* **2017**, *10*, 11063–11068.
107. Schrijver, I.T.; Théroude, C.; Roger, T. Myeloid-derived suppressor cells in sepsis. *Front. Immunol.* **2019**, *10*, 327. [CrossRef] [PubMed]
108. Arlt, W.; Hammer, F.; Sanning, P.; Butcher, S.K.; Lord, J.M.; Allolio, B.; Annane, D.; Stewart, P.M. Dissociation of serum dehydroepiandrosterone and dehydroepiandrosterone sulfate in septic shock. *J. Clin. Endocrinol. Metab.* **2006**, *91*, 2548–2554. [CrossRef]
109. Butcher, S.K.; Killampalli, V.; Lascelles, D.; Wang, K.; Alpar, E.K.; Lord, J.M. Raised cortisol:DHEAS ratios in the elderly after injury: Potential impact upon neutrophil function and immunity. *Aging Cell* **2005**, *4*, 319–324. [CrossRef]
110. De Castro, R.; Ruiz, D.; Lavín, B.A.; Lamsfus, J.; Vázquez, L.; Montalban, C.; Marcano, G.; Sarabia, R.; Paz-Zulueta, M.; Blanco, C.; et al. Cortisol and adrenal androgens as independent predictors of mortality in septic patients. *PLoS ONE* **2019**, *14*, e0214312. [CrossRef]
111. Oberbeck, R. Catecholamines: Physiological immunomodulators during health and illness. *Curr. Med. Chem.* **2006**, *13*, 1979–1989. [CrossRef] [PubMed]
112. Schedlowski, M.; Hosch, W.; Oberbeck, R.; Benschop, R.J.; Jacobs, R.; Raab, H.R.; Schmidt, R.E. Catecholamines modulate human NK cell circulation and function via spleen-independent beta 2-adrenergic mechanisms. *J. Immunol.* **1996**, *156*, 93–99. [PubMed]

113. Molina, P.E. Neurobiology of the stress response: Contribution of the sympathetic nervous system to the neuroimmune axis in traumatic injury. *Shock* **2005**, *24*, 3–10. [CrossRef] [PubMed]
114. Andreis, D.T.; Singer, M. Catecholamines for inflammatory shock: A Jekyll-and-Hyde conundrum. *Intensive Care Med.* **2016**, *42*, 1387–1397. [CrossRef] [PubMed]
115. Wu, J.; Zhang, R.; Tang, N.; Gong, Z.; Zhou, J.; Chen, Y.; Chen, K.; Cai, W. Dopamine inhibits the function of Gr-1+CD115+ myeloid-derived suppressor cells through D1-like receptors and enhances anti-tumor immunity. *J. Leukoc. Biol.* **2015**, *97*, 191–200. [CrossRef]
116. Wijnands, K.A.; Meesters, D.M.; van Barneveld, K.W.; Visschers, R.G.; Briedé, J.J.; Vandendriessche, B.; van Eijk, H.M.; Bessems, B.A.; van den Hoven, N.; von Wintersdorff, C.J.; et al. Citrulline supplementation improves organ perfusion and arginine availability under conditions with enhanced arginase activity. *Nutrients* **2015**, *7*, 5217–5238. [CrossRef]
117. Köstlin, N.; Vogelmann, M.; Spring, B.; Schwarz, J.; Feucht, J.; Härtel, C.; Orlikowsky, T.W.; Poets, C.F.; Gille, C. Granulocytic myeloid-derived suppressor cells from human cord blood modulate T-helper cell response towards an anti-inflammatory phenotype. *Immunology* **2017**, *152*, 89–101. [CrossRef]
118. Gabrilovich, D.I.; Nagaraj, S. Myeloid-derived suppressor cells as regulators of the immune system. *Nat. Rev. Immunol.* **2009**, *9*, 162–174. [CrossRef]
119. Sinha, P.; Chornoguz, O.; Clements, V.K.; Artemenko, K.A.; Zubarev, R.A.; Ostrand-Rosenberg, S. Myeloid-derived suppressor cells express the death receptor Fas and apoptose in response to T cell-expressed FasL. *Blood* **2011**, *117*, 5381–5390. [CrossRef]
120. Venet, F.; Monneret, G. Advances in the understanding and treatment of sepsis-induced immunosuppression. *Nat. Rev. Nephrol.* **2018**, *14*, 121–137. [CrossRef]
121. Ostrand-Rosenberg, S. Myeloid-derived suppressor cells: More mechanisms for inhibiting antitumor immunity. *Cancer Immunol. Immunother.* **2010**, *59*, 1593–1600. [CrossRef] [PubMed]
122. Oberbeck, R.; Kobbe, P. Beta-adrenergic antagonists: Indications and potential immunomodulatory side effects in the critically ill. *Curr. Med. Chem.* **2009**, *16*, 1082–1090. [CrossRef] [PubMed]
123. Schmitz, D.; Wilsenack, K.; Lendemanns, S.; Schedlowski, M.; Oberbeck, R. Beta-Adrenergic blockade during systemic inflammation: Impact on cellular immune functions and survival in a murine model of sepsis. *Resuscitation* **2007**, *72*, 286–294. [CrossRef] [PubMed]
124. Oberbeck, R.; Schmitz, D.; Schüler, M.; Wilsenack, K.; Schedlowski, M.; Exton, M. Dopexamine and cellular immune functions during systemic inflammation. *Immunobiology* **2004**, *208*, 429–438. [CrossRef]
125. Friese, R.S.; Barber, R.; McBride, D.; Bender, J.; Gentilello, L.M. Could Beta blockade improve outcome after injury by modulating inflammatory profiles? *J. Trauma* **2008**, *64*, 1061–1068. [CrossRef]
126. Bukur, M.; Lustenberger, T.; Cotton, B.; Arbabi, S.; Talving, P.; Salim, A.; Ley, E.J.; Inaba, K. Beta-blocker exposure in the absence of significant head injuries is associated with reduced mortality in critically ill patients. *Am. J. Surg.* **2012**, *204*, 697–703. [CrossRef]
127. Morelli, A.; Ertmer, C.; Westphal, M.; Rehberg, S.; Kampmeier, T.; Ligges, S.; Orecchioni, A.; D'Egidio, A.; D'Ippoliti, F.; Raffone, C.; et al. Effect of heart rate control with esmolol on hemodynamic and clinical outcomes in patients with septic shock: A randomized clinical trial. *JAMA* **2013**, *310*, 1683–1691. [CrossRef]
128. Macchia, A.; Romero, M.; Comignani, P.D.; Mariani, J.; D'Ettorre, A.; Prini, N.; Santopinto, M.; Tognoni, G. Previous prescription of β-blockers is associated with reduced mortality among patients hospitalized in intensive care units for sepsis. *Crit. Care Med.* **2012**, *40*, 2768–2772. [CrossRef]
129. Taniguchi, T.; Kurita, A.; Yamamoto, K.; Inaba, H. Effects of carvedilol on mortality and inflammatory responses to severe hemorrhagic shock in rats. *Shock* **2009**, *32*, 272–275. [CrossRef]
130. Huang, L.; Weil, M.H.; Cammarata, G.; Sun, S.; Tang, W. Nonselective beta-blocking agent improves the outcome of cardiopulmonary resuscitation in a rat model. *Crit. Care Med.* **2004**, *32* (Suppl. 9), S378–S380. [CrossRef]
131. Oberbeck, R.; van Griensven, M.; Nickel, E.; Tschernig, T.; Wittwer, T.; Pape, H.-C. Influence of beta-adrenoceptor antagonists on hemorrhage-induced cellular immune suppression. *Shock* **2002**, *18*, 331–335. [CrossRef] [PubMed]
132. Feinman, R.; Deitch, E.A.; Aris, V.; Chu, H.B.; Abungu, B.; Caputo, F.J.; Galante, A.; Xu, D.; Lu, Q.; Colorado, I.; et al. Molecular signatures of trauma-hemorrhagic shock-induced lung injury: Hemorrhage- and injury-associated genes. *Shock* **2007**, *28*, 360–368. [CrossRef] [PubMed]

133. Davies, M.G.; Hagen, P.O. Systemic inflammatory response syndrome. *Br. J. Surg.* **1997**, *84*, 920–935. [CrossRef]
134. Bone, R.C. Sir Isaac Newton, sepsis, SIRS, and CARS. *Crit. Care Med.* **1996**, *24*, 1125–1128. [CrossRef] [PubMed]
135. Pavlov, V.A.; Wang, H.; Czura, C.J.; Friedman, S.G.; Tracey, K.J. The cholinergic anti-inflammatory pathway: A missing link in neuroimmunomodulation. *Mol. Med.* **2003**, *9*, 125–134. [CrossRef] [PubMed]
136. Huston, J.M. The vagus nerve and the inflammatory reflex: Wandering on a new treatment paradigm for systemic inflammation and sepsis. *Surg. Infect.* **2012**, *13*, 187–193. [CrossRef]
137. Jarczyk, J.; Yard, B.A.; Hoeger, S. The cholinergic anti-inflammatory pathway as a conceptual framework to treat inflammation-mediated renal injury. *Kidney Blood Press. Res.* **2019**, *44*, 435–448. [CrossRef]

MDPI
St. Alban-Anlage 66
4052 Basel
Switzerland
Tel. +41 61 683 77 34
Fax +41 61 302 89 18
www.mdpi.com

Journal of Clinical Medicine Editorial Office
E-mail: jcm@mdpi.com
www.mdpi.com/journal/jcm

www.ingramcontent.com/pod-product-compliance
Lightning Source LLC
Chambersburg PA
CBHW061756210926
51850CB00006B/575
* 9 7 8 3 0 3 9 4 3 7 7 7 1 *